Jaypee's
Nurses'
Dictionary

WITHDRAWN

McGraw-Hill

Nurses'
Dictionary

(For Nurses and Allied Healthcare Professionals)

FOURTH EDITION

Compiled and Edited by

UN PANDA MD
Senior Physician
New Delhi, India

Jaypee Brothers

Medical

© 2009 UN Panda

Fourth Edition: **2015**

First published in India by

Jaypee Brothers Medical Publishers (P) Ltd

Corporate Office

4838/24 Ansari Road, Daryaganj, **New Delhi** - 110002, India, +91-11-43574357

Registered Office

B-3 EMCA House, 23/23B Ansari Road, Daryaganj, **New Delhi** 110 002, India

Phones: +91-11-23272143, +91-11-23272703, +91-11-23282021

+91-11-23245672, Fax: +91-11-23276490, +91-11-23245683

e-mail: jaypee@jaypeebrothers.com, website: www.jaypeebrothers.com

First published in USA by The McGraw-Hill Companies, 2 Penn Plaza, New York, NY 10121-2298. Exclusively worldwide distributor except South Asia (India, Nepal, Sri Lanka, Bhutan, Pakistan, Bangladesh, Malaysia).

NOTICE

Medicine is an ever-changing science. As new research and clinical experience broaden our knowledge, changes in treatment and drug therapy are required. The authors and the publisher of this work have checked with sources believed to be reliable in their efforts to provide information that is complete and generally in accord with the standards accepted at the time of publication. However, in view of the possibility of human error changes in medical science, neither the editors nor the publisher nor any other party who has been involved in the preparation or publication of this work warrants that the information contained herein is in every respect accurate or complete, and they disclaim all responsibility for any errors or omissions or for the results obtained from use of the information contained in this work. Readers are encouraged to confirm the information contained herein with other sources. For example and in particular, readers are advised to check the product information sheet included in the package of each drug they plan to administer to be certain that the information contained in this work is accurate and that changes have not been made in the recommended dose or in the contraindications for administration. This recommendation is of particular importance in connection with new or infrequently used drugs.

ISBN-13:   978-0-07-184548-9

ISBN-10:   0-07-184548-8

Preface to the Fourth Edition

A nursing dictionary is an effective tool of providing not only meaning of commonly used medical terms but also about procedures, investigations and pharmacological agents in brief.

The complete and concise text of the latest edition is fully revised and updated with more than 250 new entries. Around 65 new figures explaining procedures, investigations and pharmacological agents in brief have also been added.

New appendices, including Abbreviations Used Regarding the Route of Administration of Medicine, Karnofsky's Index, Normal Hematological Values, etc. would be of immense help to nursing students.

The dictionary would definitely serve as a ready reference to the entire nursing community.

UN Panda

Preface to the First Edition

Nursing is a speciality in its own right. Implementation of any health programme at community or hospital level needs active participation of nursing staff. Hence, nursing education has received a major thrust in recent times.

Medical vocabulary useful for nurses is expanding at a rapid pace. Old and obsolete words are being deleted. New procedures and investigations are being added regularly. A nursing dictionary is an effective tool of providing not only meaning of commonly used medical terms but also about procedures, investigations and pharmacological agents in brief.

In this book, I have compiled and presented the commonly used terms and their meaning without any emphasis on their pronunciation and etymon. I hope the width and depth of its coverage will be advantageous for the nursing community.

All suggestions for improvement are cordially welcome.

UN Panda

Contents

PLATE-1

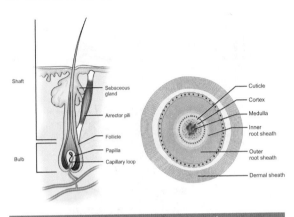

Hair in longitudinal and cross-section

PLATE-2

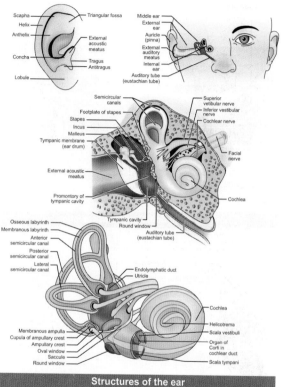

Structures of the ear

PLATE-3

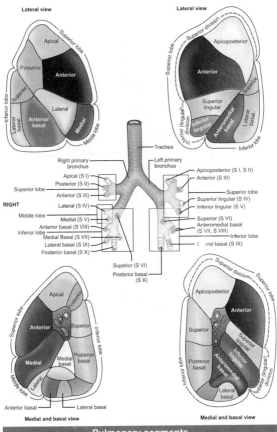

Pulmonary segments

PLATE-4

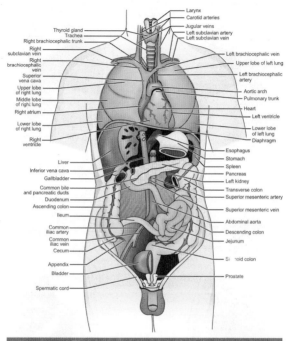

Larynx
Carotid arteries
Jugular veins
Left subclavian artery
Left subclavian vein
Thyroid gland
Trachea
Right subclavian trunk
Right subclavian vein
Right brachiocephalic vein
Superior vena cava
Upper lobe of right lung
Middle lobe of right lung
Right atrium
Lower lobe of right lung
Right ventricle
Liver
Inferior vena cava
Gallbladder
Common bile and pancreatic ducts
Duodenum
Ascending colon
Ileum
Common iliac artery
Common iliac vein
Cecum
Appendix
Bladder
Spermatic cord
Left brachiocephalic vein
Upper lobe of left lung
Left brachiocephalic artery
Aortic arch
Pulmonary trunk
Heart
Left ventricle
Lower lobe of left lung
Diaphragm
Esophagus
Stomach
Spleen
Pancreas
Left kidney
Transverse colon
Superior mesenteric artery
Superior mesenteric vein
Abdominal aorta
Descending colon
Jejunum
Sigmoid colon
Prostate

Thoracic and abdominal viscera

PLATE-5

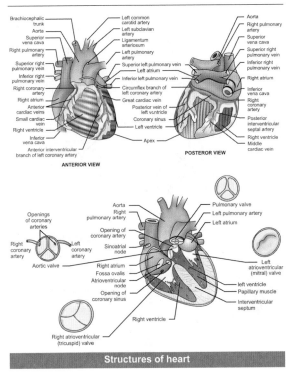

ANTERIOR VIEW

POSTEROR VIEW

Structures of heart

PLATE-6

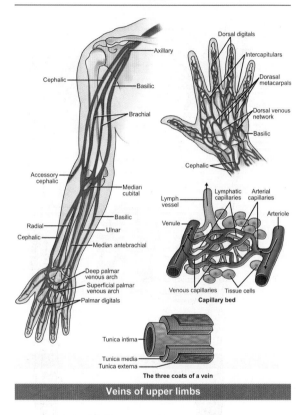

Axillary

Cephalic

Basilic

Brachial

Dorsal digitals

Intercapitulars

Dorsal metacarpals

Dorsal venous network

Basilic

Cephalic

Accessory cephalic

Median cubital

Radial

Basilic

Cephalic

Ulnar

Median antebrachial

Deep palmar venous arch

Superficial palmar venous arch

Palmar digitals

Lymph vessel

Lymphatic capillaries

Arterial capillaries

Venule

Arteriole

Venous capillaries

Tissue cells

Capillary bed

Tunica intima

Tunica media

Tunica externa

The three coats of a vein

Veins of upper limbs

PLATE-7

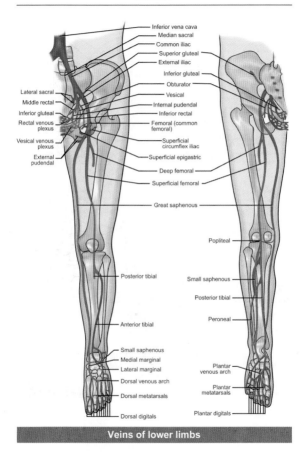

Inferior vena cava
Median sacral
Common iliac
Superior gluteal
External iliac
Inferior gluteal
Obturator
Vesical
Internal pudendal
Inferior rectal
Femoral (common femoral)
Superficial circumflex iliac
Superficial epigastric
Deep femoral
Superficial femoral
Great saphenous

Lateral sacral
Middle rectal
Inferior gluteal
Rectal venous plexus
Vesical venous plexus
External pudendal

Popliteal
Posterior tibial
Small saphenous
Posterior tibial
Peroneal
Anterior tibial
Small saphenous
Medial marginal
Lateral marginal
Dorsal venous arch
Plantar venous arch
Dorsal metatarsals
Plantar metatarsals
Dorsal digitals
Plantar digitals

Veins of lower limbs

PLATE-8

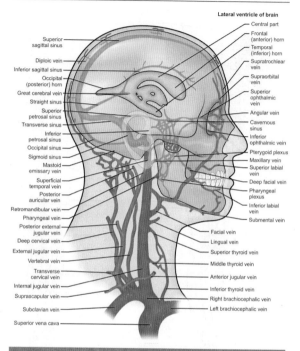

Lateral ventricle of brain

Superior sagittal sinus

Diploic vein

Inferior sagittal sinus

Occipital (posterior) horn

Great cerebral vein

Straight sinus

Superior petrosal sinus

Transverse sinus

Inferior petrosal sinus

Occipital sinus

Sigmoid sinus

Mastoid emissary vein

Superficial temporal vein

Posterior auricular vein

Retromandibular vein

Pharyngeal vein

Posterior external jugular vein

Deep cervical vein

External jugular vein

Vertebral vein

Transverse cervical vein

Internal jugular vein

Suprascapular vein

Subclavian vein

Superior vena cava

Central part

Frontal (anterior) horn

Temporal (inferior) horn

Supratrochlear vein

Supraorbital vein

Superior ophthalmic vein

Angular vein

Cavernous sinus

Inferior ophthalmic vein

Pterygoid plexus

Maxillary vein

Superior labial vein

Deep facial vein

Pharyngeal plexus

Inferior labial vein

Submental vein

Facial vein

Lingual vein

Superior thyroid vein

Middle thyroid vein

Anterior jugular vein

Inferior thyroid vein

Right brachiocephalic vein

Left brachiocephalic vein

Vein of head and neck

PLATE-9

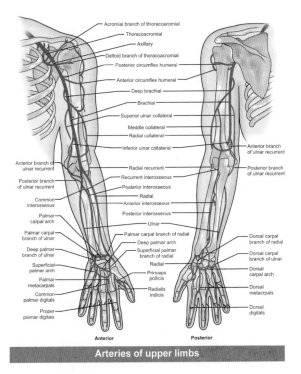

Acromial branch of thioracoaromial
Thoracoacromial
Axillary
Deltoid branch of thoracoacromial
Posterior circumflex humeral
Anterior circumflex humeral
Deep brachial
Brachial
Superior ulnar collateral
Meddle collateral
Radial collateral
Inferior uinar collateral
Anterior branch of ulnar recurrent
Posterior branch of ulnar recurrent
Anterior branch of ulnar recurrent
Radial recurrent
Recurrent interosseous
Posterior interosseous
Radial
Anterior interosseous
Posterior interosseous
Ulnar
Posterior branch of ulnar recurrent
Common interosseous
Palmar carpal arch
Palmar carpal branch of ulnar
Deep palmar branch of ulnar
Superficial palmar branch
Palmar metacarpals
Common palmar digitals
Proper palmar digitals
Palmar carpal branch of radial
Deep palmar arch
Superficial palmar branch of radial
Radial
Princeps pollicis
Radialis indicis
Dorsal carpal branch of radial
Dorsal carpal branch of ulnar
Dorsal carpal arch
Dorsal metacrpals
Dorsal digitals

Anterior   Posterior

Arteries of upper limbs

PLATE-10

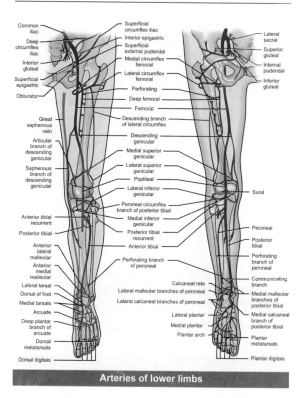

Common iliac
Deep circumflex iliac
Interior gluteal
Superficial epigastric
Obturator
Great saphenous vein
Articular branch of descending genicular
Saphenous branch of descending genicular
Anterior tibial recurrent
Posterior tibial
Anterior lateral malleolar
Anterior medial malleolar
Lateral tarsal
Dorsal of foot
Medial tarsals
Arcuate
Deep plantar branch of arcuate
Dorsal metatarsals
Dorsal digitalis

Superficial circumflex iliac
Interior epigastric
Superficial external pudendal
Medial circumflex femoral
Lateral circumflex femoral
Perforating
Deep femoral
Femoral
Descending branch of lateral circumflex
Descending genicular
Medial superior genicular
Lateral superior genicular
Popliteal
Lateral inferior genicular
Peroneal circumflex branch of posterior tibial
Medial inferior genicular
Posterior tibial recurrent
Anterior tibial
Perforating branch of peroneal
Calcaneal rete
Lateral malleolar branches of peroneal
Lateral calcaneal branches of peroneal
Lateral plantar
Medial plantar
Plantar arch

Lateral sacral
Superior gluteal
Internal pudendal
Inferior gluteal
Sural
Peroneal
Posterior tibial
Perforating branch of peroneal
Communicating branch
Medial malleolar branches of posterior tibial
Medial calcaneal branch of posterior tibial
Plantar metatarsals
Plantar digitalis

Arteries of lower limbs

PLATE-11

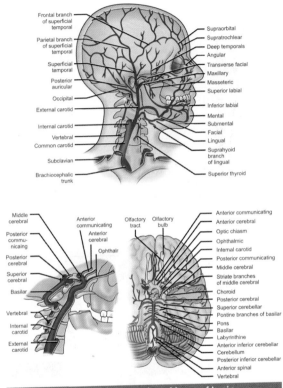

Frontal branch of superficial temporal
Parietal branch of superficial temporal
Superficial temporal
Posterior auricular
Occipital
External carotid
Internal carotid
Vertebral
Common carotid
Subclavian
Brachiocephalic trunk

Supraorbital
Supratrochlear
Deep temporals
Angular
Transverse facial
Maxillary
Masseteric
Superior labial
Inferior labial
Mental
Submental
Facial
Lingual
Suprahyoid branch of lingual
Superior thyroid

Middle cerebral
Posterior communicating
Posterior cerebral
Superior cerebral
Basilar
Vertebral
Internal carotid
External carotid

Anterior communicating
Anterior cerebral
Ophthalr

Olfactory tract
Olfactory bulb

Anterior communicating
Anterior cerebral
Optic chiasm
Ophthalmic
Internal carotid
Posterior communicating
Middle cerebral
Striate branches of middle cerebral
Choroid
Posterior cerebral
Superior cerebellar
Pontine branches of basilar
Pons
Basilar
Labyrinthine
Anterior inferior cerebellar
Cerebellum
Posterior inferior cerebellar
Anterior spinal
Vertebral

Arteries of head, neck and base of brain

PLATE-12

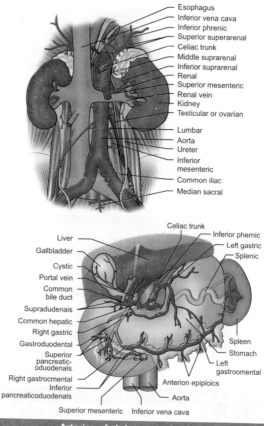

Esophagus
Inferior vena cava
Inferior phrenic
Superior superarenal
Celiac trunk
Middle suprarenal
Inferior suprarenal
Renal
Superior mesenteric
Renal vein
Kidney
Testicular or ovarian

Lumbar
Aorta
Ureter
Inferior mesenteric
Common iliac
Median sacral

Celiac trunk
Inferior phernic
Liver
Left gastric
Gallbladder
Splenic
Cystic
Portal vein
Common bile duct
Supradudenais
Common hepatic
Right gastric
Spleen
Gastroduodental
Stomach
Superior pancreatic-oduodenals
Left gastroomental
Right gastrocmental
Anterion epiploics
Inferior pancreaticoduodenals
Aorta
Superior mesenteric
Inferior vena cava

Arteries of abdomen and pelvis

PLATE-13

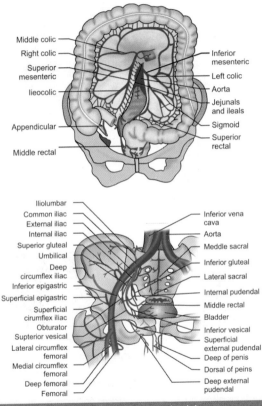

Arteries of abdomen and pelvis

PLATE-14

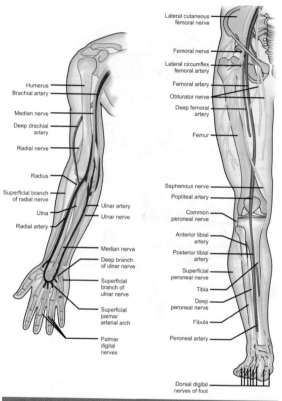

Nerves of limbs

PLATE-15

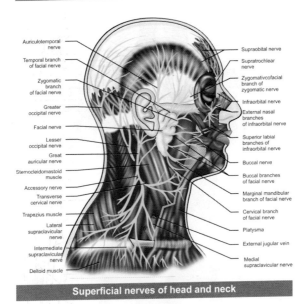

Auriculotemporal nerve

Temporal branch of facial nerve

Zygomatic branch of facial nerve

Greater occipital nerve

Facial nerve

Lesser occipital nerve

Great auricular nerve

Sternocleidomastoid muscle

Accessory nerve

Transverse cervical nerve

Trapezius muscle

Lateral supraclavicular nerve

Intermediate supraclavicular nerve

Deltoid muscle

Supraobital nerve

Supratrochlear nerve

Zygomativcofacial branch of zygomatic nerve

Infraorbital nerve

External nasal branches of infraorbital nerve

Superior labial branches of infraorbital nerve

Buccal nerve

Buccal branches of facial nerve

Marginal mandibular branch of facial nerve

Cervical branch of facial nerve

Platysma

External jugular vein

Medial supraclavicular nerve

Superficial nerves of head and neck

PLATE-16

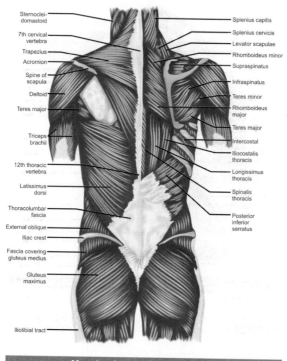

Sternoclei-domastoid

7th cervical vertebra

Trapezius

Acromion

Spine of scapula

Deltoid

Teres major

Triceps brachii

12th thoracic vertebra

Latissimus dorsi

Thoracolumbar fascia

External oblique

Iliac crest

Fascia covering gluteus medius

Gluteus maximus

Iliotibial tract

Spienius capitis

Splenius cervicis

Levator scapulae

Rhomboideus minor

Supraspinatus

Infraspinatus

Teres minor

Rhomboideus major

Teres major

Intercostal

Iliocostalis thoracis

Longissimus thoracis

Spinalis thoracis

Posterior inferior serratus

Muscle of trunk (Posterior view)

PLATE-17

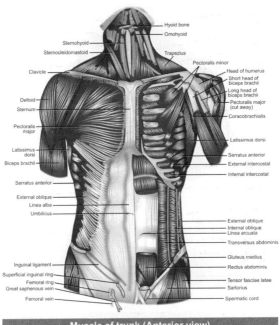

Muscle of trunk (Anterior view)

PLATE-18

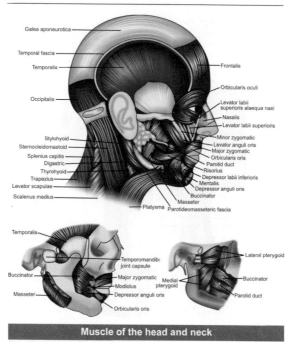

Galea aponeurotica
Temporal fascia
Temporalis
Occipitalis
Stylohyoid
Sternocleidomastoid
Splenius capitis
Digastric
Thyrohyoid
Trapezius
Levator scapulae
Scalenus medius
Frontalis
Orbicularis oculi
Levator labii superioris alaequa nasi
Nasalis
Levator labii superioris
Minor zygomatic
Levator anguli oris
Major zygomatic
Orbicularis oris
Parotid duct
Risorius
Depressor labii inferioris
Mentalis
Depressor anguli oris
Buccinator
Masseter
Platysma   Parotideomasseteric fascia

Temporalis
Buccinator
Masseter
Temporomandibular joint capsule
Major zygomatic
Modiolus
Depressor anguli oris
Orbicularis oris

Lateral pterygoid
Medial pterygoid
Buccinator
Parotid duct

Muscle of the head and neck

PLATE-19

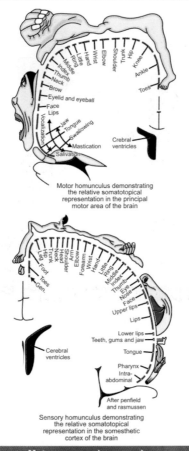

Motor homunculus demonstrating the relative somatotopical representation in the principal motor area of the brain

Sensory homunculus demonstrating the relative somatotopical representation in the somesthetic cortex of the brain

Motor-sensory homunculus

PLATE-20

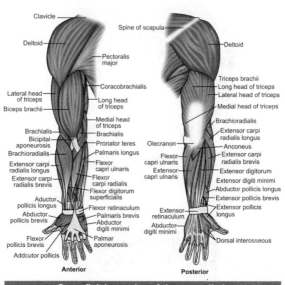

Anterior

Posterior

Superficial muscles of the upper limb

PLATE-21

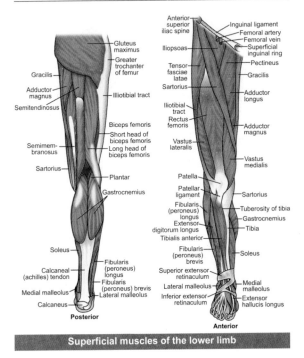

Posterior

- Gluteus maximus
- Greater trochanter of femur
- Gracilis
- Adductor magnus
- Semitendinosus
- Illiotibial tract
- Biceps femoris
- Short head of biceps femoris
- Semimem- branosus
- Long head of biceps femoris
- Sartorius
- Plantar
- Gastrocnemius
- Soleus
- Calcaneal (achilles) tendon
- Fibularis (peroneus) longus
- Fibularis (peroneus) brevis
- Medial malleolus
- Lateral malleolus
- Calcaneus

Anterior

- Anterior superior iliac spine
- Inguinal ligament
- Femoral artery
- Femoral vein
- Superficial inguinal ring
- Iliopsoas
- Pectineus
- Tensor fasciae latae
- Gracilis
- Sartorius
- Adductor longus
- Iliotibial tract
- Rectus femoris
- Adductor magnus
- Vastus lateralis
- Vastus medialis
- Patella
- Patellar ligament
- Sartorius
- Fibularis (peroneus) longus
- Tuberosity of tibia
- Extensor digitorum longus
- Gastrocnemius
- Tibialis anterior
- Tibia
- Fibularis (peroneus) brevis
- Soleus
- Superior extensor retinaculum
- Lateral malleolus
- Medial malleolus
- Inferior extensor retinaculum
- Extensor hallucis longus

Superficial muscles of the lower limb

A

Abacavir An anti-HIV drug.

Abadie's sign 1. A sign in tabes dorsalis in which there is loss of pain from squeezing the calcaneal tendon 2. Spasm of the levator palpebrae superioris muscles occurring frequently in thyrotoxicosis but also seen normally especially with tension and fatigue.

A band A dark band in muscle representing overlapping of actin and myosin filaments.

Abasia Inability to walk because of motor incoordination; compare astasia.

Abate To lessen in force or intensity; to moderate or subside.

Abattoir A slaughter house or an establishment for the killing and dressing of animals.

ABC The mnemonic used for remembering the correct protocol, in order of priority, for cardiopulmonary resuscitation. A refers to airway, B to breathing and C to circulation.

Abdominal angina An acute attack of severe abdominal pain, commonly occurring after eating and often associated with weight loss, nausea, vomiting and diarrhoea. It is caused by narrowing or obstruction of the mesenteric arteries, primarily atherosclerotic in origin.

Abdominal aponeurosis The wide tendinous expanse by which the external oblique, internal oblique, and transverse muscles are inserted.

Abdominal apoplexy Infarction of an abdominal organ, usually the small intestine, resulting from vascular stenosis or occlusion.

Abdominal epilepsy A convulsive equivalent in which abdominal pain, a sense of nausea and often headache are the most prominent symptoms.

Abdominal migraine Abdominal pain, nausea, vomiting or diarrhea associated with migraine. See also convulsive equivalent.

Abciximab An antiplatelet agent.

Abdominal muscles A group of four pair of muscles making up in abdominal wall: The external oblique, internal oblique, rectus abdominis and transversus abdominis.

Abdominal reflex Contraction of the abdominal muscles induced by stroking the overlying skin; a superficial or cutaneous reflex.

Abdominal regions The nine regions of the abdomen artificially delineated by two horizontal and two parasagittal lines. The horizontal lines are tangent to the cartilages of the ninth ribs and iliac crests, respectively, and the parasagittal lines are drawn vertically on each side from the middle of the inguinal ligament. The regions thus formed are 1. above—the right hypochondriac, the epigastric and the left hypochondriac. 2. in the middle—the right/left lateral or lumbar, umbilical and, 3. below—the right inguinal or iliac, the pubic or hypogastric, and the left inguinal or iliac. Also called regions abdominis (*see* Figure).

Abdominal respiration A type of respiration caused by the contraction of the diaphragm and the elastic expansion and recoil of the abdominal walls.

Abdominal ribs 1. The floating ribs. 2. Ossifications of the intersections tendineae.

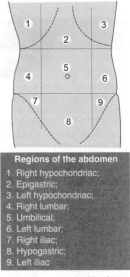

Regions of the abdomen
1. Right hypochondriac;
2. Epigastric;
3. Left hypochondriac;
4. Right lumbar;
5. Umbilical;
6. Left lumbar;
7. Right iliac;
8. Hypogastric;
9. Left iliac

Abdominoposterior In obstetrics, designating a fetal position in which the belly is forward.

Abdominovesical pouch A pouch formed by the reflection of the peritoneum from the anterior abdominal wall onto the distended urinary bladder, it contains the lateral and medial inguinal fossae.

Abducent nerve The sixth cranial nerve, whose fibres arise from the nucleus in the dorsal portion of the pons near the internal genu of the facial nerve and runs a long course to supply the lateral rectus muscle which moves the eyeball outward; also called nerves abducens.

Abducent nucleus A nucleus lying under the floor of the fourth ventricle at the junction of the pons and medulla which gives origin to the abducent nerve.

Abduct To draw away from the median line.

Abduction 1. A movement whereby one part is drawn away from the axis of the body or of an extremity. 2. In ophthalmology (a) Turning of the eyes outward beyond parallelism (*see* Figure).

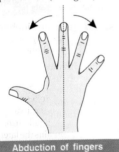

Abduction of fingers

Abduction cap An orthopedic appliance of canvas or leather to maintain abduction in case of subdeltoid bursitis.

Abductor A muscle which on contraction, draws a part away from the axis of the body or of an extremity.

Abductor A muscle found in tailed animals corresponding to the coccygeal muscle in man.

Abductor digiti minimi The abductor muscle of the little finger or little toe. Also called musculus abductor digiti-minimi.

Abductor hallucis A muscle of the medial side of the foot inserted into the base of the first metatarsal. Also called musculus abductor hallucis.

Abductor hallucis longus A muscle of the anterior region of the leg inserted into the base of the first metatarsal.

Abductor indicis The first dorsal interosseous muscle of the hand.

Abductor paralysis Paralysis of abduction especially of the posterior cricoarytenoid muscle and, thus of the vocal cords.

Abductor pollicis brevis The short abductor muscle of the thumb. Also called musculus abductor pollicis.

Abductor pollicis longus The long abductor muscle of the thumb. Also called musculus abductor pollicis longus.

Aberdeen formula A method (developed in Aberdeen in

1974) of estimating the number of nurses needed on a ward, based on the number and dependency of the patients. The formula is W = N (B + T) + A + D + E where: W = average weekly nursing workload in hours; N = average number of patients in ward; B = time in hours per week required to maintain the standard of basic nursing care for a totally helpless bedfast patient; T = time required for technical nursing of the ward speciality expressed as a percentage of the time spent on basic nursing; A = time per patient per week for administrative duties; D = time per patient per week for domestic work; E = patient dependency factor for ward speciality.

Aberrant Varying or deviating from the normal in form, structure or course.

Aberration 1. Deviation from the normal or usual. 2. Unequal refraction or focalization of a lens. *Chromatic aberration*: unequal refraction of light rays of different wavelengths, producing a blurred image with fringes of color. *Chromosomal aberration*: loss/gain/or exchange of genetic material in the chromosomes of a cell resulting in a deletion, duplication, inversion or translocation of genes.

Abetalipoproteinemia A disease entity due to almost total absence of β-lipoproteins, characterized by the predominating presence in blood of acanthocytes, hypocholesterolemia, the celiac syndrome in early childhood and later ataxia, peripheral neuropathy and frequent retinitis pigmentosa and muscular atrophy; an autosomal hereditary trait.

Abeyance 1. A cessation of activity or function 2. A state of suspended animation.

Abiogenesis A theory that living organisms can originate from nonliving matter; spontaneous generation.

Abiosis 1. Absence of life 2. Nonviability.

Abiotrophy Progressive loss of vitality of certain tissues or organs leading to disorders or loss of function applied especially to degenerative, hereditary diseases of late onset e.g., Huntington's chorea.

Abirritant An agent such as a cream or powder, that relieves irritation.

Ablatio placentae Abruptio placenate.

Ablation The removal of part of a tumor by amputation,

excision or other mechanical means.

Ablepsia Loss or absence of vision.

Abluent Detergent, Cleansing.

Abnormal 1. Not normal. 2. Deviating in form, structure or position, not conforming with the natural or general rule.

ABO blood group That genetically determined blood group system defined by the agglutination reaction of erythrocytes exposed to the naturally occurring antibodies anti-A and anti-B and to similar antiserums. The serum of normal individuals contains isoantibodies against the antigens lacking in their erythrocytes giving the following arrangement of antigens (isoagglutinogens) and antibodies.

Group (Land-steiner)	Erythrolyte Antigen (Agglutinogen)	Serum Antibody (Agglutinin)
0	A and B absent	Anti-A anti-B
A	A	Anti-B
B	B	Anti-A
AB	A,B	None

Sub Groups of A are recognised and designated by subscripts as A_1, A_2, etc.

Abort 1. To miscarry; to bring forth a nonviable fetus. 2. To terminate prematurely or stop in the early stages, as the course of a disease. 3. To check or fall short of maximal growth and development.

Aborticide 1. The killing of an unborn fetus. 2. An agent that destroys fetus and produces abortion.

Abortifacient A drug or agent inducing expulsion of the fetus.

Abortion 1. The giving birth to an embryo or fetus prior to the stage of viability i.e., 20 weeks of gestation (fetus weighs less than 400 gm). A distinction is made between abortion and premature birth. Premature infants are those born after the stage of viability has been reached but before full term, 2. The product of such nonviable birth. 3. The arrest of any action or process before its normal completion. *a. accidental* Due to a fall, blow or other injury. *a. complete* One in which the embryo including the membranes is expelled entirely and identified. *a. criminal* Induced termination of pregnancy without medical or legal justification. *a. habitual* A condition in which a woman has had three or more consecutive spontaneous abortions. *a. insipient* Threatened or imminent or impending abortion in which there is copious vaginal bleeding, uterine contractions and cervical dilation. *a. incomplete* In which part of the product of conception has been passed but part (usually the placenta) remains in uterus. *a inevitable* One signalled by rupture of the membranes in the presence of cervical dilation that has advanced beyond any hope of preventing complete abortion. *a. missed* One in which the fetus dies in utero but the product of conception is retained in utero for two months or longer.

Abortive poliomyelitis An early form of poliomyelitis, characterized clinically by relatively mild symptoms of upper respiratory infection, headache, gastrointestinal disturbances, nausea, and vomiting but which does not progress to involve the central nervous system. Definite diagnosis rests upon isolation of the virus and serologic reactions.

Abrachia Armlessness.

Abrachius An armless individual.

Abrasion 1. A spot denuded of skin, mucous membrane or superficial epithelium by rubbing or scraping as of corneal abrasion, an excoriation. 2. The mechanical wearing down of teeth, as from incorrect brushing, appliances or bruxism. Compare attrition, erosion.

Abreaction In psychoanalysis, the mental process by which repressed emotionally charged memories and experiences are brought to consciousness and occur in hypnosis and narcoanalysis.

Abrosia Abstinence from food, fasting.

Abruptio Abruption, a tearing away.

Abruptioplacentae Premature separation of the placenta prior to delivery of the infant (*see* Figure on page 7).

Abscess A circumscribed collection of pus. *a. amebic* An abscess of the liver that contains ameba, and may follow amebic dysentery. It may occur independently also without intestinal infection. *a. Bezold's* A deep abscess in the neck associated with suppuration of the middle ear and purulent sinus thrombosis. *a. Brodie's* A chronic inflammation, sometimes tuberculus, of the head of a bone especially of the tibia. *a. cold* Abscess without heat or other usual signs of

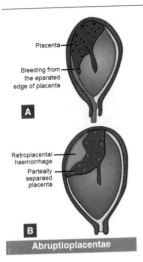

Placenta

Bleeding from the eparated edge of placenta

A

Retroplacental haemorrhage

Parteally separaed placenta

B

Abruptioplacentae

inflammation commonly tuberculous (*see* Figure on page 8).

Abscissa 1. The horizontal of the two coordinates used in plotting the interrelationship of two sets of data. The vertical line is called the ordinate. 2. In optics, the point where a ray of light crosses the principal axis.

Absence 1. Inattention to one's environment. 2. Temporary loss of consciousness, as in absence attacks or psycho motor seizures. 3. Fleeting loss of consciousness occurring in hysterical attacks or at the climax of completed or very intense sexual gratification (Freud).

Absence attack or seizure A form of epilepsy characterized by a sudden transient lapse of consciousness, by a blank stare as in a state of "Suspended animation", sometimes accompanied by minor motor activities such as blinking of the eyes, smacking of lips, stereotyped hand movements and automatism, often there is indistinct vision.

Absolute refractory period The refractory period in which no stimulus, however, strong can excite a response.

Absolute scotoma Scotoma with perception of light entirely absent.

Absolute temperature Temperature reckoned from the absolute zero estimated at approximately – 273° C or – 459° F.

Absolute threshold The lowest intensity as measured under optimal experimental conditions. At which a stimulus is effective or perceived.

Absolute zero A temperature of approximately –273.2° C or –459.8° F; the complete absence of heat.

Absorb 1. In physiology to suck; take, imbibe as fluids

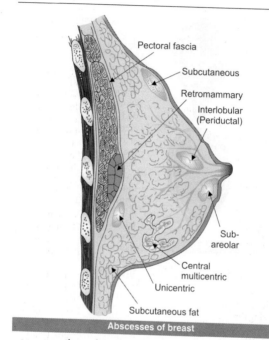

Pectoral fascia

Subcutaneous

Retromammary

Interlobular
(Periductal)

Sub-
areolar

Central
multicentric

Unicentric

Subcutaneous fat

Abscesses of breast

or gases through osmosis and capillarity. 2. To infiltrate into the skin as ultraviolet rays. 3. To incorporate into the body via the blood and lymph. 4. To receive radiant energy and convert it to another form often with rise of temperature.

Absorbable ligature A ligature composed of animal tissue

such as catgut which can be absorbed by the tissues.

Absorbed dose In radiology the amount of energy imparted by ionizing particles to a unit mass of irradiated material at a place of interest.

Absorbefacient Any agent that promote absorption.

Absorbent 1. Anything capable of absorbing or sucking up fluids, faeces or light waves. 2. A drug application or dressing that promotes absorption of diseased tissues.

Absorption 1. In physiology and pharmacology the passage by one or more processes of various body constituents or of medicinal agents through body membranes from one tissue compartment to another, e.g., products of digestion through gastrointestinal mucosa or of drugs through the skin. 2. In physics, and chemistry the taking up by one or more physical or chemical processes of a gas by a solid or liquid or of a liquid by a solid. 3. In physics, radiology and spectrophotometry the process whereby the intensity of a beam of any electromagnetic radiation is attenuated in passing through any material by conversion of the energy of radiation to an equivalent amount of energy which appears within the medium, the radiant energy is converted to heat or some other form of molecular energy. 4. In psychology inattention to all but a single thought or activity.

Absorption atelectasis Obstructive atelectasis.

Absorption band A region of the absorption spectrum in which the absorptivity passes through maximum or inflection.

Absorption coefficient A constant in the law of absorption for homogeneous radiations.

Absorption curve In radiobiology a curve showing variation in absorption of radiation as a function of wave length.

Absorption spectrum A spectrum of radiation which has passed through some selectively absorbing substance as white light after it has passed through a vapor.

Absorptive Absorbent.

Abstergent 1. Having cleansing or purgative properties. 2. A cleaning lotion. 3. A purgative.

Abstinence Voluntary self denial of or forbearance from indulgence of appetites, especially from food, alcoholic drink or sex relations.

Abstinence delirium Delirium occurring on withdrawal of alcohol or of a drug from one addicted to it.

Abulia Loss or defect of the ability to make decisions.

Abulomania Mental disorder characterized by lack of will power and indecisiveness.

Abuse Misuse, maltreatment, or excessive use. *Child a.* The non-accidental use of physical force or the non-accidental act of omission by a parent or other custodian responsible for the care of a child. *Drug a.* Use of illegal drugs or misuse of prescribed drugs. *Solvent a.* The deliberate inhalation of volatile chemicals with the aim of inducing intoxication.

Acalcerosis Calcium deficiency of the diet or of the body as a result of the loss of the mineral in the excreta.

Acalculia Loss of the power to work out any mathematical problems even the simplest.

Acanthion The tip of the anterior nasal spine (*see* Figure below).

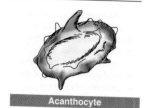

Acanthocyte

cells are acanthocytes 'throny erythrocytes', i.e., peculiar spherocytes with irregularly placed broad or coarse pseudopodia like projections; the abnormal cells manifest a greatly increased mechanical fragility and content of lipolecithin A; is thought to result from a mutant recessive allele for a gene that controls normal structure of redblood cells.

Acanthoid Spine shaped, spinous.

Acantholysis A term used in dermal pathology to denote dissolution of the layers of the epidermis. It is seen in such conditions as pemphigus vulgaris and keratosis follicularis.

Acanthoma Well differentiated keratinizing cornifying squamous cell (or epidermoid) carcinoma, term sometimes used especially with reference to such neoplasms in the skin with little or no histologic evidence of invasion. Regarded by some observers as benign

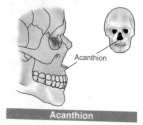

Acanthion

Acanthocyte A throny or peculiarly spiny erythrocyte characterized by multiple spiny cytoplasmic projections (*see* Figure).

Acanthocytosis A rare condition in which as many as 70 to 80 percent of the redblood

neoplasms. *a. nigricans* An eruption of warty growths and hyperpigmentation occurring in the skin of the axillae and in the groins. In adults it is indicative of abdominal malignancy. A benign type occurs in children. In the benign or juvenile type the subjects are obese and the skin condition is self limited.

Acapnia Absence of carbon dioxide in blood and tissues.

Acarbia Pronounced reduction in bicarbonate of the blood.

Acardia Congenital absence of the heart, a condition sometimes present in the parasitic members of conjoined twins.

Acardiacus A conjoined twin parasitic on its mate or utilizing the placental circulation of its mate and having no heart.

Acardiotrophia Atrophy of heart.

Acariasis Any disease caused by an acarid.

Acarid A member of the order Acarina, a mite.

Acaroid 1. Resembling a mite 2. An acarus or mite.

Acarophobia Fear of small parasites or small particles

Acatalepsia, catalepsy 1. Mental deficiency characterized by a lack of understanding 2. Uncertainty in diagnosis or prognosis.

Acataleptic Deficient in comprehension. 2. Uncertain.

Acataphasia A loss of the power of correctly formulating a statement.

Acataposis Difficulty in swallowing liquids; strictly inability to do so.

Acathexia An abnormal loss of the secretions.

Acathexis A mental disorder in which certain objects or ideas fail to arouse an emotional response in the individual.

Accessory Supplementary. *A. nerve* The 11th cranial nerve. It is made up of two portions: the cranial and the spinal.

Accident A sudden unexpected event or injury occurring without omen or forewarning or developing in the course of a disease.

Accommodation Adjustment of the eye for various distances specifically alteration of the covexity of the crystalline lens in order to bring light rays from an external object to a focus on the retina.

Accoucheur Obstetrician.

Accretion 1. Increase by addition to the periphery or material of the same nature as that already present e.g., the manner of growth of crystals. 2. In dentistry foreign material collecting on the surface of a tooth or in a cavity. 3. A growing together.

ACE inhibitors A group of drugs used in the treatment of hypertension. Their name, angiotensin converting enzyme inhibitors, explains part of their mode of action, although it is thought that some of their other actions may also be important in reducing blood pressure.

Acebutolol Betadrenergic blocking agent used in hypertension.

Aceclidine A synthetic compound resembling acecholine, used in glaucoma 0.5-4%.

Acenesthesia Absence of the normal sensation of physical existence or of the consciousness of visceral function.

Acecainide A metabolite of procainamide.

Acenocoumarol (NND) An orally effective synthetic anticoagulant of the coumarin type and with similar action.

Acestoma Exuberant granulations that are forming a cicatrix.

Acetabulum Cup shaped cavity on lateral wall of pelvic bone in which head of femur articulates.

Acetabuloplasty An operation performed to improve the depth and shape of the hip socket in correcting congenital dislocation of the hip or in treating osteoarthritis of the hip (*see* Figure below).

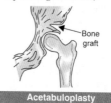

Bone graft

Acetabuloplasty

Acetal A clear liquid made by the imperfect oxidation of alcohol. Has been used as hypnotic.

Acetal dehyde $CH_3 CHO$, a colourless liquid of irritating odor; it is polymerized into paraldehyde in presence of sulphuric acid. It is an intermediate in yeast fermentation of carbohydrate and in alcohol metabolism in man.

Acetamide Acetic acid amide formed by the action of ethyl acetate on ammonia, occurs in colourless deliquescent crystals of a mousy odor.

Acetaminophen N-Acetyl-p-aminophenol, P-acetamido-phenol, a white odorless crystalline slightly bitter powder used as an antipyretic and analgesic.

Acetanilide Made from aniline by the action upon it of acetyl chloride. Occurs in the form of white scales or crystalline powder, very slightly soluble in water but soluble in 5 parts of alcohol, used as an analgesic and antipyretic. Toxic, continued use causes cyanosis.

Acetarsone Acetarsol(BP) acetyl amino hydroxy phenyl arsenic acid, N acetyl-4hydroxy-Marsanilic acid; stovarsol, Used in amebiasis and as a local application in vincents angina and in trichomonas vaginalis.

Acetate A salt of acetic acid.

Acetazolamide Diamox, the heterocyclic sulfonamide. 2. Acetylamino-1.3.4, thiadiazole 5 sulfonamide. It inhibits the action of carbonic anhydrase in the kidney causing an increase in the urinary excretion of sodium, potassium and bicarbonate, reduced excretion of ammonium, a rise in the pH of the urine and a fall in the pH of the blood. Has been used in respiratory acidosis for diuresis and control of fluid retention in epilepsy and in glaucoma.

Acetic Relating to vinegar, sour.

Acid-acetic Diacetic acid, CH_3 COOH, a product of the oxidation of alcohol and of the destructive distillate of wood, the official acid is a liquid containing 36 percent (B.P. 33%) of absolute acetic acid (hydrogen acetate). Used locally as a counterirritant and occasionally internally. Used also as a reagent.

Acetoacetic acid Diacetic acid, CH_3 $COCH_2$ COOH, one of the ketone bodies formed in excess and appearing in the urine in starvation or diabetes.

Acetobacter A genus of the family pseudomonadaceae, containing rodshaped organisms frequently found in elongated, branched or swollen forms, polarly flagellate when motile, energy secured by oxidation of alcohol in wine cider or beer to acetic acid.

Acetohexamide A sulfonylurea, used in diabetes.

Acetokinase An enzyme found in *Escherichia coli* catalyzing the formation of acetylphosphate from acetate in the presence of ATP.

Acetolactic acid An intermediate in pyruvic acid catabolism in yeast.

Acetolase An enzyme that catalyzes the oxidation of alcohol to acetic acid.

Acetomeroctol An organic mercurial antibacterial agent.

Acetomorphine Heroin, see diacetylmorphine.

Acetonaphthone Naphthyl-methyl ketone occurs as yellow needles.

Acetone A colourless volatile inflammable liquid dimethyl ketone. Extremely small amounts are found in normal urine but large quantities occur in urine and blood of diabetic persons, it sometimes imparts an ethereal odor to urine and breath of such patient.

Acetonuria The excretion in the urine of large amount of acetone, an indication of incomplete oxidation of large amount of fat, commonly occurs in diabetic acidosis.

Acetophenazine maleate Tindal maleate, phenothiazine dimaleate, a tranquilizing agent with antiemetic hypotensive, spasmolytic and antihistaminic actions.

Acetophenone A coal tar derivative, phenylethyl ketone, a colorless liquid crystalizing to white needles at low temperatures with an odor of bitter almond. Has been used as a hypnotic or mild depressant.

Acetrizoate A radio-opaque compound used in urography, injected intravenously.

Acetrizoic acid A radio-opaque medium.

Acetyl-p-aminophenylsalicylate Salicylic acid ester of acetyl-p-aminophenol, used as an analgesic, antipyretic, and intestinal antiseptic.

Acetylcholine The acetic acid ester of choline isolated from ergot. Also liberated from preganglionic and postganglionic, endings of parasympathetic fibers and from preganglionic fibers of the sympathetic. Causes cardiac inhibition, vasodilation, gastrointestinal peristalsis and other parasympathetic effects. It is hydrolized into choline and acetic acid by the enzyme cholinesterase that is present in blood and other tissue.

Acetylcholinesterase Cholinesterase, that breaks down acetyl choline into choline and acetic acid.

Acetylcoenzyme A Condensation product of coenzyme A and acetic acid, an intermediate in transfer of two carbon fragment notably in its entrance into the tricarboxylic acid cycle.

Acetylcysteine Mucomyst, a mucolytic agent that reduces the viscosity of mucous secretions.

Acetyldigitoxin Acylanid, same actions and uses as digitoxin but of more rapid onset and shorter duration of action.

Acetylene A colorless gas of a disagreeable odor that burns with an intense white flame. It is prepared commercially by the action of water on calcium carbide.

Acetylsalycylic acid An odorless white crystalline powder soluble in 300 part of water or 5% alcohol readily absorbed from mucous membranes and excreted in urine within 6 hours, widely used as an analgesic, antiinflammatory agent and in the treatment of rheumatism.

Achalasia Failure to relax, referring especially to visceral openings such as the cardia or any other sphincter muscles (*see* Figure).

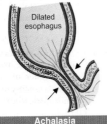

Achalasia

Acheilia Congenital absence of the lips.

Achilles A mythical greek warrior who was vulnerable only in the heel.

Achilles tendon Largest and strongest tendon of the body, formed by the union of gastrocnemius and soleus mus-

cles at the lower end of the calf and inserts into calcaneus (*see* Figure).

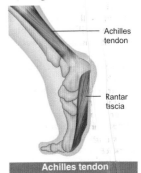

Achilles tendon

Achilles tendon reflex Reflex that occurs after the Achilles tendon is tapped while the foot is dorsiflexed. It is exaggerated in upper motor neuron disease and not present in lower motor neuron disease.

Achiria 1. Congenital absence of the hands. 2. Anesthesia with loss of the sense of possession of one or both hands, a condition sometimes noted in hysteria. 3. A form of dyschiria in which the patient is unable to tell on which side of the body a stimulus has been applied.

Achirus A malformed individual without hands.

Achlorhydria Absence of hydrochloric acid from the gastric juice.

Achluophobia Fear of darkness.

Acholia Suppressed secretion of bile.

Acholic Without bile.

Acholuria Absence of bile pigments from the urine in certain cases of jaundice.

Acholuric Without bile in urine

Achondroplasia Chondrodystrophy, diaphysial aclasis, abnormality in conversion of cartilage into bone resulting in an asymmetrical dwarf.

Achondroplasty Chondrodystrophy.

Achorion A genus of parasitic fungi, proper term now Trichophyton.

Achromasia 1. Cachectic pallor, pallor associated with the Hipocratic facies of extremely severe and chronic illness often heralding the moribund state 2. Absence of the ordinary staining reaction in a cell or tissue. 3. Achromatopsia.

Achronate An absolutely color blind person.

Achronatic 1. Colorless. 2. Not decomposing white light 3. Not staining readily.

Achromatopsia Complete colorblindness.

Achromatosis Absence of natural pigmentation as in albinism.

Achromaturia The passage of colorless or very pale urine.

Achylia 1. Absence of gastric juice or other digestive ferment. 2. Absence of chyle.

Achylous 1. Lacking in gastric juice or other digestive secretion. 2. Having no chyle.

Acid 1. A compound of an electronegative element or radical with hydrogen; it forms salts by replacing all or part of the hydrogen with electropositive elements or radical. An acid containing one displaceable atom of hydrogen in the molecule is called monobasic; one containing two such atoms dibasic and one containing more than two-polybasic. 2. In popular language any chemical compound which has a sour taste.

Acid-base Acid is a substance which generates hydrogen ions $[H^+]$ in the solution whereas base is a substance which generates hydroxyl ions $[OH^-]$ in the solution. In the body an equilibrium occurs between the acid and base elements of blood and body fluids. The normal pH of the serum is between 7.35 and 7.45. Acid- base equilibrium in the body is maintained through the regulatory systems of the kidney, lungs, skin, adrenals, pituitary and the buffer systems present in the blood. When there is a loss of balance between the acidic and alkaline components of blood and body fluids, acid-base imbalance can occur. Metabolic disorders like gastrointestinal diseases diabetes mellitus, renal diseases, etc. can commonly result in acid-base imbalance in the body.

Acidemia An increase in the H-ion concentration of the blood–a fall below normal in pH not withstanding alterations in content of bicarbonate.

Acid-fast A term denoting bacteria that are not decolorized by mineral acids after having been stained with aniline dyes; the leprosy, tubercle and hay bacilli are examples.

Acid phosphatase An enzyme found in many tissues and fluid in the body. Acid phosphatase liberated from prostate gland serves as a marker for cancer prostate. It may also be sometimes elevated in conditions like Paget's disease, oesteomalacia, hepatitis, obstructive jaundice, etc.

Acidosis A condition of reduced alkali reserve (bicarbonate) of the blood and other body fluids with or without an actual decrease in pH.

a. carbondioxide Acidosis resulting from retention of CO_2, it is an exception to the definition in the main heading, for the bicarbonate of the body fluids is usually increased. *a. compensated* Reduced alkali reserve in which compensatory mechanisms maintain the pH of the body fluids at the normal value; in compensated acidosis Co_2 and bicarbonate usually increases although pH remains within normal range. *a. renal tubular* Inability to excrete acid urine with hyperchloremia due to congenital defect in carbonic anhydrase, causing deficient formation of bicarbonate. *a. respiratory* Reduced alkali reserve of the body fluids with a fall in pH resulting from the failure of adequate compensatory mechanisms; bicarbonate may be within normal range in uncompensated acidosis from CO_2 retention.

Acid rain Rain contaminated with sulfur dioxide and nitrogen oxide. By reducing pH, it is harmful for aquatic and plant life.

Acid reflux disorder A condition in which acid comes from the stomach into esophagus causing discomfort and damage to the esophageal lining.

Aciduria Presence of excessive acid in the urine.

Acinetobacter Nonpathogenic genus of microorganism.

Acinus 1. One of the minute sac like secretory portions of an acinous gland. Some authorities use the terms acinus and alveolus interchangeably with reference to glands whereas other differentiate them by the constricted openings of the acinus into the excretory duct. 2. In the lung territory supplied by one terminal bronchiole (an absolute usage) (*see* Figure).

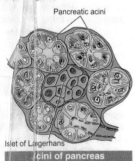

Pancreatic acini

Islet of Langerhans

cini of pancreas

Acivics A pyrimidine analog that blocks conversion of UTP to LTP.

Aclusion Lack of contact of opposing surface of molar and bicuspid teeth when jaws are closed.

Acme The peak, the time of greatest intensity of symptoms.

Acne A papular and pustular eruption due to inflammation with accumulation of secretion involving the sebaceous glands. *a. atrophica* Vulgaris in which the lesions leave a slight amount of scarring. *a. ciliaris* Follicular papules and pustules on the free edges of the eyelids. *a. keratosa* An eruption of papules consisting of horny plugs projecting from the hair follicles accompanied by inflammation. *a. neonatorum* A rare condition in infants characterized by papules and comedones on forehead and cheeks. *a. rosacea* Erythematosa, rosacea, acne of the cheeks and nose associated with papules, pustules, dilated blood vessels in the nasolabial folds and dilated follicles. *a. syphilitica* Pustular syphilides, a rare type of secondary syphilis. *a. telangiectodes* An acniform eruption associated with tuberculosis. *a. urticata* An eruption beginning as small urticarial wheals and followed by slight scarring. *a. vulgaris* Acne simplex, acne disseminata, simple uncomplicated acne, an eruption of papules and pustules on an inflammatory base; condition occurs primarily during puberty and adolescence due to overactive sebaceous apparatus, probably affected by hormonal activity.

Acnegenic Pertaining to substances thought to be responsible for causing acne vulgaris.

Acnemia 1. Atrophy of the calf muscles. 2. Congenital absence of legs.

Acognosia, acognosy A knowledge of remedies.

Acology Therapeutics.

Acomania Servile submission to those in authority while being overdomineering at home.

Acomia Alopecia, baldness.

Aconative Without the desire or wish to act.

Aconite The dried root of *Aconitum napellus*, Antipyretic, diuretic, diaphoretic anodyne, cardiac and respiratory depressant, externally analgesic.

Acorea Congenital absence of the pupil of the eye.

Acoria Absence of the feeling of satiety after eating.

Acoustic Relating to hearing or the perception of sound.

Acoustic apparatus Auditory apparatus; the anatomical structures that help in hearing.

Acoustic area Part of the brain which lies over the vestibular and cochlear nuclei.

Acoustics The science of sounds and their perception.

Acquired Denoting a disease predisposition, that is not congenital but has developed after birth.

Acrania Lack of a cranium.

Acriflavine An acridine dye, a mixture of 2:8 diamino-10 methylacaridinium chloride and 2,8 diaminacridine. A brownish red odorless powder soluble in water. A powerful antiseptic. *a. hydrochloride* Acid acriflavine, acid trypaflavine, used as a wound antiseptic. It has been administered intravenously in brucellosis, tularemia, blastomycosis, and trypanosomiasis.

Acrimony The quality of being intensely irritant; biting or pungent.

Acrisorcin Antifungal agent available as 0.2% cream.

Acrocephaly Malformation of the head consisting in a high or pointed cranial vault due to premature closure of the sagittal, coronal and lamboid sutures.

Acrocyanosis A circulatory disorder in which the hands and less commonly the feet are persistently cold, blue, and sweaty. Milder forms are closely allied to chillblains.

Acrodynia 1. Peripheral neuritis of the fingers or toes 2. A condition caused in rats by a deficiency of pyridoxine (B6) characterized by redness and swelling of the tips of the ears and nose leading to necrosis of these parts.

Acromegaly Acromegalia; Marie disease, a trophic disorder marked by progressive enlargement of the head and face, hands and feet and thorax due to excessive secretion of growth hormone by the anterior lobe of the pituitary gland (*see* Figure).

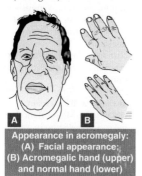

Appearance in acromegaly:
(A) Facial appearance;
(B) Acromegalic hand (upper) and normal hand (lower)

Acromelalgia A vasomotor neurosis marked by redness, pain and swelling of the fingers and toes, headache and vomiting, probably the same as erythromelalgia.

Acromion Acromial process, the outer end of the spine of the scapula which projects as a broad flattened process overhanging the glenoid fosssa; it articulates with the clavicle and gives attachment to the deltoid and some fibers of the trapezius muscles.

Acropachy Hypertrophic pulmonary osteoarthropathy.

Acropathy Simple hereditary clubbing of the digits without associated pulmonary or other progressive disease; often more severe in males, autosomal dominant inheritance.

Acrophobia A morbid dread of elevated places.

Acrosome The juxtanuclear body at the anterior extremity of a spermatid derived from the Golgi apparatus.

Acrotism Absence or imperceptibility of the pulse; pulselessness.

Actin One of the protein components into which actomyosin can be split. Can exist in a fibrous form (f-actin) or a globular form (G-actin).

Actinobacillus A genus of the family Bricellacea, Gram negative nonmotile small rods or coccoid forms characterized by the tendency to form aggregates in tissues or culture which resemble the sulfur granules of actinomycosis. Pathogenic for animals, some species attack man.

Actinomyces Ray fungus so called because it occurs in the form of aggregation of radiating clubshaped rods; a genus of the family *Actinomycetaceae,* containing nonmotile branching filamentous organisms forming a mycelium and fragmenting into elements of irregular sizes. They are mostly anaerobic but some are microaerophilic. A few of the species are pathogenic for man; several cause scab and other potato diseases but the greater number of them are nonpathogenic soil organisms.

Actinomycin An antibacterial crystalline substance isolated from Actinomyces (streptomyces) antiboiticus. Active against Gram positive bacteria e.g., *Bacillus subtilis;* slightly active against Gram negative bacteria. It is also fungicidal and toxic to animal tissues. There are three close similar compounds termed A, B and D.

Actinomycosis A disease of cattle and swine, sometimes communicated to man, caused by the ray fungus Actinomyces (Nocardia). It affects the jaw most commonly (lumpy jaw) but it may invade the brain, lungs or gastroenteric tract. It is characterized by the formation of granulomas of sluggish growth which eventually breakdown and discharge a viscid pus containing minute yellowish granulles; the constitutional symptoms are of a septic character.

Activated partial thromboplastin time (APTT) The time required for a fibrin clot to form after addition of calcium and phopholipids, normally 16-40 seconds.

Activation 1. The act of rendering active. 2. An increase in the energy content of an atom or molecule. 3. Techniques of altering the physiologic environment of the brain by stimulating it by light sound or electricity in order to produce hidden or latent abnormal activity in the electroencephalogram. 4. Stimulation of cell division in an ovum by fertilization or by artificial means.

Activator 1. A substance that renders another substance such as an enzyme active. 2. Internal secretion of the pancreas. 3. An apparatus for impregnating water with radium emanation.

4. A catalyst or accelerator for the polymerization of resins.

Active 1. Production effect; not passive. 2. More than usually likely to undergo some chemical reaction. *a. transport* The name given to the passage of ions or molecules across a cell membrane not by passive diffusion but by an energy consuming process. Active diffusion can take place against a concentration gradient.

Activities of daily living Activities performed by individuals in a normal day that allow independent living.

Actomyosin A protein complex composed of the globulin myosin and actin in the micellae of the muscle fiber. It is the essential contractile substance of muscle.

Acuity Sharpness, clearness, distinctness. *a. visual* Acuteness of vision; it is indicated by a fraction in which numerator is a number expressing the distance in feet at which the patient sees a line or typed on the chart (usually 20 feet) and the denominator a number expressing the distance in feet at which the normal eye would see the smallest letters which the patient sees at the distance at which he is; thus if at 20 feet he sees only the letters which the normal eye would see at 50 feet the formula of his vision will be V = 20/50.

Acupuncture Puncture made with long fine needles for diagnostic or therapeutic purposes.

Acute care Medical treatment given in a hospital to the patients suffering from an acute illness or injury or recovering from surgery.

Acute mountain sickness Headache, vomiting, breathlessness, insomnia occurring on ascent to high altitude without proper acclimatization.

Acute phase reactants Proteins released from liver to blood in response to cytokines like 1L-6 and C-reactive protein.

Acute respiratory distress syndrome Respiratory insufficiency due to damage to alveolocapillary membrane. The oxygen lack does not improve with nasal oxygen therapy.

Acute urethral syndrome Dysuria, urgency, frequency in women in absence of significant bacteriuria.

Acyclovir Antiviral agent used in herpes.

Acyesis 1. Sterility in the woman. 2. The nonpregnant condition.

Adalimumab Monoclonal antibody for autoimmune diseases.

Adamantine Exceedingly hard specifically relating to the enamel of the teeth.

Adamantinoma A tumor of jaw, arising from enamel cells. May be benign or of low grade malignancy. *SYN* – ameloblastoma.

Adams-Stokes syndrome Black out due to sudden fall in cerebral circulation commonly after heartblock.

Adapalene A newor tretinoin anti-acne drug.

Addict A person who finds it difficult to stop some practice especially the taking of drugs or excessive use of alcohol.

Addiction Habituation to some practice, withdrawal from which causes symptoms.

Addison's disease A disease due to deficient adrenocortical hormone secretion with asthenia, weight loss, fatigue, dehydration and shock.

Additive A substance not essentially part of a material such as food, fuel etc., but which is deliberately added to fulfill some specific purpose.

Additive effect The effect of a combination of two or more drugs that is equal to the sum of the individual drug effects.

Adducent To draw toward the median line.

Adduction 1. Movement of a limb toward the central axis of the body or beyond it. 2. A position resulting from such movement (*see* Figure).

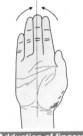

Adduction of fingers

Adductor A muscle drawing a part towards the medianline.

Adefovir Antiviral agent, used in hepatitis B.

Adenase A deaminating enzyme in the liver, pancreas and spleen that converts adenosine into hypoxanthine.

Adenine One of the two purines found in both ribonucleic acid and deoxyribonucleic acid; found also in various nucleotides of importance to the body e.g., adenylic acid adenosine triphosphate (ATP) coenzymes I and II, Q-nitrogen.

Adenitis Inflammation of a lymphnode or of a gland.

Adenoacanthoma A malignant neoplasm consisting chiefly of glandular epithelium (adenocarcinoma) usually well differentiated with foci of metaplasia to squamous (or epidermoid) neoplastic cells.

Adenoblast An embryonic cell destined to proliferate into cells that will enter into the formation of a gland.

Adenocarcinoma A malignant neoplasm of epithelial cells in glandular or glandlike pattern; frequently with infiltration of adjacent tissue, metastases, recurrence after removal etc; a malignant adenoma.

Adenocyst A cystic tumor developing from glandular epithelium, adenocystoma.

Adenocystoma Adenoma in which the neoplastic glandular epithelium forms cysts or cysts like structures.

Adenohypophysis Anterior lobe, pars anterior or pars glandularis of the pituitary gland.

Adenoid Gland like, adeniform, lymphoid; denoting a form of connective tissue found in the lymph nodes, spleen, tonsils, solitary and aggregated nodules of the intestine, red bone marrow and elsewhere; it consists of a connective tissue frame work or reticulum; containing masses of round cells (lymphocytes) in its interstices (*see* Figure).

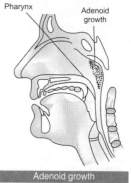

Adenoid growth

Adenoidectomy Surgical removal of adenoid glands.

Adenoma A neoplasm of glandular epithelium. *a. chromophobe* A tumor of the chromophobe cells of the anterior pituitary body associated with hypopituitarism, the cells do not stain well with acid or basic dyes. *a. eosinophilic* A tumor of the eosinophilic chromophil cells of the anterior pituitary associated with gigantism and acromegaly. *a. islet cell* A benign neoplasm of the pancreas composed of tissue similar in structure to that of the islets of Langerhans. It may contain functioning beta cells and may cause hypoglycemia, sometimes termed insulinoma or Langerhansian a. **a. racemose** A benign neoplasm composed of epithelial tissue resembling racemose gland. **a. sebaceum** A neoplasm occurring on the face composed of a mass of sebaceous glands and appearing as an aggregation of red yellow and yellow papules; the patients are sometimes mentally retarded with seizure.

Adenomyosis The ectopic occurrence or diffuse implantation of adenomatous tissue in muscle (usually smooth muscle) as in benign invasion of myometrium by endometrial tissue.

Adenomyxoma A benign neoplasm with histologic characteristics of adenoma and myxoma.

Adenosarcoma A malignant neoplasm of mesodermal tissue with adenomatoid element, sometimes applied to sarcoma originating in connective tissue of a gland.

Adenosine A condensation product of adenine and D-ribose a nucleoside which can be found among the hydrolysis products of all nucleic acids and of the various adenine nucleotides used in PSVT and stress testing.

Adenosine diphosphate A condensation product of adenosine with pyrophosphoric acid, ADP, formed from adenosine triphosphate (ATP) by the hydrolysis of the terminal phosphate group of latter compound.

Adenosis A more or less generalized glandular disease especially one involving the lymphatic nodes.

Adenotome An instrument for the removal of adenoids in the nasopharynx.

Adenovirus A group of viruses infecting upper respiratory tract.

Adenylate cyclase An enzyme that synthesizes c-AMP.

Adiaphoresis Absence or deficiency of perspiration.

Adiaphoretic A drug that causes repression of perspiration.

Adipocere A fatty substance of waxy consistency into which dead animal tissue are sometime converted when kept from the air under certain favouring conditions of temperature; it is believed to be produced by the conversion into fat of the proteins of the tissues.

Adiposis An excessive local or general accumulation of fat in the body, liposis. *a. dolorosa* Dercum's disease, an affection characterized by a deposit of symmetrical nodular or pendulous masses of fat in various regions of the body attended with more or less pain. *a. tuberosa simplex* Anders disease, an affection resembling A. dolorosa in which the fat occurs in small more or less circumscribed masses on the abdomen or confined to the extremities; these masses are sensitive to the touch and may be spontaneously painful.

Adipsia Absence of thirst.

Adjuvant That which aids or assists; denoting a remedy that is added to a prescription to assist or increase the action of the main ingredient; synergist.

Adolescence Period of attaining complete growth and maturity.

Adolescent Pertaining to the period or state of adolescence.

Adrenal Adrenal glands are small triangular paired glands which lie on the superior surface of each kidney. Each adrenal gland consists of two parts :

1. An inner zone medulla which secretes catecholamines like adrenaline and noradrenaline 2. An outer part cortex which secretes mineralocorticoids (aldosterone), glucocorticoids (cortisone) and sex steroids (testosterone). The secretions of the cortex play an important role in controlling many body functions including growth, regulation of metabolism, weight changes, neuromuscular activity, gastrointestinal function, maintenance of body fluid balance and reproduction. Catecholamines, on the other hand, are involved in mediating the fright, flight or fight response (*see* Figure).

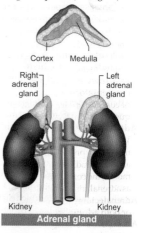

Cortex   Medulla

Right adrenal gland   Left adrenal gland

Kidney   Kidney

Adrenal gland

Adrenal cortical hyperplasia Comprises of a group of autosomal recessive disorders associated with a deficiency of an enzyme envolved in the synthesis of cortisol, aldosterone or both. The clinical manifestations are thus related to the degree of deficiency of either cortisol or aldosterone. The most common from of congenital adrenal hyperplasia is the deficiency of the enzyme 21-hydroxylase. Salt wasting may be present due to inadequate aldosterone synthesis. The sex of a neonate with congenital adrenal hyperplasia is often unclear because of genital ambiguity. Excessive production of androgens can result in female virilization, clitoromegaly, excessive facial/pubic hair, etc. Deficiency of cortisol results in compensatory hypersecretion of corticotrophins and subsequent adrenal hyperplasia.

Adrenal cortical insufficiency When the adrenal cortex is unable to produce sufficient amounts of adrenal cortical hormones, the condition is termed as adrenal cortex insufficiency.

Adrenalectomy Excision of one or both adrenal glands.

Adrenaline Trade name for epinephrine.

Adrenalism A condition resulting from abnormal function of the adrenal (suprarenal) glands, suprarenalism.

Adrenergic Relating to nerve fibers that liberate adrenaline.

Adrenochrome The red oxidation product of epinephrine, was used therapeutically in Germany during the second world war to increase efficiency of diabetic laborers. It is said to produce psychic changes.

Adrenocorticotrophin Adrenocorticotrophic hormone.

Adrenogenital syndrome A condition caused by excess secretion of androgenic hormones by adrenal gland or excess medications with male hormones. In congenital form, the female baby, due to presence of enlarged clitoris and fused labia may be mistaken as male.

Adrenoleukodystrophy A hereditary disease with white matter atrophy of brain and atrophy of adrenal glands.

Adrenosterone An androgen isolated from the adrenal cortex, also known as adrenosterone and as Reichsteins compound G.

Adriamycin Doxorubicin, an anticancer antibiotic.

Adson's maneuver Test for thoracic-outlet syndrome in which there is loss of radial pulse in the arm by rotating the head to the unaffected side with extended neck following deep inspiration.

Adsorb To attach atoms or molecules to the surface of a substance by means of unsatisfied valence bonds.

Adsorbent A substance which adsorbs e.g., ADTE, carbon, clay, magnesia, etc.

Adult Fully grown and mature, a fully grown individual.

Adulterant Impurity, additive that is considered to have an undesirable effect.

Adulteration The alteration of any substance by the deliberate addition of a component not ordinarily part of that substance, usually used to imply that the substance is debased as a result.

Advanced cardiac life support (ACLS) Use of adjuctive measures like monitoring arrhythmia control, defibrillation, and ventilatory support in patients of shock.

Adventitia The outer most covering of any organ or structure which does not form an integral part of such organ or structure specifically the outer coat of an artery; the tunica adventitia.

Adventitious 1. Coming from without; extrinsic. 2. Accidental. 3. Relating to the adventitia of an artery or an organ.

Adynamia Weakness, vital debility, asthenia.

Aerobacter A genus of the tribe Escherichia, family Enterobacteriacea, containing rod shaped Gram negative organisms, found chiefly in the intestine.

Aerobe An organism that can thrive only in presence of oxygen.

Aerocele Refers to a cavity or pouch filled with air or gas. Aeroceles are commonly seen in connection with trachea or larynx resulting in formation of eracheocele and laryngocele respectively. An epidural aerocele is a collection of air between the dura mater and walls of the spinal column.

Aerodynamics The study of air and other gases in motion, the forces that set them in motion, and the result of such motion.

Aerometer An apparatus for determining the density of or for weighing air.

Aerophagia Swallowing of air.

Aeropholia Abnormal and extreme dread of fresh air or of air in motion.

Aeroscope An instrument for the examination of air for visible impurities.

Aetinolol Cardioselective beta-blocker used in hypertension.

Afebrile Nonfebrile, apyretic.

Affect 1. Feeling 2. The sum of an emotion.

Afferent Bringing to or into, denoting certain arteries, veins, lymphatics and nerves.

Affinity 1. Attraction. 2. In chemistry the force that attracts certain atoms to unite with certain others to form compound 3. The selective staining of a tissue by a dye or the uptake of a dye chemical or other substance selectively by a tissue.

Affusion The pouring of water upon the body or any of its parts for therapeutic purposes.

Afibrinogenemia The absence of a detectable amount of fibrinogen in the blood, a relatively rare cause of hemorrhages.

Afterbirth The placenta and membranes that are extruded after the birth of the fetus and most other mammals.

Aftercare The care and treatment of a patient after operation, or of one convalescing from an acute or serious illness.

After discharge The prolongation of reflex response after cessation of stimulation.

After image 1. After vision, Spectrum. 2. Ocular spectrum, the image of an object of which the subjective sensation persists after the object has disappeared. It is called positive when its colors are the same as in the original, negative when the complementary colors are perceived

After pains Painful cramplike contractions of the uterus occurring after childbirth.

After potential The small changes in electrical potential in a stimulated nerve which follow the main potential change. They follow the "spike" potential of the oscillographic record and consists of an initial negative deflection followed by a positive deflection in the oscillograph record.

Agalactia Absence of milk in the breasts after child birth.

Agammaglobulinemia A condition characterized by 1. A lack or extremely low levels of gamma globulin in the blood (and lymphoid tissue) 2. Defective formation of antibody, and 3. Frequent occurrence of suppurative and nonsuppurative infectious disease observed in 2 clinical forms, i.e., primary and secondary. *a. acquired* A type of primary agammaglobulinemia occurs in both sexes at various ages probably resulting from pathological alteration or destruction of normal lymphoid tissue. Level of gamma globulin likely to be from zero to 100 or 125 mg per 100 ml. *a. congenital* A type of primary agammaglobulinemia occurs chiefly in male infants more than 4 to 6 months of age probably resulting from sex linked recessive gene; level of gamma globulin likely to be from zero to 20 or 30 mg per 100 ml. *a. primary* As distinguished from hypogammaglubulinemia; includes transient, congenital and acquired forms, probably results from decrease synthesis of gamma globulin with levels usually less than 100 or 125 mg per ml. *a. secondary* Probably results from increased rate of catabolism or unusual loss of gamma globulin; levels of gamma globulin usually range from 200 to 400 mg per 100 ml. *a. transient* A type of primary agammaglobulinemia occurs in infants of both sexes usually during the second to sixth months of life probably resulting from immaturity of lymphoid tissue, level of gamma globulin likely to be less than 100 to 150 mg per 100 ml.

Agamogony Asexual reproduction.

Aganglionosis The state of being without ganglia, absence of ganglion cells from Auerbach plexus in eye, distal colon in congenital hypertrophic dilation of the colon.

Agar A gelatinous substance prepared from seaweed in Japan and India, used in constipation to increase the bulk of the feces and in bacteriology as a base for culture media; when unqualified it is usually called agar-agar.

Agent An active force or substance capable of producing an effect. *a. antifoaming* Chemicals such as ethylalcohol or 2-ethylhexanol administered with oxygen to patients in pulmonary edema to relieve the respiratory obstruction aggravated by the foam of edema fluid. *a. chelating* A compound such as calcium-disodium ethylene diamine tetra accetic acid which forms a complex with a metal. The medicinal use of these agents is to render poisonous metal compounds innocuous. The resulting chelate complex is unionizable, stable and nonpoisonous and is excreted in the urine. *a. eaton* A living organism of a coccobacillary type 125 to 150 μ that is grown on living cells and on official media and produces a characteristic cold agglutinin. *a. reducing* Any substance that has the power of initiating a reaction involving the gain of electrons. *a. sclerosing* A compound such as sodium ricinoleate used in the treatment of varicose veins.

Ageusia Loss of the sense of taste.

Agglutinate Pertaining to a specific activity of antibody in an antigen antibody reaction, as a specific hemagglutin as certain red blood cells (*see* Figure).

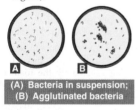

(A) Bacteria in suspension;
(B) Agglutinated bacteria

Agglutination Aggregation into clumps or masses of microorganisms or other cells upon exposure to a specific immune serum or other source of appropriate antibody. *a. cold* Agglutination of red blood cells by their own serum or by any other serum when the blood is cooled below

body temperature but is most pronounced below 25° C. The phenomenon results from cold agglutinins. Although it is seen occasionally in the blood of apparently normal persons it is more frequent in scarlet fever, staphylococcal infections, pneumonia, certain hemolytic anemias and trypanosomiasis.

Agglutinin Antibody that causes clumping or agglutination of the bacteria or other cells which either stimulate the formation of the agglutinaion or contain immunologically, similar reactive material. *a. cold* Agglutinin that agglutinates human group 0 erythrocytes at zero to 5° C but not at 37° C, found in the serum of less than half of patients with primary atypical pneumonia and also in certain other diseases especially trypanosomiasis, titer is usually at a peak relatively early during recovery.

Agglutinogen An antigenic substance that stimulates the formation of specific agglutinin.

Aggregate 1. To unite or come together in mass or cluster. 2. The total of individual units making up a mass or cluster.

Agitophasia Abnormally rapid speech in which words are

imperfectly spoken or dropped out of a sentence.

Aglossia Congenital absence of the tongue.

Aglutition Inability to swallow or great difficulty in swallowing, aphagia, dysphagia.

Agnathia Absence of the lower jaw.

Agnosia Lack of sensory ability to recognize objects. *a. auditory* Central auditory inappreciation of sound, ability to perceive sound at the end organ with inability to interpret it centrally. *a. optic* Inability to interpret visual images. *a. tactile* Inability to recognize objects by touch. *a. visual spatial* Disturbance in spatial orientation and in understanding of spatial relations; apractognosia.

Agonal Relating to the process of dying or the movement of death so called because of the former erroneous notion that dying is a painful process.

Agonist Denoting a muscle in state of contraction with reference to its opposing muscle or antagonist.

Agony Extreme mental or physical suffering; struggle for death.

A:G ratio *See* Albumin:globulin ratio.

Agrammatism Loss, through cerebral disease, of the power to construct a grammatical or intelligible sentence, words are uttered but not in proper sequence, a form of aphasia.

Agranulocytosis Acute condition characterized by pronounced leukopenia with great reduction in the number of polymorphonuclear leucocytes, infected ulcers likely to develop in the throat, intestinal tract and other mucous membranes as well as in the skin. Termed also sepsis agranulocytica, malignant leukopenia, agranulocytic angina, mucocytis necroticans agranulocytica and schultz angina.

Agraphia Loss of the power of writing due or to an inability to phrase thought. Acoustic agraphia is acquired inability to write from dictation. In amnemanic agraphia, letters and words can be written but not connected sentences; in verbal agraphia single letters can be written. Musical agraphia is the loss of power to write musical notation.

AHF Antihaemophilic factor (clotting factor VIII).

AHG Antihaemophilic globulin (clotting factor VIII).

AID Artificial insemination of a woman with donor semen.

AIDS Acquired immune deficiency syndrome. It is the extreme end of the spectrum of disease caused by human immunodeficiency virus (HIV) infection, and impairs the body's cellular immune system. This may result in infection by organisms of normally no or low pathogenicity (opportunistic infections), principally *Pneumocystis carinii* pneumonia (PCP), or the development of unusual tumours, namely Kaposi's sarcoma (KS). *A. related complex* (ARC) recurrent symptoms such as lymphadenopathy, night sweats, diarrhoea, weight loss, malaise and chest infections. Examination of the blood may show abnormally low platelet and neutrophil counts as well as low lymphocyte counts (*see* Figure on page 34).

Air A mixture of gases that make up the earth's atmosphere. It consists of: non-active nitrogen 79%; oxygen 21%, which supports life and combustion; traces of neon, argon, hydrogen, etc.; and carbon dioxide 0.03%, except in expired air, when 6% is exhaled as a result of diffusion that has taken place in the lungs. Air has weight and exerts pressure, which aids in syphonage from body cavities. *A. bed* a rubber mattress inflated with air. *Complemen-*

tal a. additional air that can be inhaled with inspiratory effort. *A. embolism* an embolism caused by air entering the circulatory system. *A. encephalography* radiological examination of the brain after the injection of air into the subarachnoid space. *A. hunger* A form of dyspnoea in which there are deep sighing respirations, characteristic of severe haemorrhage or acidosis. *Residual a.* Air remaining in the lungs after deep expiration. *Stationary a.* That retained in the lungs after normal expiration. *Supplemental a.* The extra air forced out of the lungs with expiratory effort. **Tidal a.** That which passes in and out of the lungs in normal respiratory action.

Airway 1. The passage by which the air enters and leaves the lungs. 2. A mechanical device (tube) used for securing unobstructed respiration during general anaesthesia or on other occasions when the patient is not ventilating or exchanging gases properly. It may be passed through the mouth or nose. The tube prevents a flaccid tongue from resting against the posterior pharyngeal wall and causing obstruction of the airway (*see* Figure on page 35).

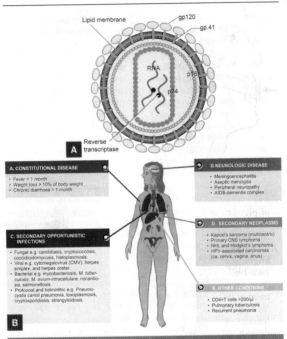

A. CONSTITUTIONAL DISEASE

- Fever > 1 month
- Weight loss > 10% of body weight
- Chronic diarrhoea > 1 month

B. NEUROLOGIC DISEASE

- Meningoencephalitis
- Aseptic meningitis
- Peripheral neuropathy
- AIDS-dementia complex

C. SECONDARY OPPORTUNISTIC INFECTIONS

- Fungal e.g. candidiasis, cryptococcosis, coccidioidomycosis, histoplasmosis.
- Viral e.g. cytomegalovirus (CMV), herpes simplex, and herpes zoster.
- Bacterial e.g. mycobacteriosis, M. tuberculosis, M. avium-intracellulare, nocardiosis, salmonellosis.
- Protozoal and helminthic e.g. Pneumocystis carinii pneumonia, toxoplasmosis, cryptosporidiosis, strongyloidosis.

D. SECONDARY NEOPLASMS

- Kaposi's sarcoma (multicentric)
- Primary CNS lymphoma
- NHL and Hodgkin's lymphoma
- HPV-associated carcinoma (ca. cervix, vagina, anus)

E. OTHER CONDITIONS

- CD4+T cells >200/µl
- Pulmonary tuberculosis
- Recurrent pneumonia

HIV virus

Akathisia Motor restlessness.

Akinesia Loss of muscle power. This may be the result of a brain or spinal cord lesion or, temporarily, to anaesthesia.

Alalia Loss of impairment of the power of speech due to muscle paralysis or a cerebral lesion.

Alanine aminotransferase An intracellular enzyme involved in protein and carbohydrate metabolism. Increased enzyme level in blood indicate necrosis of liver, muscle or brain (formerly called SGOT).

Albinism A condition in which there is congenital absence

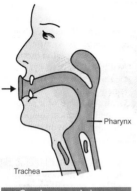

Oropharyngeal airway

of pigment in the skin, hair and eyes. It may be partial or complete.

Albright's syndrome *F. Albright, American physician, 1900-1969.* Condition in which there is abnormal development of bone, excessive pigmentation of the skin and, in females, precocious sexual development.

Albino A person with very little or no pigment in the skin, hair or choroid. A congenital diffuse absence of melanin in the skin and hair.

Albumen 1. White of egg, egg **albumin ovalbumin** 2. Albumin.

Albumin A simple protein widely distributed through-

out the tissues and fluids of plants and animals, it is soluble in pure water, precipitable from a solution by mineral acids and coagulable by heat in acid or neutral solution. Varieties of it are found in blood, milk and muscles. *a. native* Protein existing in its natural state in the body, it is soluble in water and not precipitated by diluted acids, the two principal forms are serum albumin and egg albumin. *a. normal human serum* A sterile preparation of serum albumin obtained by obtaining blood plasma proteins from healthy persons. Used as a transfusion material and to treat edema due to hypoproteinemia.

Albumin-globulin ratio Often abbreviated as A:G ratio. Albumin and globulin are different types of proteins found in the serum. Albumin is mainly synthesized by liver. This protein helps in creating an osmotic force which maintains fluid volume within the vascular space. Globulins, on the other hand, are synthesized in various other parts of the body. Globulins include: gamma globulins (antibodies), beta globulins, alpha-2-globulins and alpha-

1-globulins. Optimal range of A:G ratio is 1.7. A:G ratio may get altered in presence of a pathology.

Albuminuria The presence of protein in urine chiefly albumin (but also globulin) usually indicates disease but sometimes results from a temporary or transient dysfunction. *a. adolescent* Functional albuminuria occurring at about the time of puberty, it is usually cyclic or orthostatic albuminuria. *a. of athletes* A form of functional albuminuria following excessive muscular exertion. *a. cyclic* A functional form sometimes observed intermittently in cycles of 12 to 36 hours duration chiefly in younger persons, the degree of albuminuria is usually slight. *a. dietetic* The excretion of protein in the urine following the ingestion of certain foods, also termed digestive albuminuria. *a. functional* A collective term designating any albuminuria in which there is no detectable, associated pathologic condition in the kidneys or other tissues; may be observed intermittently during pregnancy or adolescence, in athletes etc. *a. orthostatic* A condition characterized by the appearance of albumin in the urine when the patient is in the erect posture and its disappearance when he is recumbent.

Albuterol A sympathomimetic drug used in bronchial asthma.

Alcaine Proparacaine, a local anaesthetic.

Alcohol 1. One of a series of organic chemical compounds in which the hydrogen (H) in a hydrocarbon is replaced by hydroxyl (OH), the hydroxide of a hydrocarbon radical reacting with acids to form esters as a metallic hydroxide reacts to form salt. 2. Any beverage containing ethyl alcohol. 3. Ethanol a liquid containing 92.3 percent by weight corresponding to 94.9 percent by volume of C_7H_5OH. *a. absolute* With a minimum admixture of water at most 1 percent. *a. dehydrogenase* A pyridinoenzyme of the liver catalyzing the dehydrogenation of ethyl alcohol to acetaldehyde. *a. dehydrated* Absolute alcohol; ethyl hydroxide C_2H_5-OH. Containing not more than 1 percent by weight of water. *a. denatured* Methylated spirit, ethyl alcohol that has been made undrinkable by the addition of one ninth of its volume of methyl alcohol and a small quantity of benzine or the pyridine bases. *a. dilute* Eight concentration are official, 90, 80, 70, 50, 45, 25 and 20 per cent V/V.

Alcoholism Poisoning with alcohol.

Alcoholophilia The craving for alcohol.

Alcuronium A neuromuscular blocking agent; non depolarizing.

Aldolase Zymohexase, an enzyme involved in the glycolytic chain catalyzing the splitting of fructose-1, 6-disphosphate to 3-phosphoglyceraldehyde and phosphodihydroxyacetone.

Aldose A monosaccharide containing the characterizing group of the aldehydes (CHO).

Aldosterone A steroid principle of the adrenal cortex which is more potent than deoxycorticosterone in causing sodium retention and potassium loss. It possesses little or no antirheumatic property. Chemically it differs from corticosterone in having an aldehyde group at C-18.

Aldosteronism Excessive production or excretion of aldosterone. Two forms are recognized 1. True or Primary, characterized by persistent hypokalemia (with alkalosis), hypertension, polyuria, exacerbation of muscular weakness and normal or elevated serum sodium 2. So-called secondary form that is characterized by conspicuous edema (in contrast to primary) and is associated with congestive cardiac failure, cirrhosis, nephrosis and so on.

Alendronate Bisphosphonate for osteoporosis.

Aleukia 1. Absence or extremely decreased number of leukocytes in circulating blood, sometimes also termed aleukemic myelosis. 2. Absence or extremely decreased number of blood platelets. (See also thrombopenia).

Alexia Loss of the power to grasp the meaning of written or printed words, sentences, also called optical, sensory or visual alexia in distinction to motor alexia (aphemia or anarthria) in which there is loss of the power to read aloud although the significance of what is written or printed is understood; musical blindness is loss of the power to read musical notation.

Alfacalcidol Active vit D_3.

Alfentanil Newer more potent opioid analgesic with shorter duration of action.

Alfuzosin Alfa-blocker, used in prostatic hypertrophy.

Algesia State of increased sensitivity, to pain some times provoked by stimuli not normally painful.

Alegesimeter, algesiometer An instrument for measuring the degree of sensitivity to a painful stimulus.

Algesthesia The appreciation of pain especially hypersensitivity to painful stimuli, a form of hyperesthesia.

Algid Chilly cold.

Algogenesis (*Greek:* algos+ genesis = pain + origin). Algogenesis thus refers to the origin or production of pain.

Algogenic Producing pain or lowering the body temperature.

Algolagnia (*Greek:* algos + lagnia = pain + lust). Sexual tendency in which the person derives sexual gratification either by inflicting pain to the partner or by experiencing the pain, particularly involving the erogeneous zone.

Algophily A desire to suffer from pain because one derives sexual pleasure from it.

Algophobia An abnormal and persistent fear of experiencing pain.

Algor (*latin:* algor-coolness) Algor mortis is defined as reduction in body temperature following death.

Alimentary Relating to food or nutrition.

Aliphatic 1. Fatty. 2. Denoting the open chain compounds most of which belong to the fatty series.

Alkalies A strongly basic substance alkaline in reaction and capable of saponifying fats, i.e., sodium hydroxide, potassium hydroxide.

Alkaloid A basic substance found in the leaves, barks, seeds and other parts of plants usually constituting the active principle of crude drug. A substance of similar nature is formed in animal tissues. Alkaloids are usually bitter in taste and alkaline in reaction and unite with acids to form salts.

Alkalosis A normally high alkali reserve (biocarbonate) of blood and other body fluids with a tendency for an increase in pH of the blood although it may remain normal. It may result from persistent vomiting, hyperventilation or excessive ingestion of sodium bicarbonate.

Alkaptonuria Urinary excretion of alkaptone bodies (e.g., homogentisic acid) which cause a dark color if the urine is permitted to stand or is alkalinized; Represents a defect in the metabolism of tyrosine and phenylalanine; some times associated with ochronosis.

Alkylating agents Cell cycle nonspecific anticancer drugs.

Alkylating agents
Amsacrine
Nitrogen mustard
Cyclophosphamide
Ifosamide
Melphalan
Chlorambucil
Busulfan
Thiotepa
Carboplatin
Cisplatin

Alkylation The substitution of an aliphatic hydrocarbon radical for a hydrogen atom in a cyclic or ring compound.

Allantoin Ureidohydantoin, glyoxyidiureide, a nitrogeneous crystalline substance present in the allantoic fluid, the urine of the fetus and elsewhere. Used externally to promote wound healing. It is the oxidation product of purine metabolism in animals other than man and other primates.

Allele Any one of a series of two or more different genes that may occupy the same position or locus on a specific chromosome. As autosomal chromosomes are paired each autosomal locus is represented twice in normal somatic cells. If the same allele occupies both loci the individual or cell is homozygous for this allele, if the two loci are different the individual or cell is heterozygous for both.

Allelism State of two or more genes that must occupy the same position or locus on a specific chromosome.

Allergen A substance (usually protein but may be non- protein material) that stimulates an altered cellular response in the animal or human body thereby resulting in manifestation of allergy as the protein (S) of certain foods, bacteria, pollen and so on. *a. bacterial* The specific protein (or other material) in the bacterial cell that may stimulate an allergic response e.g., tuberculin which is prepared from tubercle bacilli. *a. pollen* The material in pollen that may stimulate an allergic response.

Allergic Relating to a recognizable condition of allergy or to any response stimulated by an allergen.

Allergy 1. Any abnormal or altered reaction to an antigen or allergen including greater (hyper) or less sensitivity, the term is now used almost invariably to indicate hyper- sensitivity of the body cells to a specific substance (antigen, allergen) that results in various types of reaction. The exciting material or antigen may be protein, lipid or carbohydrate in nature. The allergic reaction is basically an antibody reaction and includes anaphylaxis, atopic diseases, serum sickness, contact dermatitis. 2. That branch of medicine which embraces the study, diagnosis and treatment of allergic manifestation. 3. An acquired hypersensitivity to certain drugs and biologic preparations. *a. bacterial* Increased sensitivity to various substance of certain species of bacteria. Usually result from previous infection with a specific organism but under special condition may occasionally develop after injection of antigenic materials not related to antibody in circulating blood. *a. bronchial* Asthma and similar conditions that are allergic in origin. *a. cold* Physical allergy produced by exposure to cold. *a. contact* Cutaneous reaction caused by direct contact with an allergen to which the person is hypersensitive. *a. delayed* Allergic response that is not apparent until several hours or a few days have passed as in hypersensitivity to tuberculin, coccidioidin, and other extracts from microorganism. *a. drug* Unusual sensitivity to a drug or other chemical or to combination products of such compounds with various substances in the body.

Alloantigen An antigen present in the blood or tissue of a donor, i.e. it is not present in the recipient. It can trigger an immune response.

Alloarthroplasty Surgical creation of a new joint in the body using materials other than the cells and tissues from human body. E.g. use of hip prosthesis. In other words it can be defined as surgical construction of an artificial joint.

Allocheiria A sensation or stimulus is perceived at a point on the body which is opposite to the point where the stimulus was actually applied. This is also known as allachesthesia, allesthesia or allochiria. This condition is usually due to the lesions in the central nervous system, particularly the parietal lobe.

Allochezia Either defecation from an opening other than the anus or expulsion of non-faecal matter from the anus.

Alloeroticism Sexual attraction toward another person, as opposed to autoeroticism.

Allogamy The fertilization of the ova of one individual by the spermatozoa of another; the opposite of autogamy.

Allograft Tissue transplanted from one person to another. *Non-viable a.* Skin, taken from a cadaver, which cannot regenerate. *Viable a.* Living tissue transplanted.

Allopath One who practises medicine according to the system of allopathy.

Allopathy A therapeutic system in which disease is treated by producing a morbid reaction of another kind or in another part by method of substitution.

Alloploidy The condition of a hybrid individual or cell having two or more sets of chromosomes derived from two different ancestral species.

Allopurinol Xanthine oxidase inhibitor, used in gout and hyperuricemia.

Allosome One of the chromosomes differing in appearance or behaviour from the ordinary

chromosomes or autosomes and sometimes unequally distributed among the germ cell, heterotypical chromosome.

Allylestrenol Progestational agent.

Alma-Ata declaration A declaration made in 1978 at in conference on Primary Health Care at Alma-Ata in USSR for attaining health for all by year 2000.

Almetrine Respiratory stimulant used in COPD.

Alochia Absence of lochia.

Alopecia Acomia, baldness. *a. areata* Condition of unknown etiology producing of circumscribed, noninflamed areas of baldness on the scalp, eyebrows and bearded portion of the face. *a. dynamica* Hair loss due to some destructive disease process affecting the hair follicles. *a. follicularis* A papular or postular inflammation of the hair follicles of the scalp resulting in scarring and loss of hair in the affected area (*see* Figure on page 42).

Alveolus A small angular cavity; bony socket of a tooth; air sac of the lungs.

Alovera Skin texture enhancer and emollient.

Alpha 1 antitrypsin An inhibitor of trypsin deficient in patients of emphysema.

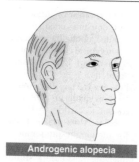

Androgenic alopecia

Alpha fetoprotein An antigen present in fetus, increased in adults with hepatic cancer.

Alprazolam A benzodiazepine, anxiolytic agent.

Alprostadil Prostaglandin used in congenital heart disease esp. PDA.

ALP test ALP (alkaline phosphatase) is an enzyme found in various body tissue. Various types of this enzyme (also known as isoenzymes) are present in different body structures, e.g. Liver and bone ALP isoenzyme. E.g. Liver and bone ALP isoenzyme. ALP isoenzyme test aims at measuring the amounts of different types of ALP present in the body. Elevated levels of ALP can occur in conditions like liver disease, biliary disease (jaundice), kidney disease, bone disease, various types of cancers, oesteogenesis imperfecta, etc.

Alternative medicine Methods other than scientific to diagnose and treat diseases like homeopathy, ayurveda, acupuncture, acupressure, aromatherapy, naturopathy, faith healing, yoga.

Altitude sickness A pathological condition occurring at high altitudes due to presence of a low air pressure. It can result in symptoms like headache, dyspnoea, lassitude, weakness, fatigue, breathlessness, insomnia, dizziness, anorexia, nausea, abdominal pain, diarrhoea, usual disturbances, mental confusion, depression, etc. The exact pathogenesis of altitude sickness is not yet understood. Though it occurs at low atmospheric pressure, it is not necessarily related to low partial pressure of oxygen.

Aluminium A white silvery metal of very light weight. Symbol Al. atomic no 13, atomic weight 26.97 melting point 660°, inhalation of the finely divided dust has been proposed to bind silica, to prevent silicosis. *a. hydroxide* Hydrated alumina a light white powder. Soluble in water, used as an astringent dusting powder. Also used internally as a mild astringent, antacid. *a. oleate* A yellow mass insoluble in water. Used locally, on mucous membranes as an astringent antiseptic. *a. phosphate* A white infusible powder insoluble in water but soluble in alkali hydroxides. Used for dental cement with calcium sulfate and sodium silicate. *a. subacetate* Used in solution as an astringent, and in embleming fluids. Diluted to about 0.5 percent with water it is used as an ingradient in mouth washes. *a. sulfate* Cake alum, a white crystaline powder soluble in water, used as an astringent, detergent in skin ulcers. *a. tannate* A basic salt of varying composition, a brownish powder insoluble in water. Used as astringent solution for local applications. *a. torotannate* A brownish powder. Used as an antiseptic and dusting powder. The tartarte is soluble in water, it is used as a local astringent.

Alveolitis Inflammation of alveoli. *a. allergic* Diffuse granulomatous lung disease caused by hypersensitivity to organic dusts (*see* Figure).

Alzheimer's cells *A. Alzheimer, German neurologist, 1864-1915.* 1. Giant astrocytes with large

Alveoli pulmonis (pulmonary alveoli), with cross-section showing the alveolar ducts and sacs

prominent nuclei found in the brain in hepatolenticular degeneration and hepatic comas. 2. Degenerated astrocytes.

Alzheimer's disease A disease of unknown etiology causing presenile dementia.

Amalgam A solution of metal in mercury. In dentistry the metal consists mainly of intermetallic compound Ag_3Sn, Zinc and copper are useful but not essential.

Amanita A genus of fungi, Agaricus. *a. phallaoides* deadly agaric, contains a poisonous principle that causes severe gastrointestinal symptoms and is hemolytic and injurious to the kidneys.

Amantidine An agent used in Parkinsonism, and influenza.

Amaurosis A total loss of vision. *a. fugax* Temporary blindness in airplane pilots when making a circular manoeuvre with head toward the centre of the circle due to centrifugal force causing cerebral ischemia, flight blindness, blackout. *a. burn's* Postmarital amaurosis; blindness following sexual excess. *a. toxic* Blindness due to optic neuritis excited by tobacco, alcohol, wood alcohol, lead, arsenic, quinine or other poisons.

Ambenoniam An anti-cholinesterase agent.

Amblyacousia Hearing dullness.

Amblyopia Uncorrectable decrease in vision in one or both eyes, which occurs commonly due to asymmetric refractive error or strabismus.

Amblygeustia Temporary or permanent diminution in the sense of taste.

Amblyoscope An instrument resembling a stereoscope used in training the fusion sense and habituating an amblyopic eye to bear its share of vision.

Ambroxol A mucolytic.

Ambu bag A hand operated, self-rainflating bag used during resuscitation. It is connected by tubing and non-rebreathing valve to a face mask or endotracheal tube and is used for artificial ventilation.

Amebiasis Infestation with *Entamoeba histolytica* or other pathogenic amoebas. *a. hepatic* Infection of the liver with entamoeba histolytica, may occur with or without antecedent amebic dysentery.

Amebocyte A cell such as a neutrophil leukocyte having the power of ameboid movements.

Ameboid 1. Resembling an ameba in appearance or characteristic 2. Of irregular outline with peripheral projections.

Ameboma An amebic granuloma, a nodular tumorlike focus of proliferative inflammation sometimes developing in chronic amebiasis especially in the wall of colon.

Ameiosis A cell division resulting in formation of gametes without reduction in chromosome number.

Amelia Congenital absence of a limb or limbs.

Amelioration Improvement, moderation in the intensity of symptoms.

Amelobastoma A neoplasm originating from epithelial tissue. Related to the enamel organ.

Amenorrhoea Absence or abnormal cessation of the menses.

Amentia 1. Idiocy 2. A form of confusional insanity marked especially by apathy, disorientation and more or less stupor.

Amethocaine A local anaesthetic for mucous membranes. *A. pastille* A lozenge that, when dissolved slowly in the mouth, will aid the passage of a bronchoscope or gastroscope.

Amethopterin Methotrexata, a cytotoxic drug.

Amifostine Cytoprotective agent in cancer chemotherapy.

Amiloride A potassium sparing diuretic.

Amikacin An aminoglycoside antibiotic.

Aminacrine Antibacterial, antitrichomonad agent used in vaginal preparations.

Amino acid A chemical compound containing both NH_2 and COOH groups. The endproduct of protein digestion. *Essential a. a.* One required for replacement and growth but which cannot be synthesized in the body in sufficient amounts and must be obtained in the diet (*see* Table). *Nonessential a. a.* One necessary for proper growth but which can be synthesized in the body and is not specifically required in the diet.

Essential amino acids
1. Threonine
2. Lysine
3. Methionine
4. Valine
5. Phenylalanine
6. Leucine
7. Tryptophan
8. Isoleucine
9. Histidine
10. Arginine

Amino caproic acid Antifibrinolytic agent used for vascular plugging in haemorrhage.

Aminoglutethimide Adrenocortical suppressant used in breast cancer.

Aminopterin 4-Aminopteroylglutamic acid, a folic acid antagonist, yellow crystals, soluble in alkali. Used in treatment of acute leukemia and other neoplastic diseases.

Aminosalicylic acid p-Aminosalicylic acid, 4-amino-2hydroxybenzoic acid, small crystals slightly soluble in water. Melting point 150° C. A bacteriostatic agent against tubercle bacilli, used as an adjunct to streptomycin. Abbreviated AS or PAS.

Amiodarone Antiarrhythmic agent.

Amitryptyline hydrochloride Chemically and pharmacologically related to imipramine hydrochloride. An antidepressant agent with mild tranquilizing properties, used in the treatment of mental depression and maniac depressive states.

Amlodipine Calcium channel blocker for hypertension.

Ammonia A volatile alkaline gas, NH_3, very soluble in water combining with acids to form a number of salts.

Ammoniemia The presence of ammonia or some of its compounds in the blood, thought to be formed from the decomposition of urea with weak pulse, gastroenteric symptoms and coma.

Ammonium A group of atoms, NH_4 that behaves as a univalent metal in forming ammonical compound; it has never been obtained in a free state. *a. acetate* White, deliquescent, crystals, soluble in water, melting point 112° C. Mild diaphoretic and refrigerant, used in preserving meat. *a. carbonate* A mixture of carbon dioxide and carbonate soluble in water, occurs in white masses with ammonical odor. Cardiac and respiratory stimulant and expectorant. *a. chloride* White crystallin powder soluble in water. Stimulant-expectorant and cholagogue. Used to relieve alkalosis, also promotes lead excretion. *a. nitrate* A white deliquescent crystalline salt, soluble in water. Used in making nitrous oxide gas in freezing mixtures and in fertilizers. *a. salicylate* White crystalline powder soluble in water. Used in rheumatism.

Amnesia Loss or impairment of memory, inability to recall past experiences. *a. anterogradea* In reference to events occurring after the trauma or disease that cause the condition. *a. retrograde* In reference to events that occurred before the trauma or disease that caused the condition. *a. visual* Inability to recall to mind the appearance of objects that have been seen or to recognize printed words.

Amniocentesis The withdrawal of fluid from the uterus through the abdominal wall by means of a syringe and needle (*see* Figure on page 47). It is primarily used in the diagnosis of chromosome disorders in the fetus and in cases of hydramnios.

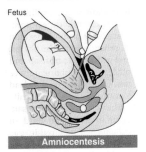

Amniocentesis

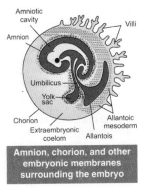

Amnion, chorion, and other embryonic membranes surrounding the embryo

Amnioinfusion Infusion of normal saline into the amniotic sac to increase the amniotic fluid volume.

Amnion The innermost or the membranes enveloping the embryo in utero. It consists of a layer of splanchnopleure with its ectodermal components toward the embryo and its somatic mesodermal component external (*see* Figure).

Amnioscope An endoscope which is passed through the uterine cervix to visualize the fetus and amniotic fluid.

Amniotomy Surgically breaking the amniotic sac to induce or expedite labor.

Amobarbital White crystalline powder of a bitter taste slightly soluble in water, melting point 156°C. A central nervous system depressant, has an intermediate duration of action.

Amodiaquine hydrochloride Camoquine hydrochloride, as the dihydrochloride hemihydrate, yellow crystals soluble in water. A synthetic antimalarial drug, effective against plasmodium vivax in the erythrocytic phase of malaria, less effective against *P.vivax* falciparum and *P. malaria* infections. Also used in treatment of amebic hepatitis, rheumatoid arthritis.

Amoeba A genus of unicellular protozoan organisms of microscopic size existing in nature in large numbers, many living as parasites, some species pathogenic for man.

Amoebiasis Infection with amoeba, particularly *Entamoeba histolytica*.

Amoebic Pertaining to, caused by, or of the nature of an amoeba. *A. abscess* an abscess cavity of the liver resulting from liquefaction necrosis due to entrance of *Entamoeba histolytica* into the portal circulation in amoebiasis; amoebic abscesses may affect the lung, brain and spleen. *A. dysentery* a form of dysentery caused by *Entamoeba histolytica* and spread by contaminated food, water and flies; called also amoebiasis. Amoebic dysentery is mainly a tropical disease by many cases occur in temperate countries. Symptoms are diarrhoea, fatigue and intestinal bleeding. Complications include involvement of the liver, liver abscess and pulmonary abscess. Several drugs are available for treatment, for example, emetine hydrochloride and chloroquine, which may be used singly or in combination.

Amoxapine Tricyclic antidepressant.

Amoxicillin Ampicillin group of antibiotic with better GI. absorption.

Ampere Unit of strength of an electrical current representing a current having a force of one volt and passing through a conductor with a resistance of one ohm.

Amphetamine An acrid liquid racemic synthetic preparation slightly soluble in water, closely related in its structure and action to ephedrine and other sympathomimetic amines. Central nervous system stimulant.

Amphoric Denoting the sound heard in precussion and auscultation resembling the noise made by blowing across the mouth of a bottle.

Amphoteric Having two opposite characteristics especially the capacity of reacting as either acid or base.

Amphotericin B An antibiotic substance derived from strains of streptomyces nodosus, used for the treatment of deep seated mycotic infections.

Ampicillin Semisynthetic broad spectrum penicillin, acid resistant.

Ampoule A hermetically sealed container usually made of glass containing a sterile medicinal solution or powder to be made up in solution, to be used for subcutaneous, intramuscular, or intravenous injection.

Ampulla A sacular dilation of canals, is seen in the semicircular canals of the ear or the lactiferous ducts of the mammary glands.

Amputation 1. The cutting off of a limb or part of a limb, the breast or other projecting part. 2. In dentistry amputation may be of the root of a tooth or of the pulp or even of a nerve root or ganglion e.g., the Gasserian ganglion.

Amrinone Bipyocidine derivative with positive inotropic effect, used in heart failure.

Amyelia Congenital absence of spinal cord.

Amyostasia Tremors of the muscle causing difficulting in standing or in coordination. This condition is commonly seen in the cases of locomoter ataxia.

Amygdala A nugget like mass of gray matter in the anterior portion of temporal lobe.

Amylase A starch splitting or amyloytic enzyme that causes hydrolytic cleavage of the starch molecule.

Amylnitrate A vasodilator used in angina and cyanide poisoning.

Amylocaine hydrochloride Benzoyl ethyldimethyl— aminopropanyl hydrochloride, a local anaesthetic. Its action is slightly stronger than that of cocaine less toxic but more irritant. It has been used for spinal anesthesia. Side effects and after effects are frequent.

Amyloid A protein (probably combined with chondrotin sulfuric acid) that is microscopically homogeneous hyaline and acidophilic and frequently manifests great affinity for congored; occurs characteristically as pathologic extracellular deposits beneath the endothelium of capillaries or sinusoids in the walls of arterioles and especially in association with reticulo endothelial tissue.

Amyloidosis Deposits of amyloid in various organs tissues. Four types of conditions are recognized i.e. primary secondary, a localized masses or nodules, and associated with multiple myeloma. *a. primary* A form of amyloidosis not associated with other recognized disease, tends to involve diffusely the mesenchymal tissues in the tongue, lungs, intestinal tract, skin, skeletal muscles, and myocardium, the amyloid in this condition frequently does not manifest the usual affinity for congored and sometimes provokes a foreign body type of inflammatory reaction in the adjacent tissue. *a. secondary* The most frequent form of amyloidosis occurs in association with another chronic disease, e.g., tuberculosis, osteomyelitis, pyelonephritis and so on; organs chiefly involved are the liver, spleen, and kidneys and the adrenal glands less frequently (*see* Figure).

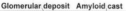

Glomerular deposit Amyloid cast

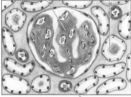

Deposit in interstitial vessel

Amyloidosis

Amylopectin A polysaccharide found in the outer layer of the starch granule, characterized by glucose residues arranged in branched chains.

Amyotonia Loss of muscular tone. Amyotonia congenita is a congenital disease associated with absent tone and reflexes in the voluntary muscles. Due to reduced muscular tone, the muscles often remain underdeveloped.

Amyotrophy Muscular wasting or atrophy.

Amyotrophic lateral sclerosis Also known as Lou Gehrig's disease. It is a progressive, neurodegenerative disease associated with degeneration of motor neurons and the nerve cells in the CNS which are responsible for controlling voluntary muscular activity. The disorder results in extreme weakness and atrophy of muscles both in upper and lower limbs. Eventually the patient loses the ability to control and initiate voluntary movements in the entire body except for the eyes. Cognitive function usually remains unimpaired. The disease has no cure. However, recently the FDA (Food and Drug Administration) has approved the use of the drug riluzole (rilutek) for treatment of this condition.

Anabolism The process of assimilation of nutritive matter and its conversion into living substances. This includes synthetic processes and requires energy.

Anaerobe A microorganism that can live and thrive in the absence of free oxygen. These organisms are found in body cavities or wounds where the oxygen tension is very low. Examples are the bacilli of tetanus and gas gangrene. *Facultative a.* A microorganism that can live and grow with or without molecular oxygen. *Obligate a.* An organism that can grow only in the complete absence of molecular oxygen.

Analgesia Loss of sensibility to pain.

Analgia Freedom from pain.

Analogous Resembling functionally but having a different origin or structure.

Analogue 1. One of two organs or parts in different species of animals or plants which differ in structure or development but are similar in function. 2. In chemistry one of two or more compounds with similar structure but different atoms e.g., nitrogen and carbon monoxide.

Analysis 1. The breaking up of a chemical compound into its simpler elements, a process by which the composition of a substance is determined. 2. The separation of any compound substance into the parts composing it. 3. Applied in electroencephalography to the estimation or recording of the components of a complex wave form in terms of their frequency and amplitude. *a. gastric* Analysis of the contents of the stomach after the ingestion of a test meal. The gastric contents are aspirated through a specially designed stomach tube, and the free and total acidities, the

pH and the peptic activity are determined. They may also be examined for food residue, bile, blood, mucus etc.

Anamnesis 1. The act of remembering. 2. The medical history of a patient.

Anandria Absence of masculinity.

Anaphase The stage of mitosis or meiosis in which the chromosomes move from the equatorial plate toward the poles of the cell. In mitosis a full set of daughter chromosomes (46 in man) moves towards each pole. In the first division of meiosis one member of each homologous pair (23 in man) now consisting of two chromatids united at the centromere, moves towards each pole. In the second division of meiosis the centromere has divided and the two chromatids separate one moving to each pole.

Anaphrodisiac A drug or a chemical substance which blunts the libido or sexual desire. It is the opposite of aphrodisiac which enhances sexual desire.

Anaphylactoid Resembling anaphylaxis. A shock may result from intravenous injection of 1. serum that is pretreated with kaolin or starch 2. Trypsin 3. organic colloids. 4. peptone or 5. several other materials. The pathologic changes in a shock are different from those of true anaphylaxis.

Anaphylatoxin According to the humoral hypothesis of the mechanism of anaphylaxis, anaphylaxis results from the in vivo combination of specific antibody (anaphylactin) and the specific. Sensitizing material, when the latter is injected at a shock dose in a sensitized animal.

Anaphylaxis The antithesis of prophylaxis; anaphylaxis is an exaggerated or extreme hypersensitivity that may be induced in various animal species as a result of the injection of even a small dose of foreign material (anaphylactogen) this is usually termed the sensitizing dose. Anaphylaxis develops during an incubation period of 10 to 14 days and then the injection of a second larger dose of the same material (usually termed the shocking dose) promptly results in anaphylatic shock.

Anaplasia 1. A reversion in the case of a cell to a more primitive embryonic type, i.e., to one in which reproductive activity is marked. 2. Loss of structural differentiation.

Anasarca Severe generalized edema.

Anastrozole Aromatase inhibitor for breast cancer.

Anastomosis 1. A natural communication direct or indirect between two blood vessels or tubular structures. 2. An operative union between of two hollow or tubular structures (*see* Figure).

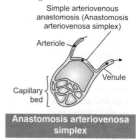

Simple arteriovenous anastomosis (Anastomosis arteriovenosa simplex)

Arteriole

Venule

Capillary bed

Anastomosis arteriovenosa simplex

Anatomy 1. The structure of an organism; morpholgy. 2. The science of the morphology or structure of organisms. 3. Dissection. 4. A work describing the form and structure of an organism and its various parts. *a. applied* Anatomical knowledge utilized in the diagnosis of disease and in treatment especially surgical treatment. *a. comparative* 1. Anatomy of the lower animals 2. The comparative study of the human body with those of other animals and observation of analogous and homologous parts. *a. surface* The study of the configuration of the surface of the body especially in its relation to deeper parts.

Ancylostoma A genus of Nematoda, the old world hookworm the members of which are parasitic in the duodenum where they attach themselves to the mucous membrane sucking the blood and causing a state of anemia and mental and physical inertia. The eggs are passed with the feces and the larvae develop in moist soil, they enter the body of man through the skin of the feet and ankles, possibly also in the drinking water and reach maturity in the intestine. *a. caninum* A species with three pairs of ventral teeth in the oral cavity infesting dogs, cause of kennel anemia, it occurs also although rarely in man. *a. duodenale* A reddish worm with two pairs of hooklike teeth on the ventral surface and one rudimentary minor pair. These species and *A. braziliense* (with only one pair of ventral teeth) are found in man, the latter in dogs and cats also (*see* Figure).

Androgen A generic term for an agent usually a hormone,

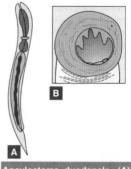

Ancylostoma duodenale, (A) Larval form; (B) mouth of adult, showing two pairs of teeth

e.g., testosterone or androsterone that stimulates the activity of the accessory sex organs of the male; encourages the development of the male sex characteristics.

Androgynoid A man with hermaphroditic sexual characteristics who is mistaken for a woman, a pseudohermaphrodite. Possession of masculine characteristics by a genetically pure female.

Androgynus Female pseudohermaphrodite.

Andropathy Any disease such as prostatitis peculiar to the male sex.

Androstenedione A testosterone precursor.

Anemia (Anaemia) Qualitative or quantitative in reduction in red blood cells. *a. ellipto-cytic* Anemia characterized by elliptical erythrocytes (ovalocytes) resembling those observed normally in camels; 1 to 15 percent of erythrocytes in nonanemic persons may be oval but greater proportions are observed in certain patients with microcytic anemia, latter conditions frequently termed symptomatic ovalocytosis. *a. hyperchromic* Characterized by an increase in the ratio of the weight of hemoglobin to the volume of the erythrocyte, i.e., the mean corpuscular hemoglobin concentration is greater than normal with the exception of some instances of hereditary spherocytosis such "supersaturation" does not occur although the weight of hemoglobin per cell may be greater in the macrocytes of pernicious anemia, the increase is proportional to larger volume and such cells are not truly hyperchromic. *a. hypochromic* Characterized by a decrease in the ratio of the weight of haemoglobin to the volume of the erythrocyte, i.e., the mean corpuscular hemoglobin concentration (MCHC) is less than normal; the individual cells contains less hemoglobin than they could have under optimal conditions. *a. hypochromic microcytic* A type of anaemia caused by a deficiency of iron; the amount of haemoglobin is reduced to a greater degree than the blood red cell count as a result of 1. less than the normal percentage of haemo-globin per cell and 2. the smaller than the normal size of most of the erythrocytes. The mean corpuscular volume (MCV), mean corpuscular haemoglobin (MCH) and mean corpuscular haemoglo-bin concentration (MCHC) are less than normal. *a. Iron deficiency* Any hypochromic microcytic anemia with the exception of that occurring in thalassemia and anemia pro-duced in certain experimental animals that are deficient, in vitamin B_6 or copper. *a. macro-cytic* Any anaemia in which the average size of circulating erythrocytes is greater than normal, i.e., the mean corpus-cular volume (MCV) is 94 cu or more (normal range 82 to 92 cu) includes such syndromes as pernicious anemia, celiac disease, anaemia of pregnancy etc. *a. megaloblastic* Any anaemia in which there is a predominant number of megaloblasts and relatively few normoblasts among the hyperplastic erythroid cells in the bone marrow (as in pernicious) *a. normochromic* Anemia in which the concentration of hemoglobin in the erythrocytes is within the normal range, i.e., the mean corpuscular haemoglobin concentration (MCHC) is around 32 to 36 percent.

Anergia Lack of activity.

Anergy Impaired ability to react with antigens.

Aneroid Equipment that does not utilize liquid medium for measurement of pressure, e.g., aneroid barometer.

Anesthesia Partial or complete loss of sensation with or without loss of consciousness (depending upon stage of anaesthesia) induced by administration of an anaesthetic agent. *a. caudal* Injection of anaesthetic agent into caudal epidural space. *a. dissociative* A type of anaesthesia characterized by amnesia, analgesia and cataplexy. The patient is dissociated from environment. *a. infiltration* Local anaesthesia produced by injecting the local anaesthetic solution directly into tissue. *a. inhalational* General anesthesia produced by inhalation of vapor or gas anaesthetic like ether, nitrous oxide, halothane, trilene etc. *a. pudendal* The pudendal nerve near the spinous process of ischium is blocked; used in perineal and obstetric surgery. *a. spinal* Anaesthesia produced by injection of anaesthetic agent into subarachnoid space. *a. surgical* Depth of anaesthesia of which relaxation of muscles and loss of sensation and consciousness are adequate for performance of surgery. *a. twilight* State of light anaesthesia.

Anesthesiologist Physician specializing in anaesthesiology.

Anesthetize To induce anesthesia.

Aneuploidy Possession of abnormal number of chromosomes.

Aneurysm Localized abnormal dilatation of a blood vessel due to congenital weakness or defect in the wall (*see* Figure on page 56). *a. atherosclerotic* Aneurysm due to degeneration of arterial wall by atherosclerosis. *a. berry* Small saccular congenital aneurysm of cerebral

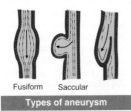

Fusiform   Saccular

Types of aneurysm

vessel. *a. cirsoid* A dilatation of network of vessels, forming a pulsating subcutaneous tumor, usually on the scalp. *a. compound* Aneurysm in which some of the layers of vessel wall are ruptured and others dilated. *a. dissecting* Aneurysm in which following interruption of wall of a blood vessel, blood enters in between the walls separating them for variable distance and often obstructing the vessel lumen. *a. fusiform* Aneurysm in which all the walls of blood vessel dilate more or less equally, forming a tubular swelling. *a. mycotic* Aneurysm due to bacterial infection of vessel wall. *a. saccular* The dilatation does not involve the entire circumference of vessel.

Angel dust Phencyclidine, a psychodelic.

Angel's trumpet A flowering shrub producing alkaloids like atropine, hyoscyamine and hyoscine.

Angel's wing Posterior projection of scapula caused by paralysis of serratus anterior.

Anger The emotion of extreme displeasure to a person, a situation or an object.

Angiectasia Dilatation of blood and lymph vessel.

Angiitis Inflammation of blood vessels.

Angina Severe pain. *a. abdominis* Abdominal pain due to ischaemia of gut. *a. cruris* Leg pain due to vascular obstruction. *a. decubitus* Attacks of angina pectoris occurring in recumbent position. *a. Ludwig* Deep infection of tissues in the floor of the mouth. *a. pectoris* Ischemic pain of cardiac origin manifesting as constriction around heart, faintness; radiation of pain occurring to jaw, neck, left shoulder, upper abdomen and along inner border of left arm. *a. prinzmetal's* Angina pectoris with ST elevation due to coronary spasm. *a. unstable* Angina of recent onset, abrupt progression; occurring at rest; is due to superadded coronary thrombosis, a fore runner of impending infarction. *a.*

variant Angina occurring at rest in absence of cardiac acceleration (*see* Figure).

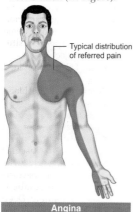

— Typical distribution of referred pain

Angina

Angioblast The mesenchymal cell derivative which ultimately develops into blood vessels.

Angioblastoma Tumor involving blood vessels of brain and meninges.

Angiocardiogram Serial X-rays of heart after intraventricular injection of radio opaque dye.

Angioedema An allergic condition characterized by urticaria and edematous areas of skin and mucus membrane or viscera. The reaction is IgE dependent, but is often complement mediated as in hereditary angioedema.

Angioendothelioma A tumor with endothelial cells predominance occurring in bone.

Angiogenesis Development of blood vessels.

Angiogenic factors A group of polypeptides that either stimulate vascular endothelium to proliferate or stimulate macrophages to secrete endothelial growth factors.

Angiography X-ray of blood vessels after injection of radio opaque material. *a. cerebral* X-ray picture of cerebral circulation to evaluate stroke, tumor, AV malformation, aneurysm or abnormal vascular pattern. *a. coronary* X-ray of coronary circulation to evaluate ischaemic disease. *a. digital subtraction* A computer aided "subtraction" technique that subtracts images of surrounding tissue from the contrast image to give better resolution and minor details.

Angioid streaks Dark wavy anastomosing striae lying beneath the retinal vessels.

Angiokeratoma Thickening of epidermis of feet with telangiectases warty growths.

Angiolipoma A mixed tumor containing blood vessels and fatty tissue.

Angiolith Calcareous deposits in walls of blood vessels.

Angiology Science of blood vessels and lymphatics.

Angioma A tumor containing blood vessels (hemangioma) or lymph vessels (lymphangioma), considered to be misplaced fetal tissue undergoing abnormal development. *a. capillary* Congenital superficial hemangioma appearing as irregular red discolouration due to overgrowth of capillaries. *a. cavernous* Elevated dark red tumor consisting of blood filled vascular spaces; involves submucous and subcutaneous tissue and is pulsatile. *a. senile* Hemangioma in elderly due to capillary wall degeneration, producing a compressible mass. *a. serpiginous* A skin disorder characterized by appearance of small, red vascular dots arranged in rings due to proliferation of capillaries. *a. stellate* Hemangioma in which telangiectatic blood vessels radiate from a central point *SYN* – spider nevus.

Angiomalacia Softening of wall of blood vessels.

Angiomatosis Multiple angiomas.

Angiomyolipoma A benign growth containing vascular, muscular and fatty elements.

Angiopathy Any disease of blood or lymph vessel.

Angioplasty Dilatation of obstructed vessel by an angiographic procedure (*see* Figure).

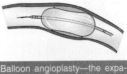

Balloon angioplasty—the expanded balloon pressing against a stenotic site in an artery

Angiotensin A vasopressor substance formed by interaction of renin on a serum globulin called angiotensinogen. *a. I* Physiologically inactive form of angiotensin. *a. II* Physiologically active form of angiotensin; a potent vasopressor and stimulant of aldosterone secretion.

Angiotensinogen A serum globulin fraction formed in the liver; hydrolyzed to angiotensin by renin.

Angle The space outlined by two diverging lines from a common point or by the meeting of two planes. *a. acromial* Angle formed by junction of lateral and posterior borders of acromion. *a. alpha* Angle formed by intersection of visual line with optic axis. *a. alveolar* Angle between the horizontal plane and a line drawn through the base of nasal spine and the midpoint of alveolus of upper jaw. *a. cardiophrenic* The angle formed by diaphragm and heart outline. *a. carrying* Angle made at the elbow by extending the long axis of fore arm and the upper arm. Normally it is around 15° in male and 18° female. *a. costophrenic* Angle formed by lateral end of diaphragm with the rib cage. *a. facial* Angle made by the lines from the nasal spine and external auditory meatus meeting between upper middle incisor teeth. *a. gamma* Angle between line of vision and visual axis. *a. of Treitz* Sharp curve at duodeno jejunal junction. *a. sphenoid* Angle formed at the top of sella turcica by intersection of lines drawn from nasal point and tip of rostrum of sphenoid bone. *a. visual* Angle formed by the line drawn from nodal point of eye to the edges of the object being viewed.

Angor animi The feeling that one is dying as in angina pectoris.

Angstrom unit Unit for measurement of wavelength equal to 10⁻¹⁰ meter.

Angular artery Artery at inner canthus of eye.

Anhedonia Lack of pleasure in normally pleasurable acts.

Anhidrosis Absence of sweat secretion.

Anhydrase Enzyme that helps in removal of water from a chemical compound.

Anhydride Compound formed by removal of water from a substance, especially an acid.

Anhydrous Lacking water.

Anicteric Without jaundice.

Aniline The simplest aromatic amine, an oily liquid derived from benzene, used for dyes.

Anilism Chronic aniline poisoning manifesting with vertigo, cardiac conduction defects, muscular weakness.

Anima Soul, individual's innerself.

Animal A living organism. *a. cold blooded* An animal whose body temperature changes with that of environment. *a. warmblooded* Animals that maintain constant body temperature irrespective of change in environmental temperature.

Animation State of being alive. *a. suspended* State of apparent death.

Anion An ion carrying negative charge being attracted to positive pole, anode.

Anion gap It is calculated from subtracting $HCO_3^- + Cl^-$ from plasma sodium. Normal value is 8-12 mEq/L.

Aniridia Congenital absence of a part of iris.

Anisindione Anticoagulant agent.

Anisocoria Inequality in size of pupils.

Anisocytosis Marked inequality in size of cells.

Anisodactyly Unequal length of the coresponding fingers or digits.

Anisogamy Sexual fusion of two gametes of different form and size.

Anisognathous A condition of having different sizes of maxillary (upper) and mandibular (lower) dental arches or jaws. The upper jaw is usually larger than the lower one.

Anisoleukocytosis Various forms of leukocytes are present in an abnormal ratio in the blood.

Anisomastia Condition of unequal size of breasts.

Anisometropia Condition in which refractive powers of each eye are different.

Anisophoria Muscular imbalance in eye so that horizontal visual plane of one eye is different from other.

Anisopiesis Inequality in arterial blood pressure between the two sides of the body.

Anisotropine A belladona alkaloid derivative, spasmolytic.

Anisuria Characterized by marked alteration in the amount of urine produced; alternating between oliguria and polyuria.

Ankle The hinge joint formed by articulation of tibia, fibula and talus. *a. clonus* Repeated contraction and relaxation of leg muscles following mild extension of ankle in patients of corticospinal disease, an evidence of increased muscle tone.

Ankle jerk Plantar flexion of foot due to contraction of calf musculature following a brisk tap to tendo achilis tendon.

Ankyloblepharon Adhesion of upper and lower eyelids at lid margin.

Ankylocolpos Imperforated or atretic vaginal canal.

Ankyloglossia Poor tongue protrusion due to abnormally short frenulum.

Ankylosis Immobility of a joint, due to fibrous tissue growth or bony fusion within joint. *a. dental* Fusion of root cementum with adjacent alveolar bone.

Annular Circular.

Annuloraphy Closure of hernial ring by suture.

Annulus A ring shaped structure.

Anococcygeal body The muscle and fibrous tissue lying in between anus and coccyx; giving attachment to.

Anococcygeal ligament A band of fibrous tissue joining coccyx to external sphincter ani.

Anode The positive pole.

Anodontia Absence of teeth.

Anomaloscope Device for detection of color blindness.

Anomaly Deviation from normal, irregularity.

Anomia Inability in naming objects.

Anopheles A genus of mosquito, vector for plasmodia, the causative agent of malaria.

Anorchism Congenital absence of one or both testes.

Anorexia Loss of appetite. *a. nervosa* A psychological malade of young girls who are anorexic for fear of becoming obese.

Anorexigenic Causing loss of appetite

Anoscope Speculum for examining anus and lower rectum.

Anosmia Loss of sense of smell.

Anovulatory Not associated with ovulation.

Anovulatory cycle Menstrual cycle not preceded by ovulation.

Anoxemia Insufficient oxygenation of blood.

Anoxia Reduced oxygenation of tissues from various causes. *a. altitude* Insufficient oxygen content of inspired air in high altitude causing anoxia. *a. anemic* Anoxia due to decreased oxygen carrying capacity of blood. *a. anoxic* Anoxia due to defective pulmonary mechanism of oxygenation, i.e., pulmonary fibrosis, edema, bronchial obstruction, emphysema etc. *a. stagnant* Tissue anoxia due to stagnant peripheral circulation as in cardiac failure, shock.

Ansa Any structure in the form of a loop or arc. *a. cervicalis* A nerve loop in the neck formed by fibres from first three cervical nerves. *a. lenticularis* Fibre tract from globus pallidus to ventral nucleus of thalamus that winds round in internal capsule. *a. peduncularis* Fibre tract from anterior temporal lobe to medio dorsal nucleus of thalamus, extending around internal capsule. *a. sacralis* Nerve loop connecting sympathetic trunk with coccygeal ganglion.

Ansamycin A rifamycin derivative, used in tuberculosis.

Ansiform Shaped like a loop.

Antabuse Disulfiram, used to cause aversion in alcoholics by increasing acetaldehyde concentration.

Antacid Agent that neutralizes gastric HCl.

Antagonism Mutual opposite or contradictory action.

Antagonist Agent or any other thing that counteracts the action of something else. *a. narcotic* A drug that reverses action of a narcotic hence producing withdrawal symptoms in some (*see* Figure).

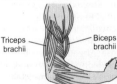

Triceps brachii

Biceps brachii

Antagonist—The triceps brachii extends the forearm at the elbow while the biceps brachii and its antagonist—flexes the elbow

Antalgesic *SYN* – analgesic, i.e., pain reliever.

Antaphrodisiac Agent that suppresses sexual desire.

Antasthenic Invigorating, strengthening, relieving weakness.

Antazoline An antihistamine used for allergic conjunctivitis.

Ante Prefix meaning before.

Antecedent Some thing coming before; precursor.

Antecibum Before meals.

Ante cubital At the bend of elbow.

Ante cubital fossa Triangular area lying anterior to and below the elbow, bounded medially by pronator teres and laterally by brachio-radialis.

Anteflexion Abnormal bending forward, e.g., especially of uterine body at its neck (*see* Figure).

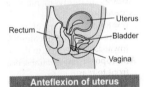

Rectum — Uterus — Bladder — Vagina

Anteflexion of uterus

Antegrade Moving forward or in the direction of flow.

Ante mortem Before death.

Antenatal Occurring before birth.

Antenatal diagnosis Diagnostic procedures done to determine the health and genetic status of foetus, e.g., ultrasound, amiocentesis, chorionic villi sampling, biophysical profile, non-stress test.

Antepar Piperazine citrate.

Antepartum Before onset of labor.

Anterior In anatomy refers to ventral portion of body.

Anterior chamber The front chamber of eye bounded infront by cornea, behind by iris and lens; contains aqueous humor.

Anterior horn cell The nerve cells in anterior horn of spinal cord whose axons form the efferent fibres innervating the muscles.

Anterograde Moving frontward.

Anteroinferior Infront and below.

Anterolateral Infront and to one side.

Anteromedian Infront and towards midline.

Anteroposterior Passing from front to rear.

Anterosuperior In front and above.

Anteversion A tipping forward of an organ as a whole, without bending (see Figure).

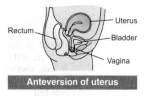

Anteversion of uterus

Anthelmintic Agents against intestinal worms.

Anthracosis SYN – black lung; accumulation of carbon deposits in lungs due to smoking or coal dust.

Anthralin A synthetic hydrocarbon used as ointment to treat fungal infections and eczema.

Anthrax Disease caused by bacillus anthracis, a disease primarily of animals. In man it may occur as cutaneus pustule with black eschar, or a pulmonary form (wool sorter's disease) with pulmonary edema, necrotizing mediastinal lymph adenitis, pleural effusion etc.

Anthropogeny Origin and development of man.

Anthropology The study of man; physical, cultural, linguistic and archaeologic.

Anthropometry Science of measuring human body, including craniometry, osteometry, skin fold thickness, height and weight measurement.

Anthropomorphism Attributing human qualities to nonhumans.

Anthropophilic Parasites that prefer human host rather than other animals.

Anti Prefix meaning against.

Antiadrenergic Counter acting or preventing adrenergic actions.

Antiagglutinin A specific antibody opposing the action of agglutinin.

Antiamebic A medicine used to treat amebiasis.

Antiandrogen Substances antagonizing action of androgen, e.g., ciproterone acetate.

Antibiosis Relationship between two organisms where one is harmful to the other.

Antibiotic Substances that inhibit or destroy micro organisms; can be bactericidal or bacteriostatic (only inhibit growth).

Antibody A protein substance developed on challenge by an antigen. Antibodies may be present due to previous infection, vaccination, transplacental transfer (IgG only) or unknown idiopathic antigenic stimulation. *a. acetylcholine receptor* present in 85% cases of myasthenia gravis. *a.anticardiolipin* present in SLE causing vessel thrombosis. *a. antiglindin* present in celiac disease; non-specific *a. antimicrosomal* directed against a thyroid microsomal antigen in patients of Hashimoto's thyroiditis. *a. antimitochondrial* directed against inner mitochondrial antigen seen in primary biliary cirrhosis. *a. antimyosin* (Indium III tagged) binds to irreversibly damaged myocardium; used in infarct avid scintigraphy. *a. antinuclear* antibodies against nuclear antigens present in SLE, rheumatoid arthritis, etc. *a. blocking* Antibody that reacts with other antigens and blocks its effects. *a. cross-reacting* Antibody that reacts with other antigens functionally similar to its specific antigen. *a. anti SSA, anti SSB* antinuclear antibodies present in SLE and Sjogren's syndrome. *a. antithyroglobulin* present in 50-75% cases of Hashimoto's disease. *a. Donath Landsteiner* IgG antibody directed against P blood group antigen, responsible for haemolysis in paroxysmal haemoglobinuria. *a.fluorescent* Antigen antibody reaction made visible by incorporating a fluorescent material into the reaction and their examination under fluorescent microscopy. *a. OKT3* mouse monoclonal antibody against T_3 lymphocytes, used to treat transplant rejection. *a. phospholipid* include anticardiolipin antibodies and lupus anticoagulants. *a. Prausnitz Kustner's* IgE antibodies causing cutaneous anaphylaxis. *a.*

warm IgG antibody that reacts with antigen at 37°C.

Antibody coated bacteria Bacteria coated with antibody present in urine. Analysis of antibody pattern can localize the site of invasion of bacteria in urinary tract. *a. warm.* IgG antibody that reacts with antigen at 37°C.

Antibromic Deodorant.

Antiburn scar garment A garment made of stretchable filaments worn to provide uniform pressure over burn graft sites inorder to reduce scarring during healing.

Anticholinergic Agents that prevent parasympathetic transmission e.g., belladona, tricyclic antidepressants, thereby causing dryness of mouth, constipation, urinary retention, blurring of vision and tachycardia.

Anticholinesterase Substance opposing action of choline sterate which causes breakdown of acetylcholine.

Anticoagulant Agents that prevent/delay clot formation, e.g., sodium citrate heparin.

Anticodon A triple arrangement of bases in tRNA that complements the triplet on corresponding MRNA.

Anticonvulsant Agents that prevent or control seizure.

Antidepressant Agents that prevent, cure or alleviate mental depression.

Antidiuretic hormone Vasopressin.

Antidote Agents that neutralize poisons or their effects. *a. chemical* Antidote that reacts with poison to produce harmless chemical compound, e.g., common salt precipitates silver nitrate to produce silver chloride. *a. mechanical* Antidote that prevents absorption of poison, e.g., charcoal, egg albumin, milk casein and fats (fats contraindicated in camphor, phosphorus poisoning). *a. universal* Two parts of activated charcoal, one part tannic acid, one part magnesium oxide; given orally mixed with water. Charcoal adsorbs, tannic acid precipitates and magnesium oxide neutralizes poisons. This antidote like chemical antidotes should be removed from stomach after some time.

Antidromic Nerve impulse travelling in opposite direction than normal.

Antiemetic Agent that prevents or relieves vomiting and nausea.

Antiestrogen Substances that block or modify action of estrogen e.g., clomifene citrate.

Antigen Substance that induces antibody production and interacts with it in a specific way. *a. Australia* hepatitis B surface antigen. *a. CA 125* antigen of epithelial ovarian carcinoma. *a. carcinoembryonic* elevated in carcinoma colon, pancreas, stomach, breast, IBD, pancreatitis; primarily used in monitoring response to treatment in colorectal cancer. *a. class I* major histocompatibility antigen found on every cell except RBC. *a. Class II* histocompatibility antigen found principally on B lymphocytes (HLAD, DR, DT, MT). *a. class III* non-histocompatibility antigens. *a. CALLA* occur in lymphoblasts of ALL. *a. Forssman* heterogenous antigen inducing production of antisheep haemolysis. *a. HbeAg* present in blood during active replication of HBV *a. K* bacterial capsular antigen, e.g. salmonella V₁ antigen. *a. Kveim* prepared from sorcoid tissue.

Antigen-antibody reaction Combination of antigen with specific antibody that may result in agglutination, precipitation, neutralization, complement fixation or increased susceptibility to phagocytosis.

Anti G suit A garment designed to maintain uniform pressure in lower extremities and abdomen; used by aviators.

Antihelix Inner curved ridge of external ear parallel to helix.

Anti-histamine Agents that weaken the actions of histamine by blocking its receptors.

Anti-inflammatory Counteracting inflammation.

Antiluetic Agent that cures or relieves syphilis.

Antilymphocytic serum Serum used in certain autoimmune disorders and in transplant patients to reduce chances of rejection.

Antimetabolite 1. A substance structurally similar to metabolite, opposes or replaces a metabolite 2. a class of antineoplastic drugs used to treat cancer.

Antimetabolites
Cytarabine
5-Fluorouracil
FUDR
Methotrexate
Hydroxy urea
6 mercaptopurine
6 thioguanine
5 azacytidine
Pentostatin
Leustatin
Edatrexate

Antimony A metal whose compounds are used to treat trypanosomiasis.

Antineoplastic Agents that prevent the development, growth and proliferation of malignant cells.

Antinuclear antibody A group of antibodies that react against normal components of cell nucleus. They are present in SLE, PSS, scleroderma, polymyositis, etc.

Antioxidants Agents that prevent or inhibit oxidation e.g. vit E, A,C.

Antipathy Antagonism, strong aversion.

Antiperistalsis Reverse peristalsis.

Antiplasmin An inhibitor of fibrinolysis; its deficiency causes bleeding.

Antiplastic Preventing or inhibiting wound healing.

Antiprostaglandins Agents that interfere with prostaglandin activity; used for treatment of arthritis, dysmenorrhoea.

Antiprostate Cowper's gland.

Antipruritic Preventing or relieving itching.

Antipyretic Agent that reduces fever.

Antishock garment Inflatable garment that compresses lower extremity and abdomen to prevent pooling of blood. Useful in aviation and in treating hypotension.

Antiseptic Agent preventing sepsis by inhibiting growth of micro-organisms.

Antisudorific Agent that inhibits perspiration.

Antithrombotic Preventing thrombosis or blood coagulation.

Antithrombin III A protein synthesized in liver. Its concentration is lowered in nephrotic syndrome leading to renal veins thrombosis.

Antitoxin Antibody capable of neutralizing a toxin.

Antitrypsin A substance that inhibits action of trypsin. *a. alpha I* A low molecular weight glycoprotein whose deficiency is associated with early onset emphysema and neonatal hepatitis.

Antitussive Agent preventing or relieving cough.

Antivenin Serum that contains antibodies against animal or insect venom. *a. black widow spider* Horse antivenin against black widow spider. *a. polyvalent* Antisnake venom against common snakes.

Antivitamin A vitamin antagonist, agents that oppose action of vitamins.

Antrectomy Excision of walls of an antrum.

Antroatticotomy Operation to open the maxillary sinus and the attic of tympanum.

Antrocele Fluid accumulation causing a cystic swelling of antrum.

Antrostomy Opening up of antral wall by surgery.

Antrum Any nearly closed cavity or chamber especially in a bone (*see* Figure).

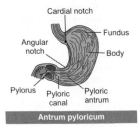

Cardial notch
Fundus
Angular notch
Body
Pylorus Pyloric canal
Pyloric antrum

Antrum pyloricum

Anulus A ring shaped structure. *a. fibrosus* The tough outer portion of intervertebral disk (*see* Figure on page 69).

Anuresis Absence of urination.

Anus The lower external opening of GI tract, lying between the folds of buttocks.

Anxiety A feeling of apprehension, worry, uneasiness.

Anxiety neurosis A mental disorder with excessive anxiety not restricted to specific situation or objects and is associated with somatic symptoms like palpitation, tremor, dryness of throat, headache.

Anxiolytic Agents that diminish or counteract anxiety.

Aorta The main arterial trunk arising from left ventricle and lying to the right and anterior to pulmonary artery. The aortic arch ends at level of fourth thoracic vertebra. The branches of aorta are 1. ascending aorta—two coronary arteries, right and left 2. arch of aorta-right innominate, left subclavian 3. thoracic aorta-bronchial arteries, esophageal arteries, intercostal arteries 4. abdominal aorta-celiac artery, renal arteries, mesenteric arteries (superior and inferior) (*see* Figure on page 69).

Aortic bodies Chemoreceptors present in wall of aorta to monitor oxygen saturation.

Aortic regurgitation Leakage of blood from aorta into left ventricle during diastole (*see* Figure on page 70).

Aortic stenosis Narrowing of aortic valve. Normal valve diameter-2 cm/m^2

Aortic valve The valve between left ventricle and ascending aorta, consists of three semilunar cusps that appose

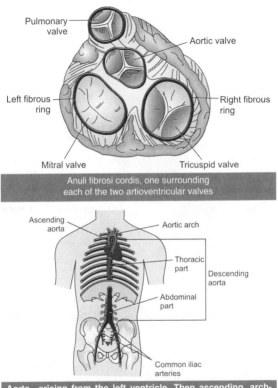

Pulmonary valve

Aortic valve

Left fibrous ring

Right fibrous ring

Mitral valve

Tricuspid valve

Anuli fibrosi cordis, one surrounding each of the two artioventricular valves

Ascending aorta

Aortic arch

Thoracic part

Descending aorta

Abdominal part

Common iliac arteries

Aorta—arising from the left ventricle. Then ascending, arching and descending through the thorax to the abdomen, where it divides into the common iliac arteries

during diastole, thus preventing backflow of blood from aorta to left ventricle.

Aortitis Inflammation of aortic wall, commonly syphilitic or of unknown origin.

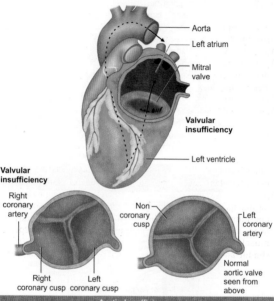

Right coronary artery

Aorta

Left atrium

Mitral valve

Valvular insufficiency

Left ventricle

Valvular insufficiency

Right coronary artery

Non coronary cusp

Left coronary artery

Right coronary cusp   Left coronary cusp

Normal aortic valve seen from above

Aortic Insufficiency

Aorto coronary bypass Surgical procedure to direct blood from root of aorta to coronary vessels by putting a saphenous vein graft or internal mammary arteries; a modality of treatment for coronary obstruction.

Aortography X-ray of aorta after contrast injection.

Aortolith Calcareous deposits in the aortic wall.

APACHE II score *Acute Physiology and Chronic Health Evaluation* II is a severity-of-disease classification, applied within 24 hours of admission of the patient to the ICU.

Apareunia Inability to accomplish sexual intercourse.

Apathetic Indifferent, disinterested.

Apathism Slowness to react to stimuli, (opposite of erethism).

Apatite The deceptive stone, a mineral containing calcium and phosphorus ions.

Aperient A very mild laxative.

Aperitive Appetite stimulant.

Apert's syndrome Congenital disorder with peaked head, webbed fingers and toes.

Aperture An orifice or opening.

Apex The pointed end of any cone shaped structure.

Apex beat The systolic movement of left ventricular apex against chest wall, felt in 5th intercostal space 1/2" inside midclavicular line.

Apgar score A system of assessing infants' physical condition one minute after birth. The heart rhythm, respiration, muscle tone, response to stimuli and skin colour are assigned a score of 0, 1 or 2. Total score is 10. Those with very low score require immediate attention. Apgar score at birth has a prognostic bearing on ultimate neurological development (*see* Table).

Aphakia Absence of lens of eye.

Aphasia Impairment of speech; may be motor or sensory (Wernicke's). *a. amnestic* Loss of memory for words. *a. anomic* Forgetful for naming. *a. Broca's* Motor aphasia with intact comprehension. *a. global* Failure of comprehension as well as speech production. *a. jargon* Use of disconnected words. *a. motor* Inability to use muscles controlling speech production. *a. semantic* Inability to understand meaning

Table: Apgar score

Sign	Score		
	0	1	2
Colour	Blue, pale	Body pink, limbs blue	Completely pink
Respiratory effort	Absent	Slow, irregular, weak cry	Strong cry
Heart rate	Absent	Slow, less than 100 bpm	Over 100 bpm
Muscle tone	Limp	Some flexion of limbs	Active movement
Reflex response to flicking foot	Absent	Facial grimace	Cry

of words. *a. syntactic* Lack of proper grammatical composition.

Aphemia Motor aphasia.

Aphephobia Morbid fear of being touched.

Apheresis Technique of separating blood into its components.

Aphonia Peripherial failure of speech production; commonly due to a laryngeal lesion.

Aphrasia Inability to speak or understand phrases.

Aphrodisiac Sex stimulant.

Aphthae Small ulcer on mucus membrane.

Aphthous Pertains to aphthae, i.e., recurrent stomatitis.

Apicectomy Excision of apex of petrous part of temporal bone.

Apicitis Inflammation of tooth/lung apex.

Aplanatic lens A lens that corrects spherical aberration.

Aplasia Failure of an organ or tissue to develop normally.

Aplastic Having deficient or arrested development.

Aplastic anemia A bone marrow disorder characterized by marrow hypoplasia and peripheral pancytopenia. Bone marrow transplantation is the choice of treatment.

Apnea Temporary cessation of breathing.

Apneumatosis Congenital atelectasis.

Apneusis Abnormal respiration with sustained inspiratory effort; caused by pontine lesion.

Apochromatic lens Lens that corrects both spherical and chromatic aberration.

Apocrine Secretory cells that contribute part of their protoplasm to the matter secreted.

Apocrine sweat glands Sweat glands of axilla and pubic region that open into hair follicles rather than directly onto surface.

Apoenzyme The protein portion of an enzyme.

Apoferritin The protein that combine with iron to form ferritin.

Apolipoprotein The nonlipid protein portion of lipoprotein named as B100, A1, AII, B and E.

Apomorphine A grayish white powder; derivative of morphine, used as emetic and cough suppressant.

Aponeurosis A flat fibrous sheet of connective tissue serving to attach muscle to bone (*see* Figure on page 73).

Apophysis An outgrowth from bone without as independent center of ossification.

Apophysitis Inflammation of apophysis.

Apoplexy Bleeding into an organ; sudden loss of consciousness with paralysis due to haemorrhage into brain.

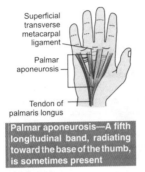

Superficial transverse metacarpal ligament

Palmar aponeurosis

Tendon of palmaris longus

Palmar aponeurosis—A fifth longitudinal band, radiating toward the base of the thumb, is sometimes present

Apoptosis Disintegration of cells into membrane bound particles, that are then phagocytosed by other cells, an important process for limitation of tumor growth.

Apparatus 1. A mechanical device or appliance used in operations or experiments. 2. A group of structures or organs that work together to perform function, e.g., *a auditory*, *a biliary*, *a juxtaglomerular*, *a lacrimal*.

Appendectomy Surgical removal of vermiform appendix.

Appendicitis Inflammation of vermiform appendix. Characterized by pain in right iliac fossa, nausea and vomiting, tenderness and rigidity over right rectus muscle or Mc Burney's point, mild fever, leukocytosis. *a.*

chronic follows acute attack with inflammatory adhesions, and formation of a lump. *a. gangrenous* Acute appendicitis involving blood vessels with their occlusion and development of gangrene and its vulnerability for rupture.

Appendicolysis Operation to free appendix from adhesions.

Appendicostomy Operation in which opening is made in vermiform appendix to irrigate cecum and colon.

Appendix An appendage. *a. atrial* Muscular pouch attached to left and right atria; the sites for atrial thrombi. *a. epiploica* Numerous pouches of peritoneum on colon filled with fat (*see* Figure on page 74).

Appestat Area of brain controlling appetite.

Appetite Strong desire for food in contrast to hunger which is a painful condition due to lack of food. *a. perverted* Desire to eat unnatural substances *SYN* – pica.

Appetizer Substance that promotes appetite.

Applanometer Device for measuring intraocular pressure.

Apple Adam's The laryngeal prominence formed by two laminae of thyroid cartilage.

Apple picker's disease Respiratory involvement due to

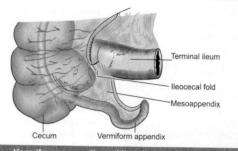

Terminal ileum

Ileocecal fold

Mesoappendix

Cecum   Vermiform appendix

Vermiform appendix and its adjacent structures

fungicides used in apple harvesting.

Appliance In dentistry a device used to correct bite such as artificial dentures.

Applicator A rod with cotton swab on end for making local applications.

Apposition Being positioned side by side.

Approach 1. Surgical procedures for exposing any organ or tissue 2. draw near.

Apraxia Inability to perform purposive and learned movements even though there is no motor/sensory loss. *a. amnestic* Patient cannot understand the action asked to perform even though ability to perform the act is intact. *a. constructional* Inability to construct two or three dimensional figures due to lack of ability to integrate percep-

tion into kinesthetic images. *a. dressing* Patient's inability to dress due to lack of knowledge about spatial relations of body. *a. ideational* Incorrect use of objects due to inability in perceiving their correct use. *a. motor* Inability to perform an action although the components of it are understood.

Apron Outergarment for protection of clothing inside.

Aprosody Absence of normal variations in pitch, rhythm and stress in the speech.

Aprotinin Protease inhibitor used in pancreatitis, carcinoid syndrome and during surgery to reduce blood loss.

Aptitude Inherent ability or skill in learning or performing.

Aptyalism Deficient secretion of saliva.

APUD cells Amine precursor uptake and decarboxylation

cells; the class of cell producing hormones like ACTH, insulin, glucagon, thyroxin dopamine, serotonin, histamine etc.

Aqua Water. *a.aerata* Carbonated water. *a.calcariae* Lime water. *a. fervens* Hot water *a.fontana* Spring water.

Aquanant Persons working under water for carrying research.

Aquaphobia Morbid fear of water.

Aquapuncture Subcutaneous injection of water to produce counter irritation.

Aqueduct Canal or channel. *a. cerebral* Canal in midbrain joining third and fourth ventricles. *a. vestibular* Passage from vestibule to petrous part of temporal bone. *a. cochleae* Canal connecting subarachnoid space and

the cochlear perilymphatic space.

Aqueous Watery

Aqueous humor Transparent liquid produced by ciliary processes and filling the posterior and anterior chambers of eye and finally absorbed into venous system by canals of Schlemm.

Arabinose A pentose plant sugar, gum sugar.

Arachidonic acid An essential fatty acid, precursor for prostaglandins, thromboxane and leukotrienes.

Arachnoid A thin membrane surrounding brain and spinal cord, lying in between dura mater and pia mater; subarachnoid space contains CSF.

Arc A structure or projected path having a curved or bow like outline (*see* Figure).

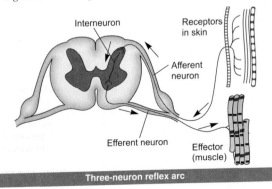

Three-neuron reflex arc

Arch Any anatomic structure with a curved or bow like outline, e.g., aortic arch. *a. axillary* An anomalous muscular slip across the axilla between pectoralis major and latissimus dorsi. *a. crural* The inguinal ligament extending from anterior superior iliac spine to pubic tubercle. *a. longitudinal* The anteroposterior arch of the foot; the medial portion is formed by calcaneus, talus, navicular, cuneiform and first three metatarsals and the lateral portion by calcaneus, cuboid and 4th and fifth metatarsals. *a. mandibular* The first branchial arch from which upper and lower jaw bones and associated structures develop, so also malleus and incus. *a. palmar* The superficial arch is formed by termination of ulnar artery and the deep arch by communicating branch of ulnar and the radial artery. *a. plantar* Arch formed by external plantar artery and deep branch of dorsalis pedis artery. *a. transverse* Transverse arch of foot formed by navicular, cuboid cuneiform and metatarsals. *a. zygomatic* Arch formed by malar and temporal bones.

Archipallium Olfactory cortex.

Architis Inflammation of anus.

Arcuate Shaped like an arc.

Arcus An arch. *a. juvenalis* Opaquering at the periphery of cornea in young, may be due to hypercholesterolemia, corneal irritation/inflammation. *a. senilis* Opaque white ring at periphery of cornea due to deposit of fat granules or hyaline degeneration.

Ardor A burning sensation during urination.

Area Well-defined space with defined boundaries. *a. association* Area of cerebral cortex that is neither sensory nor motor but seat of higher mental processes. *a. Brodman's* Division of cerebral cortex into 47 areas inrespect to their different functions. *a. Kiesselbach's* Area in anterior portion of nasal septum, with rich capillaries, a site of frequent bleed. *a. of Rolando* Area in front of fissure of Rolando in anterior central convolution governing motor function of body. *a. silent* Any area of brain whose destruction does not produce detectable motor or sensory loss (*see* Figure on page 77).

Areflexia Absence of reflexes.

Areola 1. A small space or cavity in a tissue. 2. Circular area of different pigmentation, e.g., around nipple.

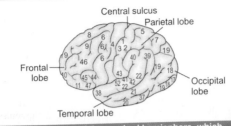

Lateral view of the cerebral hemisphere, which shows some of Brodmann's areas

Arenavirus A group of viruses that include lymphocytic choriomeningitis viruses and lassa fever viruses; mostly arthropod borne.

Areolar glands (Montgomery's glands). Large modified sweat glands beneath the areola secreting a lipoid material that lubricates the nipple.

Areometer Device for measuring specific gravity of fluids.

Arformeterol Betagonist for inlation in asthma.

Argentaffinoma An Argentaffin tumor secreting serotonin that may arise in intestinal tract, bile ducts, pancreas, bronchus or ovary.

Arginine Amino acid obtained from decomposition of vegetable matter, protamines and proteins. On hydrolysis it yields urea and ornithine.

Arginosuccinic acid Formed from citruline and aspartic acid.

Argon An inert gas occupying 1% of atmosphere.

Argyl Robertson pupil Absence of light reflex with preservation of accommodation reflex as in tabes.

Argyria Bluish discolouration of skin and mucus membranes from prolonged administration of silver.

Argyrol Mild silver protein used as an antiseptic for eye, nose, throat and urethral irrigation.

Argyrophil Cells that bind to silver salts producing brown or black stain.

Aristogenics *SYN*-eugenics. The science dealing with genetic and prenatal influences affecting expression of certain characteristics in offspring.

Arithmetic mean In statistics, the number obtained by addition of all the values listed in a group divided by total values.

Arm *a. chromosome* the two segments of chromosome, short arm P and long arm Q, joined at centromere (*see* Figure).

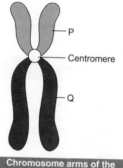

P

Centromere

Q

Chromosome arms of the segment

Arm board Board placed under the arm for stabilization during I.V. administration.

Armamentarium The total utilities at disposal like drugs, instruments, books, supplies.

Armature 1. A part of an electric generator consisting of a coil of insulated wire. 2. In biology a structure that serves to protect.

Arnold-Chiari deformity A condition in which the inferior poles of cerebellar hemispheres and medulla protrude through foramen magnum causing hydrocephalus. It is commonly associated with spina bifida and meningo myelocele.

Aroma Pleasant odor.

Aromatic 1. Having an aggreable odor. 2. Belonging to a series of compounds in which the carbon atoms form a closed ring (as in benzene) in comparison to aliphatic series where carbon atoms form straight or branched chains.

Aromatic ammonia spirit Solution of ammonium carbonate in diluted ammonia solution, fragrant oils, alcohol and water. It acts as a reflex stimulant on inhalation. Also acts as an antacid and carminative.

Arousal 1. Alertness. 2. Sexual excitement.

Arrectores pilorum Involuntary muscle in skin connected to hairfollicle whose contraction due to cold, fright causes erection of hair and "goose flesh" appearance of skin.

Arrest Cessation of function. *a. cardiac* Cessation of heart function. *a. epiphyseal* Arrest in growth of long bones. *a. pelvic* The foetal presenting part is arrested in its descent in maternal pelvis. *a. respiratory* Stoppage of spontaneous respiration. *a. sinus* The SA node does not initiate the impulse formation, a feature of sick sinus syndrome.

Arrhenoblastoma An ovarian tumor secreting male sex hormones, causing virilization in females.

Arrhythmia Variation in the normal rate or rhythm of the heart beat either in force or in time usually occurs as a result of irregularities in heart's conduction system.

Arsenic poisoning Accidental or deliberate ingestion causes acute gastroenteritis with shock, convulsion, paralysis and death.

Arsphenamine A light yellow powder containing about 30% arsenic previously used for treatment of syphilis. *SYN –* Salvarsan.

Artemether An antimalarial for resistant falciparum malaria.

Arterial line A method of haemodynamic monitoring where catheter is put into an artery for recording blood pressure, arterial gas analysis.

Arteriogram X-ray of an artery after injection of radio opaque material.

Arteriole A minute artery that leads into capillary.

Arterioplasty Repair or reconstruction of an artery.

Arteriosclerosis Thickening and hardening of an artery with loss of elasticity and contractility. Risk factors for arteriosclerosis include ageing, hyperlipidemia, obesity, diabetes mellitus, smoking etc.

Arteritis Inflammation of an artery. *a. nodosa* Widespread inflammation of adventia of small and medium sized arteries with impaired function. *a. temporal* Chronic inflammation of temporal and often occipital and ophthalmic arteries with presence of giant cells and occlusion of vascular lumen.

Artery (from Greek *arteria* meaning windpipe). The ancient Greeks believed that air travelled through them. Arteries carry oxygenated blood from heart to distant body parts: exceptions are pulmonary artery and umbilical artery. *a. end* Artery whose branches do not anastomose with those of other arteries, e.g., arteries of brain and spinal cord.

Artesunate An antimalarial for resistant falciparum malaria.

Arthralgia Joint pain.

Arthritide A skin eruption caused by arthritis.

Arthritis Inflammation of a joint usually following trauma, due to degeneration, infection (gonococcal, tubercular, brucella, pneumococcal), rheumatic fever, ulcerative colitis, collagen disorders, SLE, rheumatoid arthritis, gout, synovioma, para or periarticular infections, denervation, e.g. tabes dorsalis.

Arthrocentesis Puncture of a joint to drain joint fluid for analysis.

Arthrodesis The surgical immobilization of joint, ankylosis.

Arthrogram Visualisation of interior of a joint after injection of radio opaque dye into joint space.

Arthrogryposis Fixation of a joint in a flexed position.

Arthrolysis Restoration of mobility of an ankylosed joint.

Arthropathy Any joint disease.

Arthroplasty Reconstruction or reshaping of a diseased joint, even by replacement of joint components.

Arthroscope An endoscope for examination of interior of a joint.

Arthroscopy Visualization of interior of a joint by arthroscope.

Arthrospore A bacterial spore formed by segmentation.

Arthrotome Knife for making incision into joint.

Arthus reaction An immediate hypersensitivity reaction due to preformed antibody to injected antigen.

Articulate 1. To join together as a joint. 2. To speak clearly.

Articulation 1. A joint, classified, being synarthrosis (immovable), amphiarthrosis (slightly movable) and diarthrosis (freely movable) 2. Utterance of words and sentences. *a. apophyseal* The joint between superior and inferior articulating process of vertebra. *a. confluent* Speech in which syllables run together.

Artefact Anything artificially produced; as in histology/radiology a feature produced by the technique but not occurring naturally.

Artificial Not natural, formed by imitation of nature. *a. insemination donor* Artificial insemination of a woman with sperms of anonymous donor. *a. insemination husband* Use of husbands sperms for insemination of wife. *a. intelligence* Computer performance of cognitive tasks. *a. pneumothorax* Introduction of air into pleural cavity to induce collapse of lung as to control haemoptysis in tuberculosis.

Artisan's cramps Muscle cramp involving muscles used in prolonged spells of writing, sewing, telegraphing etc.

Aryepiglottic Pertaining to arytenoid cartilage and epiglottis.

Asafetida A gum resin with strong odor and garlic taste.

Asbestos Fibrous incombustible form of magnesium and calcium silicate used to make insulating material.

Asbestosis A form of pneumoconiosis due to inhalation of asbestos dusts, also responsible for pleural mesothelioma.

Ascariasis Infestation with ascaris lumbricoides.

Ascaris lumbricoides A species of ascaris inhibiting human intestine, often producing dyspepsia, intestinal obstruction, biliary colic and appendicitis (*see* Figure below).

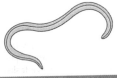

Ascaris lumbricoides

Aschheim-Zondek test A pregnancy test where patient's urine is injected into female mice to induce ovulation.

Aschner's phenomenon Slowing of pulse following carotid sinus massage or pressure on eye ball.

Aschoff's cells Large multinucleated cell with vesicular nucleus and basophilic cytoplasm (*see* Figure below).

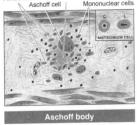

Anitschkow cells Necrotic debris
Aschoff cell Mononuclear cells
ANITSCHKOW CELL

Aschoff body

Aschoff's nodule Small nodules composed of central fibrinoid necrosis surrounded by giant cells and leukocytes, seen in interstitial tissues of heart in rheumatic myocarditis.

Ascites Accumulation of fluid in peritoneal cavity. *a. chylous* Milky ascites resulting from rupture of thoracic duct.

Ascorbic acid Vit C.

Aseptic Sterile, free from germs.

Aseptic technique Techniques that prevent contamination of operative wounds.

Asparagine Amino succinic acid; a non essential amino acid.

Aspartame An artificial sweetener, 180 times sweeter than sugar; synthesized from aspartic acid and phenyl alanine. Unsuitable for cooking as the flavor changes on eating.

Aspartic acid A nonessential amino acid, product of pancreatic digestion.

Aspergillin A pigment produced by *A. niger* which also produces black spores and commonly infects ear canal.

Aspergillosis Granulomatous inflammation of skin, lungs, ear canal and mucous membrane by A. fumigatus.

Aspermia Lack of or failure to ejaculate semen.

Aspersion Sprinkling of an affected part with water, a form of hydrotherapy.

Asphyxia Suffocation caused by lack of oxygen due to failure of breathing, tracheo bronchial obstruction, drowning, environmental oxygen lack, edema of the lungs.

Asphyxiant An agent, especially gas producing asphyxia.

Asphyxiate To cause asphyxia.

Aspirate To draw in or out by suction.

Aspirator Apparatus for evacuating fluid contents of a cavity.

Aspirin Acetyl salicylic acid.

Assault Violent physical attack on an individual. In legal sense any procedure on an individual without proper permission. *a. sexual* Sexual intercourse without consent/against will.

Assay The analysis of a substance or mixture to determine its constituents or the relative proportion of each.

Assimilate To absorb digested food.

Assimilation 1. The processes whereby the products of digestion are absorbed and utilized in the body. 2. In psychology, the absorption of newly perceived information into the existing conscious structure.

Association Relationship; interrelationship of conscious and unconscious; in genetics the occurrence together of two characteristics at a frequency greater than would be predicted by chance.

Association cortex Areas other than motor and sensory cortex which serve to integrate brain functions.

Astasia Inability to stand or sit erect due to motor incoordination. *a. abasia* A form of hysterical ataxia with inability to stand or walk although all leg movements can be performed while sitting or lying down.

Astemizole H_1 receptor blocker antiallergic.

Astereognosis Inability to recognize objects or forms by touch.

Asterion The junction of lambdoid, occipitomastoid and parietomastoid sutures (*see* Figure).

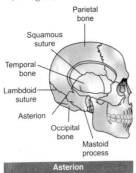

Asterion

Asterixis Transient lapses of muscle tone with involuntary jerky movements especially of hands as in hepatic failure.

Asteroid Star shaped.

Asthenia Loss of strength, debility. *a. neurocirculatory* A psycho-somatic disorder characterizes by mental and physical fatigue, dyspnea, giddiness, etc.

Asthma Paroxysmal dyspnea and wheezing caused by bronchospasm, bronchial mucosal swelling and retention of viscid sputum.

a. cardiac Asthma secondary to left ventricular failure. *a. extrinsic* Asthma due to environmental allergens. *a. intrinsic* Asthma where no external cause is identifiable.

Astigmatism A form of ametropia where the curvature of cornea or lens differ in different meridians so that an object is not sharply focussed on retina. *a. compound* The horizontal and vertical curvatures are abnormal. *a. simple* Only one meridian is defective.

Astraphobia Fear of thunder and lightening.

Astringent An agent that has constricting or binding effect, i.e., that causes coagulation of proteins and thus contracts organic tissue; there by checks haemorrhages and secretions. Common example are salts of lead, iron, zinc, tannic acid.

Astrocyte Star-shaped neuroglial cell with many branching processes (*see* Figure on page 84).

Astrocytoma A tumor of astrocytes; classified in order of increasing malignancy as grade I—consisting of fibrillary or protoplasmic astrocytes—Grade II composed of astroblasts Grade III-IV—called glioblastoma multiforme composed of spongioblast,

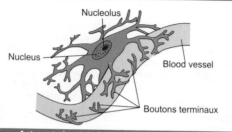

Nucleolus

Nucleus

Blood vessel

Boutons terminaux

Astrocyte in association with a blood vessel

astroblast and astrocyte in varying proportion.

Astrophobia Morbid fear of stars and celestial bodies.

Asylum An institution for mentally ill.

Asymmetry Without symmetry.

Asymptomatic Without any symptoms.

Asynclitism An oblique presentation of foetal head during labor.

Asynergia Lack of coordination between body parts or muscles that normally act in unison.

Ataraxia A state of complete mental relaxation and tranquility.

Atavism The appearance of characteristics presumed to be present in some ancestors.

Ataxia Defective muscular control and coordination. *a. alcoholic* Ataxia due

to loss of proprioception in chronic alcoholism. *a. Brun's* Ataxia of bilateral frontal lobe lesions with a tendency to stagger and fall backwards. *a. cerebellar* Motor ataxia of cerebellar disease. Often with nystagmus, tremor, scanning speech and dysmetria. *a. Friedreich's* An inherited disease manifesting in childhood or adolescence. There is degeneration of lateral and dorsal columns of spinal cord. Peripheral neuropathy, high arch palate, kyphoscoliosis are often associated. *a. sensory* Ataxia due to loss of proprioceptive impulses. *a. telangiectasia* IgA deficiency state of congenital origin manifesting with cerebellar ataxia, telangiectasia and recurrent sinopulmonary infections.

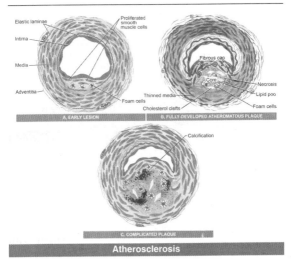

Elastic laminae
Intima
Media
Adventitia
Proliferated smooth muscle cells
Foam cells

A, EARLY LESION

Fibrous cap
Core
Thinned media
Cholesterol clefts
Necrosis
Lipid poo
Foam cells

B, FULLY-DEVELOPED ATHEROMATOUS PLAQUE

Calcification

C, COMPLICATED PLAQUE

Atherosclerosis

Atelectasis Collapsed or airless condition of lungs; the affected lungs are often unexpanded since birth, can be caused by bronchial obstruction, or compression.

Atherogenesis Formation of atheromata in the walls of arteries.

Atheroma Fatty degeneration of arterial wall with cholesterol deposit and smooth muscle hyperplasia.

Atherosclerosis A sclero degenerative disease of arterial wall marked by intimal lipid deposit, fibrous tissue accumulation and smooth muscle cell proliferation (*see* Figure above).

Athetosis Slow irregular twisting involuntary movement of hand and fingers (*see* Figure).

Athlete's foot Fungus infection of foot particularly in betweeen toes.

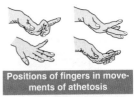

Positions of fingers in movements of athetosis

Atlantoaxial Pertaining to first and second cervical vertebrae.

Atlas This is the first cervical vertebra of the human spine. It is named after a character of Greek mythology. Atlas was the name of a powerful deity who carried the earth on his shoulders. The bone atlas articulates with the occipital bone of the cranium above and with the second cervical vertebra (axix) below (*see* Figure).

Atom The smallest form of an element consisting of protons, neutrons and electrons.

Atopy An allergy with a genetic predisposition. Principal forms of atopy are bronchial asthma, urticaria, eczema and rhinitis.

Atorvastatin Lipid lowering agent.

Atracurium Nondepolarizing muscle relaxant.

Atresia Congenital absence or closure of any tubular structure.

Atrial fibrillation Randomized irregular arhythmic atrial contractions giving rise to irregularly irregular pulse.

Atrial flutter Rapid regular atrial contraction with a varying but regular ventricular response due to fixed or varying A-V block.

Atrial natriuretic factor A hormone secreted by dilated atria that helps in natriuresis.

Atrichosis Congenital absence of hair.

Atrioventricular bundle The conducting system extending from A-V node till division into left and right bundles.

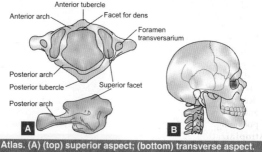

Atlas. (A) (top) superior aspect; (bottom) transverse aspect. Note the absence of the body and spinous process. (B) Position

Atrioventricularis communis Persistence of the common atrioventricular canal manifesting with atrio ventricular septal defects and A -V valve incompetence.

Atrium A chamber or cavity in communication with another. *a. of ear* Portion of tympanic cavity lying below the malleolus.

Atrophy Decrease in size of tissue or wasting. *a. acute yellow* Extensive necrosis of liver cells with jaundice, haemorrhage and mental obtundation. *a. optic* Degeneration of optic nerve head, primary or secondary (MS, glaucoma, trauma etc). *a. disuse* Atrophy resulting from lack of use of muscle. *a. peroneal muscular* A hereditary disease involving peroneal nerves with progressive atrophy of peroneal muscles. *a. Sudeck's* Acute atrophy of bone at the site of injury, possibly due to local vasospasm.

Atropine sulfate A parasympatholytic agent used for preanesthetic medication to decrease bronchial secretions and in organophosphorous poisoning.

Atropinization Administration of atropine till desired effect is obtained.

Attack The sudden onset of an illness, e.g., heart attack.

Attention-deficit-disorder A disease of infancy or childhood, mainly boys characterized by inappropriate attention, hyperactivity and impulsivity.

Attenuate To render thin, weak or less virulent.

Attic The middle ear cavity above the tympanic membrane.

Attitude 1. Behavior towards a person, thing or situation 2. Bodily posture or position assumed, e.g., catatonic posture.

Audible sound Sound with frequency of 15-15000 Hz.

Audiologist A specialist in the evaluation and rehabilitation of persons with hearing disorder.

Audiometry Testing of hearing by audiometer.

Audito-oculogyric reflex Sudden turning of eyes and head towards direction of loud sound.

Auditory bulb The membranous labyrinth and cochlea.

Auditory evoked response An objective method of assessing hearing where the hearing stimulus as traverses along its path to auditory cortex produces characteristic electric potentials recorded across the cortex. It is useful in childrens, in malingerers, and in psychiatric patients. It can pin point as to the site of lesion along the auditory pathway.

Auditory reflex Any reflex produced by stimulation of auditory nerve like blinking of eyes in response to sudden sound.

Auer bodies Rod shaped intracytoplasmic structure present in myeloblasts in acute myeloblastic leukemia.

Auerbach's plexus A plexus formed by sympathetic nerve fibers in muscular coats of GI tract.

Augmentin Amoxycillin-clavulanic acid.

Aura A subjective sensation preceding an attack of epileptic seizure or migraine; epileptic aura may be psychic in nature or sensory in the form of auditory, visual, olfactory or taste hallucinations.

Auranofin Gold preparation for rheumatoid arthritis.

Aureomycin Chlortetracycline hydrochloride.

Auricle 1. Left and right atria 2. Pinna of the ear.

Auriculopalpebral reflex Closure of eye resulting from tactile or thermal stimulation of external auditory meatus. Synonym : Kisch's reflex.

Auriscope Instrument for examination of ear.

Aurotherapy Treatment with gold salts, e.g., rheumatoid arthritis.

Auscultation The technique of listening to sounds produced within body, e.g., passage of air in bronchi, blood in occluded vessels, and A-V malformation, bowel movement, beating of heart, murmurs and adventitious heart sounds etc.

Austin Flint murmur Diastolic mitral regurgitation in a aortic insufficiency mimicking mitral stenosis but without the opening snap or presystolic accentuation.

Australia antigen Hepatitis B surface antigen, existing in serum as part of Dane particle (40-400 nm) or as free particles and rods (22 nm).

Autacoids Generic name for histamine and antihistamine like agents in body.

Autism Mental introversion with attention centered around own ego. *a. infantile* A syndrome appearing in childhood with self absorption, aloneness, inaccessibility, rage reactions and behavioral-language problems; a form of childhood psychosis.

Autoagglutinin Agglutinins that agglutinate individuals own red blood cells.

Autoanalyzer Device that analyzes multiple samples automatically.

Autoantibody Antibody acting against the host antigens.

Autoclave A device used for sterilization by steam pressure.

Autodigestion Digestion of a tissue by tissue's own products, e.g., pancreatic digestion in acute pancreatitis.

Autoerotism Sexual arousal or gratification by using one's own body as in masturbation.

Autograft A graft transferred from one part of body to another.

Autohemolysis Hemolysis of ones blood by person's own serum.

Autohemotherapy Injection of patient's own blood.

Autoimmunity Condition in which antibodies are produced against body's own tissues.

Autoimmune disease Diseases in which antibodies are produced against body's own tissues to cause organ damage, e.g., rheumatoid arthritis, SLE, glomerulonephritis, rheumatic carditis, myasthenia gravis.

Autoinfection Infection produced by an agent already present within the body.

Autoinfusion Forcing blood from extremities to body core by applying tight bandages.

Autoinoculation Inoculation of a person by organisms obtained from the same individual .

Autologous blood transfusion Use of patient's own blood for transfusion, the blood being collected prior to operation or during operation from wound site; thus avoiding dangers of mismatch and transfusion associated infections like HBV, AIDS.

Automatism Behavior without conscious volition or knowledge, the individual appearing normal but amnesic for the events.

Autonomic nervous system The part of nervous system controlling involuntary functions like heart beat, glandular secretions, bowel and bladder contraction and other smooth muscle function. It is divided into parasympathetic or craniosacral system and sympathetic or thoracolumbar system (*see* Figure on page 90).

Autopsy Postmortem examination to ascertain cause of death.

Autoregulation A phenomena where the involved tissue regulates events like blood flow into/through it according to its requirement. e.g., as in brain.

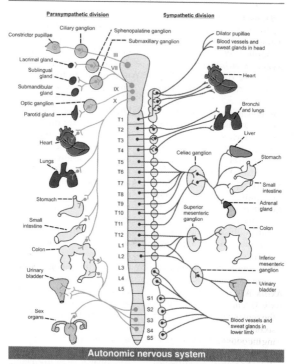

Parasympathetic division

Constrictor pupillae
Ciliary ganglion
Sphenopalatine ganglion
Submaxillary ganglion
Lacrimal gland
III
Sublingual gland
VII
Submandibular gland
IX
Optic ganglion
X
Parotid gland
T1
Heart
T2
T3
T4
Lungs
T5
T6
Stomach
T7
T8
Small intestine
T9
T10
T11
Colon
T12
L1
Urinary bladder
L2
L3
L4
L5
Sex organs
S1
S2
S3
S4
S5

Sympathetic division

Dilator pupillae
Blood vessels and sweat glands in head
Heart
Bronchi and lungs
Liver
Stomach
Celiac ganglion
Small intestine
Adrenal gland
Superior mesenteric ganglion
Colon
Inferior mesenteric ganglion
Urinary bladder
Blood vessels and sweat glands in lower limb

Autonomic nervous system

Autosomes Any of the chromosomes other than sex chromosomes.

Autosplenectomy Multiple infarcts of spleen that cause it to shrink as in sickle cell anaemia.

Autotrophic Self nourishing, e.g., green plants and bacteria forming protein and carbohydrate from inorganic salts and bicarbonates.

A-V block A block in atrio ventricular node whereby impulses arising from atria cannot reach ventricles or are delayed; divided into first degree (prolonged PR), second degree (mobitz type I and II) and third degree (A-V block).

Avascular Having poor blood supply.

Aversion therapy A form of behavior therapy where unpleasant and undesired (e.g., alcohol) stimuli are presented to patient simultaneously so that patient associates the undesired stimulus with the unpleasant one and thus discontinues the undesired stimulus.

Avidin A protein of egg white inhibiting biotin.

Avulsion A tearing away forcibly of a part or structure.

Axanthopsia Yellow blindness.

Axial line A line running in the main axis of body. The axial line of hand runs through second digit.

Axilla Armpit.

Axis 1. A line running through the center of the body. 2. The second cervical vertebra bearing the odontoid process about which atlas rotates. *a. cardiac* A graphic representation of the main conduction vector of the heart. Normal axis is 0 to + 90°. *a. visual* The line passing from object through center of cornea and lens to the fovea (*see* Figures on page 92).

Axis deviation Deviation of cardiac axis, like left axis deviation −10° to −90°, right axis deviation + 91 to −90°.

Axis traction Traction made on the fetus in the direction of long axis of birth canal (*see* Figure on page 93).

Axon A process of nerve cell conducting impulse away from the cell body.

Axoneme Axial thread of a chromosome.

Axonometer Device for determining axis of astigmatism.

Axonotmesis Nerve injury disrupting nerve impulse transmission but without severing the nerve.

Avidin A glycoprotein that binds to biotin, preventing its absorption.

Azapropazone A pyrazolon, aspirin like agent, potent uricosuric.

Azaserine Glutamine antagonist, potent inhibitor of purine nucleotide biosynthesis.

Azatidine An antiallergic agent.

Azathioprine An immunosuppressant.

Azauridine A pyrimidine analog.

Azelastine Topical vasoconstrictor for nasal allergy.

Azithromycin Antibiotic of macrolide group better than erythromycin.

Azoospermia Complete absence of sperms in the semen.

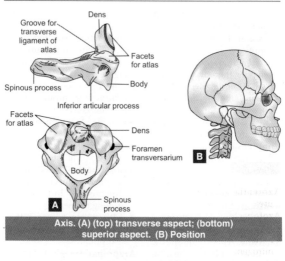

Axis. (A) (top) transverse aspect; (bottom) superior aspect. (B) Position

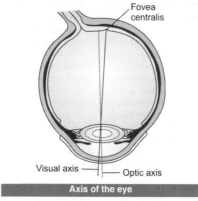

Axis of the eye

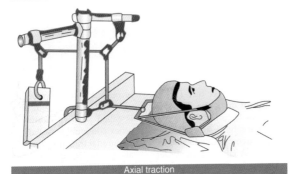

Axial traction

Azotemia Increased blood urea.

Azotobacter Gram-negative, rodshaped, nonpathogenic bacteria that fix atmospheric nitrogen.

Aztreonam An antibiotic for gram-negative sepsis.

Azygos Occurring singly, not in pairs.

Azygos vein The thoracic continuation of ascending lumbar vein through aortic hiatus in diaphragm entering superior vena cava at the level of D4 vertebra.

B

Babcock sentence test This is a test for dementia. This test aims at testing the patient's memory by asking him to repeat a complicated sentence.

Babesia A genus of the order Haemosporidia found in the cattle, sheep, horse, dogs and other vertebrate animals, transmitted by tick.

Babesia microti Principally manifesting with fever, chills and hemoglobinuria.

Babesiosis A disease caused by intraerythrocytic protozoan parasite.

Babinski's reflex Dorsiflexion of great toe and fanning out of other toes on stimulation of lateral part of sole of foot is called positive Babinski's reflex; commonly results from pyramidal tract interruption; also positive in infants below 6 months (before myelination).

Bacampacillin A long acting ampicillin given in twice daily dose.

Bacillemia Presence of bacilli in blood.

Bacillus Any rod shaped micro-organism (*see* Figure).

Bacillus Calmette-Guérin A strain of *Mycobacterium bovis* made avirulant by serial cultivation on bile glycerol

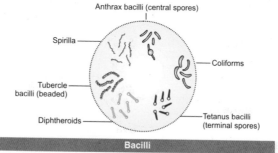

Bacilli

potato medium, used in BCG vaccine for prevention of human tuberculosis.

Bacitracin Topically used antibacterial agent.

Backache Any pain in back; due to muscle spasm, disease of disk, ligaments, vertebral body, nerve roots, and meninges.

Baclofen GABA inhibitor used to reduce muscle spasticity.

Bacteria Any microorganism of the class Schizomycetes; can be spherical or ovoid (cocci); rod shaped (bacilli) or spiral (*see* Figure).

Bacteriocin Protein produced by certain bacteria which is lethal to other bacteria.

Bacteriocinogen A plasmid that produces bacteriocin.

Bacterioclasis Fragmentation of bacteria.

Bacteriophage A virus that infects bacteria.

Bacteriuria Presence of bacteria in urine, significant if concentration exceeds 10^5/ml.

Bacteroides A genus of non-spore forming, gram negative, anaerobic bacteria frequently found in necrotic tissue.

Bagasosis Hypersensitive pneu-monitis due to inhalation of bagasse dust, the moldy fibrous waste of sugarcane.

Brainbridge reflex An increase in the heart rate caused by an increase in right atrial pressure.

Baker's cyst Synovial cyst in popliteal fossa.

Balanitis Inflammation of the glans penis and mucous membrane beneath it.

Balantidiasis Infestation with *B. coli.*

Balanoplasty Plastic surgery repair of glans penis.

Balanoposthitis Inflammation of glans and prepuce.

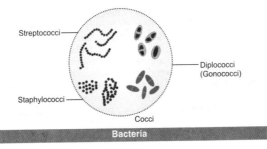

Bacteria

Balanus This is the glans of the penis or clitoris.

Ballance's sign This is a sign indicative of ruptured spleen. In this sign there is presence of a dull percussion note in both the flanks. The dullness on the left side is due to the presence of coagulated blood, whereas that on the right side is due to the fluid blood. Dullness on the left flank remains constant. However, with the change of position to the right side, the haemorrhagic fluid moves to the right flank resulting in dullness.

Ballottment Palpatory technique for examining floating objects, e.g., foetus in uterus, hydronephrotic kidney.

Balneology Science of baths and bathing.

Balser's fatty necrosis Gangrenous pancreatitis with fatty necrosis of pancreas and often of bone marrow.

Bamboo spine Spinal column in radiograph resembling bamboo stalk as in ankylosing spondylitis.

Bandage A piece of gauze to be wrapped around a body part as dressing. *b. barton* Double figure of eight bandage for the lower jaw. *b. butterfly* Adhesive bandage used to hold wound edges together. *b. but-tocks* T or double T bandage or open triangle bandage for buttocks. *b. cravat* Triangular bandage folded to form a band around any injured bony part, e.g., knee, elbow, hand, wrist, head, clavicle. *b. figure of eight* Bandage in which turns cross each other like the figure 8 used to fix and elevate the shoulders in fracture clavicle, to fix splints for the foot or hand. *b. spica* Bandage in which a number of figure of 8 turns are applied, each a little higher or lower with some overlapping. Used for breasts, shoulders, great toe etc. *b. suspensory* used for support of breast and scrotum (*see* Figure on page 97).

Bandl's ring Ring like thickening at the junction of upper and lower uterine segments.

Banti's syndrome A combination of anaemia, cirrhosis and splenic enlargement.

Barber's itch Folliculitis of face mostly by *Staph. aureus*.

Barbotage Repeated injection and withdrawal as in withdrawal of CSF and injection of drugs into SA space.

Baresthesia Pressure sense.

Baritosis Barium dust induced pneumoconiosis.

Barium An alkaline metallic compound used as barium

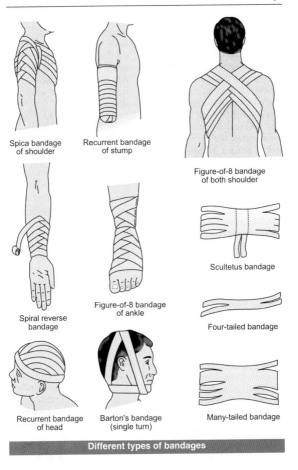

Spica bandage
of shoulder

Recurrent bandage
of stump

Figure-of-8 bandage
of both shoulder

Spiral reverse
bandage

Figure-of-8 bandage
of ankle

Scultetus bandage

Four-tailed bandage

Recurrent bandage
of head

Barton's bandage
(single turn)

Many-tailed bandage

Different types of bandages

sulphate for upper GI studies, colon and GI tract.

Barium enema Enema in which a suspension of barium sulfate is injected into the rectum to render the lower GI tract radio-opaque, in order to diagnose the intestinal (colonic or small intestinal) lesions.

Barium meal Solution of barium sulfate that is swallowed by a patient in order to aid the radiographic diagnosis of stomach and duodenum.

Barium swallow Solution of barium sulfate swallowed by the patient for the radiographic diagnosis of the esophagus.

Barlow's disease Vit. C deficiency state.

Barrette's esophagus Metaplasia of the lower esophageal squamous epithelial lining to goblet cells (usually found in the lower gastrointestinal tract).

Barognosis The ability to estimate weight.

Baroreflex Reflex mediated by pressure changes within great vessels through stimulation of mechanoreceptors.

Barotrauma Trauma due to changes in atmospheric pressure.

Barr body Sex chromatin mass seen within the nuclei of normal female somatic cells, representing inactivated X-chromosome.

Barrel chest Rounded chest due to air trapping as in emphysema. In normal chest, AP diameter is more than transverse, hence elliptical shape.

Barthel index A widely used index for the functional assessment of a person's ability to perform the daily activities like feeding, grooming, controlling bowel and bladder functions, etc.

Bartholin's duct Duct of sublingual salivary gland that runs parallel with Wharton's duct and opens with it.

Bartholin's gland A compound mucus gland lying in lateral wall of vestibule of vagina, at the junction upper and middle one third.

Bartonellosis Infection due to bartonella bacilliformis (oroya fever) characterised by fever and haemolysis; transmitted by females and flies and treated with chloramphenicol.

Bartter's syndrome Hyperplasia of Juxtaglomerular cells with hypokalemia, hyperaldosteronism but without a rise in blood pressure.

Basal body temperature chart Daily temperature charting to predict ovulation.

Basal ganglia Four masses of gray matter (caudate, lentiform, amygdaloid and claustrum) lying deep in cerebral hemispheres.

Basal metabolic rate (BMR) Normal value is 40 kcal/m^2/hour, a test of thyroid function.

Base Any substance that accepts hydrogen ion; strong bases feel slippery and are corrosives.

Base pair In double stranded helical DNA the connecting chemicals, i.e., base pairs adenine-thymine, guanine-cytosine bind the strands.

Basion Mid point of anterior border of foramen magnum.

Basiphobia Fear of walking.

Basisphenoid An embryonic bone that becomes the lower portion of sphenoid.

Bassini's operation Surgical repair of inguinal hernia.

Battered child syndrome Physical injuries inflicted upon children.

Battery Unlawful touching of a patient without consent, justification; battery occurs if a surgical or medical procedure in done without prior consent.

Battery sign Swelling behind the ear in fracture base of skull.

Baxter's formula This is a commonly used formula to calculate the fluid requirements, particularly in case of burn victims. According to this formula 4 ml of ringer lactate solution is administered per kilogram body weight percent of body surface area burnt.

Bazin's disease Erythema induratum.

B cells Bone marrow derived lymphocytes, which when stimulated by antigen, transform to antibody producing plasma cells.

BCG vaccine Bacille Calmette - Guérin, indicated for vaccination of tuberculin negative children.

Beaker Wide mouthed glass vessel.

Beau's line White lines on finger nails.

Beclomethasone Synthetic corticosteroid.

Becquerel (BQ) A measure of radioactivity of radionuclides equal to 3.7×10^{10} curies.

Bedlam Asylum for insane.

Bedsore Pressure Sore. i.e., ischaemic necrosis of tissue esp. over bony prominences.

Behçet's syndrome A symptoms complex of recurrent orogenital ulceration, uveitis and joint pains, 5 times more frequent in males.

Belching Expulsion of stomach gas through mouth and nose.

Bell's palsy Sudden unilateral lower motor facial palsy due to swelling/ischemia of the nerve in bony canal.

Bellini's tubule The straight connecting tubule of the kidney.

Bence-Zones protein A low molecular weight protein that disappears when urine is boiled to above 60°C but reappears once urine is cooled, commonly seen in multiple myeloma.

Benedict's sol A solution of copper sulfate, sodium citrate and sodium carbonate, used for testing presence of reducing sugars in urine.

Benedict's test 8 drops of urine is added to 5 ml. of Benedicts Sol. and boiled to see for green, yellow, red precipitate.

Benedipine A calcium channel β–blocker for hypertension.

Benign Not recurrent, nor progressive.

Benign prostatic hypertrophy (BPH). Prostatic enlargement in elderly due to hyperplasia causing obstruction of prostatic urethra.

Benoxynate HCl Topically used ophthalmic local anaesthetic.

Benserazide Inhibitor of amino acid decarboxylase, used in parkinsonism.

Bentonite Hydrated alumino silicate, used as a suspending agent.

Benzapril An ACE inhibition for hypertension.

Benzafibrate Lipid lowering agent.

Benzalkonium chloride An antimicrobial preservative, used as detergent and germicide.

Benzene A volatile liquid used in synthesis of dyes and drugs.

Benzidine Used for test of occult blood in stool (to a solution of benzidine in glacial acetic acid is added 3% H_2O_2 and the stool sample. Appearance of blue colour indicates presence of blood).

Benznidazole A nitroimidazole for Chaga's disease.

Benzobromarone Uricosuric agent used in gout.

Benzocaine Topical anaesthetic.

Benzodiazepine Psychotropic agents with potent hypnotic and anti anxiety effects.

Benzoic acid Antifungal agent.

Benzoin A plant resin used as inhalant, or protective coating for ulcers.

Benzoyl peroxide Keratolytic agent (for acne).

Benzthiazide Diuretic of thiazide group.

Benztropine mesylate Antiparasympathomimetic agent for treatment of parkinsonism.

Benzyl benzoate Scabicide.

Bephenium hydroxynaphthoate Anthelmintic for hookworm and mixed infestation.

Beraud's valve A fold of mucus membrane at the mouth of lacrimal duct in the lid.

Beri beri A disease due to thiamine deficiency characterized by cardiac failure (wet type) or fatigue, neuritis, poor memory, anorexia (dry type).

Berylliosis Beryllium induced pulmonary fibrosis.

Bestiality Sexual intercourse with animals.

Beta adrenergic receptors Specific receptors in blood vessels, heart, bronchi intestine etc for action of adrenaline and noradrenaline.

Beta adrenergic receptor blockers Drugs that block both Beta$_1$ and Beta$_2$ receptors.

Betadine Povidone-iodine.

Betahistine Drug used for vertigo.

Betaine An alkaloid from beet, used orally as a source of HCl.

Betalactamase An enzyme produced by certain bacteria that inactivates antibiotics.

Beta methasone Synthetic glucocorticoid.

Betatron Electron accelerator that produces high energy electrons or X-rays.

Bethanicol Choline ester used for relief of urinary retention.

Betz cells Giant pyramidal cells in the motor cortex whose axons form pyramidal tract.

Bezoar A hard mass of entangled material found in stomach or intestine, hair ball (trichobezoar), hair and vegetable fiber (trichophyto bezoar).

Bevacizumab Monoclonal antibody for colon cancer.

Biblio mania Obsession with collection of books.

Biceps A muscle with two heads. *b. brachii* Flexor of elbow and supinator. *b. femoris* Muscle on posterior lateral side of thigh, flexor of knee and rotates it outwards.

BCNU Carmustine, an antineoplastic agent.

Biconcave Concave on each side (*see* Figure A on page 102).

Biconvex Convex on both sides (*see* Figure B on page 102).

Bicornis Uterus with two horns due to incomplete union of mullerian ducts.

Bicuspid Having two cusps or leaflets mitral, often aortic.

Bicuspid tooth Permanent premolars are bicuspid.

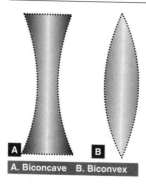

A. Biconcave   B. Biconvex

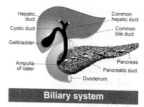

Biliary system

Bicycle ergometer Stationary bicycle used for cardiac exercise, i.e., MUGA testing/intra operative exercise test.

Bifid Cleft or split into two parts.

Bifocal Eye glasses with lenses for distant and near vision.

Bifonazole An imidazole with antifungal activity.

Bigemini Group of two beats separated by a long pause. Commonly due to regular extrasystoles, (e.g., digitalis toxicity).

Bile A thick viscid fluid with bitter taste secreted by liver. The bile when secreted in liver is straw coloured but down below is yellow-brown or green in colour (*see* Figure).

Bile acids Cholic, taurocholic and glycocholic acids that exist as salts in bile and are helpful for intestinal fat absorption (micelle formation).

Bile pigment Bilirubin and biliverdin, imparting brown colour to urine and faeces and give positive reaction in Vandenberg's test.

Biticyanin A blue or purple pigment, an oxidation product of biliverdin.

Biligenesis Formation of bile.

Bilirubin Bile pigment; yellow to orange coloured, can be direct acting when conjugated to glucuronic acid or indirect acting when unconjugated.

Biliverdin Greenish pigment, formed by oxidation of bilirubin.

Biling's ovulation method A method for estimating the time of ovulation in a woman on the basis of analysis of the colour and consistency of the cervical mucous during various phases of menstrual cycle. This method is often adopted as a method for natural family planning. At the time of ovulation, the cervical mucus becomes thick and tenacious which fractures easily on stretching.

Billroth's operation BI: Excision of pylorus and gastroduodenal anastomosis BII: Partial gastrectomy followed by side to side gastrojejunal anastomosis.

Bimanual Examination by both hands.

Bimodal Means a graphic presentation with two peaks.

Bioassay Determination of strength of a drug in live animal/humans.

Bioavailability The rate and extent to which an active drug or metabolite enters the general circulation to be available at the acting site.

Biochemistry Chemistry of living things.

Biodynamics The science of force or energy of living matter.

Biofeedback A training programme aimed at controlling in function of autonomic nervous system.

Biogenic amines Chemical compounds important in neuro- transmission, e.g., dopamine, norepinephrine, serotonin and histamine.

Biokinetics Study of growth changes and movements in developing organisms.

Biometry Computation of life expectancy, application of statistics to biological science.

Biophysics Application of physical laws to biological processes and function.

Biopsy Removal of tissue for examination *b.aspiration*–tissue removed by needle and syringe; *b. brush*- tissue removal by use of brush; *b. cone*- removal of cone shaped tissue *b.punch* tissue removal by a hollow punch.

Biostatistics Application of statistical processes and methods to the analysis of biological data e.g., morbidity rate, mortality rate etc.

Biot's breathing Short breaths in succession followed by long apnea as seen in raised intracranial pressure.

Biotin Otherwise known vit. H; deficiency manifests with poor mental and physical development, alopecia, impaired immunity etc.

Biparietal Distance between both parietal eminences important for foetal descent and delivery.

Bipolar In bipolar disease patient has alternating mania and depression.

Birefringence It is also known as double refraction. It is the decomposition of a ray of light into two rays: ordinary ray and the extraordinary ray due to the polarization of light.

Birenberg bow This is an effective intrauterine contraceptive device.

Birth mark Nevus, pigmentation or vascular tumor.

Birth rate Number of live births per 1,000 of the population per year. Syn Natality.

Bisacodyl A laxative that acts directly on the rectum. Given as tablets or in the form of suppositories.

Bisacromial Pertains to two acromial processes.

Bisexual 1. Having gonads of both sexes. 2. Hermaphrodite. 3. Having both active and passive sexual interests or characteristics. 4. Capable of the function of both sexes. 5. Both heterosexual and homosexual. 6. An individual who is both heterosexual and homosexual. 7. Of, relating to or involving both sexes as in bisexual reproduction.

Bismuth Silvery metallic element whose salts are astringent, protective, soothing and antidiarrhoeal.

Bisoprolol Betablocker.

Bite In dentistry denotes the angle and manner at which upper and lower teeth meet when jaw is closed.

b. closed lower incisors lie behind upper incisors. *b. open* gap existing between upper and lower incisors. *b. over* upper incisors overlap lower ones. *b. under* lower incisors pass in front of upper ones.

Bite wing radiograph X-ray showing crown and upper third of root of upper and lower teeth.

Bitot's spots Triangular, shiny, gray spots on conjunctiva seen in vit A deficiency.

Bjerrum's screen Used for mapping the field of visions esp. central and paracentral scotomas.

Black eye Bruising, discoloration and swelling of eyelids following trauma.

Blackhead A plug of dried sebum in a sebaceous gland (Acne).

Black measles Also called haemorrhagic measles implying a severe hemorrhagic measle eruption.

Blackout Sudden loss of consciousness.

Black water fever Haemoglobinuria following *P. falciparum* induced hemolysis.

Black widow A species of poisonous spider: Latrodectus mactans, whose bite causes severe abdominal cramps.

Bladder Receptacle to hold secretions. (urinary bladder, gallbladder). *b. autonomous* Bladder with loss of both efferent and afferent limbs of reflex arc, constant dribbling with large amount of residual urine. *b. exstrophy* Congenital eversion of bladder. *b. neurogenic* Any bladder dysfunction due to interruption of its innervation. *b. worm* Larval form of tape worm with a rounded cyst or bladder into which scolex is invaginated.

Blalock-Taussig operation *A. Blalock, American surgeon, 1899-1964; H.B. Taussig, American paediatrician, 1898-1986.* Operation in which the subclavian artery is anastomosed to the pulmonary artery. Performed in Fallot's tetralogy.

Blanch To lose colour. In blanching test, the nail is pressed quickly and then released. When circulation is good, colour returns within 5 seconds.

Bland diet Diet without irritant foods. e.g., milk, cream, prepared cereals, eggs, lean meat, fish, cheese, custard, cookie etc.

Blandin's glands Glands on each side of frenulum of tongue.

Blastocyst A stage of mammalian embryo next to morula and consists of outer trophoblast to which is attached an inner cell mass. The enclosed cavity is blastocele (*see* Figure).

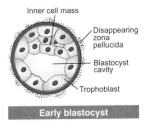

Early blastocyst

Blastoma Neoplasm composed of immature undifferentiated cells.

Blastomere One of the cells resulting from cleavage of a fertilized ovum.

Blastomyces A genus of yeast like budding fungi pathogenic to man.

Bleaching powder Calcium hypochlorite or chlorinated lime.

Bleeding time Time required for blood to stop flowing from a pin prick. Normal range 1-3 minutes (Dukes) or 1-9 minutes (Ivy).

Blennorrhagia A discharge from mucous membranes.

Bleomycin Anti tumor agent used for carcinoma of skin, lungs, head and neck.

Blepharitis Inflammation of lid margins including hair follicles and the glands.

Blepharoconjunctivitis This is the inflammation of both the conjunctiva and eyelids.

Blepharodiastasis Excessive separation of eyelids.

Blepharospasm Twitching or spasm of orbiculares oculi muscle.

Blindness Amauresis.

Blindspot Physiological scotoma situated 15° to outside of visual fixation point, corresponding to optic disc.

Blister Collection of fluid within epidermis.

Blood brain barrier A barrier membrane, i.e. endothelium and basement membrane, that prevent entry of damaging substances into CNS.

Blood group A genetically determined system of antigens located on surface of RBC. AB, and O system is the commonly accepted one. There are 30 Rh antigens too (*see* Figure on page 107).

Blood pressure Pressure exerted by moving blood on the vessel wall. A value beyond 140/90 mmHg in those below 50 years and 160/95 mmHg in those above 60 years is abnormal.

BP diastolic BP in between heart beats; depends upon elasticity of arteries and peripheral vascular resistance.

Blumenbach's sign Sign indicative of peritonitis, pain is experienced while pressure is relieved, on the abdomen by examining hand.

Boa's point A tender spot left of 12th dorsal vertebra, in patients with gastric ulcer.

Bochdalek's ganglion Ganglion of plexuses of dental nerve in the maxilla above the canine tooth.

Body-ketone They are acetone, acetoacitic acid and betahydroxy butyric acid. *b. amygdaloid* Almond shaped gray matter in the lateral wall and roof of third ventricle of brain concerned with memory. *b. Aschoff* Microscopic areas of central fibrinoid degeneration with sorrounding chronic inflammatory cell infiltration seen in rheumatic fever. *b. carotid* Flat structure at bifurcation of common carotid, containing baroreceptors. *b. Donovan* chlamydia granulomatis, causative organism of granuloma inguinale. *b. Negri* Inclusion bodies in nerve cells of CNS in patients of rabies.

Body mass index Body weight in kg divided by height in

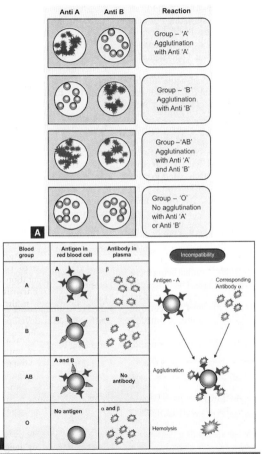

Blood group

meters squared (W/H²), an index for estimating obesity.

Body rocking Rhythmic purposeless body movements.

Boeck's sarcoid Older name for sarcoidosis.

Boil A furuncle, acute inflammation of subcutaneous tissue including glands and hair follicles.

Bombesin A neuropeptide present in gut and brain.

Bone Bone can be defined as a rigid hard connective tissue which forms part of the endoskeleton of the vertebrates. The bones help in supporting and protecting various organs in the body. The inner part of the bone is known as bone marrow which is the site for haematopoiesis. In an adult human being there are 206 bones. The bones can be of two types: compact (cortical) and cancellous (spongy) bone. Compact bone can be called as dense bone which is responsible for giving smooth, white and solid appearance to the bone. This type of bone accounts for about 80% of total bone mass in an adult skeleton. Cancellous bone comprises of a trabecular meshwork found in the interior of the bone. It accounts for the remaining 20% of the total bone mass. Depending on their shape and size, bones can be classified into five categories: long bones, short bones, flat bones, irregular bones and sesamoid bones. Each long bone is composed of three parts: epiphysis, metaphysis and diaphysis (*see* Figure).

Bone alveolar Bone of maxilla and mandible supporting the teeth. *b. sesamoid* Bone found embedded in tendons and joint capsule.

Bone age Estimation of biological age based on development of ossification centers of wrist and long bones.

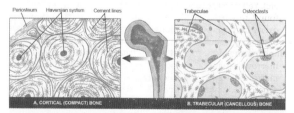

A, CORTICAL (COMPACT) BONE   B, TRABECULAR (CANCELLOUS) BONE

Bone densitometry Method of determining bone density by radiographic or ultrasonic means for diagnosis of osteoporosis.

Bone marrow Bone marrow is highly vascular, pulpy, network of reticular tissue found in the hollow interior of bones. The major function of the bone marrow in adult bones is haematopoiesis or production of new blood cells. Bone marrow is primarily of two types: red marrow and yellow marrow. Red marrow is mainly composed of myeloid tissue and is responsible for synthesis of RBC's, WBC's and platelets. Yellow marrow is mainly composed of fat cells and is responsible for synthesis of a few white blood cells. Red marrow is mainly found in the flat bones like hip bone, skull bones, rib, vertebrae, scapula and in the canellous material at the ends of long bones (femur, humerus, tibia, etc). Yellow marrow is mainly found inside the medullary cavity in the middle portions of the long bones.

Bone marrow aspiration Bone marrow aspiration or bone marrow biopsy is a medical procedure in order to obtain the bone marrow sample for the purpose of pathological examination. Bone marrow aspiration is used for the diagnosis of numerous haematological conditions including leukaemia, multiple myeloma, anaemia, haematological malignancies, etc. The common sites for bone marrow aspiration include the sternum and posterior iliac crest.

Bone marrow transplantation autologous Cryopreservation of patient marrow and its reinfusion for marrow hypoplasia following cancer chemotherapy.

Bone marrow transplantation Used in treatment of aplastic anaemia thalassemia, immune deficiency, sickle cell disease.

Bonnevie-Ullrich syndrome This is another name for Turner's syndrome. The individuals suffering from this syndrome have only one X Chromosome and no second sex chromosome (either X or Y). The phenotype of such individuals is female due to absence of Y chromosome. The individuals may show the following features: Growth retardation, webbed neck, infertility, short stature, development delay, learning disabilities, lymphedema, etc.

The external genitalia is of female type. Though uterus and fallopian tubes are present, both ovaries and testis are absent.

Borax Sodium borate, used as water softner, and weak antiseptic.

Borborygmus A gurgling, splashing sound heard in abdomen caused by passage of gas.

Boric acid An odourless white crystaline powder used as a mild antiseptic solution especially for eyes, mouth and bladder.

Bornholm's disease Pleurodynia caused by coxackie B. virus.

Bottle mouth syndrome Dental caries caused in infants when they take a bottle filled with liquid other than water.

Botulin The neurotoxin responsible for botulism.

Botulism A severe form of food poisoning due to botulinous toxins A, B, C, D, E, F and G.

Bougie A slender flexible instrument for dilating tubular organs, e.g., urethra (*see* Figure).

Boutonniere deformity Proximal IP joint flexion and DIP hyperextension, characteristic of rheumatoid deformity.

Bowleg Outward bending of lower limbs (genu varum, due to rickets).

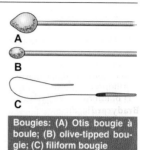

Bougies: (A) Otis bougie à boule; (B) olive-tipped bougie; (C) filiform bougie

Bowman's capsule A bilayered membrane closely applied to glomerulus. Functioning as a filter for formation of urine.

Bowman's membrane Thin homogeneous membrane separating corneal epithelium from corneal substance.

Boyle's law The law states that at a constant temperature, the volume of gas varies inversely with pressure.

Brachium pontis Middle cerebellar peduncle.

Brachycheilia Abnormally short lips.

Brachydactylia Abnormally short fingers and toes.

Brachytherapy Radioactive material implant (radium, cesium, iridium or gold) at the malignancy site.

Bradford frame This is a rectangular metallic frame having canvas or webbing straps used for immobilizing the spine and pelvis. It is often used to support individuals with diseases or fractures of the spine, hip or pelvis. This device is named after its inventor, an American orthopaedic surgeon Edward H Bradford.

Bradycardia Sinus rhythm, <60/minute in adult, 100/minute in a child and 120/minute in fetus.

Bradyarrhythmia Slow and irregular heart rate.

Bradykinesia Slownes of movement (parkinsonism).

Bradyphrasia Slowness of speech.

Bradypnea Abnormally slow respiration.

Braille Raised dots system for education of blind.

Brain Composed of neurones and neuroglia, average weight 1350-1400 gm of which 2% in spinal cord and 85% is cerebrum, divided into 1. diencephalon (thalamus, hypothalamus, epithalamus) 2. mesencephalon (tegmentum, crura cerebri, medulla) 3. metencephalon (cerebellum, pons) and 4. telencephalon (cerebral cortex) (*see* Figure).

Brain death Isoelectric EEG for atleast 30 minutes with no change in response to sound and pain stimuli; absent respiration and all reflexes, (barbiturate, diazepam, methaqualone can produce short periods of isoelectric EEG).

Bran Outer layer or husk of grains/cereals composed of

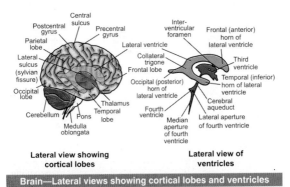

Lateral view showing cortical lobes

Lateral view of ventricles

Brain—Lateral views showing cortical lobes and ventricles

undigestible cellulose, adding bulk to stool.

Branchial arches Five pairs of arched structure that form lateral and ventral walls of pharynx of the embryo from which structures of face and neck are formed.

Branchial clefts Openings between branchial arches.

Brandt-Andrews maneuver Expulsion of placenta from uterus during third stage of labour by gentle traction on cord by one hand, the other hand pressing uterus backwards and upwards.

Braxton Hicks sign Painless intermittent uterine contractions occurring after 3rd month of pregnancy.

Break bone fever Dengue fever (group B arbovirus).

Breast cancer Malignant neoplasm of breast, leading cause of death in women. Breast self examination in useful for early detection.

Breathing Act of inhaling and exhaling air. *b. bronchial* Prolonged high pitched expiration with often a tubular quality.

Breech presentation Foetal buttocks present at pelvic inlet (*see* Figure).

Bregma That point on skull where coronal and sagittal sutures join (*see* Figure on page 113).

Breisky's disease Kraurosis vulvae.

Brennerman's ulcers This can be described as meatitis, meatal ulceration and meatal stenosis of the urinary

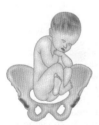
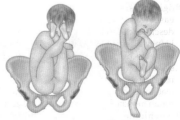

Complete breech   Frank breech   Fooiling breech

Breech presentation

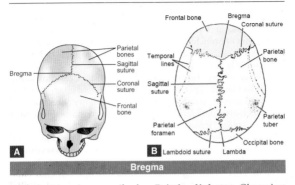

Frontal bone · Bregma · Coronal suture · Parietal bones · Sagittal suture · Coronal suture · Frontal bone · Bregma · Temporal lines · Parietal bone · Sagittal suture · Parietal tuber · Parietal foramen · Occipital bone · Lambdoid suture · Lambda

A   **B**

Bregma

meatus in circumscribed males. Circumcision results in removal of foreskin which makes the meatus prone to infection, thereby resulting in the development of ulceration.

Brenner's tumor Benign fibro-epithelioma of ovary.

Bretylium Antiarrhythmic agent.

Bright's disease Bright's disease was a term used to describe different forms of kidney disease in accordance with the older classification system of renal diseases. This usually referred to the inflammation of kidneys, what is now commonly known as nephritis.

Brimonidine Anti-glaucoma eye drop.

Briquet's syndrome A personality disorder with alcoholism and somatization disorder.

Brittle diabetes Changing and unpredictable response to insulin leading to ketosis, particularly in childhood diabetes.

Broca's area Posterior end of left inferior frontal gyrus which contains motor speech area controlling movements of lips, tongue and vocal cord.

Brodie's abscess Subacute osteomyelitis usually due to tuberculosis or *Staph. aureus* infection.

Brodmann's area Division of cerebral cortex into 47 areas, now classified according to their function.

Bromhexine Mucolytic agent.

Bromocryptine mesylate A dopaminergic ergot derivative that is used in hyper-prolactinemia.

Bronchiectasis Chronic irreversible and permanent dilatation of bronchi, may be congenital or acquired.

Bronchiocele Circumscribed dilatation of bronchus.

Bronchiole Respiratory bronchiole is the last division of bronchial tree and continues as alveolar duct into alveolus. Terminal bronchiole is next to last subdivision of a bronchiole.

Bronchiolitis Inflammation of bronchioles, commonly in small children.

Bronchitis Inflammation of mucous membrane of bronchi (*see* Figure).

Bronchodilator An agent that dilates the air passages and relaxes the bronchial smooth muscles in order to aid breathing.

Bronchogram Radioopaque material opacification of bronchi.

Broncholith A calculus in the bronchus.

Bronchophony The voice as heard over normal bronchus by use of stethoscope.

Bronchopneumonia Inflammation of terminal bronchioles and alveoli.

Bronchoscope An endoscope for visualization of tracheobronchial tree, biopsy and foreign body removal (*see* Figure on page 115).

Bronchoscopy Examination of bronchial tree by a bronchoscope.

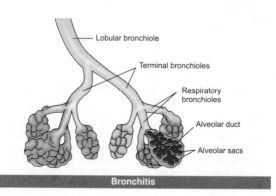

- Lobular bronchiole
- Terminal bronchioles
- Respiratory bronchioles
- Alveolar duct
- Alveolar sacs

Bronchitis

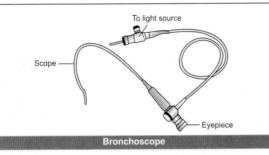

Bronchoscope

Bronchovesicular Sounds intermediate between bronchial and alveolar sounds.

Bronchus The hollow tubes formed by division of trachea at the level of D_4.

Brooke's formula This is one of the most commonly used formula for calculating the amount of fluid to be administered within the first twenty-four hours following burns injury in a patient with burns involving more than 50% of the surface area. It calls for administration of ringer's lactate solution at the rate of 2 ml /kg/% burn.

Brown-Séquard syndrome Hemisection of spinal cord with loss of pain and temperature on opposite side, motor paralysis on the same side with loss of position and vibratory sense.

Brucellosis Infection caused by Brucella organism (*B. abortus, suis* and *melitensis*).

Bruch's membrane The membrane lying between choroid membrane and the pigmented epithelium of retina.

Bruck's disease A combination of muscle atrophy and skeletal disorder like multiple fracture, ankylosis.

Bruise Injury with effusion of blood into subcutaneous tissue and skin discolouration with intact skin.

Bruit An adventitious sound of arterial or venous obstruction narrowing.

Brunner's glands Compound glands of duodenum and upper jejunum secreting mucus.

Brush border Hollow microvilli in the renal tubules and intestinal epithelium.

Brushfield spots Gray or pale yellow spots present at the periphery of iris in Down's syndrome.

Bruxism Grinding of teeth particularly during sleep.

Bryant's traction Traction applied to lower leg vertically in treating femur fracture in children.

Buck's traction Traction of lower extremity applied in line with long axis of the leg.

Buclizine Antihistamine used for motion sickness.

Budesonide A corticosteroid used as bronchial spray in asthma.

Buerger's disease Thromboangitis obliterans, a vasospastic disease, often nicotine induced, responding to sympathectomy, revascularization and vasodilators.

Buffalo hump Excess fat deposition in cervical and upper thoracic region due to cortisone excess.

Buffer A substance that maintains hydrogen ion concentration in blood. Principal blood buffers are: bicarbonates, carbonates, carbonic acid, dibasic phosphates, Hb and plasma proteins.

Buffy coat A light coloured layer containing white cells that forms when blood is centrifused or is allowed to stand in a test tube.

Bufotenine A hallucinogen from plant, N-methylation product of - 5HT.

Bulb Any rounded or globular structure; *bulbar paralysis*-paralysis due to disease of medula oblongata.

Bulbitis Inflammation of urethra in its bulbous portion, e.g., posterior portion of corpus spongiosum found between the two crura of penis.

Bulbocavernosus reflex Contraction of bulbocavernosus muscle on percussing of dorsum of penis.

Bulbomimic reflex Contraction of facial muscles following pressure on eyeball.

Bulbourethral glands Cowper's glands: Two small glands about the size of a pea, one on each side of prostate gland secreting a viscid fluid adding to semen.

Bulimia Excessive and insatiable appetite. Bouts of over eating followed by vomiting in young girls.

Bulla A large blister or skin vesicle filled with fluid.

Bullaquine An antimalarial.

Bumetanide A diuretic.

Bunion Inflammation and thickening of the bursa of the joint of great toe often with lateral displacement of the toe (*see* Figure).

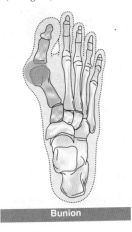

Bunion

Buphthalmos Infantile glaucoma with uniform enlargement of eye esp. cornea.

Buprenorphine Semisynthetic morphine analog, very potent analgesic.

Burkitt's lymphoma Undifferentiated lymphoblastic lymphoma involving sites other than lymph nodes and RE system, with strong association with EB virus infection.

Burn An injury to tissues caused by: (a) physical agents, the sun, excess heat or cold, friction, nuclear radiation; (b) chemical agents, acids or caustic alkalis; (c) electrical current. Burns are described as being partial thickness (involving only the epidermis) or full thickness (involving the dermis and underlying structures). Clinically, emphasis is placed on the percentage of the body affected by the burn. The treatment of shock and prevention of infection and malnutrition need special attention.

Burnett's syndrome Milk - alkali syndrome.

Burning foot syndrome Burning in the sole of feet due to vitamin deficiency and chronic renal failure.

Burr or Bur A device that rotates at high speed, used by dentist or surgeon to make holes in cranium (*see* Figure).

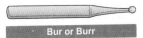

Bur or Burr

Bursa A pad like cavity in the vicinity of joint lined with synovial membrane, acting to reduce friction between tendon and bone (*see* Figure on page 118).

Bursitis Inflammation of a bursa.

Bursolith Calculus formed in bursa.

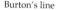

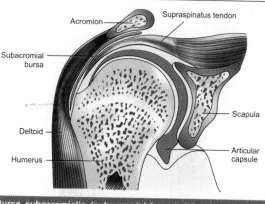

Acromion

Supraspinatus tendon

Subacromial bursa

Deltoid

Humerus

Scapula

Articular capsule

Bursa subacromialis (subacromial bursa), lying between the acromion and supraspinatus tendon and extending between the deltoid and greater tubercle

Burton's line A blue line along the margin of the gum visible in chronic lead poisoning.

Buspiron Antianxiety agent.

Busulphan A cytotoxic drug that depresses the bone marrow and may be used to treat myeloid leukaemia.

Butenafine An antifungal.

Butorphanol Morphine conzener, acts like pentazocine.

Butterfly rash Skin rash on both cheeks joined by an extension across the bridge of nose (*see* Figure on page 119).

Butoxamine Beta$_2$ adrenergic antagonist.

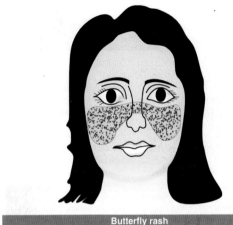

Butterfly rash

Butyric acid A fatty acid used in disinfectants, emulsifying agent.

Butyrophenone A class of chemicals of which haloperidol is a member, antipsychotic agents.

Byler's disease Inherited disease with cirrhosis and mental retardation in children.

Byssinosis Pneumonoconiosis of cotton and textile workers.

C

Cabergoline Dopamine receptor agonist used in hyperprolactinemia.

Cachet Used for administering medicines with a bitter taste.

Cachexia A state of ill health, malnutrition, wasting.

Cacogenesis Abnormal development or growth.

Cacogeusia Unpleasant taste in the mouth.

Cacosmia Unpleasant odor (olfactory hallucination).

Cadaver Dead body, corpse cardaverine-malodorous substance, cadaverous; resembling corpse.

Cadence Rythmic movements.

Cadwell luc operation Also known as maxillary antrostomy, this procedure involves opening the maxillary sinus by giving an incision in the buccal cavity over the canine teeth. This procedure helps in the drainage of this sinus.

Cafe-au-lait spots Spots of patchy pigmentation of skin, usually light brown in color-characteristic of neurofibromatosis.

Caffeine An alkaloid of tea, coffee. CNS stimulant, analgesic.

Caffey's disease This disease is also known as infantile cortical hyperostosis and is characterized by subperiosteal new bone formation over many bones. The bones most commonly involved include mandible, clavicle and shafts of long bones. There could be appearance of fever.

Caisson's disease A condition that develops in divers when air pressure is rapidly reduced while ascent to the surface. Symptoms are due to bubbling out of dissolved nitrogen.

Calabar A parasitic infection mainly seen in Africa, characterized by presence of lumps in the subcutaneous tissue, particularly anterior chamber of eyes.

Calamine A pink powder containing zinc oxide and little ferric oxide, used as protective, astringent.

Calcaneus The heel bone articulating with talus and cuboid.

Calciferiol Vit D$_2$, ergocalciferol.

Calcitonin Calcium lowering hormone, used in hypercalcemia, pagets disease secreted by D cells thyroid.

Calcitriol A sterol of vit D activity, very potent.

Calcium channel blockers A group of drugs that act by slowing the influx of calcium ions into muscle cells resulting in decreased arterial resistance and decreased myocardial O$_2$ demand.

Calcium dobesilate Endothelium stabilizer for haemorrhoid.

Calculus Any abnormal concretion in the body.

Calf Fleshy muscular back part of leg formed by gastrocnemius and soleus.

Caliper A two-pronged instrument that may be used to exert traction on a part. *Walking c.* An appliance fitted to a boot or shoe to give support to the lower limb. It may be used when the muscles are paralysed or in the repair stage of fractures.

Calisthenics An exercise programme to bring suppleness and gracefulness of body combined with music.

Callosity Localized hypertrophy/thickening of skin at friction/pressure points.

Callus See callosity.

Calmodulin Intracellular proteins that combine with calcium and activate a variety of cellular responses.

Caloric test A test for vestibulo-ocular reflex. In involves irrigating cold or warm water into the external auditory canal. In a patient with intact cerebrum, the irrigation of cool water causes the eyes to turn towards the ipsilateral ear with horizontal nystagmus in the contralateral ear. Warm water, on the other hand, causes the eyes to turn towards the contralateral ear with horizontal nystagmus in the ipsilateral ear. In patients with absent vestibulo-ocular reflex, the nystagmus component of the test would be absent with both hot and cold water.

Calvaria The dome like superior portion of cranium (*see* Figure on page 122).

Calorie A unit of heat. Used to denote physiological values of various food substances, estimated according to the amount of heat they produce on being oxidized in the body. *See* Oxidization. A Calorie (or kilocalorie) represents the heat

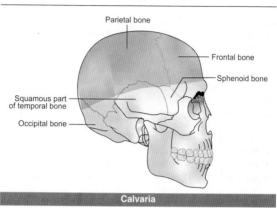

Calvaria

required in raising 1 kg (1000 g) of water by 1°C. A small calorie equals the heat produced in raising 1 g of water by 1°C. In the SI system the calorie is replaced by the joule (1 cal = 4.18 kJ).

Calvé-Perthes disease Aseptic necrosis of femoral head epiphysis.

Calyx Any cuplike organ or cavity.

Canal Channel, passage way. *c. femoral* The medial division of femoral sheath, containing some lymphatic vessel and a lymph node. *c. inguinal* 1½″ long oblique passage extending from internal inguinal ring to external inguinal ring transmitting spermatic cord, and ilioinguinal nerve in male and round ligament of uterus and ilioinguinal nerve in female.

Canaliculus Small channel or canal.

Cancer Malignant tumor which is invasive and metastasizes to new sites by lymph/blood (*see* Table on page 123).

Cancrum A rapidly spreading ulcer.

Candida A genus of yeast like fungi that develop a pseudomycelium and reproduce by budding (*see* Figure on page 123).

Candidiasis Infection of skin and mucus membrane by candida.

Cane sugar Sucrose.

Table: Early warning signs of cancer

- Any lump or thickening, especially in the breast, lip or tongue.
- Any irregular or unexplained bleeding. Blood in the urine or bowel movements. Blood or bloody discharge from the nipple or any body opening. Unexplained vaginal bleeding or discharge, or any bleeding, after the menopause.
- A sore that does not heat, particularly around the mouth, tongue or lips, or anywhere on the skin.
- Noticeable changes in the colour or size of a wart, mole or birthmark.
- Loss of appetite or continual indigestion.
- Persistent hoarseness, cough or difficulty in swallowing.
- Persistent change in normal elimination (bowel habits).

Special note: Pain is not usually an early warning sign of cancer.

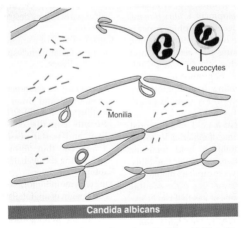

Candida albicans

Canker Ulceration of mouth and lips.

Cannabis Dried flowering tops of the cannabis sativa.

Cannibalism Eating of human flesh (kuru)

Cannon waves These refer to the large 'a' waves present

on jugular venous pulse. These waves usually result when the right atrium has to contract against an increased resistance, e.g. tricuspid atresia or stenosis or right atrial myxoma.

Canthoplasty Enlargement of palpebral fissure by division of external canthus.

Canthridin Keratolytic for removal of warts.

Cap Protective covering. *c. enamel* cap like structure of enamel organ developed during third month of fetal development. *c. phrygian* the cholecystographic appearance of gallbladder showing kinking between body and fundus. *c. ofzinn* a prominence of pulmonary arc representing dilated pulmonary artery in PA view in patent ductus arteriosus.

Capacity a. Volume or potential volume of material. b. power or ability to hold, retain or contain. *c. diffusion* the ability of alveolo capillary membrane to transfer gas. *c. forced vital* volume of gas that can be expelled with maximum effort. *c. functional residual* volume of gas in the lungs after quiet expiration. *c. iron binding* capacity of serum transferin to bind iron. *c. total lung* volume

of air in the lungs at the end of maximal inspiration. *c. vital* volume of gas that can be expelled after full inspiration (*see* Figure on page 125).

Capitulum Rounded articular end of a bone.

Caplan's syndrome Rheumatoid arthritis with progressive massive lung fibrosis in pneumoconiosis.

Capreomycin A second line tuberculostatic drug.

Capsid Protein covering around the central core of virus particle protecting the virus particle from destructive enzymes.

Capsofungin Potent antifungal.

Capsule Gelatin enclosure for drug delivery. *c. articular* A two layered covering for sinovial joints. The inner layer is sinovial and outer layer is fibrous. *c. Glisson* Outer fibrous capsule covering liver and portal vessels. *c. Tenon* The thin fibrous sac enveloping the eyeball.

Captopril Angiotensin converting enzyme inhibitor, blocking conversion of angiotensin I to angiotensin II. A vasodilator useful for hypertension and congestive failure.

Caput succedaneum Swelling on presenting part of foetal head during labour.

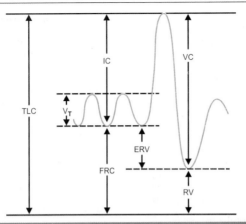

Subdivisions of total lung capacity: TLC, total lung capacity; VT, tidal volume; IC, inspiratory capacity; FRC, functional residual capacity; ERV, expiratory reserve volume; VC, vital capacity; RV, risidual volume

Table: Black's classification of dental caries

Class	Dental caries
Class I	Cavities occurring in pit and fissure defects in occlusal surfaces of bicuspids and molars, lingual surfaces of upper incisors, and facial and lingual grooves sometimes found on occlusal surfaces of molar teeth.
Class II	Cavities in proximal surfaces of bicuspid and molars.
Class III	Cavities in proximal surfaces of incisors and cuspids not requiring removal of incisal angle.
Class IV	Cavities in gingival third of labial, lingual, or buccal surfaces.
Class VI (Not a true Black classification)	Cavities in incisal edges and smooth surfaces of teeth above the height of contour.

Caramel Flavoring and colouring agent made by heating sugar or glucose, destroying the sweet taste in the process.

Carbachol Cholinergic drug for producing miosis, also used for emptying bladder.

Carbamate Ester of carbonic acid–the insecticides and parasiticides that act by inhibiting choline esterase. e.g. Aldicarb, Aminocarb, Carbaril, Carbofuran, Dimetilan, Methomyl, Propoxur.

Caries The decay or death of bone which becomes soft discoloured and porous.

Carbamazepine Antiepilepsy drug used for temporal lobe epilepsy and trigeminal neuralgia.

Carbasone Contains 28% arsenic, antiamoebic agent.

Carbenicillin Broad spectrum antibiotic, penicillin derivative.

Carbenoxolone Oleandane derivative used in peptic ulcer.

Carbidopa Dopa decarboxylase inhibitor, used in combination with levodopa for parkinsonism.

Carbimazole Antithyroid drug.

Carbocistine Beta lactamase inhibitor.

Carbohydrate Chemical substances containing carbon, oxygen and hydrogen e.g., sugar, glycogen, starches, dextrin and celluloses. Sucrose is glucose + fructose; maltose is 2 D glucose; lactose is glucose + galactose.

Carbon ^{14}C is radioactive isotope of carbon with halflife of 5600 years. Used in archeology dating and as tracer element in metabolic studies.

Carbon dioxide Final metabolic product of carbon compounds present in food. CO_2 combining power is a test of buffer capacity of blood. Solid CO_2 (–80ºC) used for removal of naevi, telangiectasis, warts, haemorrhoids, etc.

Carbon monoxide Present in automobile exhaust fumes, displaces O_2 from haemoglobin, hence diminishing O_2 transport.

Carbon tetrachloride A colourless toxic anesthetic liquid, previously used for ankylostomiasis but toxic to liver and kidney.

Carboplatin Antineoplastic agent.

Carboxyhemoglobin Compound formed by CO and Hb.

Carboxylase An enzyme that catalyzes the removal of carboxyl group (COOH) from amino acids in the presence of Vit. B_1 acting as an coenzyme.

Carboxylation Replacement of hydrogen by a carboxyl (COOH) molecule.

Carboxylic acid Organic acid with COOH group.

Carbuncle Spreading inflammation of deeper skin.

Carbutamide An oral hypoglycemic agent.

Carcinoembryonic antigen A class of antigen in fetus and expressed by colonic tumors. CEA level returns to normal after complete removal of colonic tumor.

Carcinogen Carcinoma inducing chemicals e.g., benzpyrines.

Carcinoid Tumor of Argentaffin cells in the GI tract, bronchi, ovary, secreting serotonin.

Carcinoid syndrome Syndrome due to metastatic carcinoid tumors secreting serotonin, bradykinin, histamine and prostaglandin. Symptoms are diarrhoea, flushing, hypotension and heart valve lesions.

Carcinoma Malignant growth of epithelial tissue; *basal cell c.* is from basal layer of skin, rarely metastasizes (rodent ulcer). *epidermoid c.* tumor on the surface either wartlike or infiltrating. *Medullary c.* Carcinoma that is soft because of predominance of cells and paucity of fibrosis. *Squamous cell c.* Cancer from squamous epithelium with rolled out everted edges. *Scirrhous c.* A form of cylindrical carcinoma with a firm, hard structure. *Cylindrical c.* Carcinoma of glands usually entodermal origin.

Carcinophilia Having affinity for cancer cells.

Cardarelli's sign Pulsating movement of trachea with aortic aneurysm.

Cardiac arrest Abrupt cessation of heart beat (temporary or permanent), that results in the loss of effective circulation. It is usually caused by ventricular fibrillation.

Cardiac cirrhosis Cirrhosis of liver secondary to a cardiac cause. Commonly constructive pericarditis.

Cardiac cycle The period from beginning of one heart beat to beginning of next beat. It comprises atrial systole 0.1 second, ventricular systole 0.3 second and ventricular relaxation of 0.5 seconds.

Cardiac failure Condition resulting from inability of heart to pump sufficient blood to meet the body needs.

Cardiac output Blood ejected from left/right ventricle per minute, usually 3 lit/m^2.

Cardiac plexus Branches of vagus and sympathetic trunk encircling base of heart.

Cardiac position A position of comfort for the patients of asthma and cardiac diseases, who are unable to breathe easily in lying-down position. The patient is propped up in sitting position with the means of back rest and pillows and an overbed table is placed in front with a pillow on it, so that the patient can lean forwards and take rest.

Cardiac reflex Slowing of heart rate from stimulation of sensory nerve endings in the walls of carotid sinus from a rise in arterial blood pressure. (Marey's law).

Cardiac reserve The capacity of heart to increase cardiac output and raise blood pressure to meet body requirements.

Cardiectasis Dilatation of heart.

Cardiff count-to-ten chart Method of evaluating the intrauterine wellbeing of the fetus in which the pregnant woman records fetal movements during her normal activities. If the count is less than 10, further medical evaluation is recommended.

Cardinal Important or of primary importance.

Cardiocele Herniation of heart through an opening in diaphragm or chest wall.

Cardiocentesis Puncture of heart.

Cardiodynia Pain in the region of heart.

Cardioesophageal reflux Reflux of gastric contents into esophagus.

Cardiogenesis Formation and growth of embryonic heart.

Cardiogenic In relation to heart itself.

Cardiogram Recording of electrical activity of heart.

Cardiograph Machine that picks up electrical activity of heart.

Cardiolipin An extract of beef heart used for test of syphilis.

Cardiomegaly Enlargement of heart.

Cardiomyopathy Primary disease of heart muscle.

Cardiomyopexy Stitching of pectoral muscle to cardiac muscle inorder to augment vascular supply to heart muscle.

Cardiomyoplasty Reinforcement of cardiac muscle contractility by transfer of lattismus dorsi to surround the heart and to contract synchronously with cardiac muscle.

Cardiomyotomy Surgical therapy of achalasia in which the muscle surrounding cardio esophageal junction is cut but the mucus membrane is left intact.

Cardioplegia Deliberate arrest of cardiac function by use of hypothermia, potassium, etc.

Cardiopulmonary resuscitation Emergency medical care to a person whose heart and lung function is going to stop or has recently stopped. Artificial respiration and cardiac massage are the two principal components of CPR (*see* Figure).

Cardiorrhexis Rupture of heart.

Cardioverter Defibrillator that delivers electric shockwaves for treating cardiac arrhythmia/ventricular standstill.

Caries The decay or death of bone which becomes soft discoloured and porous.

Cariogenic Conducive to dental caries formation.

Carisoprodol A muscle relaxant, acting through CNS.

Carminative Agent that helps to get rid of gas in intestine.

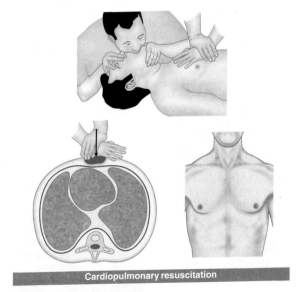

Cardiopulmonary resuscitation

Carmustine Antineoplastic agent.

Carnal Related to desires or appetite of flesh.

Carnett's sign Method of determining the source of pain while evaluating a surgical abdomen, when the patient raises his head after being in supine position. It is positive, if the pain increases or remains the same and indicates that the source of origin lies in the abdominal wall and not the viscera.

Carnitine A chemical important in metabolism of palmitic and stearic acid. Used therapeutically in treatment of myopathy due to carnitine deficiency.

Carnivorous Flesh eating.

Carotene Yellow cristalline pigments of plant and animal tissue, converted to Vit A in liver.

Carotenemia A benign condition with high blood caroten level causing yellow colouration of skin but not of conjuctiva.

Carotid body A pressure and hypoxia sensitive flat structure present at carotid bifurcation.

Carotid sinus A dilated area at the bifurcation of common carotid, richly supplied with sensory nerve endings, responding to changes in concentration of O_2 and blood pressure.

Carotid siphon The S shaped terminal portion of internal carotid artery.

Carotidynia Pain elicited by pressures on common carotid artery.

Carotinase Enzyme that converts carotine into Vit A.

Carpal tunnel The canal beneath flexor retinaculum of wrist in which flexor tendons and median nerve pass.

Carpal tunnel syndrome Pain, tenderness and weakness of muscles of thumb caused by pressure on median nerve in carpal tunnel.

Carphology Involuntary picking at bed clothes, muttering etc. the signs of impending end.

Carpopedal spasm Spasms of hand and feet seen in tetany and hyperventilation (see Figure).

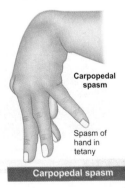

Carpopedal spasm

Spasm of hand in tetany

Carpopedal spasm

Carpus Wrist (*see* Figure).

Carrier A person who harbors a pathogenic organism without any sign or symptom of disease but is capable of spreading the organism to others.

Cartilage A type of dense connective tissue capable of withstanding high pressure and tension. Cartilage is avascular and is without nerve supply. *c. hyaline* Bluish - white glassy translucent cartilage, e.g., semilunar cartilage of knee, thyroid cartilage.

Caruncle Small fleshy growth.

Carvedilol Betablocker.

Cascara A laxative prescribed from the bark of the Californian buckthorn. It may be prepared as an elixir or tablets.

Casein The principal protein in milk derived from casinogen.

Casoni's test Appearance of wheal surrounded by erythematous zone following intradermal injection of sterile hydatid fluid. The test is false positive in 40% cases in diagnosis of *Echinococcus granulosus.*

Cast 1. A solid mold of a part, usually applied for immobilization of fracture, dislocation and severe injuries. 2. In dentistry a positive copy of tissues of jaw over which denture base is to be made. 3. Pliable or fibrous matter which

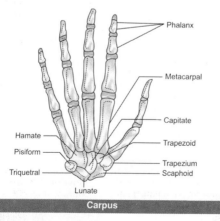

Phalanx

Metacarpal

Capitate

Trapezoid

Trapezium

Scaphoid

Hamate

Pisiform

Triquetral

Lunate

Carpus

mould to the shape of the part in which they accumulate. According to source they can be classified as bronchial, intestinal, nasal, esophageal, renal, vaginal etc. According to constituents casts can be bloody, fatty, hyaline, granular, waxy etc.

Castellani's paint Composed of phenol, resorcinol, used as a disinfectant for skin and as an antifungal.

Castle factor Also known as Castle's intrinsic factor, it is a small mucoprotein secreted by the gastric parietal cells. This factor is required to facilitate adequate absorption of vitamin B_{12} by the stomach. Deficiency of this factor can result in pernicious anaemia.

Castor oil Obtained from the plant *Ricinus communis*, hydrolyzed in intestine to ricinoleic acid that acts as laxative.

Castrate To remove or inactivate ovaries or testes.

Casuality Accident/injury/death.

Catabolism Breakdown of complex substances into simpler substances with consumption of energy; opposite of anabolism.

Catagen Intermediate phase of hair growth lying between anagen (growing) and telogen (Resting phase).

Catalase An enzyme that helps in breakdown of hydrogen peroxide into water and oxygen.

Catalepsy A trance like state with diminished responsiveness but often intact perception.

Catalysis Enhancement of a chemical reaction by a catalyst.

Catalyst A substance that speeds up chemical reaction without itself being permanently altered, e.g., HCl catalyzes hydrolysis of sucrose.

Catamenia Menstruation.

Cataphasia Involuntary repitition of same word.

Cataphoria Tendency of visual axes to incline below the horizontal plane.

Cataphylaxis The process of carrying antibodies and leukocytes to the site of an infection.

Cataplexy The brief sudden loss of muscle control brought on by strong emotion i.e., excitement, anger.

Catapres Clonidine, an antihypertensive agent.

Cataract Opacity of lens nucleus, capsule or both. *Immature stage.* Lens swollen, anterior chamber shallow *Mature stage.* Lens shrinks, no iris shadow on transillumination, cataract can be polar, lamellar, nuclear, cortical, congenital, traumatic, diabetic but senility is the single most common cause.

Catarrh Inflammation of mucous membranes esp. of head and throat.

Catatonia A phase of schizophrenia in which patient is unresponsive and tends to assume fixed posture.

Catecholamine Biologically active amines like epinephrine and nor epinephrine derived from amino acid tyrosine.

Catgut Suture made-up of sheep's intestine. Chromium trioxide treatment enhances strength of the suture.

Catharsis Purgation.

Cathartic Agent causing purgation.

Catheter A hollow tube for evacuation and injection of fluids. Arterial and venous catheters for recording of pressure, pacing catheter for atrial/ventricular pacing; self-retaining bladder catheter; Tenckoff peritoneal catheter for peritoneal dialysis.

Cathexis The emotional or mental energy used in concentrating on an object or idea.

Cathode Negative electrode, opposite of anode.

Cation An ion with positive charge that travels onto cathode.

CAT scan Computerized axial tomography : computerized X-ray picture of any body part.

Cat scratch fever Febrile disease with lymphadenopathy transmitted by cats.

Cauda Tail or tail like structure. Terminal portion of spinal cord—cauda equina. Inferior portion of epididymis—cauda epididymidis (*see* Figure).

Caudate Possessing a tail.

Causalgia Intense burning pain accompanied by trophic skin changes, due to injury to sympathetic innervation.

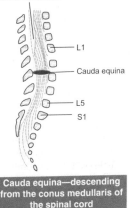

Conus medullaris

L1

Cauda equina

L5

S1

Cauda equina—descending from the conus medullaris of the spinal cord

Caustic An agent particularly an alkali that destroys living tissue.

Cauterization Destruction of tissue by caustic, electric current, freezing etc.

Cautery The means of destroying tissue.

Cavalry bone Sesamoid bone in adductor longus of thigh in riders.

Cavernitis Inflammation of corpus cavernousum of penis.

Cavernoma Cavernous haemangioma.

Cavernous Containing a hollow space.

Cavitis Inflammation of venacava.

Cavity A hollow space in a viscus or tooth.

Cavity preparation Artificial cavity prepared in teeth for tooth restoration e.g., root canal treatment.

Cecectomy Surgical removal of cecum.

Cecopexy Surgical fixation of cecum to abdominal wall.

Cecum The first portion of large intestine, 6 cm in length, 7.5 cm in width, with appendix arising at its lower end.

Cefadroxyl Longacting oral cephalosporin.

Cefadinir Oral cephalosporin.

Cefotaxime A third generation cephalosporin antibiotic having a broad spectrum of activity, used to treat intra-abdominal infections, bone and joint infections, gonorrhoea, and other infections due to susceptible organisms, including penicillinase-producing strains.

Cefoxitin A semisynthetic cephalosporing antibiotic, especially effective against Gram-negative organisms,

Table: Major groups of cephalosporin

First generation	Second generation	Third generation	Fourth generation
Cephalothin	Cefamandole	Cefotaxime	Cefepime
Cephapirin	Cefuroxime	Ceftizoxime	
Cefazolin	Cefonicid	Ceftriaxone	
	Ceforanide	Ceftazidime	
Cephalexin	Cefaclor	Cefoperazone	
Cephadrine	Cefoxitin	Moxolactam	
Cephadroxyl	Cefotetan	Cefixime	
	Cefuroxime	Ceftibutane	

with strong resistance to degradation by β-lactamase.

Cefpodoxime Oral third generation cephalosporin.

Celiac disease Intestinal malabsorption syndrome mostly gluten induced.

Celiac plexus Sympathetic plexus near origin of celiac artery.

Celiocentesis Abdominal puncture.

Cell The basic structural unit of all plants and animals containing protoplasm and nucleus. *c. Alzheimer's* giant astrocytes with large prominent nuclei found in hepatic coma and hepatolenticular degeneration. *c. antigen presenting* group of dendritic cells that process antigen and present them to lymphocytes. *c. APUD* amine precursor uptake and decarboxylation cells, that include melanocytes, chromaffin cells, and cells in thyroid, parathyroid, hypothalamus, adrenals secreting epinephrine, serotonin somatostatin, dopamine etc. *c. argentaffin* Epithelium of digestive tract containing granules that stain with silver. *c. basket* found in cerebellar cortex whose axon gives off brushes of fibrils. 1. Branching basal cell of salivary gland 2. Certain cells of cerebellar cortex.

c. beta Insulin secreting cells of pancreas (islets of Langerhans). *c. Betz* Large pyramidal cells of motor cortex. *c. chief* Parathormone secreting cells, pepsin secreting gastric cells, chromophobe cells of pituitary. *c. columnar* Cells with height breadth. *c. cuboid* Cell with height equal to width and depth. *c. Downey's* atypical lymphocytes of three types invariably present in infectious mononucleosis. *c. endothelial* Flat cells outlining blood vessels, peritoneum and pleura-pericardium. *c. Fanana's* type of neuroglical cell found in cerebellar cortex. *c. gitter* polymorphonuclear leukocytes with granules showing brownian movement; their presence in urine may indicate pyelonephritis. *c. Hela* Cells cultured from patients of carcinoma of cervix. *c. Kupffer* Fixed phagocytic cells in sinusoids of liver. *c. Langerhan's* stellate dendritic cells found in epidermis and are antigen presenting cells. *c. Leydig* Interstitial cells of testes. *c. littoral* Macrophages in sinuses of lymphatic tissue. *c. mast* Cells containing heparin and histamine. *c. Merkel* specialized cell at epithelial dermal junction acting as

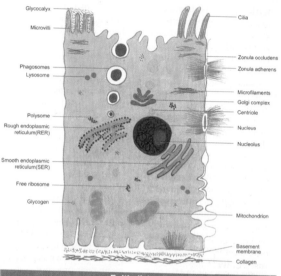

Glycocalyx	Cilia
Microvilli	Zonula occludens
	Zonula adherens
Phagosomes	
Lysosome	Microfilaments
	Golgi complex
Polysome	Centriole
Rough endoplasmic reticulum(RER)	Nucleus
	Nucleolus
Smooth endoplasmic reticulum(SER)	
Free ribosome	
Glycogen	
	Mitochondrion
	Basement membrane
	Collagen

Epithelial cell

touch receptors. *c. Mikulicz's* cells in rhinoscleroma that contain the bacillus. *c. Mott* abnormal plasma cells containing Mott/Russel bodies in multiple myeloma. *c. natural killer* A line of B lymphocytes that kill the virus infected and tumor cells. *c. neuroglia* Supporting cells in CNS and retina. *c. Niemann-Pick* A foamy lipid filled cell present in spleen and bone marrow in Nieman and Pick's disease. *c. Owl's eye*

degenerated renal epithelial cell. *c. Paneth's* epithelial cells seen in crypts of Lilberkuhn. *c. parafollicular* lie along thyroid follicles and secrete calcitonin. *c. plasma* antibody secreting cells of B lymphocyte lineage. *c. Purkinje* Cells of cerebral cortex whose axon extend to brainstem nuclei, cerebellum or anterior horn cells of spinal cord.
c. Roji cells from cultured lymphoblast cell line of Burkitt's

lymphoma, used for detection of immune complexes. *c. Reed Sternberg* giant histiocyte, multinucleated seen in Hodgkin's lymphoma. *c. Schwann* large nucleated cell whose cell membrane wraps around myelinated neurone thus augmenting conduction. *c. Sertoli's* supporting cells in seminiferous tubules. *c. Sezary* abnormal mononuclear cell in cutaneous T-cell lymphoma. *c. stem* a precursor or progenitor cell. *c. target* thin RBC with dark center and a peripheral ring of haemoglobin seen in thalassemia, liver disease. *c. Vero* a cell line derived from African green monkey kidney cells used in isolation of viruses. *C. Warthin Finkeldey's* multinucleated giant cells in intranuclear inclusions seen in measles (*see* Figure on page 136).

Cell kinetics The study of growth and division of cells.

Cell membrane The envelop surrounding cell, composed of carbohydrate, lipid and protein.

Cell organelle Structures in the cytoplasm like mitochondria, golgi complex, endoplasmic reticulum, ribosomes etc.

Cellophane Thin transparent water proof sheet of cellulose acetate, used as dialysis membrane.

Cellular immunity T-cell mediated immune reaction, basis of organ transplant rejection, lepromin test and BCG vaccination.

Cellulitis Inflammation of cellular or connective tissue.

Celsius scale Temperature scale where boiling point of water is $100°$ and melting point is of ice is $0°$.

Cement Material that makes one substance bind to another.

Cementitis Inflammation of dental cementum.

Cementoblast Cells lining the developing tooth depositing cementum.

Cementoclast Multinucleated large cells that remove cementum (i.e., odontoclasts).

Cementoma A benign fibrous connective tissue growth usually at root of tooth containing small masses of cementum.

Cementum Thin layer of calcified tissue formed by cementoblast covering the root of tooth (*see* Figure on page 138).

Center A group of nerve cells in CNS subserving special function. *c. apneustic* Center in brainstem regulating breathing. *c. auditory* Center for hearing in the anterior part of transverse temporal

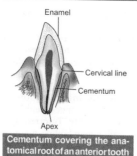

Enamel

Cervical line

Cementum

Apex

Cementum covering the anatomical root of an anterior tooth

gyri. *c. autonomic* Center controlling autonomic functions located in hypothalamus, brainstem and spinal cord. *c. cardioaccelerator and c. cardioinhibitory* Both present in medulla oblongata, innervating the heart through sympathetic and parasympathetic fibers. *c. Broca's* Center in inferior frontal gyrus (area) controlling speech. *c. ciliospinal* Center in spinal cord giving rise to sympathetic fibers dilating the pupil. *c. defecation* Two centers located in medulla oblongata and in S_2-S_4 segments of spinal cord. *c. deglutition* Center in medulla oblongata on the floor of fourth ventricle that controls swallowing. *c. heat regulating* A heat loss and a heat production center located in medulla. *c. micturition* Located in S_2-S_4, medulla

and hypothalamus controlling micturition. *c. pneumotaxic* Center in pons that rhythmically inhibits inspiration. *c. respiratory* The inspiratory, expiratory and pneumotaxic centers in medulla oblongata controlling the respiratory movements. *c. satiety* An area in ventromedial thalamus that modulates eating behavior.

Centigram Hundredth of gram, 10 mg.

Centiliter Hundredth of liter, 10 ml.

Centimeter Hundredth of meter, 10 mm.

Centepede Arthropod with long flat segmented body each with a pair of legs.

Central core disease A form of benign familial polymyopathy characterized by hypotonia, and nonprogressive muscle weakness.

Central line A venous access device to give fluids and to monitor venous pressure in vena cava and atrial chamber.

Central venous pressure Pressure in superior vena cava and right trium, normally 5-10 cm of H_2O.

Centrifugal Force directed outwards from center of rotation.

Centrifuge A machine that spins test tubes at high speed, causing heavy particles to settle down to the bottom.

RBCs settle down at bottom, and WBCs form a thin layer between RBC and plasma.

Centrilobular Concerning the center of a lobule.

Centriole A minute organelle consisting of a hollowed cylinder closed at one end and open at the other. During mitosis the centrioles migrate to opposite poles of the cell to which spindle fibers are attached.

Centripetal Directed towards the axis, i.e., center.

Centromere The constricted central portion of chromosome that divides chromosome into two.

Cephalexin Analog of antibiotic cephalosporin.

Cephalgia Headache, pain in the body.

Cephalhematoma Subcutaneous swelling containing blood found on the head of a newborn baby disappearing within 2-3 months.

Cephalic index Maximal length of head divided by maximal breadth × 100.

Cephalometry Measurement of the head using various bony points used to assess growth and in determining orthodontic or prosthetic treatment.

Cephaloridine An analogue of the antibiotic cephalosporin.

Cephalotomy Perforating the foetal head to facilitate delivery.

Cercaria A free swimming stage in the development of fluke or trematode.

Cerclage Encircling of a part with a ring or loop as in incompetent cervix.

Cerebellum Largest portion of rhombencephalon lying dorsal to pons and medulla oblongata; involved in coordination of fine movements, maintenance of posture, equilibrium, muscle tone, etc.

Cerebromalacia Softening of cerebrum.

Cerebroside A lipid constituent of nerve tissue.

Cerebrospinal fever Inflammation of brain and meninges.

Cerebrospinal fluid The cushioning fluid formed in the choroid plexuses of the lateral and third ventricle. Normal amount 100-140 ml, specific gravity 1003-1008 (*see* Figure on page 140).

Cerebrovascular accident (CVA) Ischemic or haemorrhagic cerebral events due to embolism, thrombosis, vasculitis, aneurysm, A.V. malformation, etc.

Cerebrum Consists of two hemispheres united by two commissures; corpus callosum, anterior and posterior hippocampal commissures (*see* Figure on page 140).

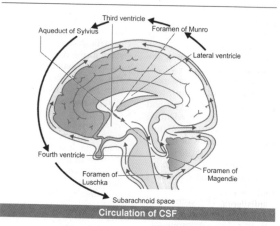

Third ventricle
Aqueduct of Sylvius
Foramen of Munro
Lateral ventricle
Fourth ventricle
Foramen of Luschka
Foramen of Magendie
Subarachnoid space

Circulation of CSF

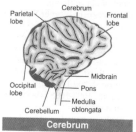

Parietal lobe
Cerebrum
Frontal lobe
Occipital lobe
Midbrain
Pons
Cerebellum
Medulla oblongata

Cerebrum

Ceruloplasmin Copper transporting glycoprotein in blood.

Cerumen The wax like, soft brown secretion in external auditory canal.

Ceruminosis Excessive secretion of cerumen.

Cervical plexus The plexus formed by joining of anterior rami of first 4 cervical nerves, communicating with sympathetic ganglia.

Cervical spondylosis Osteoarthritis of cervical vertebra with osteophytic growths often causing nerve root compression.

Cervical vertebra First seven bones of spinal column.

Cervicitis Inflammation of uterine cervix.

Cervicodynia Pain in the neck, cervical neuralgia.

Cervix The neck or part of an organ resembling neck. *c. uteri* The lower tubular part of uterus, 1" long protruding into vaginal valt.

Cesarean section Delivery of foetus by giving incision on uterus, either extraperitoneal or intraperitoneal. Commonly done in cephalopelvic disproportion, breech presentation and foetal distress.

Cesium ^{137}Cs an radioactive isotope of metal cesium is used for radiation of cancer tissue.

Cestoda A subclass that includes tapeworms that have a scolex and a chain of segments (proglottids).

Cetirizine H_1 receptor blocker antiallergic.

Chaddock's reflex 1. Extension of great toe when outer edge of dorsum of foot is stroked. 2. Flexion of wrist and fanning of fingers when tendon of palmaris longus is pressed; positive in corticospinal tract lesions.

Chadwick's sign Also known as Jacquemier's sign, this is a sign of pregnancy. This sign is associated with bluish discolouration of cervix, vagina and vulva due to venous congestion.

Chafing Erythema, maceration and fissuring of skin due to friction of clothing in axilla, groin, between digits.

Chaga's disease African trypanosomiasis.

Chalasia Relaxation of sphincters.

Chalazion Distention of a meibomian gland of eyelid with hard secretions, resembling tumor.

Chalicosis Pneumonoconiosis associated with inhalation of dust produced during stone cutting.

Challenge In immunology, administration of specific antigen to an individual known to be sensitive to that antigen in order to produce an immune response.

Chamber Closed space or compartment. *c. anterior, posterior* Anterior and posterior chambers of eye containing aqueous humor, lying between cornea and iris, iris and lens respectively. *c. Boyden* Chamber used to measure chemotaxis. *c. hyperbaric* Closed chamber with high internal air pressure, e.g., hyperbaric oxygen chambers for treatment of frost bite, gangrene decompression sickness. *c. pulp* The chamber within crown of tooth containing nerve endings and blood vessels (*see* Figure on page 142).

Chancre Hard painless syphilitic primary ulcer on exposed part with slough leather base.

Chancroid Non-syphilitic venereal ulcer due to *Haemophilus ducreyi*.

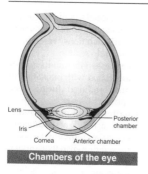

Chambers of the eye

Charcoal Activated charcoal used for adsorption of gas and poisonous alkaloids in GI tract.

Charcot's joint Denervated degenerating joint in syringomyelia, tabes dorsalis or spinal cord injury with hypermobility.

Charcot-Leyden crystal Colourless, hexagonal, double pointed and often needle like crystals found in sputum of asthmatic patients and in faeces of patients of intestinal amoebiasis.

Charcot-Marie-Tooth disease A form of hereditary progressive neuro-muscular atrophy usually developing in childhood, commonly males. (SYN-peroneal muscular atrophy).

Charcot's triad Combination of nystagmus, intention tremor, and scanning speech; frequently associated with multiple sclerosis.

Charle's law At constant pressure, a given amount of gas will expand in direct proportion to absolute temperature.

Charting The process of making a tabulated record of the progress of patient during hospital stay in relation to temperature, blood pressure, intake, etc.

Chédiak-Higashi syndrome AR disease in which neutrophils contain peroxidase positive inclusion bodies. Partial albinism, photophobia and pale optic fundi are the clinical features. Children usually die between 5 - 10 years of age due to lymphoma like disease.

Cheilitis Inflammation of lips.

Cheilosis Red lips, with fissured angles of mouth commonly due to riboflavin deficiency.

Chelation The process of chelating; meaning to hold ionic metallic compounds preventing their absorption or action at target sites, e.g. calcium disodium edetate.

Chemabrasion Use of chemicals to destroy superficial layers of skin to treat scars, tatoos, abnormal pigmentation.

Chemical warfare Warfare with toxic-chemical/biological agents. The chemicals used are nerve gases/disease producing organisms.

Chemiluminescence Light produced by chemical reactions without production of heat, e.g. light production during bacterial killing by neutrophils, fire flies.

Chemodectoma Tumor of chemoreceptor system, e.g. para ganglioma.

Chemoprophylaxis Use of drugs to prevent occurrence of disease.

Chemoreceptor A sense organ or sensory nerve ending that is stimulated by and reacts to certain chemical stimuli; usually located outside CNS, e.g., carotid and aortic bodies, taste buds olfactory cells of nose.

Chemosis Edema of conjunctiva.

Chemotaxis Movement of cells in response to a chemical stimulus or message, e.g. movement of neutrophils to site of injury.

Chemotherapeutic index The ratio of the toxicity of the drug, expressed as maximum tolerated dose/kg body weight to the minimal curative dose/kg of body weight.

Chemotropism Ability of impulse to progress or turn in certain direction in response to certain stimuli.

Chenodeoxycholic acid Used for dissolution of gallstones.

Cherry red spots Red spot in retina of Taysach's disease.

Chest The body part accommodating heart and lungs. *c. emphysematous* Short and round thorax with AP diameter equal to transverse diameter, horizontal ribs (barrel chest). *c. flail* Paradoxical chest movement due to multiple rib fracture. *c. flat* Chest deformity with short AP diameter, long thorax, oblique ribs and prominent scapula. *c. pigeon* Prominent sternum with prominent sternal ends of the ribs.

Chest thump A sharp blow to chest in precordial area in order to revert a VT or restore normal rhythm in cardiac arrest.

Cheyne-Stokes respiration Breathing pattern in which period of apnea is followed by gradually increasing depth and frequency of respiration. Common in diencephalic and frontal lobe dysfunction.

Chiari-Frommel syndrome Persistent amenorrhoea and

lactation following child birth due to hyperprolactinemia.

Chiasm A crossing or decussation. *c. optic* An incomplete crossing of the optic fiber (*see* Figure).

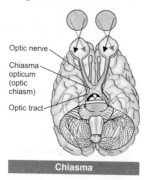

Optic nerve

Chiasma opticum (optic chiasm)

Optic tract

Chiasma

Chikungunya An arboviral infection with fever, joint pain and rash.

Chilblain A form of cold injury characterized by local erythema, itching and often blistering.

Child abuse Emotional, physical and sexual injury to a child.

Chill Shivering with sensation of coldness and pallor of skin.

Chimpanzee An intelligent ape native to parts of Africa.

Chinese Restaurant Syndrome Headache, perspiration and chest pain after eating monosodium glutamate.

Chiropodist Podiatrist

Chiropractic A system of health care which emphasizes on good relationship between organs for proper functioning.

Chi-square (χ^2) A statistical test to determine the similarity of the number of occurrences being investigated to the expected occurrences.

Chlamydia A genus of microorganisms causing ornithosis, lymphogranuloma venereum, trachoma and genital infection.

Chloasma Skin pigmentation (localized) following trauma, idiopathic or pregnancy.

Chloral hydrate Colourless, caustic, hypnotic agent.

Chlorambucil Cytotoxic agent used to treat C.L.L., Hodgkin's disease, etc.

Chloramphenicol Antibiotic isolated from *Streptomyces venezuelae*, specific for treatment of enteric fever.

Chlorbutanol Antiseptic and local anaesthetic used in dentistry and as a preservative.

Chlordane An insecticide.

Chlordantion Topical antifungal agent.

Chlordiazepoxide A benzodiazepine, used to treat anxiety, alcohol withdrawal syndrome, etc.

Chloremia Increased chloride concentration in blood.

Chlorhexidine Topical anti-infective agent.

Chlorinated lime Calcium hypochlorite and calcium chloride, used as bleaching agents and antiseptic.

Chlorite A salt of chlorous acid, used as disinfectant and bleaching agent.

Chlormezanone Antianxiety sedative agent.

Chloroguanide Antimalarial agent.

Chloroma Sarcoma of periosteum of cranial bones (green cancer).

Chlorophane Green-yellow pigment in retina.

Chlorophenothane An insecticide known as DDT.

Chlorophyll The green pigment in plants.

Chlorphene A phenol, disinfectant.

Chlorpheniramine An antihistamine agent.

Chlorphenoxamine Drug for parkinsonism.

Chlorpromazine Tranquiliser used in psychosis.

Chlorpropamide Oral hypoglycemic agent of sulfonyl urea group.

Chlorprothixene Anti-depressant.

Chlortetracycline Bacteriostatic antibiotic of tetracycline group.

Chlorthalidone Diuretic.

Chlorthiazide A diuretic.

Chlorzoxazone Muscle relaxant.

Choana Funnel shaped opening esp. on the posterior nares.

Choking Obstruction within respiratory passage or constriction in the neck obstructing breathing and circulation to brain.

Cholagogues An agent which promotes increased bile flow.

Cholangiectasis Dilatation of bile ducts.

Cholangiography Radiography of biliary system.

Cholangioma Tumor of bile ducts.

Cholangitis Inflammation of the bile ducts.

Cholecystectomy Excision of gall bladder.

Cholecystitis Inflammation of gall bladder manifesting with fever, chills, upper abdominal pain and mild jaundice; nearly always caused by gall stones.

Cholecystokinin Hormone secreted by duodenum that stimulates gall bladder contraction and pancreatic secretion.

Cholelithiasis Stone formation within gall bladder.

Cholemia Hyperbilirubinemia.

Cholera Profuse watery diarrhoea and vomiting with

dehydration caused by vibrio cholerae.

Choleriform Resembling cholera.

Cholesteatoma An epithelial pocket filled with keratin debris.

Cholesterol A monohydric alcohol, principal constituent of gall stones and constituent of cell membrane, percursor of hormones.

Cholesterosis Cholesterol deposition in tissues.

Cholestyramine An ion exchange resin to treat itching of hyperbilirubinemia.

Cholic acid A bile acid.

Choline An amine, constituent of lecithin and other phospholipids; involved in protein metabolism.

Cholinergic Nerve endings that liberate acetyl choline.

Cholinergic fibers They include all preganglionic fibers, all post-ganglionic parasympathetic fibers, postganglionic sympathetic fibers to sweat glands and, efferent fibers to skeletal muscle.

Cholinesterase Enzyme that catalyzes the hydrolysis of choline esters, i.e. acetyl cholinesterase breaks down acetylcholine into acetic acid and choline.

Choluria Presence of bile salts and/or pigments in the urine and is usually indicative of jaundice.

Chondrin Gelatin like material obtained by boiling of cartilage (the basic substance of cartilage).

Chondritis Inflammation of cartilage.

Chondrodysplasia Multiple exostoses of epiphysis esp. of long bones, metacarpals, and phalanges.

Chondrogen Basal substance of cartilage and corneal tissue, which changes to chondrin on boiling.

Chondroitin Substance present in connective tissue, including cornea and cartilage.

Chondroma A painless, slow growing tumor of cartilage.

Chondromalacia Softening of articular cartilage, usually involving patella.

Chondrosarcoma Cartilaginous sarcoma.

Chorda A cord or tendon. *c. tympani* Branch of facial nerve whose efferent fibers innervate submandibular and sublingual glands and afferent fibers convey taste sensation from anterior two thirds of tongue.

Chordae tendinea Tendinous cords connecting free edges

of A-V valves to papillary muscles.

Chordee A condition associated with downwards (ventral) or upwards (dorsal) curvature of the head of penis. The condition is most commonly associated with hypospadias. Chordee develops due to the presence of fibrous tissue between the glans and urethral opening.

Chorditis Inflammation of vocal/spermatic cord.

Chordoma A tumor along vertebral column composed of embryonic nerve tissue.

Chorea A movement disorder due to extrapyramidal damage characterized by quasipurposive, involuntary, non repititive limb movements, e.g., Sydenham's (rheumatic) chorea, chorea gravidarum, Huntington's chorea.

Choreoathetosis Jerky bizarre involuntary muscle contraction, usually more proximal than distal.

Chorioadenoma Adenoma of chorion, the outer membrane enclosing the foetus.

Chorioamnionitis Inflammation of membranes covering foetus, i.e., amnion & chorion.

Choriocarcinoma Malignant neoplasm of chorion usually following hydatid mole,

abortion or often normal pregnancy.

Choriomeningitis Inflammation of meninges. *c. lymphocytic* is of viral origin.

Chorion An extraembryonic membrane that covers outer-wall of blastocyst from which develop chorionic villi.

Chorionic villus sampling The procedure of obtaining samples of chorionic villi for prenatal evaluation of foetus.

Chorioretinitis Inflammation of choroid and retina.

Choroid Dark brown vascular layer of eye in between sclera and retina (*see* Figure).

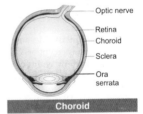

Choroid

Choroideremia X-linked choroid degeneration manifesting as nightblindness progressing to absolute blindness.

Choroiditis Inflammation of the choroid.

Christian-Weber disease Nodular, nonsuppurating panniculitis with fever.

Christmas factor A thromboplastin activator present in plasma.

Chromaffin cells Pigment cells of adrenal medulla and paraganglia containing granules that stain with chromium salts.

Chromatin It is a DNA structure present in the cell nucleus. Males are chromatin negative and females are chromatin positive (inactivated X-chromosome).

Chromatography A method of separating two or more chemical compounds in solution by passing across the surface of an absorbent paper.

Chromatophore A pigment bearing cell.

Chromatoptometry Measurement of color perception.

Chromoblasts An embryonic cell that becomes a pigment cell.

Chromolysis Dissolution of chromophil substance (Nissle bodies) in neurons in certain pathological conditions.

Chromomycosis Fungal infection of skin marked by warty plaques.

Chromophil Easily staining cell of anterior pituitary which is usually secretory.

Chromosome The structures containing DNA that store genetic information. There are 22 pairs of autosomes and one pair of sex chromosome in every cell.

Chronic fatigue syndrome It can be described as a debilitating disorder or disorders of uncertain causation. Symptoms usually include muscle and joint pain, cognitive difficulties and severe mental or physical exhaustion in a previously healthy and active person. It is also sometimes known as myalgic encephalomyelitis.

Chronic granulomatous disease A disease of children characterized by inability of neutrophils to kill ingested organisms.

Chronic obstructive lung disease (COLD) Included in this group are chronic asthma and bronchitis with dyspnoea, poor FEV_1, and maximum breathing capacity.

Chronological Description of an event in natural sequence according to time.

Chvostek's sign Spasm of facial muscle by tapping over area of facial nerve, a sign of tetany.

Chyle The protein and fat rich fluid of lymphatic channels drained to left subclavian vein via thoracic duct.

Chylemia Chyle in peripheral circulation.

Chylomicron Small particles of fat rich in triglycerides.

Chyluria Presence of chyle or fat globules in urine.

Chyme Thick semifluid mass consisting of partly digested food and digestive secretions that is passed from stomach to duodenum during digestion.

Chymopapain An enzyme related to papain.

Chymotrypsin A proteolytic enzyme present in the intestine that hydrolyses proteins to peptones.

Cicatrix Scar left by a healed wound.

Cicatrization Healing by scar formation.

Ciclesonide Topical steroid for rhinitis.

Ciclopirox Locally applied antifungal agent.

Cilia Hair like processes projecting from epithelial cells of bronchi propelling up mucus and foreign particles. *c. immotile syndrome* A group of inherited conditions characterized by immotility of cilia of respiratory mucosa and sperms. *SYN*-Kartagener's syndrome.

Ciliary body An annular structure on the inner surface of anterior wall of eyeball, composed of ciliary muscles and secretes aqueous humor.

Ciliary ganglion The ganglion in orbital fossa receiving preganglionic fibers from Edinger-Westphal nucleus and giving rise to 6 short ciliary nerves that innervate ciliary muscles, sphincters of iris and smooth muscles of blood vessels.

Ciliary muscles Smooth muscles of ciliary body, by contraction loosen suspensory ligament of lens allowing lens to become more spherical for accomplishing near vision.

Ciliary process About 70 folds arranged meridionally so as to form a circle, secrete nourishing fluid for cornea, lens and vitreous.

Ciliary reflex Normal contraction of pupil during process of accommodation.

Ciliospinal center Center in spinal cord that controls dilatation of pupil.

Ciliospinal reflex Dilatation of pupil following stimulation of the skin of the neck.

Cilostazol A vasodilator.

Cimetidine H_2 receptor antagonist inhibiting gastric acid secretion.

Cinchona Dried bark of cinchona tree containing quinine, cinchonine.

Cinchophen Old agent for gout frequently producing fatal hepatitis.

Cineangiocardiography Graphic record of heart and blood flow dynamics after constrast injection.

Cingulotomy Excision of anterior half of cingulate gyrus for control of intractable pain.

Cingulum A band of association fibers in the cingulate gyrus extending from anterior perforated substance to hippocampal gyrus.

Cinnarazine Drug used for vertigo.

Cinoxacin A quinolone, antibacterial agent.

Ciprofloxacin A quinolone with broad spectrum antibacterial activity.

Circadian Pertains to events that occur approximately at 24 hours interval.

Circle of Willis The anastomosis at base of brain where posterior cerebral and middle cerebral vessels meet (*see* Figure).

Circulatory failure Inadequate cardiac pump action to meet oxygen demand of body tissues. Peripheral circulatory failure means pooling of blood in expanded vascular space consequent to vasodilatation resulting in decreased venous return to heart.

Circumcision Removal of extra prepucal skin covering glans penis.

Circumduction Circular movement performed by the limb,

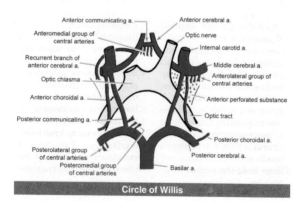

Anterior communicating a.
Anteromedial group of central arteries
Recurrent branch of anterior cerebral a.
Optic chiasma
Anterior choroidal a.
Posterior communicating a.
Posterolateral group of central arteries
Posteromedial group of central arteries

Anterior cerebral a.
Optic nerve
Internal carotid a.
Middle cerebral a.
Anterolateral group of central arteries
Anterior perforated substance
Optic tract
Posterior choroidal a.
Posterior cerebral a.
Basilar a.

Circle of Willis

the joint performing the movement is at the apex of the cone.

Circumflex Winding around.

Circumvallate papillae V-shaped row of papillae at base of tongue (*see* Figure).

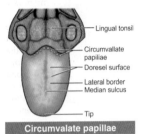

Lingual tonsil
Circumvallate papiliae
Doresel surface
Lateral border
Median sulcus
Tip

Circumvalate papillae

Cirrhosis Chronic liver disease characterized by bridging fibrosis, hepatic cell degeneration and regeneration and evidence of portal hypertension. *c. alcoholic* 20% of chronic alcoholics develop cirrhosis. *c. biliary* Cirrhosis following chronic bile stasis. *c. cardiac* Chronic heart failure leading to passive congestion of liver ending in cirrhosis. *c. infantile* Childhood cirrhosis due to protein malnutrition. *c. macronodular* Cirrhosis characterized by broad bands of fibrous tissue and large irregular regenerating nodules, e.g. post-necrotic/post hepatic cirrhosis.

Cisapride Agent to improve GI motility.

Cisplatin Antineoplastic agent for treatment of ovarian and testicular tumors.

Cisterna A reservoir or cavity.

Cisvestitism Wearing of clothes contrary to ones profession.

Citalopram An antidepressant.

Citric acid A tribasic acid present in juice of citrous fruits.

Citric acid cycle (Kreb's cycle) The cycle involving oxidative metabolism of pyruvic acid to CO_2, and H_2O, releasing energy (36 ATP).

Citrovorum factor Folinic acid used with dihydrofolate reductase inhibitors.

Citruline Amino acid formed from ornithine, present in water melons.

Clark's rule A formula for calculating pediatric dose i.e. weight of the child in lb. × adult dose/150.

Clasmatocyte A large wandering uninucleated cell with many branches, a fixed macrophage of loose connective tissue.

Claude's syndrome Third cranial nerve palsy, contralateral ataxia and tremor, caused by lesion around red nucleus.

Claudication Pain in calf muscle during walking due to inadequate blood supply.

Claustrophilia Dread of being in an open space, a morbid desire to remain within with windows shut.

Claustrophobia Fear of closed space.

Claspknife rigidity Passive flexion of the joint causes increased resistance of the extensors. This gives way abruptly if flexon is continued, a sign of pyramidal tract lesion.

Clavulanic acid Beta lactamase inhibitor.

Clawfoot Excessively high longitudinal arch of foot with dorsal contracture of toes.

Clawhand A hand characterized by hyperextension of proximal phallanges and extreme flexion of middle and distal phallanges (*see* Figure).

Clean catch method Contamination free urine specimen collection.

Cleavage Splitting a complex molecule into two or more simple ones.

Cleft A fissure or elongated opening. *c. alveolar* An anomaly resulting from lack of fusion between median na-

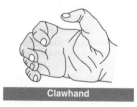

Clawhand

sal process and the maxillary process, commonly associated with cleft lip and cleft palate. *c. bronchial* An opening between branchial arches of an embryo (*see* Figure).

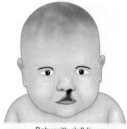

Baby with cleft lip

Cleft lips

Cleft foot A bipartite foot resulting from failure of a digit and its corresponding metatarsal to develop.

Clemastine Antihistaminic agent.

Clenching With the teeth in contact, forcible repeated contraction of jaw muscles.

Cleptomania Impulsive stealing in which motive is not related to value of stolen object.

Clidinium bromide Parasympathetic inhibitor used for treatment of peptic ulcer.

Climacteric Menopause or end of woman's reproductive ability. Male climacteric points to lessening male sexual activity.

Climax Sexual orgasm, period of greatest intensity.

Clindamycin hydrochloride An antibiotic against gram-positive cocci, implicated to produce pseudomembranous colitis due to resistant claustridium dificile.

Clinocephaly Congenital flatness or saddle-shape of the top of the head caused by bilateral premature closure of the sphenoparietal sutures.

Clinoid processes Three pairs of prominences on upper surface of sphenoid bone.

Clinoquinol Iodochlor hydroxy quine, antiamoebic agent.

Clithrophobia Morbid fear of being locked in.

Clitoridectomy This refers to partial or total removal of the clitoris. This has been defined by the WHO as type I female genital multilation (Type I FGM).

Clitoridotomy This refers to removal or splitting of the clitoralhood. This is also a type of female genital mutilation.

Clitoris Small erectile body beneath anterior labial commissure of female, homologous to penis of male.

Clitoris Crises Involuntary orgasm in female in tabes dorsalis.

Clitorism Recurring painful erection of clitoris, akin to priapism in male.

Clivulus A surface that slopes as in sphenoid bone.

Clobazam A benzidiazepine.

Clofazimine Antileprotic agent that stains skin.

Clobetasol A locally applied steroid.

Clofibrate Lipid lowering agent, may be carcinogenic and causes gall stones.

Clomiphene A nonsteroidal agent to stimulate ovulation in females and spermatogenesis in males.

Clonazepam Anticonvulsant for myoclonic seizure.

Clonidine Antihypertensive agent, also used for migraine prophylaxis.

Clonus Alternate contraction and relaxation of muscles, sign of upper motor lesion.

Clonic spasm Spasm marked by repeated muscular contraction followed by relaxation.

Clonorchiasis Liver fluke caused by chlonorchis sinensis which infects bile duct of man. Infection contacted by eating uncooked fresh water fish containing larvae. Treatment is with praziquantel.

Clopidogrel Antiplatelet agent.

Clostridium Anaerobic spore forming rods common in soil

and G-I tract of animal and man. *c. botulinum* Produces botulism. *c. difficile* Causes pseudomembranous colitis. *c. histolytium* Proteolytic, isolated from gas gangrene. *c. perfringens* Causes gas gangrene (C. welchii) *c. tetani* Produces tetanus.

Clotrimazole Antifungal agent for treatment of vulvovaginal candidiasis.

Cloxacillin Betalactamase resistant penicillin.

Clozapine Diabenzodiazepine group of antipsychotic agent.

Clubbing Bulbous enlargement of finger and toes tips with exasserated lateral and longitudinal curvatures. Most commonly found in infective endocarditis, suppurative lung disease, cyanotic heart disease and often congenital.

Clumping Thick grouping of micro organisms in a culture when specific immune serum is added.

Cluster headache Nocturnal headache, 2-3 hours after falling asleep, continuing for months associated with watering from eyes.

Clutton's joint Hydroarthrosis of knee joint often associated with interstitial keratitis, seen in congenital syphilis.

Coagulation The process of clotting, dependent upon availability of prothrombin, calcium, fibrinogen and thromboplastin. Prothrombin is converted to thrombin by the action of thromboplastin in the presence of calcium ions. Thrombin then converts soluble fibrinogen to insoluble fibrin mesh work on which RBCs are entangled. Thromboplastin is produced from injured vessel wall or by activated platelets (*see* Figure on page 155).

Coarctation A stricture, compression of walls.

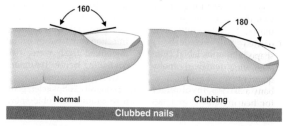

Normal

Clubbing

Clubbed nails

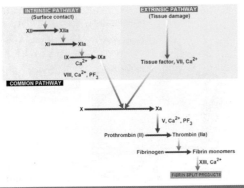

Coagulation

Coat's disease Development of large white masses in blood vessels of retina.

Cobalt 60 Radioactive isotope for treating malignancies.

Cocaine CNS stimulant, in toxic doses causes CNS depression, cardiac arrhythmia, and respiratory depression.

Coccidioidomycosis A coccidioidal granuloma.

Coccygeal body Small arteriovenous anastomosis at the level of coccyx.

Cochlea A winding cone-shaped tube resembling a snail shell, winding two and three quarter turns about a central bony axis, organ responsible for hearing (*see* Figure on page 156).

Cochlear implant An electronic device that receives sounds and transmits the resulting electric signals to implanted electrodes in cochlea so that the sound is perceived. *SYN* – Cochlear prosthesis.

Cochlear nerve 8th cranial nerve supplying cochlea with nucleus at pons and medulla.

Cochleo-palpebral reflex Contraction of orbicularis oculi from sudden noise near the ear.

Cocktail Any beverage or product containing several ingredients.

Codeine Derivative of opium used as analgesic-hypnotic.

Cod liver oil Oil extracted from liver of fish rich in vitamin A and D

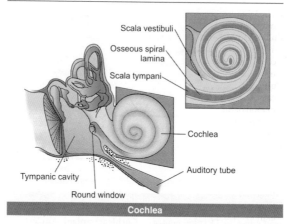

Scala vestibuli

Osseous spiral lamina

Scala tympani

Cochlea

Auditory tube

Tympanic cavity

Round window

Cochlea

Codman's exercise Mild exercises to restore the motion and function in the arms or shoulders after injury or immobilization.

Coenzyme A diffusible heat-stable enzyme which when combines with apoenzyme forms active complete enzyme, e.g. riboflavin, coenzyme I and II.

Coenzyme A A Precursor for biosynthesis of fatty acids and sterols.

Cogan's syndrome Interstitial keratitis associated with tinnitus, vertigo and usually deafness.

Cognition Awareness with perception, reasoning, judgement, memory, etc.

Cogwheel Combination of tremor and rigidity as in extrapyramidal disease, i.e., Parkinson's disease.

Coherent Sticking together, adhesiveness.

Cohort The component of population born during a period and traced through life.

Cohort study In epidemiology, a method of investigation is a cohort, q.v.; is followed prospectively or retrospectively.

Coin test A test for pneumothorax, a coin placed on chest is struck with another coin. A metallic ringing sound is heard at a distant site of the chest in pneumothorax.

Coitus Sexual intercourse between male and female.

Colchicine Antigout medicine, may produce GI side effects.

Cold agglutinin The agglutinin agglutinating RBCs at 4°C, commonly seen in viral and mycoplasma infections.

Cold common *SYN* – nasal catarrh, acute catarrhal inflammation of mucous membrane of nasal cavity, sinuses and pharynx caused by rhinovirus.

Cold pack Wrapping patient in cold water soaked clothing to reduce fever, for relief of pain and diminution of swelling in bruise.

Colestipol Ion exchange resin akin to cholestyramine.

Colic Spasmodic pain originating from any hollow viscus. *c. biliary* Gall stone in bile duct/cystic duct causing pain. *c. intestinal* Abdominal pain due to worms, infection, spasm of intestines. *c. renal* Passage of stone, clot along ureters with pain in loin radiating to groin, genitalia and inner aspect of thigh. *c. uterine* Dysmenorrhoeic pain due to retained clots.

Colistin Polymyxin, an antibiotic effective against many organisms including pseudomonas.

Colitis Inflammation of colon. *c. ulcerative* Inflammation involving rectum with skip lesions, cobble stone appearance, friable mucosa and bloody offensive diarrhea.

Collagen Fibrous insoluble protein of skin, bone, ligaments and cartilages.

Collagen vascular diseases A group of diseases of blood vessels of unknown etiology manifesting with joint pain, skin rash, muscle ache and bleeding manifestations. Included in this group are SLE, rheumatoid arthritis, systemic sclerosis etc.

Collagenase Enzyme responsible for breakdown of collagen.

Collapse 1. An abnormal retraction of the walls of an organ 2. A sudden exhaustion, prostration or weakness due to poor circulation.

Collapse therapy Unilateral pneumothorax induced to promote healing/stop bleeding of Koch's lesion.

Collapsing pulse Pulse of aortic regurgitation.

Colles' fascia Inner layer of superficial fascia of perineum.

Colles' fracture Transverse fracture of distal end of radius with displacement of lower fragment backwards, upwards and laterally (*see* Figure).

Radius

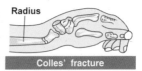

Colles' fracture

Collecting tubule Small ducts in renal medulla that receive urine from several renal tubules. These ducts form papillary ducts of Bellini that open into renal papillae.

Colloid A glue like substance; the homogeneous gelatinous substance seen in thyroid gland containing thyroid hormones.

Coloboma A cleft or fissure in iris or ciliary body of eye.

Colon The large intestine, from the caecum to the rectum (*see* Figure below). *Ascending c.* That part arising to the right of the abdomen to in front of the liver. *Descending c.* That part running down from in front of the spleen to the sigmoid colon. *Giant c.* Megacolon. *Irritable c.* [*see* Irritable (Bowel syndrome)]. *Pelvic c., sigmoid c.* That part lying in the pelvis and connecting the descending colon with the rectum. *Transverse c.* That part lying across the upper abdomen connecting the ascending and descending portions.

Colon irritable Motility disorder of colon manifesting with abdominal pain, frequent small ribbon like stools, usually triggered by anxiety.

Colonic irrigation Flushing out of colon prior to surgery of colon, colonoscopy.

Colonoscope A fibreoptic instrument, passed through

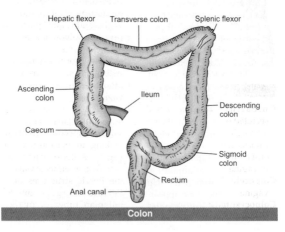

Hepatic flexor   Transverse colon   Splenic flexor

Ascending colon

Ileum

Caecum

Descending colon

Sigmoid colon

Rectum

Anal canal

Colon

the anus, for examining the interior of the colon.

Coloproctectomy Surgical removal of colon and rectum.

Color blindness Defective perception of color; color blindness in which all colors are perceived as gray is called monochromasia.

Colorimeter Instrument for measuring intensity of colour.

Colostomy Opening up of colon to exterior through abdominal wall (*see* Figure).

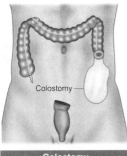

Colostomy

Colostrum Breast fluid secreted during first 2-3 days after delivery, rich in protein, calories and antibodies.

Colpectomy Surgical removal of vagina.

Colpocele A hernia into the vagina.

Colpocystitis Inflammation of the bladder and vagina.

Colpoperineoplasty Plastic repair of the vagina and perineum.

Colpoperineorrhaphy Surgical repair of the ruptured vagina and perineum.

Colpopexy Suture of a prolapsed vagina to the abdominal wall.

Colpoplasty Also called vaginoplasty. It is the plastic surgery of the vagina.

Colpoptosis This is a condition associated with the prolapse of vagina.

Colporrhaphy Repair of the vagina. *Anterior c.* Repair for cystocele. *Posterior c.* Repair for retrocele.

Colporrhexis A tearing or laceration of the vaginal vault.

Colposcopy Examination of vagina and vaginal portion of cervix by colposcope, usually to select sites of abnormal epithelium for biopsy in patient with abnormal papsmear.

Colpostenosis Narrowing of vagina.

Colpotomy Also known as vaginotomy. This is a surgical procedure involving making an incision over the vagina. Anterior colpotomy is performed either to vsualize the pelvic structures or to Perform surgery on the fallopian tubes or ovaries. Posterior colpotomy is usually performed to drain an abscess in the pouch of Douglas.

Colpoxerosis A condition characterized by unusual dryness of the vaginal mucous membrane.

Column A cylindrical supporting structure.

Coma A state from which patient cannot be aroused by painful stimuli and he does not respond to inner needs.

Coma vigil Coma with open eyes and vaccant look as in severe systemic infections.

Comedo Blackhead, discoloured dried sebum plugging an excretory duct of the skin, e.g., acne involving face, back and neck in adolescents.

Comma bacillus Vibrio comma, organism of cholera.

Comma tract of Schultze The fasciculus interfascicularis, a tract of descending fibers located between the fasciculus cuneatus and fasciculus gracilis in the posterior funiculus of spinal cord.

Commensal Organisms that live in an intimate non parasitic relationship.

Comminuted fracture A fracture where the bone is splintered or crushed.

Comminution Reducing a solid body to varying sizes by grating, pulverizing, slicing etc.

Commissure A transverse band of nerve fibers passing over the midline in the CNS. *c. anterior cerebral* Band of white fibers that passes across lamina terminalis connecting the two cerebral hemispheres. *c.posterior* Commisure just above the midbrain containing fibers that connect the superior colliculi.

Commissurotomy Surgical incision of any commisure. Commonly refers to mitral commissurotomy in mitral stenosis.

Communicable disease A disease that may be transmitted directly or indirectly from one person to another.

Compatibility Ability of two individuals or groups to live together without strife or tension.

Complement A series of enzymatic proteins in normal serum that once activated augment immune mechanisms by leukocyte chemotaxis, and bacterial opsonization.

Complement fixation Some antigen antibody reactions fix complement for completion of reaction. This process is the basis of Wasserman reaction for syphilis.

Compliance The property of altering size and shape in

response to application of force, weight or release from such force, e.g. pulmonary compliance a measure of the force required to expand the lungs. Children have higher pulmonary compliance in comparison to adults.

Compound astigmatism Myopia/hypermetropia of differing diopters in both longitudinal and vertical axes.

Compound fracture Fracture with communication to exterior by breach in the skin.

Compress A soft pad that is applied on body parts with pressure to control hemorrhage or to supply heat, cold, or medication to relieve pain.

Compulsion Repetitive stereotyped act performed to relieve fear connected with obsession; dictated by patient's subconscious mind against his wishes and if not performed causes uneasiness.

Compulsion neurosis Obsession that compels one to perform an absurd act.

Compulsive ideas An idea that continues to haunt against one's will.

Computer An electronic device for storing and retrieving numerical or textural information.

Computer assisted design Computer use to assist in designing objects, e.g. reshape body parts in plastic surgery, artificial hip implant, crown preparation.

Concanavalin A A lectin that stimulates proliferation of T lymphocyte but not B lymphocytes.

Conceive To become pregnant, to form an idea, to form a mental image.

Concentration Strength of a substance in solution, fixation of mind on one subject with exclusion of all other thoughts.

Conception Union of male spermatozoa with ovum.

Concha The outer ear or pinna; the turbinate inside nasal cavity.

Conchotomy Surgical incision of nasal concha.

Concoction Mixture of two medicinal substance aided by heating.

Concomitant Occurring at the same time.

Concussion cerebral Transient loss of consciousness from external cranial trauma.

Conditioning Improving physical capability by an exercise programme. *c. operant* Learning of a particular action or type of behavior that is followed by reward.

Conduction The transfer of electron, heat, ions or sound wave through a conducting medium or the process whereby a state of excitation is transmitted.

Condyle A rounded protuberance at the end of a bone forming an articulation (*see* Figure).

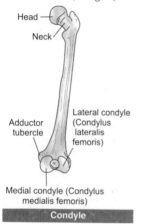

Head

Neck

Adductor tubercle

Lateral condyle (Condylus lateralis femoris)

Medial condyle (Condylus medialis femoris)

Condyle

Condyloma A wart like growth in the skin around anus/external genitalia. *c. acuminata* Usually venereal, caused by virus. *c. latum* A mucous patch on the vulva or anus characteristic of syphilis.

Confabulation A form of memory loss in which the patient fills his memory gaps with inappropriate words.

Confluent Running together, merging together.

Confusion Disorientation in respect to time, place or person.

Congener Two or more muscles with same function, or two substances with similar origin, function or structure.

Congestion The presence of excessive amount of blood or tissue fluid in an organ or tissue. *c. active* Congestion arising out of increased blood flow or vasodilatation. *c. passive* Vascular congestion due to impaired pumping action by heart. *c. pulmonary* Pulmonary vascular congestion due to increased LA pressure (MS) or LVF.

Coniology The study of dust and its effects.

Coniotomy Cricothyrotomy.

Conization Excision of a cone of tissue as in chronic cervicitis.

Conjugate Paired or joined. *c. deviation* Deviation of both eyes to either side. *c. diagonal* Distance measured from center of sacral promontory to the back of symphysis pubis. True conjugate is 1.5 to 2 cm less than diagonal conjugate. *c. true* It is anterior - posterior diameter of pelvic inlet; the distance between the midline superior point of the sacrum and the upper margin of symphysis pubis.

Conjugation A coupling together. In biology, the union of two unicellular organisms accompanied by an interchange of nuclear material.

Conjunctiva Mucous membrane that lines eyelids and is reflected onto eyeball.

Conjunctivitis Inflammation of conjunctiva. *c. actinic* Conjunctivitis from exposure to actinic (ultraviolet rays). *c. angular* Conjunctivitis involving angles of eyes, due to Morax Axenfield bacillus. *c. catarrhal* Conjunctivitis with mucoid discharge due to foreign body, allergy, heat, cold etc., *c. epidemic haemorrhagic* Viral infection of eye with swollen eyelids, and subconjunctival haemorrhage. *c. inclusion* Purulent inflammation of conjunctiva due to *Chlamydia trachomatis*. *c. phlyctenular* Nodules around limbus, particularly in allergy to Koch's bacillus. *c. vernal* Allergic spring conjunctivitis.

Conn's syndrome Primary hyperaldosteronism with muscle weakness, polyuria, hypertension, hypokalemia and alkalosis.

Consanguinity Blood relationship, i.e, being descended from a common ancestor.

Consciousness A state of awareness, i.e., orientation in time, place and person. Stupor is a state from which only intense stimulus can arouse the patient. Normal motor reflex. In coma patient does not perceive the environment and intense stimuli produce only rudimentary response if any at all.

Consensual Reflex stimulation of another or opposite part.

Consensual light reflex Contraction of opposite pupil from focussing of light on one side.

Consent Granting permission by patient for a procedure. *c. implied* Consent presumed in certain circumstances, i.e., when patient sits on a dental chair thereby implying examination. *c. informed* The understanding between the person and institution conducting an experimental medical investigation involving human subjects.

Consolidation The act of becoming solid, especially solidification of lung due to pathological engorgement of the tissue as occurring in pneumonia.

Constipation Infrequent defecation with passage of unduly hard and dry fecal material, sluggish action of bowels. *c. obstructive* Obstructive colonic/intestinal lesion causing constipation. *c. atonic* Constipation due to weakness of muscles of colon and rectum. *c. spastic* Constipation due to excessive tonicity of intestinal wall.

Consummation The completion of marriage by the first act of sexual intercourse.

Contact Mutual touching or apposition of two persons/objects or one who has recently been exposed to contagious disease.

Contact dermatitis Dermatitis due to an irritating or sensitizing chemical.

Contact lens Device, either rigid or flexible that rests on cornea to improve refractive error.

Contagious Communicable; transmitted readily from one person to another either directly or indirectly.

Contagium The agent causing infection or contagion.

Contamination 1. Introduction of disease germs, or infectious materials into normally sterile objects. 2. Radiation in or on a place where it is not wanted.

Continent Capable of controlling urination and defecation or sexual indulgence.

Continine Principal metabolite of nicotine excreted in urine.

Contortion A twisting into an unusual shape.

Contour Surface configuration of a part.

Contraception Prevention of conception.

Contraceptive Any process, device or method that prevents contraception. They include spermicides, estrogen-progesterone pills, and physical barriers like IUD.

Contract To contract a disease/infection, to shorten or reduce in size.

Contraction isometric Muscular exercise where muscle does not change its length.

Contraction isotonic Muscular contraction in which the muscle maintains constant tension by changing its length during contraction.

Contracture Permanent contraction of a muscle due to paralysis/ spasm/ischaemia. *c. Dupuytrens* Contraction of palmar fascia leading to deformity of fingers. *c. Volkmann's* Atrophy of forearm muscles with pronation and flexion of the hand resulting from constricting cast/bandage on brachial artery (*see* Figure).

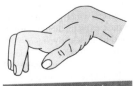

Volkmann's contracture

Contraindication Inadvisable form of therapy.

Contralateral Opposite side of body.

Contrast In radiology, radiopaque material to provide a contrast in density between tissue or organ being X-rayed.

Contrecoup injury Injury to one part of brain with lesion on opposite side. e.g., blow to the back of head causing injury to frontal lobes as they are forced against anterior portion of cranial valt.

Contusion A bruise, injury with subcutaneous hemorrhage but intact skin.

Conus Shaped like a cone. *c. arteriosus* The portion of right ventricle giving rise to pulmonary arteries. *c. medullaris* Lower conical portion of spinal cord.

Convalescence The period of recovery after an illness/ operation.

Convection Heat transfer through liquids or gases.

Convergence The moving of two or more objects at same point.

Conversion reaction Hysterical neuroses denoting a psychological conflict translated into physical ailment.

Convolution A turn, fold or coil of anything that is convoluted. In anatomy, a gyrus, one of the many folds on the surface of cerebral hemispheres that are separated by grooves, (sulci or fissures).

Convulsion Paroxysms of involuntary muscle contraction and relaxation.

Cooley's anemia Thalassemia major, an inherited disorder of hemoglobin synthesis.

Coombs' test A test for detection of antiglobulins in blood, helpful in diagnosis of autoimmune hemolytic anemia.

Coordination Working together of various muscles for performing certain movements.

Copolymer A polymer composed of two different kinds of monomers.

Copper sulfate Deep blue crystals/granules, used as algicide/ astringent.

Coprolalia The use of vulgar, obscene language as in

schizophrenia and Gilles de la Tourette syndrome.

Coprolith Hard feces.

Coprophilia Unusual preoccupation with feces, a perversion in adults.

Coproporphyria Excessive coproporphyrin excretion in feces, as in inherited porphyrias.

Coproporphyrin A porphyrin present in urine and feces.

Copula Any connecting part.

Copulation Sexual intercourse.

Coracoid Resembling in shape a crow's beak.

Coracoid process Process on anterior upper surface of scapula.

Cord A string like structure. *c. spermatic* The channel for sperms to pass from testes to seminal vesicle. *c. spinal* Extension of CNS, into the spinal canal upto upper border of first lumbar vertebra. *c. umbilical* Cord that connects fetal circulatory system to the placenta, consists of two umbilical arteries and one umbilical vein.

Cordotomy Resectional of lateral spinothalamic tracts in the cord to relieve intractable pain.

Cori cycle In carbohydrate metabolism, the breakdown of muscle glycogen with formation of lactic acid which is converted to glycogen in liver. Liver glycogen is released as glucose which is taken up by muscles being then reconverted to muscle glycogen.

Corn Hardening or thickening of skin that has a conical shape extending into dermis causing pain.

Cornea The clear, transparent anterior portion of eye covering 1/6 the surface of globe functioning as an important refractive medium. It is composed of 5 layers: epithelium, Browman's membrane, substantia propria, Descemet's membrane and layer of endothelium (*see* Figure).

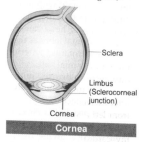

Cornea

Corneal reflex Closure of eye lid on touching the cornea: Afferent limb by trigeminal and efferent by facial nerves.

Corneal transplant Either partial thickness or full thickness transfer of cornea from a healthy cadaver, donor to treat corneal opacity obstructing vision.

Corneoblepharon Adhesion of eyelid to cornea.

Cornification The process by which squamous epithelial cells are converted into hard horny material, e.g., horns, hairs, nails, feathers etc.

Cornu Any projection like a horn.

Corona Any structure resembling a crown.

Corona radiata Ascending and descending fibers of internal capsule that above corpus collosum extend in all directions to reach cerebral cortex.

Coronal plane Plane dividing into front and back portions.

Coronary angiography Opacification of coronary arteries by injection of iohexol or urograffin or any such contrast agent.

Coronary arteries A pair of arteries, left and right arising from left and right coronary sinuses supplying blood to myocardium. The left artery is usually dominant.

Coronary bypass Surgically established shunt between root of aorta and involved coronary distal to block or diverting internal mammary to augment myocardial blood flow.

Coronary care unit A specially equipped unit in a hospital providing intensive care to patients of coronary artery disease, i.e., myocardial infarction, unstable angina, etc.

Coronary plexus A plexus of autonomic nerve fibers supplying the heart.

Coronary sinus The channel carrying venous drainage of heart into right atrium.

Coronavirus The virus particle surrounded by a crown, e.g., common cold virus.

Coronoid fossa An oval depression on anterior surface of distal end of humerus articulating with coronoid process of ulna.

Corpse A dead body; cadaver.

Corpulent Obese.

Corpulmonale Right heart failure secondary to pulmonary pathology.

Corpus The principal part of any organ or body. *c. callosum* The commissure joining two cerebral hemispheres. *c. cavernosum* Erectile tissue of penis, clitoris, bulb of vestibule etc. *c. luteum* The yellow body left on the surface of the ovary and formed from the remains of the graafian follicle after the discharge of the ovum. If it retrogresses, menstruation occurs, but it persists for several months if pregnancy supervenes. *c. striatum* The structures in cerebral hemispheres consisting of caudate and lentiform nuclei.

Corpuscle Any small rounded body, an encapsulated sensory nerve ending, blood cell. *c. malphigian* A renal corpuscle consisting of a glomerulous and Bowman's capsule. *c. Meissner's* An encapsulated touch receptor in the epidermis of skin esp of palm, hand and feet. *c. pacinian* A large ovoid sensory end organ consisting of concentric layers of connective tissue surrounding nerve ending acting as receptor of proprioception and deep pressure.

Corrigan's pulse A full bounding pulse of aortic insufficiency.

Corrosive poisoning Poisoning by strong alkalies, acid, antiseptics, e.g., hydroxides of sodium, ammonium, potassium.

Corrugator The muscle of eye drawing eyebrow medially and inferiorly, arising from frontal bone and inserted on the skin of medial half of eye-brows.

Cortex Outer layer of an organ like kidney, adrenal, ovary, lymphnode, thymus, cerebrum and cerebellum.

Corticoid Steroid hormone secreted by adrenal cortex.

Corticosterone Hormone of adrenal cortex influencing carbohydrate metabolism, Na^+ and K^+ homeostasis.

Corticotrophin (ACTH) The anterior pituitary hormone that stimulates adrenals to secrete glucocorticoids.

Corticotrophin releasing factor The hypothalamic factor regulating secretion of corticotrophin.

Cortisone Adrenal hormone, largely inactive till converted to active cortisol. Influences metabolism of fat, carbohydrate, protein, N^+ and K^+

Corynebacterium Gram-positive nonmotile drum stick shaped rod, causing diphtheria.

Coryza Acute nasal catarrh with profuse watery secretion.

Cosmetic Agents or methods of improving physical appearance (appearance promoters).

Cosmetic surgery Commonly known as plastic surgery done to improve appearance, i.e., correction of ugly burns and scars, elephantiasis, localized obesity, pendulous breast, facial wrinkles.

Cosmic Universe.

Costen's syndrome Tempromandibular arthritis.

Cotton p. A round cotton ball having 1 cm diameter. It is used for applying medicines topically.

Cotton wool spots Soft wooly exudates in retina in hypertension and uremia, probably superficial infarcts.

Couching Forcible downward displacement of lens caused to improve vision in cataract patients.

Cough Forceful expiratory effort with closed glottis, to expectorate mucous and foreign body.

Counselling Providing of advice and guideline to a patient by health professional.

Counter Geiger Device for detection and counting of ionizing radiation.

Countercurrent exchanger The exchange of chemicals between two counter current streams separated by a membrane.

Counterimmunoelectrophoresis A process in which antigen and antibodies are placed in separate wells and an electric current is passed through diffusion medium.

Antigens migrate to anode and antibodies to cathode. If the antigen and antibody correspond to each other, they upon meeting in the diffusion medium will precipitate and will form a precipitin band or line.

Counterincision A second incision made to facilitate drainage or to reduce tension on the stitches.

Counterirritant An agent applied locally to produce mild inflammatory reaction to relieve pain of adjacent or deeper structure.

Counter shock An electric shock applied to heart to correct arrhythmia.

Countertraction Application of a force in a direction opposite to the force of traction, usually in fracture reduction.

Couple To join together, to have sexual union.

Courvoisier's law Sudden obstruction of bile duct by gallstone does not cause enlargement of gallbladder as opposed to gradual obstruction as in malignancy of pancreas/ampulla of Vater which consistently causes marked enlargement of gall bladder.

Couvelaire uterus Extravasation of blood into uterine

musculature often demanding hysterectomy.

Covalent Sharing of electrons between two atoms.

Cowden's disease Multiple hamartomas.

Cowling's rule Age of child on next birth day divided by 24 to give pediatric dose.

Cowper's gland A pair of compound tubular mucous glands beneath the bulb of male urethra, akin to Bartholin glands in female.

Coxalgia Pain in the hip.

Coxiella burnetti Causative organism of Q fever.

Coxsackie virus A member of picorna virus causing herpangina, aseptic meningitis, pleurodynia, epidemic conjunctivitis, myocarditis.

Crab louse Louse infecting pubic regions (phthirus pubis)

Cracked pot sound Percussion note resembling cracked pot as in pulmonary cavity, hydrocephalus.

Cramp Spasmodic painful contraction of a muscle.

Cranioclast Instrument for crushing foetal skull to facilitate delivery of large dead foetus.

Craniocleidodysostosis A congenital condition that involves defective ossification of bones of face, head, and clavicle.

Craniometry Measurement of skull bones.

Craniostenosis Contracted skull due to premature closure of cranial sutures.

Craniostosis Congenital ossification of cranial sutures.

Craniotabes Abnormal softening of skull bones.

Cranium The skull can be divided into two parts: 1. Cranium– The bony framework which supports the brain. 2. Mandible– The bony framework which supports the jaw and the lower part of the face. The cranium is composed of 8 bones namely: Two parietal bones, one frontal bone, two temporal bones, one occipital bone, sphenoid and ethmoid.

Cravat bandage Triangular bandage folded to form a band around the injured part.

Crazybone Name for medial epicondyle of humerus, as slight trauma to it causes pain and tingling in fingers due to stimulation of ulnar nerve.

c. reactive protein Acute phase reactant, a serum globulin whose concentrations is increased in acute infections like rheumatic fever.

Creatine Methylglycocyamine, a colourless substance excreted in urine. Combines with phosphate to form creatine phosphate.

Creatine kinase Enzyme present in skeletal and cardiac muscles that acts in breakdown of ATP to ADP. Serum level is increased in myocardial infarction, skeletal muscle injury, and muscle dystrophy.

Creatinine Formed from creatine.

Crede's method Expulsion of placenta by putting downward pressure on the uterus through anterior abdominal wall and squeezing uterus but inversion is a danger.

Cremaster A fascia like muscle suspending and enveloping testicles and spermatic cord.

Cremasteric reflex Retraction of testes on stimulation of innerside of thigh, a superficial reflex mediated via L_1, L_2 segment.

Crepitation Crackling sound heard 1. in lungs in pneumonia, 2. movement of fractured bones, 3. in soft tissues in anaerobic gasforming infections and 4. in subcutaneous emphysema.

Crescent Shaped like sickle e.g., menisci of knee joint, choroid atrophy in myopics (myopic crescent).

Cresol Coal tar derivative disinfectant containing 5% phenol.

Cresomania Hallucination of possession of great wealth.

Crest Ridge or elongated prominence. e.g., alveolar crest that surrounds teeth whose resorption can be delayed by flurbiprofen.

CREST Syndrome Calcinosis, Raynaud's phenomenon, esophageal dismotility, sclerodactily and telangiectasia, a variant of systemic sclerosis.

Cretin Hypothyroidism in babies manifesting as rough skin, mental subnormality, potbelly, coarse features, hypoactivity and delayed dentition.

Creutzfeldt-Jakob disease *H.G. Creutzfeldt, German physician, 1885-1964. A. Jakob, German physician, 1884-1931.* A rapidly progressive disease of the nervous system affecting middle-aged and elderly people; caused by a 'slow' virus. Transmission between humans is very unusual, although the disease has been reported in young people treated with human pituitary extract for short stature - now no longer used.

Crevice A small fissure or crack e.g., gingival crevice: a fissure produced by the marginal gingiva with tooth surface.

Crib A small bed with high legs and sides for infants and babies.

Cribiform Sieve like e.g., 1. Cribiform plate, the thin perforated medial portion of ethmoid bone perforated by olfactory nerve fibers. 2. Cribiform fascia, the part of deep fascia of thigh covering fossa ovalis.

Cricoid Shaped like a signet ring, e.g. cricoid cartilage; the lowermost cartilage of larynx, the broad portion being posterior and anterior portion forming the arch.

Cri-du-chat syndrome A chromosomal deletion disorder characterized by cry like a cat, microcephaly, mental retardation, dwarfism and laryngeal defect.

Crisis Critical period, e.g., 1. Addisonian crisis. (acute adrenal failure) 2. Sickle cell crisis (acute bone/abdominal pain of sickle cell anemia due to thrombotic infarcts) 3. Thyroid crisis: Fever, delirium and extreme tachycardia of sudden deterioration of hyperthyroidism. 4. Sudden fall in temperature in pneumonia.

Crista A crest or ridge, e.g. 1. Crysta ampularis, the local-ized thickening of membrane lining the ampulla of semicircular canals. 2. Crista supraventricularis of heart.

Crocodile tear Production of tear during mastication in patients with facial palsy due to abnormal regeneration, so named because crocodiles are believed to weep after eating their victims.

Crohn's disease Regional enteritis, a granulomatous inflammation involving all the three coats of small intestine and often colon.

Cromolyn sodium Disodium chromoglycate, useful in bronchial asthma, mast cell stabilizer.

Cross fertilization Fusion of male and female gametes from different persons.

Crossmatching A test for compatibility in blood transfusion where donor red cells are matched with recipient plasma and vice versa.

Cross over Reciprocal exchange of genetic material between chromosomes.

Crotamiton A scabicide used as 2% ointment.

Croup Laryngitis marked by barking cough, stridor, and respiratory difficulty usually due to formation of diphtheritic membrane.

Crouzon's disease Congenital disease characterised by hypertelorism (wide spaced eyes) craniofacial dysostosis, exophthalmos, optic atrophy and divergent squint.

Crowning Showing of fetal head in vulva during parturition.

Cruciate Cross shaped as in cruciate ligament of knee.

Crura Divergent bands resembling legs. e.g., crura of diaphragm, connecting to spinal column; crura cerebri; cerebral peduncles.

Crush syndrome Renal failure following crush injury with myoglobinuria.

Crutch A device of wood or metal fitting the armpit; used for supporting body weight. *C. axillary* has long rigid vertical structure, a short padded horizontal bar fitting under axilla. *c. conadian* triceps crutch. *C. forearm* the top is at level of forearm with a hand bar as well as cuff. *c. Lofstrand* a form of forearm crutch. *c. triceps* two uprights extending halfway between elbow and shoulder, with a cross piece for the hand and a curved upper part (*see* Figure).

Crutch paralysis Crutch induced paralysis of brachial plexus/radial nerve.

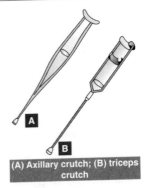

(A) Axillary crutch; (B) triceps crutch

Cryocautery Cold application for therapeutic objective.

Cryoextraction Use of liquid nitrogen/carbon dioxide probe to anterior lens aiding in its extraction.

Cryoglobulin An abnormal globulin that precipitates when cooled but dissolves on heating, found in multiple myeloma, leukemia and mycoplasma pneumonia.

Cryoprecipitate Precipitation of immunecomplexes in patients with autoimmune diseases when their serum is stored in cold.

Cryopreservation Preservation of biological material e.g., sperm, organs, tissue, plasma in subzero temperature.

Cryosurgery Tissue destruction by application of cold

probe (−20°C or below) as to control pain, bleeding, e.g., haemorrhoidectomy, tonsillectomy, conization of cervix, thalamotomy.

Crypt Small cavity, i.e. anal crypts lying behind junction of anal skin and rectal mucosa, tonsillar crypts on tonsils surrounded by lymphnodules.

Cryptitis Inflammation of anal crypts.

Cryptococcosis SYN − torulosis: Systemic fungal infection involving skin, brain, lungs caused by cryptococcus neoformans.

Cryptogenic Of unknown or indeterminate origin.

Cryptomenorrhoea Monthly subjective symptoms of menstruation without vaginal bleed usually due to unperforated hymen.

Cryptosporidiasis Acute diarrhoea caused by protozoa cryptosporidium usually in immunocompromised.

Crystal Small particles with definite pattern and angles, e.g., apatite crystals of calcium phosphate with other elements; Charcot-Leyden crystals found in sputum of patients with asthma where in there is eosinophilia.

Crystallography Study of crystals, pertains to study of renal and biliary calculi.

Crystalluria Appearance of crystals, in urine, commonly after administration of sulfa drugs. *c. terminal* The alpha carboxyl group of last amino acid.

Chemoreceptor trigger zone (CTZ) The area of medulla oblongata whose stimulation causes vomiting.

Cubital fossa The hollow anterior to elbow bounded medially by pronater teres and laterally by brachioradialis.

Cubitus Forearm *c. valgus* lateral deviation of forearms beyond 16-18°. *c. varus* medial deviation of forearm (*see* Figure on page 175).

Cuff Glove, structure encircling a part.

Cul-de-sac A blind pouch or cavity.

Culdocentesis Perforation of posterior upper vaginal wall for draining rectouterine pouch for diagnostic/therapeutic purposes.

Culdoscopy Examination of pelvic cavity by passing endoscope into posterior vaginal fornix.

Culex Mosquito responsibe for filariasis.

Culicide Agents that destroy gnats and mosquitoes.

Cullen's sign Bluish discoloration of periumbilical skin due to intraperitoneal hemorrhage,

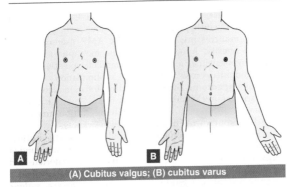

(A) Cubitus valgus; (B) cubitus varus

usually following pancreatitis, tubal pregnancy rupture.

Culmen Top or submit of a thing.

Cult People following an ideal or principle.

Culture Propagation of microorganisms or living tissue in special media.

Cumulus Small elevation.

Cupid's bow The normal bow shape of upper lip.

Cupola The dome at the apex of cochlea; the dome of pleura. covering apex of lung.

Cuprous Monovalent copper Cu$^+$; Cupric is Cu^{++}.

CUPS *Critical, unstable, potentially unstable, and stable.* Priority classification of patients used during the initial assessment of the patient.

Curarization Anticonvulsant medication, by administration of agents negating effects of acetylcholine, i.e., suxamethonium.

Curet A spoon-shaped scraping instrument used in dentistry, gynaecology and orthopedics.

Curie Unit of radiation equivalent to $10^{10} \times 3.7$ disintegration per second.

Curling ulcer Peptic ulcer following severe stress i.e., burn injury.

Current A flow, usually of electrical impulse. *c. alternating* Currrent that periodically flows in opposite directions. *c. direct* Unidirectionally flow of current.

Curriculum Course of study.

Curschmann's spirals Coiled spirals in sputum of asthmatic patients.

Curvilinear Concerning or pertaining to a curved line.

Cushing's disease Hypersecretion of ACTH with hypercortisolism manifesting with trunkal obesity, hyperglycemia, hypokalemia purplish striae and osteoporosis.

Cushing's syndrome Symptoms arising out of hypercortisolism.

Cusp Points on crown of tooth, leaf like portions constituting heart valves.

Cutis The skin.

Cyanemia Blue colour of blood.

Cyanhemoglobin Cyanide haemoglobin compound where blood appears cherry red as in cyanide poisoning.

Cyanocobalamin Vit B_{12}.

Cyanosis Bluish discolouration of skin due to raised (±4 gm%) of reduced hemoglobin in blood. *c. central* Occurring by admixture of venous and arterial blood in heart/lungs e.g.: pulmonary A-V fistula, fallot tetralogy and TGV *c. peripheral* Local cyanosis over cold parts due to increased oxygen extraction e.g. CHF *c. differential* Cyanosis of feet but not arms in Eisenmenger syndrome in patent ductus arteriosus.

Cyclamate Artificial sweetner 30 times more sweet than sugar.

Cyclandelate Vasodilator.

Cyclazocin Used in opioid addiction.

Cyclic AMP Adenosine 3'5' cyclic monophosphate, an intracellular messenger of end organ stimulation.

Cyclitis Inflammation of ciliary body.

Cyclizine Antihistamine for motion sickness.

Cyclodialysis Drainage operation for treatment of glaucoma in which communication is established between supra arachnoid space and angle of anterior chamber.

Cyclo-oxygenase Enzyme converting arachidonic acid to prostaglandin.

Cyclophosphamide Antineoplastic and immunosuppressant.

Cycloplegia Paralysis of ciliary muscles leading to dilatation of pupils.

Cyclopropane Gaseous anaesthetic agent.

Cycloserine Broad spectrum antibiotic used in tuberculosis.

Cyclosporine Immune suppressant used in transplant patients.

Cyclothymia The alteration of mood seen in manic depressive psychosis.

Cyclotron A particle accelerator in which the particle is rotated between the ends of a magnet, gaining speed with each rotation.

Cyesis Pregnancy. *Pseudo c.* Signs and symptoms suggestive of pregnancy arising when no fertilization has taken place. 'Phantom pregnancy'.

Cylindroma Malignant tumor containing a collection of cells forming cylinders.

Cyproheptadine Antiserotonin drug used in allergy and dumping syndrome.

Cyproterone An antiandrogen used to treat male hypersexuality and prostatic carcinoma.

Cyst A closed sac or pouch with a definite wall containing fluid, semisolid material. *c. alveolar* Cyst at tooth apex, air containing cyst in lungs due to ruptured alveoli. *c. colloid* Cyst with gelatinous contents. *c. dentigerous* A fluid filled cyst around crown of an unerupted tooth. *c. dermoid* Cyst containing epidermal elements like hair, nail, teeth. *c. Gartner* Cyst developing from a vestigeal mesonephric duct (Gartner's duct) in female. *c. meibomian* Cyst of meibomian gland of eyelid, usually post-inflammatory. *c. nabothian* Retention cyst of nabothian glands of cervix. *c. pilonidal* Midline cyst

over sacrum lined with stratified squamous epithelium. *c. porencephalic* Anomalous cystic cavity in cortex communicating with ventricular system.

Cystadenoma An adenoma containing cyst, may be serous when filled with clear fluid or pseudomucinous when contains thick viscid fluid.

Cystathionine An intermediate compound in the metabolism of methionine to cystine.

Cysticercosis Formation of cysts by encapsulation of larvae of tapeworm (*T. solium*).

Cystic fibrosis Inherited disease of exocrine gland affecting respiratory tract, pancreas and intestine characterized by dry viscid mucus, respiratory infection, pancreatic insufficiency, increased sodium content of sweat *SYN*– mucoviscidosis.

Cystisis Inflammation of the urinary bladder.

Cystocele A prolapse of the bladder into the vagina (*see* Figure on page 178).

Cystoscopy The method of using cystoscope for the examination of bladder.

Cystotomy Incision of the urinary bladder for removal of calculi, etc. *Suprapubic c.* Incision above the pubes.

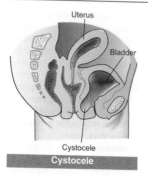

Cystocele

Cytarabine Compound of cytosine and D ribose.

Cytochrome A pigment important for cellular respiration.

Cytochrome oxidase Enzyme responsible for electron transfer from cytochromes to oxygen thus activating oxygen to combine with hydrogen to form water.

Cytochrome P450 A protein similar to Hb in the microsomes of liver cells, catalyzing metabolism of steroid hormones and detoxification of many chemicals.

Cytogenesis Origin and developments of cell.

Cytomegalic inclusion disease A viral disease that often affects fetus in utero and immunocompromised (AIDS victims) with hepatosplenomegaly, microcephaly, mental retardation.

Cytosine One of the pyrimidine bases found in Deoxyribonucleic acid. *C. arabinoside* an antimetabolite used in the treatment of acute leukaemia. Cytarabine.

D

D Symbol for *dioptre*.

Dacarbazine An alkylating agent used in treatment of malignant melanoma, Hodgkin's disease.

Dacryocystitis Inflammation of lacrymal gland.

Dacryostenosis Narrowing of lacrimal duct.

Dactylitis Chronic inflammation of phallanges and metatarsals.

Dactinomycin Antitumor antibiotic.

Dalteparin A factor Xa inhibitor, anticoagulant.

Dalton's law In a mixture of gases total pressure is equal to sum of partial pressure of each gas.

Danazol A progesterone used in endometriosis and fibroadenosis of breast.

Dance, Saint Vitus *SYN*—chorea, i.e., involuntary quasipurposive nonrepetitive jerky movements.

Dandruff Seborrhoea, exfoliation of epidermis of scalp with white greasy, dry scales.

Dandy-Walker syndrome Congenital hydrocephalus due to blockage of foramen of Luschka and Magendie.

Dane particle 42 nm sphere of hepatitis B virus.

Dantrolene A muscle relaxant.

Dapsone Diaminodiphenyl sulphone, a bacteriostatic antileprotic agent.

Daraprim Pyrimethamine, used in malaria.

Dariers disease (Keratosis follicularis) a congenital disorder characterized by verrucous papular growths that colaesce into plaques of various sizes on scalp, face, neck and trunk.

Darier's sign Burning and itching sensation in lesions of urticaria after stroking and it becomes red and raised.

Dark room Light tight room for processing X-ray films.

Dartos The subcutaneous muscle of scrotum.

Datura The plant, source of scopalamine and hyosciamine, the anticholinergic agents.

Daunorubicin Anthracycline antineoplastic antibiotic used for leukemia and malignancies.

Dawn phenomenon A phenomena in diabetes mellitus with

morning hyperglycemia due to growth hormone release.

DDT Dichlordiphenyl trichlorethane (chlorphenothane) an insecticide used in mosquito control.

Deafness Complete or partial loss of ability to hear *d. conduction* Resulting from obstruction to sound waves reaching the normal cochlea, e.g., otosclerosis, wax, eustachian catarrh. *d. perceptive* Deafness due to lesions of cochlea or cochlear nerve/nucleus.

Deamination Removal of NH_2 radicals from amino compounds. The process being oxidative or hydrolytic.

Death Permanent cessation of all vital functions including that of brain, heart, lung.

Death rate Number of deaths per 1000 population in a given time.

Death rattle Rattle sound produced by passage of air through accumulated mucous in the bronchi in terminal patients due to want of cough reflex.

Debridement Removal of foreign material along with devitalized tissue.

Debrisoquin Antihypertensive agent.

Decadron Dexamethasone, a long acting corticosteroid.

Decadurabolin Nandrolone decanoate, an anabolic steroid.

Decameter A measure of 10 meters.

Decapitation Beheading.

Decarboxylase Enzyme catalyzing release of carbondioxide from compounds like aminoacids.

Deceleration Decrease in velocity.

Decibel The unit expressing degree of intensity or loudness of sound.

Decidua Endometrium of uterus during pregnancy with outer compact layer and inner spongy layer. *d. basalis* That unites with chorion to form placenta. *d. capsularis* That surrounds chorionic sac.

Deciduoma Uterine tumor containing decidual tissue, when malignant termed choriocarcinoma.

Deciduous teeth Primary dentition of 20 teeth that erupt between 6 months and 3 years.

Deciliter 100 ml or 10 centiliter.

Decimeter 10 cm or 1/10 of meter.

Decision analysis A logically consistent approach to the common clinical problem of needing to make a decision when its consequences cannot be foretold with certainty. The biological variation, inconsistent drug response and poor clinical outcome data on many drug/therapeutic procedures make decision analysis a charter so that patient can be foretold in advance all about the possible outcome of treatment and he can choose the one he thinks best.

Decision making The process of using all the informations available about a patient and arriving at a decision concerning therapeutic plan.

Declaration of Geneva The declaration adopted in 1948 by world medical association at Geneva which reads as "At the time of being admitted as a member of medical profession I solemnly pledge my life to the service of humanity......cond..

Declaration of Hawaii The guidelines laid down by General Assembly of world psychiatric association for psychiatrists in 1976 at Hawaii.

Decline Progressively decrease.

Decoction A liquid medicinal preparation made by boiling vegetable substances with water.

Decompensation Failure of heart to maintain adequate circulation to meet oxygen demand of tissues.

Decomposition Decay, putrefaction.

Decompression illness Illness arising from rapid reduction of surrounding pressure as in sea divers suddenly coming to surface. Symptoms are due to release of dissolved nitrogen.

Decongestant Reducing congestion or swelling.

Decorticate posture The typical posture like flexed arms, clenched fists and extended legs in a comatose patient with lesion above upper brainstem.

Decortication Removal of surface layer of an organ, e.g., removal of pleura, renal capsule.

Decrudescence Decrease in the severity of symptoms of a disease.

Decubitus projection A radiographic procedure that helps in the demonstration of air-fluid levels, using decubitus position and central ray of X-ray beam placed horizontally.

Decubitus ulcer Skin ulceration due to prolonged pressure, commonly over bony prominences.

Decussation A crossing of structures in the form of X.

Dedifferentiation 1. The return of parts to a homogeneous state, 2. process by which mature differentiated cells or tissues at sites of origin of immature elements of the same type, as in some cancers.

Deduction Reasoning from general to particular.

Deep reflex Reflexes influenced by higher cortical centers, e.g., ankle, knee, supination, biceps jerks.

Deep vein thrombosis Formation of thrombus in the deep-seated veins, especially of legs, characterized by pain and tenderness in the thighs or calves; occurs primarily in patients who are immobilized for long periods, suffering from chronic debilitating diseases, cancer, or after surgery.

Defecation Bowel evacuation.

Defecation syncope Syncope occurring during or immediately after defecation.

Defeminization Loss of female sexual characteristics.

Defense Resistance to disease.

Deferens Carrying away.

Deferroxamine Iron chelating agent used in thalassaemia major, haemosiderosis.

Deferiprone Iron chelating agent.

Defibrillation Stoppage of fibrillation of heart by drugs or electrical current.

Definition The precise.

Definitive Clear and final without ambiguity.

Deformity An alteration in the natural form or alignment of an organ. *d. Akerlund* X-ray deformity of duodenal cap in duodenal ulcer. *d. boutonnière* flexion of PIP joint and hyperextension of DIP. *d. Madclung* radial deviation of hand due to overgrowth of distal ulna or shortening of radius. *d. Springel's* congenital elevation of scapula. *d. swan-neck* hyperextension of PIP joint and flexion of DIP joint (*see* Figures).

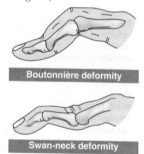

Boutonnière deformity

Swan-neck deformity

Degeneration Deterioration in organ structure or function. *d. fatty* Deposition of abnormal amounts of fat replacing normal cells. *d. calcareous* Deposition of calcium salts. *d. cystic* Degeneration with cyst formation. *d. hyaline* The degenerated tissues assume a homogeneous and glossy appearance. *d. hydropic* Appearance of water droplets in cytoplasm. *d. pigmentary* Degenerated cells change their colour. *d. spongy* Familial demyelination of deep cerebral cortex. *d. subacute combined* Degeneration of lateral and posterior columns of spinal cord as in Vit.B$_{12}$ deficiency.

Dehiscence 1. Splitting along a line or slit; 2. Separation of any suture layers of an operative wound.

Dehydration Excessive fluid loss or inadequate fluid intake resulting in haemoconcentration and renal failure.

Dehydrocholic acid A bile salt that stimulates production of bile from the liver.

Dehydrocholesterol Precursor of vit. D.

Dehydrocorticosterone Adrenal corticosteroid.

Dehydroepiandrosterone A 17 ketosteroid with androgenic activity.

Deiters' cells Supporting cells in organ of corti.

Deiter's nucleus Cell collection behind auditory nerve nucleus.

Deja entendu The illusion or experience of hearing a thing which he has previously heard.

Deja vu The illusion or experience of seeing some thing which as if has seen/experienced previously (unreasonable familiarity with person/surrounding).

Deladelaphus Twins fused above thorax, but separated below.

Deleterious Harmful.

Deletion The loss of genetic material from one chromosome.

Delinquent One with antisocial/criminal behavior.

Delirium A state of mental confusion in which patient is disoriented for time and place with illusions and hallucinations. This may occur during fever, after head injury, drug intoxication etc. *d. of persecution* Delirium in which patient feels persecuted by others. *d. tremens* Delirium in patients of chronic alcoholism following abstinence or illness. Usually benign but convulsion is a danger.

Delivery Child birth.

Deltoid ligament Internal lateral ligament of knee joint.

Deltoid muscle The prominent muscle covering shoulder—attached to deltoid ridge of humerus.

Delusion A false belief inconsistent to ones knowledge and experience, and with evidence to contrary. *d. nihilistic* Victim believes that everything has ceased to exist. *d. grandeur* Victim feels himself wealthy, rich and extraordinary and behaves so. *d. persecution* Patient feels that every body around him are against him and may persecute him. *d. reference* Delusion that causes the victim to read a meaning not intended in the acts or words of others. *d. systematized* Logical correlation with false reasoning and deduction. *d. unsystematized* Delusion without any correlation between ideas and surroundings.

Demeclocycline An antibiotic of tetracycline group.

Dementia Global impairment of intellectual function (cognition) interfering with social and occupational activities. *d. Alzheimer* dementia of gradual onset, and slow progression with delusion, delirium, depressed mood, behavioral disturbance; not due to atherosclerosis or systemic disease occurs in age below 65 (persenile). *d. subcortical* dementia due to involvement of subcortical brain structures, basal ganglia, thalamus.

Demerol Meperidine hydrochloride, opium derivative.

Demilune A crescent shaped group of serous cells forming a caplike structure over a mucous alveolus, commonly present in submandibular gland.

Demineralization Loss of minerals: calcium and phosphorus from bone.

Demography Statistical and quantitative study of characteristics of human population like size, growth, density, sex, age, etc.

Demorphinization Gradual decrease in the dose of morphine in morphine addicts.

Demulcent Soothening agent acting on mucous membrane like honey, glycerin, olive oil.

de Musset's sign Head nodding with each cardiac contraction in severe aortic incompetence.

Demutization Overcoming mutism by teaching the patient to speak or use sign language.

Demyelination Destruction of myelin sheath.

Denaturation Addition of substances to ethyl alcohol to make it toxic and unfit for human consumption.

Denatured protein A protein that has lost some of its physical and chemical properties by treatment.

Dendrite A branched protoplasmic process of a neurone that conducts impulses to cell body (*see* Figure on page 185).

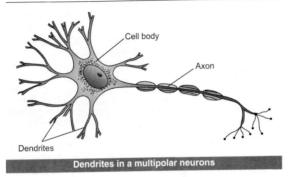

Dendrites in a multipolar neurons

Denervation Depriving a structure or organ from its nerve supply.

Dengue A group B arbovirus disease caused by bite of *Aedis egypti* mosquitoes, characterized by fever, myalgia, lymphadenopathy and often purpuric spots.

Densimeter An instrument for measuring optical density of a radiograph.

Densitometry Determining the amount of ionizing radiation to which a patient is being exposed.

Dental arch The arch formed by cutting and chewing surfaces of teeth.

Dental consonant A consonant pronounced with the tongue at or near the front upper teeth.

Dental disk The disk with abrasive powder for cutting or polishing teeth.

Dental formula A brief method of expressing the dentition of mammals.

Dental plaque A gummy mass of micro organisms and minerals that grows on the crown and causes dissolution of enamel and tooth substance.

Dental pulp The embryonic connective tissue rich in vessels and nerves occupying the central space within the tooth and its roots.

Denticle A small tooth like projection, A calcified structure within pulp of tooth.

Dental scalants Application of plastic films to the chewing surfaces of teeth to seal the pits and grooves where food and bacteria can be trapped.

Dentifrice A powder or other substance used for cleaning the teeth.

Dentin The calcified hard part of tooth surrounding the pulp chamber, covered by enamel in the crown and by cementum in the root area.

Dentinogenesis Formation of dentin in development of a tooth.

Dentition The type, number and arrangement of teeth in the dental arch (*see* Chart).

Dentulous Having one's natural teeth.

Denture Artificial teeth substituting natural teeth.

Denver development screening test Widely used assessment for screening cognitive and behavioral problems in children up to the age of 6 years.

Deodorant An agent that masks or absorbs fowl odour.

Deontology Study of professional obligations and commitments.

Chart: Eruption of deciduous (milk) teeth

Upper	Eruption	Lower	Eruption
Central incisor	5-7 Mths	Second Molar	20-30 Mths
Lateral incisor	7-10 Mths	First Molar	10-16 Mths
(Cuspid) Canine	16-20 Mths	(Cuspid) Canine	16-20 Mths
First Molar	10-16 Mths	Lateral incisor	8-11 Mths
Second Molar	20-30 Mths	Central incisor	6-8 Mths

Eruption of permanent teeth

Upper	Completed by	Lower	Completed by
Central incisor	9-10 yr	Third Molar	18-25 yr
Lateral incisor	10-11 yr	Second Molar	13-16 yr
(Cuspid) Canine	12-15 yr	Second Premolar (Bicuspid)	13-14 yr
First Premolar (Bicuspid)	12-13 yr	First Premolar (Bicuspid)	12-15 yr
Second Premolar (Bicuspid)	12-14 yr	First Molar	6-7 yr
First Molar	6-7 yr	(Cuspid) Canine	10-13 yr
Second Molar	14-16 yr	Lateral incisor	9-10 yr
Third Molar	18-25 yr	Central incisor	8-9 yr

Deoxycorticosterone A renal hormone with mineral corticoid activity.

Deoxycholic acid $C_{24}H_{40}O_4$, a bile acid.

Deoxycoformycin Anti leukemic agent.

Deoxyribonuclease Enzyme causing hydrolysis of DNA.

Deoxyribonucleic acid A protein consisting of deoxyribose, phosphoric acid, two purine bases (adenine and guanine) and two pyrimidines (thymine and cytosine), principally present in cell nucleus; principal protein of genes and chromosomes (*see* Figure).

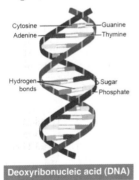

Cytosine — Guanine
Adenine — Thymine

Hydrogen bonds — Sugar
— Phosphate

Deoxyribonucleic acid (DNA)

Deoxyribose A phosphoric ester of a pentose sugar.

Dependence Psychic craving for a drug that may or may not be accompanied by physiological dependence.

Depersonalization disorder The belief that ones own reality is lost or altered.

Depilation The process of hair removal.

Depletion Removal of substances like water, electrolyte, blood from the body.

Depolarization Electrical change in excitable cell in which inside of cell becomes positive.

Depolymerization The breakdown of polymers into monomers.

Depomedrol Methyl prednisone acetate.

Depot Storage, e.g., fat depot.

Depressant Agent that depresses body function or nerve cell activity.

Depression 1. Altered mood with loss of interest in pleasurable activities, feeling of worthless, excessive guilt, self reproach, suicidal ideation. 2. lowering of a part, 3. Decrease in the activity of a vital organ. *d. bipolar* Depression with alternating periods of elation and grief. *d. endogenous* Depression without apparent cause. *d. reactive* depression Following adverse life situations. *de. Quervain's disease*

Tenosynovitis involving tendon sheaths of abductor pollicis longus and extensor pollicis brevis.

Dercum's disease SYN—Adiposis dolorosa. Painful areas of fat accumulation in menopausal women.

Dereism In psychiatry, activity and thought based on fantasy and wishes rather than logic or reason.

Derivative Derived from another.

Dermatitis Inflammation of skin, may be allergic, actinic, infective, exfoliative, etc. characterized by redness, itching etc. *d. atopic* Dermatitis of unknown etiology, usually familial mostly self limited in children, often with lichenification. *d. contact* Secondary to contact with such agents like deodorants and perfumes, usually in hypersensitive skin. *d. exfoliative* Constitutional symptoms, desquamation and extensive involvement. Pigmentation is frequent. *d. herpetiformis* Chronic inflammatory disease with vesicular, bulbous or pustular eruptions with linkage to HLA-B$_8$ and gluten. Responds to oral dapsone. *d. seborrheic* Rounded irregular or circinate lesions on scalp, eye brows, nasolabial folds with greasy, shiny yellow or yellow gray scales.

Dermatoglyphics Study of lines of hand and feet for drawing inference about one's susceptibility to disease.

Dermatome 1. Area of skin innervated by one segment of spinal cord, 2. Instrument to cut thin section of skin as in skin grafting (*see* Figure).

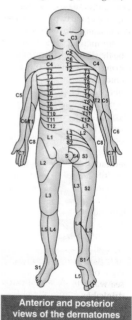

Anterior and posterior views of the dermatomes

Dermatomyositis A connective tissue disorder characterized by skin edema, dermatitis and inflammation/dysfunction of voluntary and involuntary muscles.

Dermatophobia Excessive fear about skin disease.

Dermatophyte A fungus that grows in skin or its appendage e.g., epidermophyton, trichophyton and microsporum.

Dermatophytosis Fungus infection of skin of hand and feet.

Drematosis Any disease of skin; inflammation may not be there.

Dermis The true skin below epidermis, containing nerve fibers and blood vessels.

Dermoid Resembling the skin.

Dermoid cyst A non malignant cystic tumor containing ectodermal elements like skin, hair and teeth.

Dermonosology The science of classification of skin disease.

Dermotropic Acting especially on the skin.

Dermodidymus A malformed foetus with two heads and neck but a single body and normal limbs.

Desalination Removal of salt, e.g., removal of salt from sea water to make the water drinkable.

Desaturation A process where by a saturated organic compound is converted into an unsaturated one.

Descemet's membrane Membrane between endothelial layer of cornea and substantia propria.

Desensitization Prevention of anaphylaxis usually by administering repeated small doses of the agent causing anaphylaxis/allergy.

Desert fever Coccidiodomycosis.

Desferrioxamine Iron chelating agent.

Desiccant Agent causing dryness.

Desipramine Antidepressant (tricyclic group).

Deslanoside Cardiac glycoside similar to lanatoside - C

Desmitis Inflammation of a ligament.

Desmocyte A supporting tissue cell.

Desmoid Resembling a tendon.

Desmoplasia An abnormal tendency to form fibrous tissue or adhesive bands.

Desmopressin Synthetic vasopressin analogue.

Desonide A locally acting steroid.

Desquamation Shedding of the epidermis.

Dessault's bandage Bandage for stabilizing fracture of clavicle.

Destructive Causing ruin, opposite to constructive.

Detachment Becoming separate.

Detail In radiology, the sharpness with which an image is presented on a radiograph.

Detector An instrument for determining the presence of something. *d. lie* A polygraph, an instrument for determining minor physical changes assumed to occur under stress of lying or any other emotion.

Detergent Cleansing agents, either anionic or cationic.

Deterioration Retrogression.

Determinant That which determines the character of any thing.

Determination Establishing the nature or precise identity of a substance, organism or event.

Detonation A violent noise caused by an explosive.

Detoxify To remove toxic quality of a substance. To treat toxic overdose of a drug/alcohol.

Detrition Wearing away of a part usually due to friction as that of teeth.

Detritus Degenerative matter produced by disintigration.

Detrusor External muscular coat of urinary bladder.

Detumescence Subsidence of swelling, esp. of erectile tissue like penis and clitoris.

Deuteranopia Green colour blindness.

Deuterium Heavy hydrogen with two atoms.

Developer In radiology, the solution used to make the latent image visible on the radiograph.

Developmental milestones Development of skills like crawling, sitting, laughing, walking in infants and children (*see* Table on page 191).

Deviant behavior Actions considered abnormal.

Deviation Departure from normal. *d. conjugate* Deviation of face and eyes to same side. *d. standard* In statistics, the measure of variability from the central tendency of any frequency curve. It is the square root of variance.

Device intrauterine contraceptive Devices placed in uterus to prevent contraception e.g., copper T.

Devitalization Loss of vitality; esp. anesthetizing the pulp of a tooth.

Devolution Degradation, or destructive process.

Dexamethasone Synthetic glucocorticoid.

Dexchlorpheniramine Antihistaminic (polaramine).

Dexterity Motor skill .

Table: Developmental milestones

Age	Ideal body wt.	Height	Body surface	% adult dose
Newborn	3.4 kg	50 cm	0.23 m	12.5%
1 month	4.2 kg	55 cm	0.26 m	14.5%
3 months	5.6 kg	59 cm	0.32 m	18%
6 months	7.7 kg	67 cm	0.4 m	22%
1 year	10 kg	76 cm	0.47 m	25%
3 years	14 kg	94 cm	0.62 m	33%
5 years	18 kg	108 cm	0.73 m	40%
7 years	23 kg	120 cm	0.88 m	50%
12 years	37 kg	148 cm	1.25 cm	75%

Dextrality Right handedness.

Dextran A plasma volume expander, a polysachharide fermented from sucrose.

Dextrase Enzyme splitting dextrose into lactic acid.

Dextriferron Ferric hydroxide used in treating iron deficiency.

Dextrin $(C_6H_{10}O_5)_{11}$, a carbohydrate produced during digestion of starch.

Dextroamphetamine An isomer of amphetamine, a CNS stimulant.

Dextrocardia Heart positioned in right side of thoracic cavity (*see* Figure).

Dextrocardiogram Electrocardiogram representing right ventricular forces.

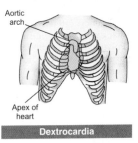

Aortic arch

Apex of heart

Dextrocardia

Dextroduction Movement of visual axis to right.

Dextromethorphan A cough suppressant.

Dextrophobia Abnormal aversion to objects on right side of body.

Dextropropoxyphene Analgesic with high addiction potency.

Dextroposition Displaced to right.

Dextrose $C_6H_{12}O_6$ (SYN-glucose), a simple monosachharose sugar.

Dextrothyroxine A thyroxine like drug used to treat type II hyperlipoproteinemia.

Diabetes A general term for diseases causing excessive urination. *d. brittle* Patient's glucose tolerance variable especially. in type I diabetes mellitus. *d. bronze* (hemochromatosis) iron storage disease with hepatomegaly, darkening of skin, pancreatic endocrine deficiency often with cardiac dysfunction. *d. insipidus* Polyuria and polydipsia due to inadequate antidiuretic hormone secretion by posterior pituitary. *d. mellitus* A disorder of carbohydrate metabolism due to either insulin deficiency, insulin resistance or insulin antibodies characterized by hyperglycemia and glycosuria. *d. nutritional* Diabetes in malnourished with pancreatic calcification.

Diabetic tabes Diabetic neuropathy with neuritic leg pain and loss of knee jerk.

Diabinese Chlorpropamide, an oral sulphonyl urea.

Diacele Third ventricle of brain.

Diacetic acid Acetoacetic acid, a ketone found in urine in diabetic ketoacidosis.

Diacerin Anti-inflammatory pain-killer.

Diacetyl morphine Heroin, strong addictive potential.

Diadochokinesia Ability to make antagonistic movements like pronation and supination in quick succession.

Diagnosis The term used to denote the name of disease or diseased process using scientific and skillful methods. *d. antenatal* Diagnostic procedures to determine the health of the fetus e.g., amniocentesis, biochemical profile (L: S ratio, estriol assay), amnioscopy, nonstress test, ultrasound, chorionic villous biopsy. *d. differential* Comparison of diseases having some what similar presentation.

Dialysate The dialysis fluid used to remove or deliver compounds or electrolytes that the failing kidney cannot excrete or retain in proper concentration.

Dialysis The process of diffusing blood across a semipermeable membrane to remove toxic materials. *d. continuous ambulatory peritoneal* Patient is put on continuous peritoneal dialysis by an implanted peritoneal catheter and attached disposable dialysate bags; a substitute to chronic haemodialysis. **d. dementia** Neurologic disturbances like speech difficulties, dementia, seizure, myoclonus, etc. after chronic dialysis, probably related to increased aluminium concentration in brain. **d. disequilibrium** The symptoms of nausea, vomiting, drowsiness, headache and seizures that appear shortly after starting hemo/peritoneal dialysis. The cause is brain edema as urea in brain remains relatively higher in comparison to serum. **d. haemo** The patient's blood and dialysate are passed in opposite directions across a semipermeable membrane (a coil, plate) in a dialysis machine. More effective than peritoneal dialysis. **d. peritoneal** Dialysis in which the lining endothelium of peritoneal cavity is used as dialysis membrane. 2 liters of dialysis fluid are introduced into peritoneal sac in 20 minutes, is retained for 20 minutes and is then drained off in 20 minutes (one cycle), 8 cycles in a day.

Diameter Distance from one point to another diagonally opposite point on the perimeter of a sphere. **d. antero-posterior of pelvic inlet** Distance between posterior surface of symphysis pubis to sacral promontory usually 11 cm in adult female. **d. antero-posterior of pelvic outlet** Distance between tip of coccyx and lower edge of symphysis pubis. **d. biparietal** Transverse diameter between parietal eminences of both sides (about 9.25 cm). **d. bitemporal** Distance between two temporal bones (about 8 cm) **d. bitrochanteric** Distance between highest point of two trochanters (useful for breech delivery) **d. bizygomatic** Distance between most prominent points of zygomatic arches. **d. cervicobregmatic** Distance between anterior frontal and junction of neck with floor of mouth. **d. diagonal conjugate** Distance from the upper part of symphysis pubis to the most distant part of brim of pelvis. **d. external conjugate** Antero-posterior diameter of pelvic inlet measured externally, i.e., distance from the skin over the upper part of symphysis pubis to the skin over a point corresponding to the sacral promontory. **d. mento bregmatic** Distance from chin to the middle of anterior fontanel. *d. occipitofrontal* Distance from posterior fontanel to the root of nose. *d. occipitomental* Greatest distance between the most prominent portion of the occiput and point of chin (13.5 cm). *d. of fetal skull* In full term fetus, the various diameters are: suboccipitobregmatic: 9.5 cm, cervicobregmatic 9.5 cm, frontomental: 8.1 cm, occipitomental: 12.7 cm. Occipitofrontal: 11.4 cm, biparietal: 9.5 cm. bitemporal: 8.1 cm (*see* Figure on page 195).

Diamox Acetazolamide, a carbonic anhydrase inhibitor.

Diapedesis Passage of blood cells esp. leukocytes by amoeboid movement through the intact wall of capillary (*see* Figure).

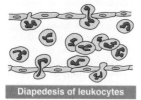

Diapedesis of leukocytes

Diaphane A very small electric light utilized in transillumination.

Diaphanography Transillumination of breast.

Diaphanometer A device for estimation of the amount of solids in a fluid by its transparency.

Diaphanoscope Device for transillumination of body cavities.

Diaphoresis Profuse sweating.

Diaphoretic Agents that increase sweating/perspiration.

Diaphragm The musculomembranous wall separating abdomen from thoracic cavity. It contracts with each inspiration permitting descent of base of lung. The attachment is to 6th rib anteriorly and 11-12th ribs posteriorly. Diaphragmatic contraction aids in defaecation, parturition and urination by increasing intraabdominal pressure. It becomes spasmodic in hiccough and sneezing. Contribution of both diaphragms to respiratory inflow is 40% and nerve supply is by phrenic nerves. *d. pelvic* Formed by levator ani and coccygeus muscles pierced in midline by vagina, urethra and rectum. *d. urogenital* Urogenital trigone or triangular ligament that lies between ischiopubic rami. It lies superficial to the pelvic diaphragm and in the male surrounds the membranous urethra; in females it

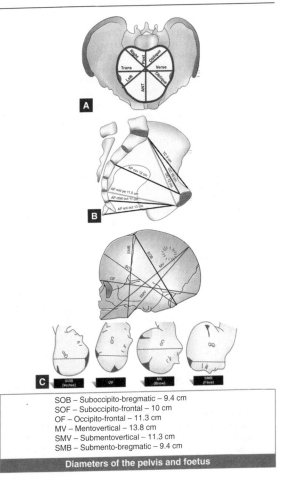

SOB – Suboccipito-bregmatic – 9.4 cm
SOF – Suboccipito-frontal – 10 cm
OF – Occipito-frontal – 11.3 cm
MV – Mentovertical – 13.8 cm
SMV – Submentovertical – 11.3 cm
SMB – Submento-bregmatic – 9.4 cm

Diameters of the pelvis and foetus

surrounds vagina. *d. contraceptive* A rubber or plastic cup that fits on to the cervix to prevent entry of sperms into uterus. *d. of microscope* The apparatus controlling illumination in the instrument.

Diaphysis The middle part of long bone (*see* Figure).

Diapophysis An upper articular surface of transverse process of vertebra.

Diarrhea Frequent passage of unformed watery stool due to inflammation, irritation, retention, emotion, etc. *d. traveler's* Diarrhoea in travellers due to *E. coli.*

Diascope A glass plate held against the skin for examining superficial lesions. Erythema-tous lesions blanch but not haemorrhagic lesions.

Diastage The enzyme converting starch to sugar.

Diastasis The last part of diastole, of 0.2 second duration and is immediately followed by atrial contraction.

Diastole That period of cardiac cycle (usually of 0.5 sec) during which the heart dilates, ventricles fill with blood.

Diastolic pressure The period of least pressure in the arterial vascular system.

Diathermy The therapeutic use of a high frequency current to generate heat within some part of body. *d. short-wave* Employs wavelengths of 3-30 meters. *d. surgical* Diathermy of high frequency

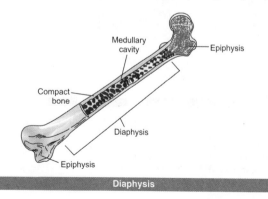

Medullary cavity

Epiphysis

Compact bone

Diaphysis

Epiphysis

Diaphysis

for electrocoagulation or cauterization.

Diathrosis A hinge joint.

Diatom One group of unicellular microscopic algae seen in lungs of patients with antemortem drowning.

Diatrizoate meglumine Radioopaque dye for arterial use (gastrograffin).

Diatrizoate sodium Radioopaque dye for visualisation of bladder, urinary tract, reproductive system.

Diaxon A neurone having two axons.

Diazepam Antianxiety benzdiazepine useful in treatment of cocaine poisoning, status epilepticus, convulsion and a variety of anxiety disorders valium.

Diazo reaction A deep red colour in urine produced by action of ammonia and p-diazobenzene sulfuric acid on aromatic substances of urine.

Diazoxide Drug used IV to treat hypertensive crisis and hypoglycemia.

Dibasic Substance with two atoms of hydrogen in each molecule replaceable by a base.

Dibenzyline Trade name for phenoxybenzamine.

Dibucaine hydrochloride Local anaesthetic similar to cocaine.

Dicalcium Phosphate Dibasic calcium phosphate, used for calcium supplement.

Dichloramine A germicide, disinfectant containing chlorine.

Dichlorphenamide Carbonic anhydrase inhibitor used for glaucoma.

Dichotomy Dividing into two parts.

Dichromation Ability to distinguish only two primary colours, i.e., red and green.

Dick test A skin test for susceptibility to scarlet fever similar to shick test for diphtheria.

Diclofenac Analgesic-anti inflammatory agent.

Dicloxacillin sodium A semisynthetic penicillin for treatment of penicillinase resistant staphylococci.

Dicophane DDT.

Dicrotic Relates to a double pulse.

Dicrotic notch The notch on descending limb of pulse wave.

Dicrotic wave The positive wave following dicrotic notch.

Dicumarol An anticoagulant that increases prothrombin time.

Dicyclomine An anticholinergic agent.

Didactic Pertains to teaching by lectures or texts as

opposed to clinical or bedside teaching.

Didactylism Congenital condition in which there are only 2 digits on a hand or foot

Didelphic Pertains to double uterus.

Didymitis Inflammation of testicle.

Didymodynia Pain in the testicle.

Dieldrin A chlorinated hydrocarbon used as insecticide.

Diencephalon The portion of brain encompassing epithalamus, thalamus, metathalamus and hypothalamus.

Dienestrol Synthetic estrogen.

Dientamoeba fragilis Parasitic ameba inhabiting small intestine and causing diarrhoea.

Diet Food substances normally consumed in the course of living. *d. balanced* Diet adequate in energy providing all tissue building materials, vitamins and proteins. *Bland d.* One that is free from any irritating or stimulating foods. *Elemental d.* One consisting of a well-balanced, residue-free mixture of all essential and non-essential amino acids, combined with simple sugars, electrolytes, trace elements and vitamins. *Elimination d.* One for diagnosis of food allergy, based on omission of foods that might cause symptoms in the patient. *High-calorie d.* One that furnishes more calories than needed to maintain weight, often more than 3500-4000 kcal/day. *High-fibre d.* One relatively high in dietary fibre, which decreases bowel transit time and relieves constipation. *High-protein d.* One containing large amounts of protein, consisting largely amounts of protein, consisting largely of meats, fish, milk, legumes and nuts. *Hospital d.* a routine diet plan, provided in a hospital, that includes general, soft and liquid diets and modifications of them to suit the needs of specific patients. *Ketogenic d.* One containing large amounts of fat (*see also* ketogenic (diet). *Liquid d.* A diet limited to liquids or to foods that can be changed to a liquid state (*see also* liquid (diet)). *Low-calorie d.* one containing fewer calories than needed to maintain weight, e.g. less than 1200 kcal/day for an adult. *Low-fat d.* One containing limited amounts of fat. *Low-residue d.* One with a minimum of cellulose and fibre and restriction of the connective tissue found in certain cuts of meat. It is prescribed for irritations of the intestinal tract, after surgery of the large intestine, in partial intestinal obstruction, or when limited bowel movements are desirable, as in colostomy patients. Called also low-fibre diet.

Dietetics The science of applying the principles of nutrition to the feeding of individuals or groups.

Diethazine hydrochloride Anticholinergic used in treatment of Parkinsonism.

Diethylcarbamazine Antifilarial agent.

Diethylpropion An adrenergic drug with actions similar to amphetamine.

Diethylstilbestrol Synthetic estrogen.

Diethyltoluamide Insect repellant.

Diethyltryptamine Hallucinogenic agent.

Dietitian A person experienced in field of nutrition and dietetic advice.

Dietl's crisis Renal colic from partial obstruction of ureter.

Dieulafoy's triad Tenderness, muscular rigidity and skin hyperesthesia at Mc Burney's point in acute appendicitis.

Differential blood count Determination of number of each variety of leukocytes in one micro litre of blood.

Diffraction The deflection that occurs when light rays are passed through crystals, prisms or other deflecting media.

Diffusion A process by which various gases intermingle as a result of incessant motion of their molecule i.e., there is always a tendency of molecule or substances (gas, liquid, solid) to move from a region of high concentration to a low concentration.

Diflunisal A salicylic acid derivative that, like aspirin, has analgesic and anti-inflammatory properties, but fewer side-effects than aspirin, does not affect bleeding time or function and has a long half-life that permits twice daily dosage.

Digestion The process by which food is broken down by enzymatic action into absorbable forms.

Digital radiography Radiography using computerized imaging instead of conventional film or screen imaging.

Digital reflex Sudden flexion of terminal phalanx when nail is suddenly tapped.

Digitalis Cardiotonic glycoside that increases myocardial contraction and refractory period of A-V node.

Digitoxin Cardiotonic glycoside.

Dihydroergotamine Vasoconstrictor used in migraine.

Dihydrosphingosine An amino alcohol present in sphingo lipids.

Dihydrotachysterol A sterol obtained by irradiation of ergosterol and functions as Vit D.

Dihydroaluminium aminoacetate An antacid.

Dihydroxycholecalciferol Sterols with hormonal properties akin to vit D e.g., calcitrol.

Diiodohydroyquin Iodoquinol.

Diktyoma Tumor of ciliary epithelium.

Dilantin A derivative of glyceryl urea (diphenyl hydantoin sodium) used as antiepileptic, best for clonic/toxic clonic seizure.

Dilatation Expansion of a vessel or an orifice.

Dilation and Curettage Cervical canal dilatation and scraping of uterine cavity.

Dilation and evacuation Cervical canal dilatation and evacuation of product of conception by suction/forcep.

Dilators Instruments used to dilate canals, cavities or openings (*see* Figure).

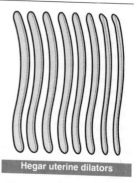

Hegar uterine dilators

Diltiazem Calcium channel blocker, useful for ischaemic heart disease.

Dimenhydrinate A drug for control of dizziness, vomiting and nausea.

Dimercaprol Used as an antidote for gold, arsenic, mercury etc. injected IM mixed with benzyl benzoate and alcohol.

Dimethicone A silicone oil used to protect the skin against water soluble irritants.

Dimethindene maleate Antihistamine.

Dimethisterone Progesterone compound.

Dimethylphthalate An insect repellant.

Dimethyl sulfoxide A solvent used to facilitate absorption of medicines through the skin.

Dimethyltryptamine An agent with properties similar to hallucinogens like LSD.

Dimple sign A sign used to differentiate dermatofibroma from malignant nodular melanoma. Upon application of lateral pressure, the dermatofibroma will dimple or become indented, but melanoma protrudes above plane of skin.

Dinoprost tromethamine A drug causing uterine contraction hence used to induce abortion.

Dioctyl calcium, sodium/potassium/sulfosuccinate A stool softener.

Diopter Refractory power of lens with focal length at 1 meter.

Diosmin Antithrombotic, anticoagulant.

Dioxybenzone Chemical for protecting skin from sun.

Dipeptidase An enzyme that catalyzes the hydrolysis of dipeptides to amino acids.

Diphemanil methyl sulfate An anticholinergic agent used for treatment of peptic ulcer.

Diphenhydramine hydrochloride Antihistamine, (Benadryl).

Diphenoxylate Antidiarrheal agent smooth muscle relaxant (Lomotil).

Diphenyl hydantoin sodium Anti convulsant.

Diphenyl pyraline An antihistamine.

Diphonia Simultaneous production of two voice tones.

2-3 diphosphoglycerate An organic phosphate that effects affinity of haemoglobin for RBC and is depleted in stored blood.

Diphtheria Acute infectious disease, characterized by fever, sore throat, cervical lymphadenopathy and formation of gray pseudomembrane at the site of infection i.e. tonsil, pharynx larynx nose etc. Causative agent is club shaped bacillus, coryne bacterium diphtheriae.

Diphtheroid Resembling diphtheria or diphtheria bacillus.

Diphyllobothrium Genus of tape worm, D-latum is fish tapeworm infesting humans, causing B_{12} deficiency.

Diplegia Paralysis of legs and hands of one side.

Diploe Spongy tissue between the two layers of compact bone.

Diploid Having two sets of chromosomes.

Diplomyelia Doubling of spinal cord due to a length wise fissure, often seen in patients of spina bifida.

Diplopia Double vision. *d. binocular* Double vision

occurring when both eyes are used due to diseases of cranial nerves, cerebrum. *d. monocular* Double vision with one eye open (hysterics). *d. uncrossed* SYN—homonymous diplopia; each image appears on the same side as the eye that sees the image. *d. crossed* Images are on the side opposite to the eye that sees the image. *d. vertical* Diplopia with one of the two images higher than other.

Dipole Two equal and opposite charges separated by a distance.

Dipsomania A morbid craving for alcohol.

Dipstic A chemical impregnated paper strip used for analysis of chemical constituents in urine.

Direct current An electric current flowing continuously in one direction only.

Direct light reflex Contraction of pupil on focussing a light beam on it.

Directly observed therapy Strategy for ensuring a patient's compliance with a therapy in which there is oral administration of a drug to a patient and observing that each dose of prescribed drug is swallowed.

Dirofilaria A genus of micro filaria.

Disaccharidase Carbohydrate composed of two monosaccharides e.g., sucrose.

Discitis Inflammation of inter vertebral disk.

Disconnection syndrome Disturbances of visual and language functions due to section of corpus callosum or occlusion of anterior cerebral artery, manifesting as inability to match an object held in one hand with that in the other when eyes are closed.

Discordance In genetics, the expression of a trait in only one of the twin pair.

Discrete Separate, distinct.

Discrimination The process of distinguishing or differentiating. *d. tonal* Ability to distinguish one tone from the other, a function dependent upon integrity of transverse fibers of the basilar membrane in organ of Corti. *d. two point* Ability to localize two points of pressure when applied to skin as separate sensations.

Disdiadochokinesia Inability to make quick alternating movements like pronation and supination common to cerebellar disease.

Disease Literally the lack of ease, or illness/suffering. *d. autoimmune* A state of immune aberration where body produces antibodies against healthy host tissues as in some cases of glomerulonephritis, haemolytic anaemia, rheumatoid arthritis, myasthenia gravis, thyrotoxicosis, SLE, scleroderma etc. *d. heavy chain* Diseases in which heavy chain production of immunoglobulins is in excess. IgA chain excess manifests with abdominal lymphoma and malabsorption, IgM with repeated bacterial infections, lymphadenopathy and Ig D chain with picture similar to multiple myeloma. *d. hereditary* Where disease is transmitted from parent to offspring. *d. motor neurone* There is degeneration of anterior horn cells of spinal cord, cranial nerve nuclei in the brain stem, and pyramidal tracts. e.g., progressive muscular atrophy, amyotropic lateral sclerosis. *d. psychosomatic* Psychological factors contribute to initiation or exacerbation of the disease e.g., asthma, tension headache, neurodermatitis, peptic ulcer, etc.

Disengagement The emergence of foetal head from within the maternal pelvis.

Disinfectant A substance that prevents infection by killing pathogenic organisms.

Disinfection The process of making rooms/linens/organs germ free. The common methods of disinfection are by autoclaving, boiling in water, ethylene oxide/formaldehyde gas, alcohol, iodine, phenols etc.

Disinfestation The process of killing infesting insects/parasites.

Disintegration The falling apart of constituents of a substance.

Disk A circular or rounded flat plate. *d. articular* pad of fibrocartilage in synovial joints. *d. Bowman's* disk like plates that make up striated muscle fibers. *d. intercalated* dense bands running between myocardial cells both transversely and longitudinally (*see* Figure on page 204).

Dislocation Displacement of any part. *d. monteggia* Dislocation of the hip in which the head of femur lies near anterosuperior spine of ileum. *d. Nelaton's* Dislocation of ankle in which talus is forced up between the end of the tibia and fibula (*see* Figure on page 205).

Dismutase superoxide An enzyme that destroys superoxide (O_2^-) formed by flavo

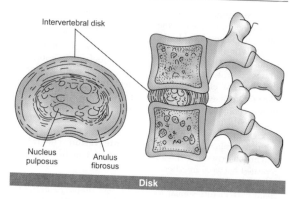

Intervertebral disk

Nucleus pulposus

Anulus fibrosus

Disk

enzymes. The enzyme protects aerobic bacteria from superoxide being present in them. Now being used for myocardial protection soon after infarction.

Disodium edetate A chelating agent used to treat hypercalcemia.

Disopyramide phosphate Antiarrhythmic agent of class II.

Disorientation Inability to be aware of time, place and person.

Dispensary Place for dispensation of drugs.

Disperate Suspension of finely divided particles in liquid.

Dispersion Dissipation or disappearance of colloid in a fluid.

Dispersonalization Mental state in which individual denies presence of some of his bodyparts or personality.

Displacement Removal from normal place. In psychiatry, transference of emotion from the original idea with which it was associated to a different idea.

Disposition Individuals aptitude, behavior as sum total of such evident characteristics.

Disproportion A part being different in size from that considered to be normal.

Dissect To split, to go into detail, to separate various parts of cadaver.

Dissection The cutting of parts for purpose of separation and study.

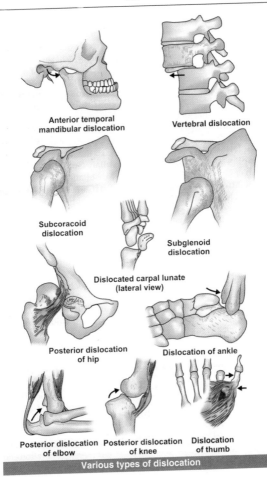

Anterior temporal
mandibular dislocation

Vertebral dislocation

Subcoracoid
dislocation

Subglenoid
dislocation

Dislocated carpal lunate
(lateral view)

Posterior dislocation
of hip

Dislocation of ankle

Posterior dislocation
of elbow

Posterior dislocation
of knee

Dislocation
of thumb

Various types of dislocation

Disseminated Scattered or widely distributed.

Disseminated intravascular coagulation A coagulation disorder with bleeding tendency due to consumption of clotting factors and platelets due to thrombin generation in blood stream (*see* Figure).

Dissipation Dispersion of matter.

Dissociation Separation of complex compounds into simpler ones.

Dissociation AV Atria and ventricles beat independently as sinus node impulse does not reach the ventricle. *d. of personality* Split in consciousness resulting in two different phases of personality, neither being aware of words, acts or feelings of others.

Dissolution Breaking up the integrity of anatomical entity.

Dissolve Dispersion of a solid within a liquid.

Dissonance Disagreement.

Distal Farthest from the center, from a medial line.

Distance Space between two objects. *d. focal* Distance from the optical center of lens to focal point.

Distend To stretch; to inflate.

Distensibility The property of being stretchable.

Distichiasis Maldirection of eye lashes, commonly directed inwards.

Distillate Substance obtained by distillation.

Distillation Condensation of vapor that has been obtained from a liquid heated to volatilization point.

Distome A fluke with two suckers.

Distomiasis Infestation with flukes.

Distortion Change from regular to irregular/altered shape.

Distractibility Inability to focus ones attention or mental wandering.

Distraction State of mental confusion.

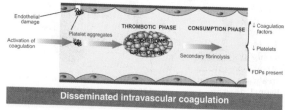

Disseminated intravascular coagulation

Distraught The mental state of being deeply troubled, having conflicting thoughts.

Distress Physical or mental agony.

Distribution The lay out pattern, or spreading/supply of nerve, blood vessels, etc.

Districhiasis Two hairs growing from the same hair follicle.

Disulfiram Drug used to create aversion from alcohol.

Diuresis Passage of large amounts of urine.

Diuretic An agent that increases formation of urine.

Diurnal Daily.

Divalent A molecule with two electric charges.

Divalproex Antiepileptic.

Divergence Separation from a common center.

Diverticulum A pouch or sac in the wall of a hollow organ. *d. false* Diverticulum without muscular coats in the wall of the pouch. *d. Meckel's* Diverticulum due to persistence of omphalomesenteric duct. *d. of colon* Most are asymptomatic and cause symptom when inflamed. *d. of jejunum and duodenum* Diverticulum commonly located near entrance of common bileduct and pancreatic duct into duodenum. Jejunal diverticula are usually symptomatic and cause

severe bleeding. *d. Zenker: See:* Zanker's diverticulum (*see* Figure).

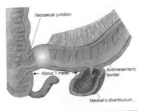

Meckel's diverticulum

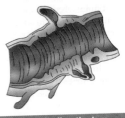

Colonic diverticulum

Diving reflex Emersion in cold water or sprinkling of cold water on body causes parasympathetic stimulation with reduced cardiac output and increasing A-V block. Hence used to treat paroxysmal supraventricular tachycardia.

Division Separation into parts.

Divulsion Forcibly pulling apart.

Dizygotic twins Twins who are products of two ova.

Dizziness A sensation of unsteadiness or whirling.

DNA probe A method of identifying defective genes and genetic constitution of a cell through employment of recombinant DNA technology.

Dobutamine A betadrenergic agonist, used in hypotension.

Doctor To teach, A person qualified to practice medicine. *d. bare foot* A practitioner of traditional or native medicine in China who have not attended any medical school.

Doctrine The system of principles taught or advocated.

Docusate sodium A stool softner.

Dohle bodies Inclusions in neutrophils as seen in burn, trauma, infection and neoplastic diseases.

Dolicocephalic Having a skull with long anteroposterior diameter.

Dolicomorphic A long and slender body (ectomorph).

Doll's head maneuver A test to know brainstem damage in comatose patients. Normally eyes more together to the opposite side of head rotation.

Dolophine hydrochloride Methadone.

Dolor Pain, principal component of inflammation. Other are rubor (redness), tumor (swelling), color (heat) and loss of function.

Dolorimeter Device for measurement of degree of pain.

Domiciliary Carried on in a house.

Dominance 1. Genetic quality through which one gene of pair of allele expresses, while the other is suppressed. 2. Preferred hand or side of body. 3. In psychiatry the tendency to control others.

Domperidone Antiemetic increases gastric motility, useful in dyspepsia.

Donath-Landsteiner phenomenon A test for paroxysmal cold haemoglobinuria where cold haemolysin combines to RBCs at 5°C and upon warming these red cells haemolyze.

Donnan's equilibrium A equilibrium is established between two solutions separated by a semipermeable membrane so that the sum of anions and cations on one side is equal to that on otherside.

Donor One who donates blood, tissue or an organ for use in another person. *d. universal* One with blood group 'O' which is compatible with blood of all other persons, though this is not universally true as there are many other blood antigens besides A, B, and O.

Donovan body Organism of granuloma inguinale. i.e., *Chlamydia trachomatis*.

Dopa 3:4 dihydroxy phenylalanine, produced by oxidation of tyrosine by tyrosinase.

Dopamine hydrochloride A vasopressor catecholamine and neurotransmitter, also implicated in some forms of psychosis and abnormal movement disorder.

Doping In sports medicine, use of drugs to improve sports performance; commonly androgenic anabolic steroids.

Doppler A method to measure blood flow in arteries and veins.

Doraphobia Aversion to touching the hair or fur of animals.

Dorllo's canal A bony canal in the tip of temporal bone enclosing abducens nerve.

Dorsal Pertains to back, opposite of ventral.

Dorsal nerves Branches of spinal nerves that pass dorsally to innervate structures near to vertebral column.

Dorsal slit A surgical method of making the foreskin of penis easily retractable. The foreskin is cut in dorsal midline but not far enough to extend to mucous membrane next to glans.

Dorsiflexion Bending a part towards posterior aspect of body (*see* Figure).

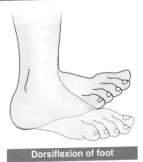

Dorsiflexion of foot

Dosage Pertains to quantity, frequency and number of doses of a drug/radiation.

Dose Amount of medicine/radiation to be given at one time. *d. absorbed* Dose of ionizing radiation imparted to a tissue or target. *d. cumulative* Total dose of radiation resulting from repeated exposures. *d. maximum permissible* The maximum amount of radiation exposure permitted to person whose occupation requires working with radioactive agents. *d. therapeutic* Dose required to produce therapeutic effect.

Dose calculation for children
Young's formula

$$\frac{\text{Age in years}}{\text{Age} + 12} \times \text{adult dose or}$$

Body surface area of child/1.7 × adult dose.

Dose response curve A graph showing the degree of effect of a drug in relation to its doses.

Dosimeter Device for measuring radiation.

Dothiepin Antidepressant.

Double blind technique A method of scientific investigation in which neither the subject nor the investigator knows what treatment the subject is receiving. The code is only broken at the end of completion of treatment.

Double contrast examination Radiographic examination in which both a radio-opaque and a radioluscent contrast medium are used simultaneously to visualize internal anatomy.

Double personality Dual personality seen in hysteria and schizophrenia.

Douche A current of vapour or - stream of hot/cold water directed against a part. *d. vaginal* Douche of vagina is used for deodorant, antiseptic, stimulating or haemostatic purposes. Douching in healthy women is not warranted as it may alter vaginal pH and flora predisposing to vaginitis.

Douglas fold The arcuate line of the sheath of rectus muscle.

Douglas pouch Peritoneal space lying between uterus and front of rectum.

Down's syndrome Congenital anomaly due to trisomy 21 manifesting with mental retardation, skeletal anomalies and light yellow spots at periphery of iris (*see* Figure).

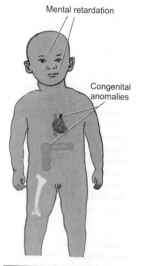

Down's syndrome

Doxapram Respiratory stimulant.

Doxepin Tricyclic-antidepressant.

Doxorubicin Anthracycline antitumor antibiotic.

Doxycycline Broad spectrum tetracycline used in b.i.d dose.

Doxylamine A sedative.

Dracontiasis *SYN* – Dracunculiasis i.e., infestation with d. medinesis.

Drain To draw off a fluid, exit or tube for discharge of body fluid.

Drainage The free flow of fluid from a wound/cavity. *d. closed* Drainage without access of air into drained site via the tube. *d. negative pressure* Drainage where negative pressure is maintained within the tube, e.g., pneumothorax drainage. *d. open* Drainage without exclusion of air. *d. postural* Drainage of sinuses and bronchi by gravity (*see* Figure on page 212).

Dramamine Diphenhydramine, an agent for vertigo.

Dramatism Dramatic behavior and lofty speech as in lunatics.

Drastic Acting strongly.

Draught A liquid medicinal dose to be gulped at once; drink.

Draw sheet The rubber cloth spread on the bed to protect the mattress and linen from drainage and soilage.

Drawer sign Sign of cruciate ligament rupture of knee.

Drepanocyte Resembling sickle cell.

Dressing Protective or supportive covering for injured part. *d. occlusive* Dressing that seals the wound completely thus preventing infection and also preventing moisture from the wound escaping through the dressing. *d. pressure* Dressing that applies pressure on the wound, e.g., following skin grafting.

Drift Movement due to an external force, in an aim less fashion.

Drill (*SYN*-burr) Device for rotating sharp cutting instrument e.g., cavity preparation in dentistry.

Drip Infusion of a liquid drop by drop. *d. post nasal* Post nasal discharge as in chronic sinusitis.

Dromostanolone An antineoplastic agent.

Dromotropic Fibers in cardiac nerves influencing conduction.

Dronabinol Synthetic tetrahydrocanabinol, a psychoactive substance.

Droperidol A neuroleptic, sedative and tranquilizer.

Droplet infection Infected particles coming as spray from patient's mouth and nose.

Dropsy Generalized edema.

Drotaverine Antispasmodic.

Drowning Asphyxiation due to immersion in liquid.

Drowsiness The state of almost falling asleep.

Drug abuse Self administered drug overuse.

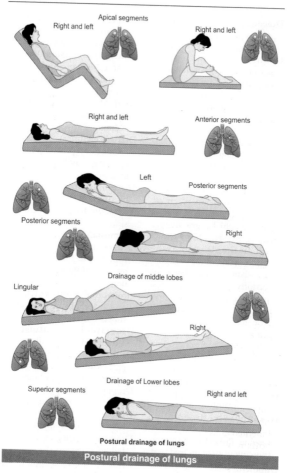

Postural drainage of lungs

Postural drainage of lungs

Drug addiction A condition caused by excessive or continued use of habit forming drugs.

Drug dependence A psychic and often physical dependence upon a drug.

Drug fever Fever caused by drugs.

Drug interaction Interaction between drugs taken concurrently.

Drug rash Rash produced in some individuals by intake or application of drugs.

Drug reaction Adverse and undesired reactions to a substance.

Drug receptors The protein molecules on cell surface that bind to a particular drug and then activate a series of reactions through which the drug produces the desired pharmacological effect.

Drunkenness Alcoholic intoxication with blood ethyl alcohol level exceeding 0.3-0.4%.

Drusen Small hyaline, globular pathological growths formed on Descemet's membrane.

Duazomycin Glutamine antagonist, anticancer drug.

Dubin-Johnson syndrome Inherited defect of bile metabolism with conjugated hyperbilirubinemia.

Dubowitz score A method to assess a newborn clinically,

up to 5 days after birth, to determine infant's maturity and gestational age by neurological and other physical criteria.

Duchenne's muscular dystrophy Most common fatal genetic disorder caused by the mutation of gene that code for dystrophin and is characterized by muscular dystrophy that worsens quickly.

Ducrey's bacillus Small rod shaped organism found in pairs, causative agent of soft sore.

Duct A narrow tubular vessel or channel to convey secretions from gland. *d. alveolar* A branch of respiratory bronchiole that leads to alveolar sacs of lungs. *d. commonbile* Duct formed by joining of hepatic duct with cystic duct and draining to duodenum at ampulla of vater. *d. endolymphaticus* Duct connecting endolymphatic sac with the utricle and saccule. *d. Gartner* A remnant of wolfian duct extending from parovarium through the broad ligament into vagina. *d. lacrymal* Two ducts, superior and inferior draining tear from eye into lacrymal sac. *d. mesonephric* Duct in embryo connecting mesonephros with the cloaca. In the male, it develops into reproductive ducts. *d.*

mullerian Ducts in the embryo that form the uterus, vagina and fallopian tubes. *d. right lymphatic* Duct draining lymph from right side of body above diaphragm into right innominate vein. *d's of Skene's* Two slender ducts of skene's glands that open on either side of female urethral orifice. *d. thoracic* The left lymphatic duct that drains the lymph from body below diaphragm and the left thorax into left innominate vein (*see* Figure).

Ductus arteriosus The channel communicating ascending aorta to left pulmonary artery in the fetus.

Ductus venosus The duct through which the umbilical vein drains into inferior vena cava in fetus.

Duffy system A blood grouping system.

Duloxetine Antidepressant.

Dumping syndrome Dumping of stomach contents into the intestine manifesting with weakness and sweating soon after food in patient's of gastrojejunostomy.

Duodenal bulb First part of duodenum beyond pylorus.

Dupuytren contracture Contracture of palmar fascia causing flexion deformity of ring and fifth fingers.

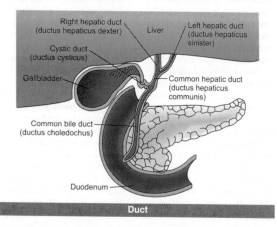

Right hepatic duct (ductus hepaticus dexter)

Liver

Left hepatic duct (ductus hepaticus sinister)

Cystic duct (ductus cysticus)

Gallbladder

Common hepatic duct (ductus hepaticus communis)

Common bile duct (ductus choledochus)

Duodenum

Duct

Dura mater The outer membrane covering the brain and spinal cord.

Duritis SYN—pachymeningitis, inflammation of dura.

Duroziez murmur Systolic and diastolic murmur heard over an artery when pressure is applied just distal to stethoscope.

Dust Minute fine particles of earth. *d. ear* Fine calcareous bodies found in gelatinous substance of otolith membrane of ear. *d. house* Matters included in house dust are mites, hairs, pollen, and smoke particles.

Dutasteride Antiandrogen for prostatic hypertrophy.

Dwarf An abnormally short or undersized person. *d. achondroplastic* Normal trunk, small extremities, large head and prominent buttocks.

Dyclonine hydrochlorides A topical anaesthetic.

Dye Any colored or colouring agent, employed for staining slides for histopathological examination or manifacturing test reagents.

Dynamic Pertains to vital force or inherent power; opposite of static.

Dynamograph Device for recording muscular strength.

Dyne Force needed for imparting acceleration of 1 cm. per second to a 1 gm mass.

Dynorphins An endogenous opioid peptide.

Dysacusis Difficulty in hearing, dycomfort caused by loud noise.

Dysarthria Difficulty in articulation or speech.

Dysautonomia A hereditary disease involving autonomic nervous system characterized by motor inco-ordination, fluctuating blood pressure, mental retardation, etc.

Dysbasia Difficulty in walking.

Dyscalculia Inability to solve mathematical problems.

Dysdiadochokinesia Inability to perform quick alternating movements.

Dysentery Inflammation of mucosal lining of GI tract with passage of blood, pus and mucus in stool. The causative agent may be chemical irritants, bacteria, protozoa, viruses or parasitic worms. *Amoebic d.* common in tropical countries; caused by protozoon *Entamoeba histolytica*. Spread is decreased in placed with high standards of hygiene and sanitation. A notifiable disease in the UK. Called also amoebiasis. *Bacillary d.* The most common and acute form of the disease, caused by bacteria of the genus *Shigella*.

Dysesthesia Abnormal sensation on the skin with

tingling, numbness, burning etc.

Dysgammaglobulinemia Disproportion in the concentration of gammaglobulins in blood.

Dysgenesis Defective development.

Dysgerminoma Malignant neoplasm of ovary.

Dysgeusia Impairment or perversion of gustatory sense so that normal taste is interpreted as being unpleasant.

Dysgraphia Difficulty in writing.

Dyshidrosis Disorder of sweating; recurrent vesicular eruption on the limbs with intense itching (pompholyx).

Dyskeratosis Altered keratinization of epithelial cells of epidermis, characteristic of many skin disorders.

Dyskinesia Defect in voluntary movement. *d. tardive* Slow rhythmical, involuntary stereotyped movements especially with use of psychotropic drugs.

Dyslexia Inability to interpret written language even though vision is normal.

Dyslogia This refers to difficulty in expression of ideas or impairment of the ability to reason or think logically. This is usually due to a lesion of central nervous system.

Dysmaturity *SYN* — small-for-date infants, intrauterine growth retardation; infant's weight is less for his length or age.

Dysmyelia This refers to a group of disorders associated with congenital malformation of the upper and lower extremities. These disorders are usually characterized by hypoplasia or partial and total aplasia of the tubular bones of the extremities or complete loss of an extremity.

Dysmenorrhoea Painful menstruation. *d. congestive* Caused by pelvic congestion. *d. membranous* Passage of uterine casts causing pain. *d. spasmodic* Spasmodic uterine contractions causing pain.

Dysmetria Rapid jerky movement as patient is unable to control range and strength of muscular contraction, as seen in cerebellar disease.

Dysmorphia Dysmorphia refers to a deformity or an abnormality in shape.

Dysostosis Defect in ossification.

Dysoxia Inability of mitochondria to utilize oxygen properly.

Dyspareunia Painful sexual intercourse.

Dyspepsia Imperfect digestion with abdominal bloating,

heart burn, flatulence, anorexia nausea etc. can be gastric, hepatic, biliary, alcoholic in origin.

Dysphagia Difficulty in deglutition, can be due to spasm of pharyngoesophageal musculature, stricture, neoplasm, paralysis.

Dysphasia Impairment of speech both articulation and comprehension.

Dysphonia Difficulty in speaking but comprehension is normal; hoarseness.

Dysphoria Excessive depression feeling without apparent cause.

Dysplasia Abnormal tissue growth/differentiation. *d. ectodermal* Absence of sweat glands, hair follicles and abnormality of nail, teeth, and mental development. *d. monostotic* Replacement of bone by fibrous tissue. *d. polyostotic fibrous* Replacement of bone by vascular fibrous tissue with bone deformity and fracture.

Dyspnea Labored or difficulty in breathing either due to vigorous physical activity, anemia, cardiac or pulmonary disease.

Dyspraxia A disturbance in the programming, control and execution of volitional movements.

Dyssynergia Difficulty in proper muscular co-ordination.

Dystocia Difficult labor, can be due to abnormal passage (small outlet), passenger (large foetus) or power (uterine inco-ordination).

Dystonia Increased muscle tone. *d. musculum deformans* Progressive disorder of childhood with distorted twisting body movements.

Dystopia Displacement of any organ.

Dystrophy Defective muscle power, nutrition and metabolism. *d. Landouzy-Dejerine* Childhood progressive muscular dystrophy involving muscles of shoulder girdle, face characterized by myopathic facies, inability to raise arms above head, inability to whistle. *d progressive muscular* Familial disease with atrophy of muscles, occurring at early childhood. *d pseudohypertrophic muscular* Affected muscles are bulky but weak at the beginning but ultimately become atrophic.

Dysuria Painful micturition either due to concentrated acid urine, urinary crystals/concretions, urinary infections, pelvic pathology and prolapse uterus.

Eales' disease Retinal vein thrombophlebitis with recurrent hemorrhages into retina and vitreous.

Ear The organ of hearing and of equilibrium (*see* Figures). It consists of three parts: (a) the *external e.*, made-up of the expanded portion, or pinna, and the auditory canal, separated from the middle ear by the drum, or tympanum; (b) the *middle e.*, an irregular cavity containing three small bones (incus, malleus and stapes) that link the tympanic membrane to the internal ear; it also communicates with the pharyngotympanic tube and the mastoid cells; (c) the *internal e.*, which consists of a bony and a membranous labyrinth (the cochlea and semicircular canals).

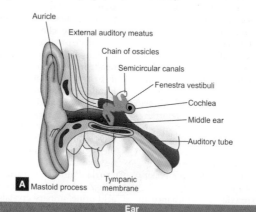

Auricle
External auditory meatus
Chain of ossicles
Semicircular canals
Fenestra vestibuli
Cochlea
Middle ear
Auditory tube
A Mastoid process
Tympanic membrane

Ear

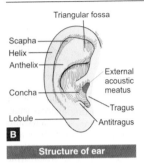

Triangular fossa
Scapha
Helix
Anthelix
Concha
Lobule
External acoustic meatus
Tragus
Antitragus

B

Structure of ear

Ear dust Calcareous concretions in the membranous labyrinth.

Ear plug Device for plugging the external auditory canal, thereby preventing access of sound to internal ear.

Earwax Sticky honey coloured cerumen secreted by glands at outer one-third of ear canal mixed with dust.

Eaton agent Mycoplasma pneumoniae.

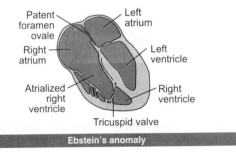

Patent foramen ovale
Right atrium
Atrialized right ventricle
Left atrium
Left ventricle
Right ventricle
Tricuspid valve

Ebstein's anomaly

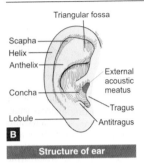

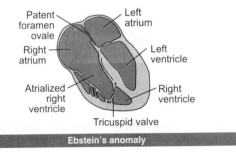

Eccrine sweat glands Sweat glands of skin with density of over 400 per sq. cm. on the palms and about 80 per sq. cm. on thigh.

Eccyclomastopathy Lesion of breast made-up of connective tissue and epithelial cells.

Echeosis Mental disturbance caused by noise.

Echinococcosis Infestation with *T. echinococcus.*

Echinococcus A genus of tape worm. Consisting of scolex and three or four proglottids. *e.granulosus* A species of tape worms infesting carnivores causing hydatid cyst in liver or lungs.

Echinocyte Abnormal erythrocyte with multiple spiny projections from surface.

Echinostoma A genus of fluke found in aquatic birds.

Echo A reverberating sound produced when sound waves are reflected back to their source.

Echocardiography The technique of imaging the cardiac structures non-invasively through passage of ultrasound.

Echoencephalogram Recording of midline shift of brain structures by ultrasound waves.

Echokinesia Involuntary repetition of another's gestures.

Echopraxia Imitation of actions of others.

ECHO virus Enterocytopathogenic human orphan virus causing viral meningitis, enteritis, pleurodynia, myocarditis, etc.

Eclampsia Coma and convulsion occurring after 28th week of pregnancy and in immediate postpartum.

Eclecticism An old system of medicine where treatment is dependent upon individual signs and symptoms rather than the disease as a whole.

Econazole A topical antifungal agent.

Economo's disease Encephalitis lethargica.

Ectasia Dilatation of any tubular structure.

Ecthyma A shallow skin lesion with crusting, often followed by pigmentation and scarring.

Ectocervix The portion of cervical canal outlined by squamous epithelium.

Ectoderm The outer layer of cells in developing embryo giving rise to skin, teeth, nervous system, organs of special sense, pituitary, pineal and suprarenal glands.

Ectomorph Linear slender body build with poor musculature.

Ectoparasite Parasite living on outer surface of body e.g., lice, fleas, ticks.

Ectopia Malposition or displacement. *e. cordis* Malposition of heart with the organ lying outside the thorax. *e. lentis* Displacement of lens in the eye. *e. vesicae* Displacement of bladder e.g., extrophy.

Ectopic In an abnormal position e.g., ectopic heart beat.

Ectopic pregnancy Implantation of fertilized ovum outside the uterine cavity; can be abdominal, tubal, or ovarian with liability for rupture and hemorrhage (*see* Figure).

Ectopic rhythm Any abnormal or irregular cardiac rhythm.

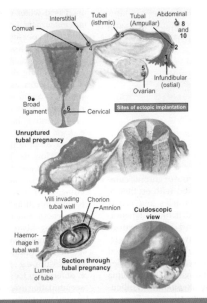

Ectopic pregnancy

Ectoplasm The outermost layer of cell protoplasm.

Ectostosis Formation of bone beneath periosteum.

Ectothrix Fungus growing on hair shafts.

Ectotrichophyton Fungi causing hair and skin infection.

Ectozoon Parasite living on another animal.

Ectromelia Hypoplasia of long bones of limbs.

Ectropion Eversion of eyelid margin (*see* Figure).

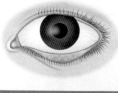

Ectropion

Eczema Acute or chronic cutaneous lesion with erythema, papule, vesicles and crusts leading to itching, lichenification and pigmentation; mostly atopic or allergic. *e. marginatum* Eczema caused by ringworms. *e. numular* Coin or oval shaped eczema lesions. *e. pustular* Follicular or impetiginous form of eczema. *e. seborrheic* Eczema

with seborrhea. *e. vaccinatum* Generalized vaccinial lesion or local lesions elsewhere in persons with eczema who receive vaccination.

Edema Excessive tissue accumulation water, either localized or generalized, can be due to poor venous drainage, lymphatic obstruction, increased venous pressure (CHF), hypoalbuminemia, or increased water retention. *e. angioneurotic* Local edema due to hypersensitivity to drugs food, physical agents (cold) or idiopathic. *e. brain* Brain swelling due to water accumulation as following injury, toxemia or infection. *e. cardiac* Dependent edema of congestive heart failure. *e. high altitude* Pulmonary edema of mountaineers related to low partial pressure of oxygen. *e. larynx* Usually of allergic origin but life threatening. *e. of glottis* Usually follows infection with cough, hoarseness and dyspnea. *e. nonpitting* Myxomatous tissue accumulation appearing as edema without any dimple on pressure, e.g., myxedema. *e. pulmonary* Increased fluid accumulation in lungs following left heart failure, toxic gas inhalation, or ARDS.

Edge A margin or border.

Edrophonium chloride A cholinergic drug (anticholinesterage).

Edrophonium test A test for myasthenia gravis. A positive test demonstrates brief improvement in the muscle strength.

Efavirenz Anti-HIV agent.

Effacement Dilatation of cervix and stretching of birth passage (*see* Figure).

Effect Result of an action or force. *e. cumulative* Drug effect on repeated administration of a drug.

Effector One of the nerve endings having the efferent process and in a gland or muscle cell. Also applied for effector organs (muscle and glands).

Effeminate A male having physical characteristic or mannerism of a female.

Efferent Carrying away from a central organ.

Efferent nerve Nerves that carry impulses away from the nerve cell (motor nerve).

Effervescence Formation of bubbles of gas rising to surface of fluids.

Effluent Fluid discharged from sewage treatment or industrial plant.

Effusion Escape of fluid/air into a cavity, e.g., hydro-pneumothorax, chylothorax, pleural effusion.

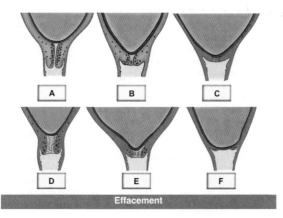

Effacement

Ego 1. In psychoanalysis, the three divisions are id, ego and superego. The ego possesses consciousness and memory and serves to mediate between the primitive instinctual or animal drives (the id), internal social prohibitions (super ego) and reality. 2. Selfishness or self love.

Egoism An inflated estimate of one's value or effectiveness.

Egophony A nasal sound like bleating of a goat, present on lung tissue above effusion.

Ehlers-Danlos syndrome An inherited disorder of elastic connective tissue characterized by fragile hyperelastic skin, hyper mobile joints.

Eicosanoids Metabolites of arachidonic acid metabolism like prostaglandins, thromboxane and leukotrienes.

Eisenmenger's complex In a case of congenital heart disease with left to right shunt (ASD, VSD, PDA etc) when the pulmonary vascular resistance equals or exceeds systemic resistance it is called Eisenmenger complex.

Ejaculation Ejection of seminal fluid from male urethra. *e. retrograde* Lax internal sphincter due to autonomic dysfunction in diabetics or following prostatectomy,

the ejaculation occurs retrogradely to bladder.

Ejaculatory duct The terminal portion of seminal duct formed by the union of the ductus deferens and excretory duct of the seminal vesicle.

Ejection fraction The percentage of blood ejected from LV into aorta with each cardiac contraction.

Elastase Proteolytic pancreatic enzyme.

Elastic Stretchable.

Elastic bandage Bandage that can be stretched to exert continuous pressure.

Elastic cartilage Yellow cartilage of epiglottis, pharynx, external ear, auditory tubes.

Elastic stocking Stocking applied to aid in return of blood from the extremity to heart. (e.g., in varicosity).

Elastic tissue Connective tissue supplied with elastic fibers as in tunica media of vessels.

Elastin The protein of elastic tissue.

Elastometry The measurement of elasticity of tissues.

Elbow Joint between arm and forearm, consisting of humeroulnar, humeroradial and proximal radioulnar articulations. *e. tennis* Tendinitis of lateral forearm muscles near their origin from lateral epicondyle of humerus (lateral epicondylitis).

Elective therapy A planned convenient therapy/operation.

Electra complex In psychoanalysis, a group of symptoms due to suppressed sexual love of daughter for father.

Electric shock Tissue injury from passage of electricity.

Electricity A form of kinetic energy having magnetic, chemical, mechanical and thermal effects; formed from interaction of positive and negative charges.

Electroanalgesia Pain relief by use of low intensity electric currents.

Electrocardiogram Record of electric activity of heart (*see* Figure).

Electrocardiograph The machine used to record electrocardiogram.

Electrocautery Cauterization by an arc heated by electric current.

Electrocoagulation Coagulation of tissue by means of a high-frequency current.

Electroconvulsive therapy The use of shock to produce convulsion, indicated for acute psychosis and depression with suicidal tendency.

Electrocution Death by electric current.

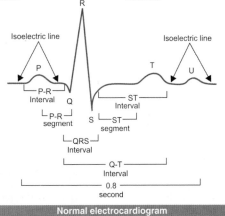

Normal electrocardiogram

Electrode A medium intervening between an electric conductor and the object to which the current is to be applied.

Electrodesiccation Drying of cells or tissues by means of high frequency electric spark used for achieving hemostasis following bleeding from small capillaries and veins during surgery.

Electrodialysis A method of separating electrolytes from colloids by passing current through the solution.

Electrodynamometer Instrument used to measure strength of current.

Electroejaculation Production of ejaculation by electrical stimulation from a probe placed in rectum, e.g. in paraplegics for artificial insemination.

Electroencephalogram (EEG) Recording of electrical activity of brain through surface electrodes.

Electroencephalograph The machine recording EEG.

Electrogoniometer Electrical device for measuring angles of joints and their range of motion.

Electrology The branch of science dealing with properties of electricity.

Electrolysis Dissolution of tissue by electric current e.g., destruction of hair follicle.

Electrolyte 1. A solution which conducts electricity. 2. Ionised salts in blood, tissue fluids and cells.

Electrometer An instrument for measuring differences in electric potential.

Electromotive force (EMF) The difference in potential that causes the flow of electricity. It is measured in volts.

Electromyography Preparation, study and interpretation of electromyograms.

Electromyogram A graphic record of the contraction of muscle on electric stimulation.

Electron The negatively charged particle of an atom.

Electronics The science of all systems involving use of electric devices e.g., communication, data control and processing.

Electronystagmography A method of recording nystagmus from electrical activity of extraocular muscles.

Electrooculogram Recording of electric currents produced by eye movements.

Electrophoresis The movement of charged colloidal particles as a result of changes in electric potential.

Electrophysiology Branch of physiology dealing with relationships of body functions to electrical phenomena.

Electroretinogram (ERG) A record of action currents of retina produced by visual or light stimuli.

Element A substance that cannot be further broken down to substances different from it, e.g. carbon, sodium, calcium, etc.

Elephantiasis Hypertrophy of skin and subcutaneous tissue due to lymphatic stasis e.g., in filariasis that involves scrotum, penis, legs, breasts and hands (*see* Figure).

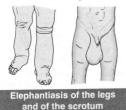

Elephantiasis of the legs and of the scrotum

Elevator Surgical instruments used to raise depressed fractures (e.g., skull), extracting teeth.

Eliminate To expel, to get rid of body waste product.

Elimination diet A diet regime used to determine which foods cause allergic response. Offending food then is discovered when one by one food is gradually introduced into diet.

Elixir Sweetened hydro-alcoholic liquid.

Ellipsoid Spindle shaped.

Elliptocyte Oval shaped red-blood cell. Normally, 15% of human RBC are oval and bird and reptiles have normally all RBC in elliptocytic form.

Elliptocytosis Benign hereditary disease, causing haemolytic anaemia.

Ellis-van Creveld syndrome Congenital syndrome consisting of polydactyly, chondrodysplasia and congenital heart defects (ASD).

Emaciation To become excessively lean.

Emasculation Castration; excision of entire male genitalia.

Embalming Use of antiseptics and preservatives to prevent premature biodegradation of dead body.

Embarrass To interfere with or compromise function.

Embden-Meyerhof pathway Anaerobic metabolism of glucose to lactic acid in humans.

Embolectomy Removal of embolus from a vessel, e.g., in stroke, pulmonary embolism.

Embolism Obstruction to blood flow by mass of red

blood cells and fibrin mesh. Atrial fibrillation and pelvic-leg vein thrombosis predispose to embolism.

Embolus A mass of undissolved matter in blood vessel, may be clot, fat, air bubble, clumps of bacteria, amniotic fluid.

Embramine Antiallergic agent.

Embryo 2nd through 8th weeks of fetal development (*see* Figure).

Embryogeny The growth and development of an embryo.

Embryology The science that deals with origin and development of an organism.

Emergency cardiac care (ECC) Care necessary to deal with an acute cardiopulmonary event like infarction, arrhythmia, pulmonary embolism.

Emesis Vomiting, due to gastric, CNS, systemic or metabolic factors.

Emetic Agent producing vomiting, e.g., apomorphine.

Emetine Ipecac derivative, used for extraintestinal amebiasis.

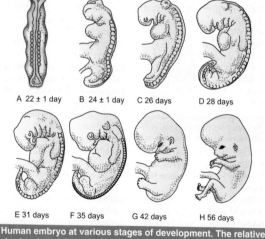

A 22 ± 1 day   B 24 ± 1 day   C 26 days   D 28 days

E 31 days   F 35 days   G 42 days   H 56 days

Human embryo at various stages of development. The relative size has been distorted to emphasize correspondence of parts

Emigration Passage of WBC through walls of capillaries.

Eminence Prominence or projection esp. on a bone.

Emissary An outlet.

Emission Discharge. *e. nocturnal* Involuntary discharge of semen during sleep.

Emmetropia When the eyes are at rest parallel rays are focussed exactly on retina; i.e., normal refraction.

Emmetropic Normal vision.

Emolient An agent that smoothens and softens the skin when applied.

Emotion A mental state or feeling such as fear, hate, grief, joy with some change in cardiorespiratory function.

Empathy Objective awareness of and insight into the feelings, emotions and behavior of another person and their meaning and significance.

Emphysema 1. Pathological distension of tissues by air/gas. 2. Chronic pulmonary disease with dilatation of airspaces beyond terminal bronchioles (*see* Figure).

Empirical Based on experience rather than scientific principle.

Emprosthotonus A form of spasm in which body is flexed forward opposite to opisthotonus.

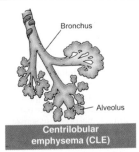

Centrilobular emphysema (CLE)

Empyesis Any pustular skin lesion.

Empyocele Suppurating hydrocele.

Emulsification Breaking down of large fat globules into smaller ones by bile acid that lower surface tension.

Emulsion A mixture of two liquids not mutually soluble.

Enalapril Converting enzyme inhibitor, used in heart failure, hypertension.

Enamel Hard dense glistening white substance forming a covering on crown of teeth.

Enamel organ A cup shaped structure that forms on the dental lamina of an embryo.

Enantiopathy Treatment of one disease by using another disease that produces symptoms antagonistic to former.

Enathem Eruption on mucous membrane.

Encapsulation The process of formation of a capsule around a structure.

Encephalagia Deep seated headache.

Encephalitis Inflammation of brain parenchyma, manifesting with changes in level of consciousness, increased intracranial pressure, sensory motor dysfunction.

Encephalocele Protrusion of brain substance through a cranial defect (*see* Figure below).

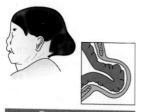

Encephalocele

Encephalogram (air) X-ray of brain with air injected into ventricular system.

Encephalomalacia Softening of brain.

Encephalomeningocele Protrusion of membrane and brain parenchyma through cranial defect.

Encephalomyelitis Inflammation of brain and spinal cord. *e. acute disseminated* That following acute exanthema but fewer symptoms.

Encephalopathy Any dysfunction of brain.

Enchondroma A benign cartilaginous tumor occurring within a bone and expanding the diaphysis.

Encopresis Condition associated with constipation and passage of watery colonic content across the hard fecal mass, mimicking diarrhoea.

Endarterectomy Surgical removal of lining endothelium of an artery.

Endarteritis Inflammation of intima of an artery resulting from syphilis, trauma, infective thrombi.

Endemic A disease occurring repeatedly in a particular population confering some immunity and hence low mortality.

Endocarditis Inflammation of endothelial lining of heart chambers and heart valves; may be due to invasion of microorganisms or abnormal immunologic response. *e. verrucous* Nonbacterial endocarditis associated with wasting diseases, e.g., SLE. *SYN* — Libman - Sack. *e. subacute bacterial* Caused by *streptococcus viridans* group. *e. ulcerative* Rapidly destructive acute bacterial endocarditis.

Endocervicitis Inflammation of mucus lining of endocervix.

Endocrine glands Glands secreting directly into blood stream.

Endocytosis A method of ingestion of a foreign substance by a cell.

Endodontics A branch of dentistry concerned with diagnosis, treatment and prevention of diseases of dental pulp and its surrounding tissue.

Endogenous Produced or arising from within a cell or organism.

Endolymph Pale transparent fluid within the labyrinth of ear.

Endometer Electronic device used to determine the length of tooth root canal.

Endometriosis Proliferation of endometrium at ecopic sites, i.e. sites other than ulterine cavity (*see* Figure).

Endometritis Inflammation of endometrium. *e. dissecans* Endometritis accompanied by development of ulcers and shedding of mucous membrane.

Endomorph Body build characterized by predominance of tissues derived from endoderm.

Endomysium A thin layer of connective that tissue surrounds each striated muscle fiber.

Endoneurium A delicate connective tissue sheath that surrounds nerve fibers.

Endonuclease Enzyme that clears ends of polynucleotides.

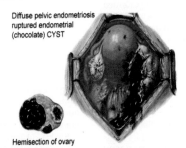

Diffuse pelvic endometriosis
ruptured endometrial
(chocolate) CYST

Hemisection of ovary

Endometriosis

Endopelvic fascia The downward continuation of the parietal peritoneum of abdomen that supports pelvic viscera.

Endopeptidase Proteolytic enzyme that cleaves peptides.

Endophthalmitis Inflammation within substance of eye.

Endorgan The expanded end of a nerve fiber in a peripheral tissue.

Endorphins Polypeptides produced in the brain tissue that bind to opioid receptors and block them, there by producing analgesia. The most important is beta endorphin.

Endosalpingitis Inflammation of lining of fallopian tubes.

Endoscope A device containing optical system for observing or conducting surgery in hollow structures like abdomen, pelvis.

Endosome The vacuole formed when material is absorbed in the cell by process of endocytosis. The vacuole fuses with lysosome.

Endosteitis Inflammation of the endosteum of medullary cavity.

Endothelioma Malignant tumor of endothelial cells lining any cavity, blood vessel lumen.

Endotheliosis Increased growth of endothelial cells.

Endothrix Fungus growth within hair.

Endotoxemia Toxemia due to presence of endotoxin in blood.

Endotoxin Bacterial toxin released after death of bacteria.

Endotracheal tube Tube that provides an airway through trachea while preventing aspiration by its inflated cuff.

Endplate The terminal end of nerve fibre to a muscle.

End product The final product of a chemical/metabolic process.

Enema Stimulation of bowel activity by introduction of soothning, cleansing and chemical agents into rectum. Drugs can be given as enema, e.g., steroids in ulcerative colitis, paraldehyde. *e. double contrast* Enema of barium and air for colonography. *e. retention* e.g., saline or steroids for purpose of nutrition/medication.

Energy The capacity of a system in doing work.

Energy Expenditure Basal (BEE) Harris Benedict equation.

For women $6.55 + (9.6 \times W) + (1.8 \times H) - (4.7 \times A)$

For men $66 + (13.7 \times w) + (5 \times H) - (6.8 \times A)$.

Where A = Age in years H = Height in cm and W = Weight in kg.

Energy expenditure is increased by 13% over basal needs for each °C rise in temperature than normal. Stress, burn, trauma increase the need of calories to the extent of 40- 100%.

Enflurane Anaesthetic agent (volatile).

Engagement In obstetric descent of presenting part into true pelvic cavity, i.e. the part is immobile.

Engorgement Vascular congestion.

Enkephalins Polypeptides produced in brain that bind to opioid receptors to produce analgesia.

Enolase An enzyme present in muscle tissue that converts phosphoglyceric acid to phosphopyruvic acid.

Enophthalmos Recession of eyeball into orbit.

Enoxaparin Factor Xa inhibitor, anticoagulant.

Enriched Addition of something extra.

Entameba A genus of parasitic ameba found in human digestive tract, e.g., *E. coli, E. gingivalis, E. histolytica E. undulans*.

Enteral tube feeding Feeding patient with a tube passed into stomach.

Enteric coated Tablet or capsule coated with special coating that only dissolves in intestine.

Enteritis Inflammation of intestine.

Enterobacteriaceae Gram -ve nonspore bearing rods which include *Shigella, Salmonella, Klebsiella, Yersinia, Proteus, Escherichia.*

Enterobiasis Infestation with pinworms.

Enterococcus Any species of streptococcus inhabiting human intestine.

Enterocolitis Inflammation of intestine and colon. *e. necrotizing* Unknown necrotizing fatal disease of newborn.

Enterocolostomy Surgical joining of small intestine to colon.

Enterocystoplasty Use of a portion of small intestine to enlarge the bladder.

Enteroenterostomy Establishing communication between two intestinal segments that are not continuous.

Enterogastrone A hormone secreted by intestinal mucosa that decreases gastric emptying. Fat stimulates its secretion.

Enterolith Concretions in intestine.

Enteromyiasis Disease caused by maggots (larva of flies) in the intestine.

Enteron The elementary canal.

Enteropathogen Microorganism that causes intestinal infection.

Enteropeptidase Enzyme of duodenal mucosa that helps conversion of trypsinogen to trypsin.

Enteropexy Fixation of intestine to abdominal wall.

Enterovirus A class of picornavirus, that includes polio, coxsackie and Echo viruses.

Enterozoon Any intestinal parasite.

Enthesis The use of metallic or other inert substances to substitute or replace lost tissue.

Enthesitis Inflammation at site of attachment of a tendon to bone.

Entoderm Innermost primary germ layer giving rise to epithelium of digestive tract, and associated glands, the respiratory tract, bladder, vagina and urethra.

Entomology Study of insects and their relationship to disease.

Entoptic phenomena Visual phenomena like seeing floating bodies, circles of light, black spots, transient flashes of light.

Entropion Inward turning of an edge, e.g., margin of eyelid. *e. cicatricial* Inversion resulting from scar tissue (e.g., trachoma) *e. spastic* Inversion resulting from spasm of orbicularis oculi.

Enucleate To remove eyeball, to remove a part of mass or entire mass.

Enuresis Involuntary passage of urine in bed after the age of 5 years, often a familial tendency.

Envenomation Introduction of poisonous venum into body by bite or sting.

Enzootic Endemic disease confined to animals.

Enzyme Complex proteins catabolizing reactions but without being changed themselves; can be synthesizing, coagulating, branching, debranching, digestive, fermenting, glycolytic, lipolytic, mucolytic. *e. mucolytic* Enzyme that depolymerizes mucus by splitting mucoproteins, e.g., mucinase, hyaluronidase. *e. respiratory* Enzymes acting within cells catalyze oxidative reactions with release of energy (ATP), e.g., cytochromes, flavoproteins.

Enzyme induction Increase in enzyme level due to its increased production or decrease degradation. Drugs commonly causing hepatic enzyme induction are barbiturates.

Enzyme-linked immunosorbent assay (ELISA) A test to detect antigen or antibody, hormones.

Eosin Synthetic rose colored dye used for staining tissues/body fluids for microscopic examination.

Eosinophil Granular leukocyte staining with acid stain eosin.

Eosinophilia Increased blood eosinophil count beyond 6-8% or 300/cmm.

Ependyma Membrane lining the cerebral ventricles and central canal of spinal cord.

Ependymitis Inflammation of ependyma.

Ependymoma A tumor of ependymal elements.

Ephebiatrics Adolescent medicine.

Ephebology Study of puberty and its changes.

Ephedrine Sympathomimetic agent used locally as decongestant and systemically for bronchodilation and raising blood pressure.

Epiandrosterone Androgenic hormone normally present in urine.

Epiblast SYN–Ectoderm; outer layer of cells of blastoderm.

Epiblepharon A fold of skin passing across either lids so that eyelashes are pressed against eye.

Epicanthus A vertical fold of skin extending from root of nose to the median end of eyebrow covering inner canthus and caruncle (*see* Figure).

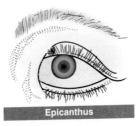

Epicanthus

Epichordal Dorsal to notochord.

Epichorion The portion of decidua of placenta that covers the ovum.

Epicondyle Bone element above the condyle, i.e. articular surface of bone.

Epidemic Appearance of a disease in a high proportion not expected for a community in a geographical area.

Epidemiology Science concerned with study and analysis of interrelationship of factors that determine disease frequency.

Epidermis Outer layer of skin, avascular, consists of 4 layers from inwards to outwards, i.e., stratum germinatum, stratum granulosum, stratum luciderm and stratum corneum.

Epidermization Conversion of deeper germinative layers of cells into outer layers of epidermis.

Epicyte An epithelial cell.

Epididymis A small long convoluted organ lying behind testes and containing the ducts of testes. It ends in spermatic duct.

Epididymitis Inflammation of epididymis, usually as a complication of gonorrhoea, syphilis, tuberculosis, mumps, filariasis, etc.

Epididymography Radiographic examination of epididymis after introduction of contrast.

Epididymoorchitis Inflammation of epididymis and testes.

Epidural Outside dura.

Epigastric reflex Contraction of upper portion of rectus abdominis when skin of epigastric region is scratched.

Epigastrium Region over pit of the stomach.

Epiglottis Leaf shaped flat membrane covering entrance of larynx during swallowing (*see* Figure).

Epiglottitis Inflammation of epiglottis, usually bacterial,

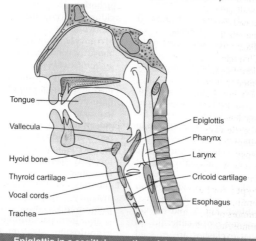

Tongue
Vallecula
Hyoid bone
Thyroid cartilage
Vocal cords
Trachea

Epiglottis
Pharynx
Larynx
Cricoid cartilage
Esophagus

Epiglottis in a sagittal secretion of the head and neck

often threatens airway obstruction if treatment is delayed.

Epilate To extract hair by the roots.

Epilation Extraction of hair.

Epilemma Neurilemma of small branches of nerve filament.

Epilepsy Recurrent, paroxysmal electrical dysfunction of brain characterized by altered consciousness and motor/sensory phenomena. *Focal* or *jacksonian e.* A symptom of a cerebral lesion. The convulsive movements are often localized and close observation of the onset and course of the attack may greatly assist diagnosis. *Temporal lobe e.* Characterized by hallucination of sight, hearing, taste and smell, paroxysmal disorders of memory and automatism. Caused by temporal or parietal lobe disease.

Epileptic Concerning epilepsy.

Epileptiform Mimicking epilepsy.

Epiloia A syndrome of mental retardation, convulsion, hypertrophic sclerosis of brain, adenoma sebaceum, tumors of kidneys.

Epimorphosis Regeneration of a part of organism by growth from cut surface.

Epimysium Outermost sheath of connective tissue surrounding a skeletal muscle.

Epinephrine Hormone of adrenal medulla, synthesized from phenylalanine having ionotropic, bronchodilator and sympathomimetic effects.

Epinephritis Inflammation of adrenal gland.

Epinephroma Lipomatoid tumor of kidney.

Epineurium Connective tissue sheath of a nerve.

Epiphora Abnormal overflow of tears either due to excess secretion or blockage of lacrimal duct.

Epiphylaxis Increase in defensive power of body.

Epiphysiolysis Separation of an epiphysis.

Epiphysis An ossification center separated from parent bone by a cartilage in infants and children; an indicator for assessment of bone age.

Epiphysitis Inflammation of an epiphysis especially that of knee, hip, shoulder in infants.

Epiplocele Hernia containing omentum.

Epiploic Pertains to omentum.

Epipygus A developmental anomaly where accessory limb is attached to the buttocks.

Epirubicin Antitumor antibiotic.

Episcleral Overlying sclera of eye.

Episiotomy Incision of perineum to facilitate delivery and avoid laceration (*see* Figure).

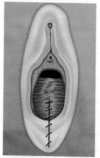

Median episiotomy closed by continuous sutures

Episiotomy

Epispadius Congenital opening of urethra on dorsal aspect of penis or clitoris (*see* Figure).

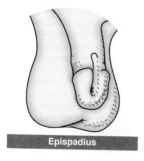

Epispadius

Episplenitis Inflammation of splenic capsule.

Epistasis Suppression of any discharge.

Epistaxis Bleeding from Kiesselbach's area of nose.

Epitendon The connective tissue holding a tendon within its sheath.

Epithelial cells Cells irregular in shape, having a single nucleus.

Epithelial tissue Those tissues covering outer surface of body and lining the internal passages or cavities. The cells lie in close proximity of each other with little intercellular substance.

Epithelioid Resembling epithelium.

Epithelioma Malignant tumor arising from epithelium. e.g., skin or mucous membrane. *e. adamantinum* Tumor of jaw arising from enamel organ usually of lowgrade malignancy, may be cystic.

Epoprostinol PGI_2.

Epsilon-aminocaproic acid Synthetic substance, antifibrinolytic, used to check bleeding.

Epsom salt $= MgSO_4$ a, cathartic.

Epulis A fibrous sarcomatous tumor of lower jaw.

Eradication Complete elimination of disease.

Erben's reflex Slowing of pulse when head and trunk are forcibly bent forward.

Erb's paralysis Paralysis of muscles supplied by C_5 and C_6.

Erectile tissue Spongy vascular tissue which when filled with blood becomes erect and rigid e.g., penis, clitoris, nipple.

Erection Swelling, hardness and stiffness of penis on sexual arousal/physical handling.

Erector spinae reflex Irrigation of skin of back causes hardening due to contraction of erector spinae.

Erethism Excessive excitation or irritation.

Erg In physics, the amount of work done when a force of 1 dyne acts through a distance 1 cm.

Ergasthenia Weakness due to overwork.

Ergocalciferol Vit D_2.

Ergocristine An ergot alkaloid.

Ergograph An apparatus for recording contractions of muscles and measuring the amount of work done.

Ergometer An apparatus for measuring amount of work performed.

Ergonomics The science concerned with how to fit a job to man's anatomical, physiological and psychological characteristics in a way that will enhance human efficiency and well-being.

Ergonovine maleate An ergot derivative used in treatment of migraine. It also stimulates contraction of uterus.

Ergosterol The sterol of plant and animal tissue that can be converted to Vitamin D_2 on irradiation.

Ergotamine tartarate Ergot alkaloid used to treat migraine or to enhance uterine contraction.

Ergotism Ergot poisoning.

Erode To wear away.

Erosion Destruction of surface layer. *e. dental* Enamel loss. *e. cervix* Alteration of the epithelium, squamous cells replacing columnar cells following low grade infection.

Erotism Sexual desire. *e. auto* Self-gratification of sexual instincts by manual stimulation of erogenous areas like penis, clitoris.

Erotology The study of love and its manifestations.

Erotomania Pathological exaggeration of sexual behavior.

Erotophobia Aversion to sexual love or its manifestations.

Erratic Fluctuating, unpredictable.

Error Mistake, miscalculation.

Eructation Belching, bringing out gas from stomach.

Eruption Appearance of a lesion such as redness or spotting on the skin or mucous membrane. *e. creeping* A skin lesion characterized by a tortuous elevated red line that progresses at one end while fading at the other usually caused by migration of larva of Ankylostomas. *e. drug* Drug ingestion causing skin eruption.

Erysipelas Spreading inflammation of skin and subcutaneous tissue accompanied by systemic disturbance.

Erysipeloid An infective dermatitis resembling erysepalas.

Erythema Diffuse macular redness of skin. *e. induratum* Chronic vasculitis of skin occurring in young adult females; often breaking down with formation of atrophic scar. *e. multiforme* A macular erruption with dark red papules or tubercles that appear as rings, disc shaped patches, figured arrangements. *e. marginatum* A form of erythema multiforme with central fading area but elevated edges.

e. nodosum Red and painful nodules on legs, often caused by drugs, toxins.

Erythrasma Red brown eruption in patches in axillae and groin caused by *Corynebacterium minitissimum.*

Erythrityl tetranitrate Anti anginal agent.

Erythroblast Nucleated red blood cell, may be pronormoblast, basophilic normoblast, polychromatic normoblast, orthochromatic normoblast (*see* Figure).

Erythroblastosis fetalis Hemolytic disease of newborn usually due to Rh incompatibity or ABO mismatching.

Erythrocyanosis Red or bluish discolouration of skin with swelling, burning and itching.

Erythrocyte The non-nucleated bi-concave disc of 7.7 micron. matured red blood cell containing hemoglobin, involved in oxygen transport. *e. crenated* RBC with serrated or crenated edge.

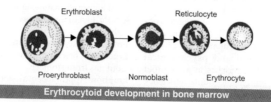

Erythroblast · Reticulocyte · Proerythroblast · Normoblast · Erythrocyte

Erythrocytoid development in bone marrow

Erythrocyte sedimentation rate The rate at which erythrocytes sediment in a given blood sample in one hour.

Erythrocythemia Increased red cell mass.

Erythrocytopenia Decrease in number of red cells.

Erythrocytosis Increase in red cell mass.

Erythrodema An infantile disease characterized by itchy lesions of hands and feet, and polyarthritis.

Erythroderma Abnormal redness of skin.

Erythrodontia Reddish-brown staining of teeth.

Erythroid Concerning red blood cells.

Erythroleukemia A variant of acute myeloid leukemia with anaemia, bizarre red cell morphology, erythroid hyperplasia in bone marrow.

Erythromelia Painless erythema of extensor surface of arm.

Erythromelalgia Burning and throbbing in feet that come and go.

Erythromycin Antibiotic from *Streptomyces erythreus* effective for many gm + ve and few gram –ve organisms.

Erythropoitin An alfaglobulin secreted by kidney that stimulates erythropoisis.

Erythropsin Pigment in external portion of rods of retina.

Erythrosine Sodium A dye (2%) used as dental disclosing agent.

Eschar Slough cast off by from the surface of skin produced after a burn, gangrene, corrosive application, or ulcer.

Esmarch's bandage Narrow hard rubber tourniquet to limit the blood flow (*see* Figure).

Esculent Suitable for use as food.

Esophagoenterostomy Making communication between esophagus and intestine following resection of stomach as in gastric malignancy.

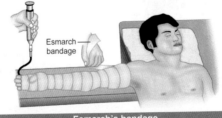

Esmarch —
bandage

Esmarch's bandage

Esophagomyotomy Incision of muscular coat of esophagus as in achalasia cardia.

Esophagoplication Reduction of dilatation of esophagus by taking tucks in its walls.

Esophagotomy Surgical incision into the esophagus as in achalasia cardia.

Esophagus The musculomembranous tube extending from pharynx to stomach (*see* Figure).

Esophoria Amount of inward turning of eye, *SYN*-esotropia.

ESP Extrasensory perception.

ESR Electron spin resonance, a newer medical technique for imaging e.g., NMR studies.

ESRD End-stage renal disease.

Essence Alcoholic solution of volatile oil.

Essential Indispensable.

EST Elctroshock therapy.

Ester Compound formed by organic acid with alcohol.

Esterase Enzyme catalyzing hydrolysis of esters.

Esthesia Perception, feeling, sensation.

Esthesiometer Device for measuring tactile sensibility.

Estradiol $C_{18}H_{24}O_2$. Steroid hormone of ovary with estrogenic properties.

Estriol $C_{18}H_{24}O_3$ Metabolic product of estrone and estradiol.

Estrogen Substance having estrogenic activity, i.e. development of female sex

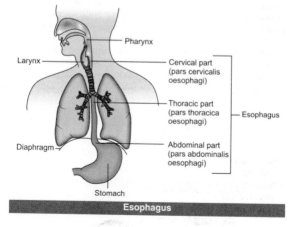

Esophagus

characteristics, cyclic changes in endometrium and vaginal epithelium, breast changes.

Estrone $C_{18}H_{22}O_2$. Natural estrogenic hormone less active than estradiol but more active than estriol.

Estrus The cyclic period of sexual activity in mammals; during estrus animal is said to be 'in heat'.

Etanercept TNFa receptor antagonist, used in rheumatoid arthritis.

Etching Application of corrosives material to a glass/metal to create a pattern or design.

Ethambutol Antitubercular bacteriostatic agent.

Ethamsylate Procoagulant agent.

Ethanol Ethyl alcohol.

Ethaverine hydrochloride Mild coronary artery dilator.

Ethchlorvynol Hypnotic agent.

Ether diethyl $C_4H_{10}O$ inflammable anaesthetic agent.

Ethics Moral principles or standards governing conduct.

Ethinamate Mild sedative - hypnotic agent.

Ethinyl estradiol An estrogenic hormone.

Ethionamide Bacteriostatic second line antitubercular drug.

Ethionine Progestational agent used in contraceptive.

Ethoheptazine Analgesic agent.

Ethomoid bone Sieve like spongy bone forming roof of nasal fossa and partly floor of anterior cranial fossa containing ethmoidal air cells.

Ethmoiditis Inflammation of ethmoidal air cells causing pain in between eyes, headache and nasal discharge.

Ethnic Groups of people with one cultural system.

Ethnology Comparative study of cultures using ethnographic data.

Ethopropazine Anticholinergic used in parkinsonism.

Ethosuximide Anticonvulsant, principally used for absence seizure.

Ethotoin Sparingly used anticonvulsant.

Ethyl chloride C_2H_5Cl. Volatile liquid used for topical anaesthesia.

Ethyl cellulose Ether of cellulose, used for drug preparation.

Ethylene glycol Antifreeze, poisonous.

Ethylene oxide C_2H_4O a fumigant. Also used for sterilizing articles that cannot withstand heat.

Ethylenediamine Solvent for theophyline.

Ethylenediaminetetra acetic acid (EDTA) A chelating agent.

Ethylmorphine Used as cough suppressant.

Ethylnorepinephrine Adrenergic drug used in asthma.

Etidronate Drug used in Paget's disease.

Etofamide An intraluminal amoebicide.

Etoposide Podophylotoxin for malignant diseases.

Etopride GI prokinatic agent.

Etoricoxib Anti-inflammatory, analgesic.

Etretinate Retinoid used for acne.

Eucalyptus oil Oil distilled from eucalyptus leaves, used as an expectorant.

Eucapnia Normal CO_2 concentration in blood.

Eudiometer Instrument for testing purity of air and making analysis of gases.

Eugenics The science dealing with genetic and prenatal influences that affect the expression of certain characteristic in offsprings.

Eugenol A topical analgesic used in dentistry. Used with zinc oxide to make temporary filling.

Eunuch Castrated male; male without secondary sexual characteristics.

Eunuchoidism Deficient male sexual characteristics.

Euphoria Exaggerated feeling of well-being.

Euploidy In genetics, a state of having complete sets of chromosomes.

Eustachian tube 4 cm long mucus lined tube extending from middle ear to pharynx.

Eustachian valve Valve at the entrance of inferior venacava.

Euthanasia Mercy killing; dying easily, quietly and painlessly; ending ones life with an incurable disease.

Euthenics The science of improvement of population through modification of environment.

Euthyroid Normal thyroid function.

Evacuate To discharge especially bladder and bowel; to transfer patient from one site to another.

Evaluation Assessment.

Evanescent Not permanent, brief duration.

Evans blue A dye used IV as diagnostic agent.

Evaporation Change from liquid to gaseous state.

Evenomation Removal of venom from biting site.

Eventration Removal of contents of abdominal cavity, partial protrusion of abdominal contents through an opening in the abdominal wall.

Eversion Turning outwards (*see* Figure).

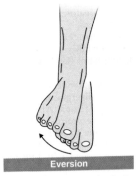

Eversion

Evisceration Removal of viscera.

Evoked response Study of function of sense organs even though patient is unconscious by giving sensory stimuli and recording the electric response along the propagation pathway to brain.

Ewing's tumor Diffuse endothelioma causing a fusiform swelling of long bone.

Exacerbation Aggravation of symptoms.

Exanthem Eruption of skin rash.

Excavator 1. an instrument for hollowing out something. 2. A scoop for surgical use. *e. dental* a hard cutting instrument for removal of carious dentia (*see* Figure).

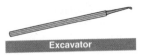

Excavator

Exchange transfusion Transfusion and withdrawal of small amounts of blood until blood volume is entirely replaced; used in autoimmune haemolytic anaemia, hyperbilirubinemia.

Excipient The vehicle for the drug.

Excise Removal by surgery.

Excitability Property of muscle or nerve fiber to contract or produce action potential on stimulation respectively.

Excitation wave The wave of irritability originating in sinoatrial node and moving across atria and conduction system to ventricular muscles.

Excoriation Abrasion of epidermis by chemicals, burns, irritation.

Exenteration Evisceration.

Exercise Performed activity of muscles. *e. isometric* Active contraction of muscle without shortening of muscle length. *e. isotonic* Active muscle contraction where muscle length is decreased. *e. static* Alternate contraction and relaxation of muscle without movement of joint.

Exercise *e. isokinetic* dynamic exercise performed at a constant angular velocity, the torque and tension remaining constant. *e. Frenkel's* movements performed by ataxic patients for improving coordination. *e. Kegel's* exercises to strengthen pubococcygeal muscles to prevent stress incontinence. *e. William's* flexion back exercises.

Exercise electrocardiogram *SYN*—Stress test.

Exercise tolerance test A test to determine the efficiency of cardiorespiratory system, e.g., treadmill testing.

Exflagellation The formation of microgametes (flagellated bodies) from microgametocytes. Occurs in plasmodia in the stomach of mosquito.

Exfoliation The shedding of cells.

Exhalation The process of breathing out.

Exhaustion Fatigue. *e. heat* A state of salt and water deficit on constant exposure to high temperature.

Exhibitionism Tendency to attract attention to oneself by any means.

Exhumation Removal of a dead body from grave.

Exner's nerve Nerve from pharyngeal plexus to cricothyroid membrane.

Exocrine Secretion of a gland to exterior/lumen.

Exodontology Branch of dentistry dealing with dental extraction.

Exoerythrocytic Occurring outside RBC.

Exomphalos Umbilical hernia.

Exophoria Tendency of visual axes to diverge outwards.

Exophthalmos Abnormal excessive protrusion of eyeballs due to thyrotoxicosis, retro orbital tumors, aneurysm, secondary to leukemic deposit (*see* Figure).

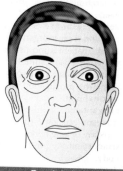

Exophthalmos

Exoplasm Outer protoplasm of a cell.

Exostosis Outgrowth from bone surface.

Exotic Not native.

Exotoxin Toxins produced by micro organism to surrounding medium.

Exotropia Divergent squint.

Expectoration The act of expulsing sputum.

Expiration Breathing out of inhaled air. It may be active or passive.

Explode To burst.

Exponent The mathematical method of indicating the power.

Exposure The amount of radiation delivered / received.

Exsanguination Excessive blood loss to the point of death.

Extrophy Congenital turning inside out of an organ.

Extension Movement by which both ends of a part are pulled apart.

Extinction The process of extinguishing or putting out.

Extirpation Excision of a part.

Extorsion Rotation of a part outward.

Extracapsular Outside the joint capsule.

Extracorporeal Outside the body.

Extracorporeal membrane oxygenator (ECMO) A device for oxygenation of blood used for patients of acute respiratory failure.

Extracorporeal shockwave lithotripsy: (ECSWL) shock wave dissolution of renal and gallstones.

Extract To pull out forcibly e.g., teeth; Active principle of a drug obtained by distillation or chemical process. It can be alcoholic, aqueous.

Extradural Outside dura matter.

Extramural Outside the wall of an organ or vessel.

Extraocular eye muscles Muscles attached to the capsule of eye controlling its movements.

Extrapyramidal Outside the pyramidal tracts of CNS.

Extrapyramidal syndrome Syndrome arising out of disease or degeneration of basal ganglia and their connections manifesting with tremor, rigidity, in coordination.

Extrasensory perception Perception of external events by other than the five senses.

Extrasystole Premature contraction of heart muscle by a stimulus originating in the conduction system or musculature. It can be atrial, junctional, nodal or ventricular. *e. atrial* Normal QRS complex with altered P waves. *e. ventricular* Wide bizarre QRS without P waves.

Extravasation Fluid escaping from vessel.

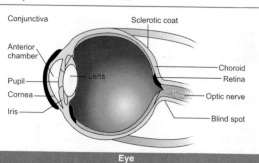

Eye

Extremity The terminal part of any thing, an arm or leg.

Extroversion Eversion, turning inside out.

Extrovert Opposite of introvert. One who is interested mainly in external objects and actions.

Extrusion In dentistry, position of a tooth when pushed forward from line of occlusion.

Extubation Removal of tube, e.g., laryngeal.

Exuberant Excessive growth of tissue, joyful, happy.

Exudate A protein rich fluid, high in cell count can be pus, catarrhal, haemorrhagic, fibrinous.

Exude To pass out slowly through the tissues.

Eye Organ of vision consisting of outer layer (cornea and sclera), middle layer (choroid, ciliary body and iris) and inner retina. *e. aphakic* Eye without lens. *e. black* Ecchymosis of tissue surrounding eye. *e. dominant* Eye which one preferentially uses as in seeing through mono-ocular microscope, while using a gun (*see* Figure above).

Eye bank An organization that collects corneas and stores them for transplantation.

Eyelids Movable protective folds closing the anterior surface of eyeball; the upper is the larger and more movable, raised by contraction of levator palpebrae superioris.

Eye muscle imbalance Incoordinate action of extraocular muscles causing esophoria or exophoria.

Eye strain Tiredness of eye due to errors of refraction, overuse, debility, anaemia.

Ezetimibe A lipid lewering agent.

F

FABERE test *Flexion, abduction, external rotation, and extension of hip* test for the identification of hip arthritis.

Fabrication Deliberately false statement told as if it were true, present in Korsakoff's syndrome.

Fabry's disease An inherited disorder of metabolism with accumulations of glycolipid in tissues.

Face Anterior part of head from forehead to chin, composed of 14 bones.

Facet A small smooth area on a bone or hard surface.

Facetectomy Excision of articular facet of vertebra.

Facial center Brain center responsible for facial movements.

Facial nerve Seventh cranial nerve supplying facial muscles, platysma, submandibular and sublingual glands, and carrying taste sensations from anterior two thirds of tongue.

Facial reflex Contraction of facial muscles following pressure on eyeball.

Facial spasm Involuntary contraction of muscles supplied by facial nerve.

Facies The expression or appearance of face (*see* Figure). *f. adenoid* Dull lethargic appearance with open mouth due to chronic mouth breathing. *f. aortica* Seen in aortic insufficiency; with bluish sclera, sunken cheeks and sallow face. *f. hepatica* Shunken eyes, yellow conjunctiva.

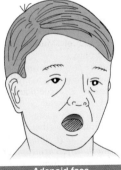

Adenoid face

f. hippocratic Face of long continued illness with hollow cheeks, sunken eyes, lead complexion and relaxed lips. *f. leonine* Lion like face of lepromatous leprosy with thick inelastic skin, depressed bridge of nose and leprosy nodules. *f. masklike* Expressionless face with little or no animation/blinking as seen in parkinsonism. *f. mitralis* Face of mitral insufficiency with dilated capillaries, pink and often cyanotic cheeks. *f. myopathic* Facies due to muscular atrophy and relaxation, lids drop and lips protrude.

Facilitation Hastening of an action.

Factitious False, not natural, artificial.

Factitious disorder Disease not genuine, produced voluntarily for gain, etc: Munchhausen syndrome.

Factor 1. any of several substances necessary to produce a result. 2. a coefficient or conversion factor 3. one of two or more quantities that multiplied together form a product. *f. B. lymphocyte growth/differentiation* factors derived form activated T-cells that stimulate B-cells to differentiate into antibody secreting plasma cells. *f. C3 nephritic* an auto-antibody that binds the C_3 causing alternative pathway activation. *f. colony stimulating* a group of glycoprotein lymphokine growth factors produced by monocytes, tissue macrophages and activated lymphocytes that induce stem cell differentiation into granulocyte and monocyte cell colonies. *f. decay accelerating* CD_{55}, a protein that protects cell membranes from attack by autologous complement. *f. endothelium derived relaxant* nitric oxide, a vasodilator. *f eosinophil chemotactic* released by basophils and mast cells in immediate hypersensitivity reactions. *f. epidermal growth* a factor essential in embryogenesis and wound healing. *f. granulocyte colony stimulating* factor secreted by endothelial cells, fibroblasts, and macrophages that stimulates production of neutrophils form precursor cells. *f. insulin like growth* include somatomedin C and A that mediate cell growth and replication. *f. myocardial depressant* a peptide produced in shock which has negative inotropic effect on heart. *f. nerve* *growth* factor that stimulates growth of sensory and sympathetic nerves. *f. osteoclast activating* a lymphokine that stimulates bone resorption. *f. platelet activating* factors (phospholipid) secreted by basophils, mast cells, macrophages and neutrophils that cause bronchoconstriction, platelet aggregation. *f. rheumatoid* IgM antibodies directed against IgG in rheumatoid arthritis (80% cases). *f. transforming growth* TFG a stimulates endothelial cell growth and TGF-beta stimulates growth of haematopoitic tissues and wound healing. *f. tumor necrosis* a macrophage secreted lymphokine that can cause necrosis of tumour cells; can induce shock when bacterial endotoxin's cause its release. *f. von Willebrand* a glycoprotein synthesized by endothelial cells and megakaryocytes promoting platelet adhesion to damaged vascular surfaces.

Facultative In biology and bacteriology, having the ability to live under certain condi–tions. Thus, a bacteria can be facultative with respect to O_2 and be able to live with or without O_2.

Faculty A normal mental attribute or sense; teaching staff.

Faget's sign A slower pulse than expected for the rise in temperature, a feature of enteric fever and viral infections.

Fahrenheit A temperature scale with freezing point of water at 32° and boiling point at 212° point.

Failure Loss of function of an organ. *f. heart* Poor pump function secondary to myocardial anoxia, necrosis, abnormal pre/after load or electrical disturbance. *f. renal* Loss of kidney function with uremia due to infection, diabetes, hypertension, glomerulo-nephritis etc. *f. respiratory* Inability of lungs to oxygenate the blood and expel carbon dioxide, occurring due to disease of diaphragms/ intercostal muscles or lung parenchyma (ARDS, COPD). *f. hepatic* Liver failure with cholemia due to cirrhosis, acute hepatic necrosis, etc.

Faint syncope About to lose consciousness.

Faith healing Healing through divine power, without medical aid.

Falciform Sickle shaped.

Falciform ligament Triangular ligament attached to sides of sacrum and coccyx by its base.

Falciform ligament of liver Sickle shaped reflection of

peritoneum attaching liver to diaphragm and separating right lobe from left lobe (*see* Figure on page 253).

Falciform process That portion of falciform ligament along the inner margin of ramus of ischium.

Fallopian tube The 4½" long tube joining peritoneal cavity near the ovary to lateral side of fundus of uterus. It serves to convey ovum from ovary to uterus. It has three parts: the infundibulum, isthmus and ampulla.

Fallot's tetralogy Congenital cyanotic heart disease characterized by overriding of aorta, infundibular stenosis, right ventricular hypertrophy and a ventricular septal defect (*see* Figure below).

Fallout Settling of radioactive fission products from

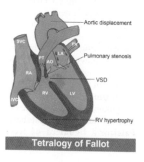

Tetralogy of Fallot

atmosphere after nuclear explosion.

False-positive A test indicating that the disease is present when in fact it is not.

False-negative A test indicating that the disease is not present when actually it is present.

False ribs The lower five pairs of ribs that do not unite directly with the sternum.

Falx Any sickle shaped structure. *f. cerebelli* A vertical fold of dura partitioning the two halfs of cerebellum. *f. cerebri* A fold of dura mater lying in longitudinal fissure, separating the two cerebral hemispheres. *f. inguinalis* The conjoint tendon that forms the origin of transverse abdominis and internal oblique muscles.

Famciclovir Antiviral agent for herpes.

Familial Disease occurring more frequently in a family than would be expected by chance.

Familial Mediterranean fever Inherited autosomal recessive disorder in persons of Irish or Italian descent manifesting with periodic fever, chest/abdominal pain and a propensity for amyloidosis.

Familial periodic paralysis Paralysis occurring at awak-

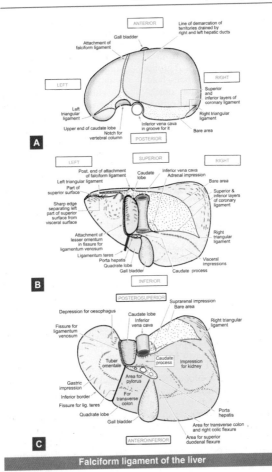

A

ANTERIOR

Attachment of falciform ligament

Gall bladder

Line of demarcation of territories drained by right and left hepatic ducts

LEFT

RIGHT

Superior and inferior layers of coronary ligament

Left triangular ligament

Right triangular ligament

Upper end of caudate lobe

Notch for vertebral column

Inferior vena cava in groove for it

Bare area

POSTERIOR

B

LEFT

SUPERIOR

RIGHT

Post. end of attachment of falciform ligament

Caudate lobe

Inferior vena cava

Adrenal impression

Bare area

Left triangular ligament

Part of superior surface

Superior & inferior layers of coronary ligament

Sharp edge separating left part of superior surface from visceral surface

Right triangular ligament

Attachment of lesser omentum in fissure for ligamentum venosum

Ligamentum teres

Porta hepatis

Quadrate lobe

Gall bladder

Caudate process

Visceral impressions

INFERIOR

C

POSTEROSUPERIOR

Depression for oesophagus

Suprarenal impression

Bare area

Caudate lobe

Inferior vena cava

Right triangular ligament

Fissure for ligamentum venosum

Tuber omentale

Caudate process

Impression for kidney

Gastric impression

Area for pylorus

Inferior border

For transverse colon

Fissure for lig. teres

Quadrate lobe

Gall bladder

Porta hepatis

Area for transverse colon and right colic flexure

Area for superior duodenal flexure

ANTEROINFERIOR

Falciform ligament of the liver

ening with hypokalemia or even normokalemia.

Family 1. A group of individuals descending from a common ancestor. 2. A group of people living in a household who share common attachments, such as mutual caring, emotional bonds, common goal, etc. 3. In biology the division between an order and genus.

Family planning Planning and spacing of childbirth according to wishes of the couple rather than to chance.

Famotidine H_2 receptor blocker, used for peptic ulcer disease.

Fanconi syndrome Rickets with aminoaciduria, hypoplastic anaemia, growth failure.

Fang A sharp pointed tooth.

Fantasy The mechanism of creating in one's mind.

Farad A unit of electrical capacity. The capacity of a condenser that charged with 1 coulomb, gives a difference of potential of 1 volt.

Faradism Therapeutic use of an interrupted current to stimu-late muscles and nerves.

Farmer's lung Hypersensitive alveolitis on exposure to moldy hay.

Farsightedness An error of re-fraction in which parallel rays are focussed at a point behind retina, so that near objects are not seen clearly.

Fartan's procedure Palliative surgical procedure in children with single effective ventricle either because of heart valve defects, abnormality in pumping of the heart, or a complex congenital heart disease where it not possible or advisable to do bi-ventricular repair.

Fascia Fibrous membrane covering, supporting or separating muscles, uniting skin with underlying tissue. *f. Buck's* Facial covering of penis derived from Colle's fascia. *f. Cloquet's* Femoral fascia. *f. cribriform* Fascia of thigh covering saphenous opening. *f. pelvic* It maintains strength of pelvic floor. *f. Scarpa's* The deep layer of superficial fascia of abdomen. *f. transversalis* Fascia located between the perineum and transversalis muscle.

Fascicle A fasciculus.

Fasciculation Involuntary contraction or twitching of muscle fibers.

Fasciculus A small bundle especially of muscle or nerve fibers. *f. cuneatus* Triangular shaped bundle of nerve fibers in the dorsal column carrying sense of proprioception and deep touch. *Syn* – column of Burdach. *f. gracilis* It lies medial to f. cuneatus SYN – Column of Goll.

Fasciectomy Excision of a portion of fascia.

Fasciolopsis buski A fluke infesting intestinal tract of certain mammals including man.

Fascitis Inflammation of fascia.

Fastigium The highest point; The most posterior portion of fourth ventricle in brain.

Fasting Accepting no food.

Fat Adipose tissue of body serving as energy reserve, providing fat soluble vitamins.

Fatigue Feeling of tiredness resulting from continuing activity.

Fatty acids Omega - 3 Unsaturated fatty acids present in fish and certain vegetables, not synthesized in body. They reduce platelet adhesiveness and lower serum triglyceride; hence used in coronary artery disease prevention.

Fatty change Abnormal accumulation of fat within the cell.

Fauces The constricted opening leading from mouth to the pharynx bounded by soft palate, base of the tongue and palatine arches.

Faucial reflex Sensation of vomiting resulting from irritation of fauces.

Favism Hereditary hypersensitivity to a kind of bean, vicia faba characterized by fever, hemolytic anemia, vomiting; common to patients of G-6-PD deficiency.

Favus Fungal infection of skin characterized by yellowish crusts over hair follicle with itching and musty odor.

Fc Fragment A part of antibody.

Fc Receptor A receptor on phagocyte that binds to Fc fragment of IgG and IgE.

Fear Emotional reaction to external or internal threat, a feature of depression.

Febrile convulsion Convulsion precipitated by fever.

Feces Excreta, stool.

Feculent Having sediment.

Fecundation Fertilization, impregnation.

Fecundity Fertility, ability to produce children.

Feedback Return to original place, can be positive or negative.

Feeder A device permitting independent eating by severe neurologically disabled person. *f. artificial* Tube feeding, the tube passed through esophagus or rectum.

Feeling The conscious phase of nervous activity. Emotions are centrally stimulated feelings.

Fehling's solution A solution for testing urine sugar; prepared by dissolving 34.66 gm of copper sulfate in 500 ml. of water to make solution A and 173 gm. potassium iodide and 50 gm of sodium hydroxide in 500 ml. of water to make solution B. When urine containing sugar is boiled after addition of both the solutions, a red precipitate of cuprous oxide is formed.

Felbamate A newer antiepileptic agent.

Felodipine A calcium channel blocker used in hypertension.

Felon Abscess of soft tissue in terminal portion of finger.

Felty syndrome Rheumatoid arthritis associated with splenomegaly, neutropenia, anemia and often thrombocytopenia.

Female Woman, sex that produces ova.

Feminism Male developing secondary sexual characteristic of female.

Feminization testicular An apparent female with genetic characteristic of male due to tissue resistance to androgenic hormones secreted by testes.

Femoral artery A branch of external iliac artery.

Femur The longest and largest bone of the body extending from pelvis to knee (*see* Figure).

Fenestra An aperture frequently closed by membrane.

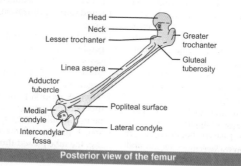

Head
Neck
Lesser trochanter
Greater trochanter
Gluteal tuberosity
Linea aspera
Adductor tubercle
Medial condyle
Popliteal surface
Intercondylar fossa
Lateral condyle

Posterior view of the femur

Fenfluramine An adrenergic agent.

Fenofibrate Lipid lowering agent.

Fenoprofen calcium Non-steroidal anti-inflammatory agent.

Fenoterol Beta-adrenergic agonist used in bronchial asthma.

Fenoverine Antispasmodic agent.

Fentanyl citrate Synthetic potent analgesic.

Ferment To decompose.

Fern A flowerless plant, whose extracts are used as anthelmintic.

Fern pattern Palm leaf (arborization) pattern of cervical mucus when allowed to dry on a glass slide; dependent on salt concentration in mucus which is further dependent upon amount of estrogen in the mucus. This test is only posi-tive in midcycle. If posi-tive in late cycle, indicates lack of progesterone.

Ferritin Iron-phosphorus protein complex containing about 23% iron, the principal tissue storage form of iron.

Ferrokinetics Study of absorption, utilization, storage and excretion of iron.

Ferroprotein Important oxygen transferring enzyme.

Ferrous Bivalent iron.

Ferric Trivalent iron, oxidized form.

Ferule A bond or ring of metal applied to the end of the root or crown of tooth in order to strengthen it.

Fertilization Union of ovum with spermatozoa or union of male and female gametes in plants (*see* Figure on page 258).

Fervescence Increase of fever.

Festinant Increase in speed, accelerating.

Fetal alcohol syndrome Birth defects and mental retardation in babies born to alcoholic mothers who continued alcohol ingestion during first trimester.

Fetal circulation Oxygenated blood from placenta passes via umbilical vein and ductus venosus to inferior vena cava bypassing liver and thence to right atrium and then via foramen ovale to left atrium, left ventricle and aorta. Some blood from right atrium also enters right ventricle and pulmonary artery to be shunted to aorta via ductus arteriosus. Blood to placental villi are returned via the two umbilical arteries which are continuation of hypogastric arteries (*see* Figure on page 259).

Feticide Killing of the fetus.

Fetish An object thought to have magical supernatural power.

Fertilization

The penetrarion of sperm through the corona radiata
and the zona pellucida is accomplished by the release
of acrosomal enzymes (acid phosphatase and acrosomase)
by many sperm

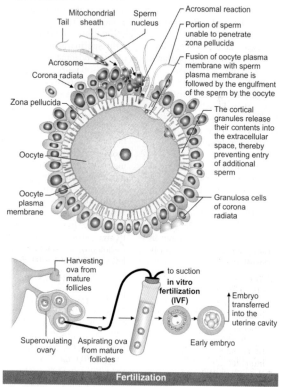

Tail — Mitochondrial sheath — Sperm nucleus

Acrosomal reaction

Portion of sperm unable to penetrate zona pellucida

Acrosome

Fusion of oocyte plasma membrane with sperm plasma membrane is followed by the engulfment of the sperm by the oocyte

Corona radiata

Zona pellucida

The cortical granules release their contents into the extracellular space, thereby preventing entry of additional sperm

Oocyte

Oocyte plasma membrane

Granulosa cells of corona radiata

Harvesting ova from mature follicles

to suction

in vitro fertilization (IVF)

Embryo transferred into the uterine cavity

Superovulating ovary

Aspirating ova from mature follicles

Early embryo

Fertilization

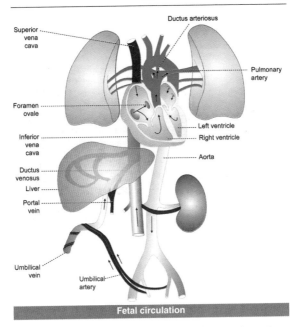

Fetal circulation

Fetoprotein A fetal antigen often present in adults. Amniotic fluid fetoprotein level can indicate about fetal wellbeing and maturity. Level is increased in defects of neuroaxis. Increased level in adults indicates hepatoma.

Fetoscope An flexible optical device of fiberoptic material used for direct visualization of fetus *in utero*.

Fetotoxic Materials toxic to developing fetus, e.g., alcohol sedatives, tetracycline, tobacco.

Fetus Child *in utero* from third month to birth. *f. amorphus* Shapeless fetus, barely recognizable as fetus. *f. calcified* Fetus dyeing *in utero* with calcification. *f. in fetu* A small imperfect fetus is contained within body of another fetus (e.g., desmoid). *f. mummified* A dead fetus that has assumed mummified form. *f. papyraceus* In twin pregnancy, the dead fetus is pressed flat by living fetus.

FEV1 Forced expiratory volume in 1 second. After full inspiration patient exhales as hard and as fast as possible into spirometer and the amount of air exhaled in 1 second is recorded. FEV_1 is reduced in obstructive lung disease.

Fever Elevation of body temperature above 37°C (98.6°F). Rectal temperature is 0.5-1°F higher than oral temperature. Body calorie expenditure is increased by 12% for each 0°C of fever. *f. continuous* Fever with diurnal variation of below 2°F as in enteric, typhus. *f. drug* Almost any drug can cause fever as a side effect. *f. of unknown origin* (FUO) Fever above 38°C on several occasions continuing for more than 3 weeks but without a diagnosis even with 1 week of hospital investigation. Common causes are neoplasms, collagen vascular diseases, pulmonary embolism, drug fever. *f. periodic* Inherited disease of unknown etiology manifesting with joint pain,

abdominal pain, pleurisy etc. *f. blister* Herpes simplex (type I) eruption of lips.

Fexofenadine H_1 receptor blocker, antiallergic.

Fiber Thread like element, can be nerve fiber, muscle fiber or a cellular product like collagen fiber, elastic fiber, reticulin fiber. *f. afferent* Fiber carrying impulses towards nerve cell. *f. dietary* Undigestible elements of food, i.e., cellulose, hemicellulose, lignin, pectin that add bulk to stool. Foods rich in fiber include whole grain, fruits, leafy vegetables, and their skin. High fiber intake prevents constipation, prevents diverticulosis, lowers cholesterol and sugar and possibly prevents colon cancer. *f. efferent* Nerve fiber carrying information away from nerve cell. *f. medullated* Nerve fiber whose axis cylinder is covered by myelin sheath.

Fibril A small fiber, often the component of a cell or a fiber; can be myofibril or neurofibril.

Fibrillation Spontaneous contraction of individual muscle fibers. *f. atrial* Rapid, irregular and incomplete contraction of atria. *f. ventricular* Similar to above, with ineffectual contraction of ventricles.

May result from mechanical injury to heart, coronary artery disease, drugs, electrocution, electrolyte imbalance, etc. Life-threatening unless immediately treated.

Fibrin Whitish filamentous protein formed by action of thrombin on fibrinogen. Fibrin entangles RBC and platelets to produce the clotting. *f. foam* A sponge like substance prepared from human fibrin used as hemostatic in surgery.

Fibrinogen A coagulation protein of plasma that is precursor of fibrin.

Fibrinogenolysis Dissolution of fibrin.

Fibrinogenopenia Reduction in blood fibrinogen.

Fibrinoid Resembling fibrin.

Fibrinoid change Change in connective tissue with immunologic injury, the tissue becoming homogeneous, swollen and band like.

Fibrinokinase Enzyme of animal tissue that activates plasminogen.

Fibrinolysin *SYN*—Plasmin that dissolves fibrin.

Fibrinolysis The process of dissolution of fibrin by plasmin.

Fibrinopeptide The substance removed from fibrinogen during blood coagulation; fibrin degradation product.

Fibrinosis Excess fibrin in blood.

Fibroadenoma Adenoma with fibrous tissue stroma.

Fibroangioma A fibrous tissue angioma.

Fibrocartilage A type of cartilage in which the matrix contains thick bundles of white or cartilaginous fibers. Found in the intervertebral disks.

Fibrocyst A fibrous tumor having undergone cystic degeneration.

Fibrocystic disease of breast Painful lump in breast, the pain and size fluctuating with menstrual cycle; 50% of women in reproductive age have this problem and carry a 2-5% greater risk of developing breast cancer.

Fibrocystic disease of pancreas Cystic fibrosis.

Fibroid Fibromyoma of uterus which may grow inwards or outwards to become subperitoneal (*see* Figure on page 262).

Fibroma Encapsulated, irregular, firm slow growing connective tissue tumor. Can arise within muscle, breast, uterus (causes menorrhagia) (*see* Figure on page 262).

Fibromatosis Simultaneous development of multiple fibromas. *f. gingivae* An inher-

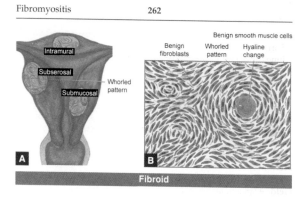

Fibroid

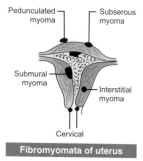

Fibromyomata of uterus

ited condition in which there is hypertrophy of gums prior to eruption of teeth.

Fibromyositis Inflammation of muscle and surrounding connective tissue, a nonspecific illness characterized by pain, tenderness, stiffness of joint capsule.

Fibromyxoma A fibroma that has undergone partial myxomatous degeneration.

Fibromyxosarcoma A sarcoma containing fibrous and myxoid tissue or sarcoma that has undergone mucoid degeneration.

Fibronectin A group of proteins whose presence in cervical secretion may act as marker for preterm labor.

Fibropapilloma Mixed fibroma and papilloma seen in bladder.

Fibrosarcoma A spindle celled sarcoma containing abundant connective tissue.

Fibrosis Abnormal fibrous tissue formation. *f. diffuse interstitial pulmonary SYN* – Hamman rich syndrome, causing respiratory distress of new born. *f. of lungs* Formation of scar tissue in lungs following pneumonia, lung abscess, tuberculosis. *f. retroperitoneal* Of unknown etiology, causes obstruction of ureter and great vessels.

Fibula The outer and smaller bone of leg, often sacrificed in bone grafting (*see* Figure below).

Fick method A method to determine cardiac output.

Field A specific area in relation to an object.

Fifth cranial nerve Trigeminal nerve, a mixed nerve with its sensory - motor nuclei in Pons - medulla.

Fifth disease Parvovirus infection with rash mimicing rubella.

FIGO staging system Staging system for gynecological cancers developed by International Federation of Gynecology and Obstetrics.

FIGLU excretion test Test for folic acid deficiency. When histidine is administered to a patient with folic acid deficiency formiminoglutamic acid excretion in urine is increased.

Filament Thread like coil of Tungsten found in X-ray tube.

Filaria A long filiform nematode found in lymphatics, serous cavities and connective tissue, e.g., *W. bancrofti*.

Filariasis A chronic disease due to filaria species.

Filiform Hair like, filamentous.

Film A thin membrane/covering; photographic film usually cellulose coated with a light sensitive emulsion. *f. bitewing* Technique used for taking film of several teeth at the same time.

Film badge A badge containing a film to calculate the total exposure of an individual to X-rays.

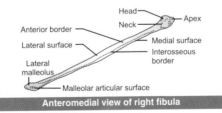

Head — Apex
Neck
Anterior border
Lateral surface — Medial surface
Interosseous border
Lateral malleolus
Malleolar articular surface

Anteromedial view of right fibula

Filter Device for filtering light, liquid, radiation, etc. *f. Berkefeld* A diatomaceous earth filter designed to remove bacteria from solutions passed through it (excepting viruses). *f. infrared* Filter that permits only passage of infrared waves of certain wave lengths. *f. optical* Device that only permits a portion of the visible light spectrum. The filter absorbs the unwanted wave length. *f. umbrella* Filter placed in blood vessels in order to prevent passage of emboli, e.g., inferior vena cava umbrella filter placement to reduce pulmonary embolism in patients of pelvic or deep leg vein thrombosis. *f. Wood's* A glass screen allowing passage of ultraviolet rays and absorbing rays of visual light, useful for diagnosis of fungus infection of hair.

Filtrate The fluid that has been passed through a filter. *f. glomerular* The protein free plasma filtered while passage of blood through glomeruli.

Filum A thread like structure. *f. coronaria* A fibrous band extending from the base of the median cusp of tricuspid valve to the aortic annulus. *f. terminale* A long slender filament at the terminal end of cord terminating in coccyx.

Fimbriate Having finger like projections (*see* Figure).

Finasteride Antiandrogen used for prostatic hypertrophy.

Fine motor skills Skills pertaining to synergy of small muscles of hand.

Finger One of the five digits of hand. *f. clubbed* Enlarged terminal phalanx of the finger. Present in cyanotic heart disease, pulmonary suppuration and malignancy, bacterial endocarditis. *f. hammer* Permanent flexion of terminal phalanx due to damage of extensor tendons. **Finger** *f. mallet* partial permanent flexion of terminal phalanx from rupture of extensor tendon. *f. trigger* momentary arrest of finger flexion/exten-

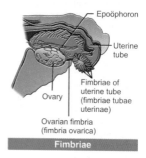

Fimbriae

sion followed by snapping into place due to stenosing tenovaginitis or nodule on flexor tendon.

Fingerprint An imprint made by the cutaneous ridges of fingers, used for the purpose of identification.

First aid Emergency assistance to injured/sick individuals prior to physician's care or transportation to hospital. Common situations necessitating first aid are: foreign body, coma, convulsion, burn, poisoning, etc.

First cranial nerve Nerve carrying smell sensation from olfactory mucosa.

First degree A.V. block Partial block of conduction in A-V node characterized by prolonged P-R interval. When occurring independently does not need treatment but if with anterior myocardial infarction or bundle branch block, it may progress to complete heart block and hence needs permanent pacemaker.

Fish skin disease A disease of skin characterized by increase of the horny layer and deficiency of the skin secretion.

Fission Splitting into two or more parts; a method of asexual reproduction in bacteria, protozoa and other lower forms of life.

Fissiparous Reproducing by fission.

Fissure A groove or natural division, cleft or slit, break in enamel of tooth, crack like sore, deep furrow in an organ like brain, liver, spinal cord. *f. anal* Linear painful ulcer at anal margin. *f. auricular* Fissure of petrous part of temporal bone. *f. Broca* Fissure encircling the third left frontal convolution of the brain. *f. inferior orbital* Fissure at the apex of orbit, through which pass the infraorbital blood vessels and maxillary branch of trigeminal nerve. *f. of Rolando* Fissure separating frontal and parietal lobes. *f. of Sylvius* Fissure separating frontal and parietal lobes from temporal lobe. *f. transverse* 1. Fissure between cerebrum and cerebellum of brain. 2. Fissure on the lower surface of liver serving as the hilum for entrance of hepatic vessels and exit of ducts.

Fistula An abnormal free passage from cavity/or inner organ to exterior/another organ. *f. arteriovenous* Direct communication between artery and vein. *f. horseshoe* Perianal fistula in which the tract goes round the rectum and communicates with skin at one or more point. *f. thyroglossal* A midline fistula about thyroid that connects the persistent embryonic thyroglossal duct to exterior.

Fixation point The fovea or the point on the retina where the visual axes meet for clearest vision. *f. external* external pin fixation, the pins connected to metal bar for maintaining alignment of open fracture. *f. internal* open reduction and fixation by plate, nail, screw or wire. *f. complement* the consumption of complement when reacting with immune complexes containing complement fixing antibodies. *f. nitrogen* traping of atmospheric nitrogen as nitrate or amino group by bacteria of genus *Rhizobium*. *f. ossicular chain* fixation of one or more auditory ossicles.

Flaccid Paralysis with loss of muscle tone, reduction or loss of tendon reflexes, atrophy of muscles, usually due to lesion of lower motor neurone.

Flagellate A protozoon with one or more flagella.

Flagellation Whipping, massage by strokes, a form of sexual aberration in which sexual urge is brought about by being whipped or whipping the partner.

Flagellin Protein of flagella, resembling myosin

Flagellum A hair like motile process on a protozoon.

Flail chest A condition arising from fracture of a number of ribs, or ribs at many points, resulting in the flail rib segment moving in paradoxically with inspiration and out with expiration.

Flail joint Joint with excessive mobility due to paralysis of acting muscles.

Flange In dentistry, the part of an artificial denture that extends from embedded teeth to the border of denture.

Flank The part of body between ribs and upper border of ilium.

Flap A mass of partially detached tissue used in plastic surgery. *f. pedicle* Flap made by suturing the edges to form a tube. Then one end of the tube is severed and sutured to another site. By use of this jump flap technique, such a flap may be moved in several stages, a great distance. *f. periodontal* Gingival flap removed or repositioned to eliminate periodontal pockets or to correct mucogingival defects.

Flare A spreading area of redness that surrounds a line made by drawing a pointed instrument across the skin. It is due to dilatation of blood vessels.

Flashbacks The return of imagery and hallucinations after the immediate effect of hallucinogens is worn off.

Flash point The temperature at which substance will burst into flames spontaneously.

Flat foot Abnormal flatness of sole and loss of arch on innerside of foot.

Flatness Resonance heard on percussion over solid organs or when there is fluid in the thoracic cavity.

Flatulence Excessive formation or passage of gas from GI tract.

Flatus Expulsion of gas from anus. Average person excretes 400-1200 cc of gas everyday, containing hydrogen, methane, skatoles, indoles, carbon dioxide, small amounts of oxygen and nitrogen. Flatulogenic foods are milk, legumes, fried items.

Flatus tube A rectal tube which is pushed to facilitate expulsion of gas.

Flavi virus Previously called group B arbo virus responsible for yellow fever, dengue fever and encephalitis.

Flavin One of a group of natural water soluble pigments occurring in milk, yeast, bacteria and some plants.

Flavism Having a yellow tinge.

Flavobacterium A group of bacteria producing orange-yellow pigments in culture. Flavobacterium meningosepticum causes virulent meningitis in prematures.

Flavoprotein A group of conjugated proteins that constitute yellow enzyme for cellular respiration.

Flavour The quality that affects the sense of taste.

Flavoxate Urinary antispasmodic.

Flaxedil Gallamine triethiodide.

Flea Wingless blood sucking insects that have legs adapted for jumping. Xenopsella species transmit plague from rats to humans. Fleas may transmit tularemia, endemic typhus and brucellosis. *f. chigger* Sand flea.

Fleccainide acetate Antiarrhythmic agent.

Fleece of Stilling Meshwork of white fibers that surrounds the dentate nucleus of cerebellum.

Fleming Alexander Scottish physician who in 1945 was awarded Nobel prize for discovering penicillin.

Flesh Soft tissues of animal body, esp. the muscles.

Fletcher factor A blood clotting factor, prekallikrein.

Flexibility Adaptibility, quality of being bent without breaking.

Flexion The act of bending forward.

Flexor Muscle that bends a part in proximal direction. *f. left colic* Bend in colon where transverse colon continues as descending colon *SYN* – splenic flexure. *f. right colic* Bend in colon where ascending colon becomes the transverse colon *SYN* – hepatic flexure.

Flicker The visual sensation of alternating intervals of brightness caused by rhythmically interrupting light stimuli.

Flight of ideas Continuous but fragmentary stream of talk may be seen in acute mania.

Floaters Translucent specks of various sizes and shapes that float across the visual field; usually small bits of protein or cells.

Flocculation The gathering together of fine dispersed particles in a solution into larger visible particles.

Flocculus 1. A small tuft of wool like fibers. 2. Lobes of cerebellum behind the middle cerebral peduncle.

Floppy-valve syndrome Mitral valve prolapse.

Floss To use dental floss or tape to remove plaque or calculus.

Flour Ground wheat powder.

Flowmeter Device for measuring flow of gas or liquid, i.e. flow of anesthetic gases.

Flow state An altered state of consciousness in which the mind functions at its peak, time may seem to be distorted and a sense of happiness seems to pervade that period.

Floxuridine An antimetabolite used in cancer treatment.

Fluconazole Benzimidazole antifungal for candidiasis, cryptococcosis.

Fluctuation A wavy impulse felt in palpation and produced by vibration of body fluid.

Flucytosine Antifungal agent.

Fludrocortisone Synthetic corticosteroid with high mineral retaining property.

Flufenamic acid Nonsteroidal anti-inflammatory agent.

Flufenazine enanthate A phenothiazine type antipsychotic drug.

Fluid amniotic Clear yellowish fluid of specific gravity 1.006 composed of albumin, urea, water mixed with lanugo, epidermal cells, vernix caseosa, and meconium.

Fluid cerebrospinal Fluid found in central canal of spinal cord, in the ventricles of brain and in the subarachnoid space.

Fluid synovial Fluid contained within synovial cavities, bursae and tendon sheaths.

Fluid Balance Regulation of water homeostasis in body.

Fluke A parasite belonging to class trematoda. *f. blood* Schistostoma hematobium, *S. mansoni, S. japonicum* belong to this group inhabiting mesenteric and pelvic veins. *f. hepatica Fasciola hepatica,* chlorosis sinensis. *f. intestinal Fasciolopsis buski. f. lung Paragonimus westermani.*

Flumethasone Synthetic corticosteroid.

Flunarizine Calcium channel blocker for migraine.

Fluocinolone acetonide Synthetic corticosteroid.

Fluorescein sodium A red crystalline powder, used for corneal staining and angiography.

Fluorescence Property of certain substances to emit light when exposed to ultraviolet radiation.

Fluorescent Luminous when exposed to other light rays.

Fluorescent antibody A body tagged with fluorescent material, for diagnosis of various kinds of infections.

Fluorescent treponemal antibody absorption test (FTA-ABS) Test for syphilis using fluorescent anti-body.

Fluoridation Addition of fluorides to water to prevent dental caries in the concentration of 1 mg/1000 ml of water drinking to assure daily fluoride intake of 0.25 to 0.5 mg.

Fluoroapatite A compound formed when the enamel of teeth is treated with appropriate concentration of fluoride to form hydroxyapatite which is less acid soluble, hence resistant to caries.

Fluorometer Device for determining amount of radiation produced by X-rays.

Fluoroscope A radiological tool consisting of a fluorescent screen by means of which the shadows of objects interposed between the tube and screen are made visible.

Fluoroscopy Patient examination by fluoroscope.

Fluorosis Chronic flourine poisoning causing mottling of tooth enamel, and hyperluscency of bone.

Fluorouracil Antimetabolite, anticancer agent.

Fluoxetine 5HT antagonist, antidepressant.

Fluoxymesterone An anabolic and androgenic hormone.

Flupenthixol Antipsychotic agent.

Flurandrenolide A corticosteroid.

Flurazepam Sedative - hypnotic agent.

Flurbiprofen Propionic acid derivative NSAID.

Flurogestone A progestational drug.

Fluroxene An anesthetic agent administered by inhalation.

Flush 1. Sudden redness of skin. 2. Irrigation of cavity with water. *f. hot* Flush accompanied with sensations of heat, common in menopausal syndrome and neuroses.

Flutamide Antiandrogen used for BPH.

Fluticasone Steroid inhaler for asthma.

Flutter A tremulous movement. *f. atrial* Rapid atrial contraction (200-400/ min.) but with a regular heart beat due to 1:2/1:3 AV block. *f. diaphragmatic* Rapid diaphragmatic contraction. *f. mediastinum* Abnormal side to side motion of diaphragm.

Fluvoxamine SSRI antidepressant.

Flux An excessive flow or discharge from an organ or cavity of body.

Foam Production of gas bubble interspersed with fluid.

Foam solubility test Procedure for determining the presence or absence of surfactant active material in amniotic fluid. Surfactant deficit is diagnostic of respiratory distress syndrome.

Focus The point of convergence of light rays or waves of sounds.

Fog Water droplets in air.

Fogging 1. A method of testing vision used particularly in testing astigmatism and in postcycloplegic examination. 2. Unwanted density on the radiographic film resulting from exposure to secondary radiation, light, chemicals, heat, etc.

Foil A thin pliable sheet of metal. Gold foils are used in dental restoration work.

Fold A doubling back. *f. aryepiglottic* The ridge like lateral walls of the entrance to larynx. *f. gastric* Gastric mucosal folds; mostly longitudinal. *f. rectum* Transverse mucosal folds of rectum, *SYN*—valves of Houston.

Foley's catheter A urinary tract catheter with balloon attachment at the end (*see* Figure).

Foliaceous Resembling leaf.

Folic acid $C_{19}H_{19}N_7O_6$, chemically pteroyl glutamic acid, found in green plant tissue, liver and yeast. Deficiency causes megaloblastic anemia.

Folinic acid The active form of folic acid.

Follicle A small secretory sac or cavity. *f. aggregated Syn*—Peyer's patch. An aggregation of solitary nodules or group of lymph nodules at the junction of ileum with colon at the anti- mesenteric border. *f. graffian* Developing primary oocyte in the cortex of ovary. *f. hair* An invagination of the epidermis from which hair develops. *f. lymphatic* The densely packed collection of lymphocytes and lymphoblasts that make up cortex of a lymph node. *f. nabothian* Dilated cyst of glands of uterine cervix. *f. ovarian* A spherical structure in the cortex of ovary consisting of an oocyte and surrounding follicular cells. *f. primordial* Follicle of ovary with ovum enclosed in a single layer of cells. *f. of thyroid* Spherical structure lined with a single

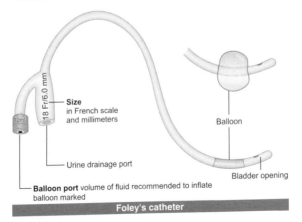

Foley's catheter

Follicle-stimulating hormone (FSH) Hormone of anterior pituitary stimulating spermatogenesis in male and maturation of graffian follicle in female.

Follicular tonsillitis Inflammation of follicles on surface of tonsils which become filled with pus.

Folliculitis barbae Ringworm of beard.

Folliculoma A tumor of ovary originating in graffian follicle in which cells resemble the cells of stratum granulosum.

Folliculosis Presence of an abnormal quantity of lymph follicles.

Follow-up The continued care or monitoring of a patient after the initial visit or examination.

Fomentation A hot, wet application for the relief of pain or inflammation.

Fomes (fomite) Any substance that adheres to and transmits infectious material.

Fontana's spaces Spaces between the processes of ligamentum pectinatum of iris, conveying aqueous humor.

Fontanel Unossified space lying between cranial bones of the skull. *f. anterior* Lying at the junction of coronal, frontal and sagittal sutures. *f. posterior* Lying at the junction of sagittal and lambdoid sutures (*see* Figure).

Food additives Substances other than basic food stuffs that are present in food during production, processing, storage or packaging.

Food adulterants Substances making food impure or toxic like toxic organisms, pesticide residues, poisonous substance or substances added to increase weight or bulk of food.

Food allergies Allergic reaction resulting from ingestion of food to which one has become

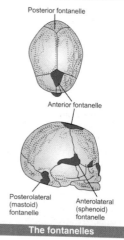

Posterior fontanelle

Anterior fontanelle

Posterolateral (mastoid) fontanelle

Anterolateral (sphenoid) fontanelle

The fontanelles

sensitized. Common offenders are: milk, egg, shellfish, chocolate, oranges.

Food and drug administration (FDA) In USA, an official regulatory body for food, drugs, cosmetics, and medical devices, a part of Department of Health and Human Services.

Foodball Gastric stone made up of fruit and vegetable skins, seeds and fibers. *SYN* – phytobezoar.

Food chain Sequential transfer of food energy from green plants to herbivorous animals and then to man through animal flesh. Interruption of this chain can result in ecological disaster.

Food poisoning Illness resulting from ingestion of foods containing poisonous substances, e.g., mushroom poisoning, insecticides contaminating food, milk from cows that have eaten some poisonous plants, ingestion of putrefied or decomposed food.

Food requirement Requirement of calorie and protein depending upon age, muscular work and environment. Average active healthy (70 kg) man requires 2700 cal/day and average healthy woman 2000 cal/day. Persons in sedentary work require less calories. Protein requirement of adult is 1 gm/kg of their ideal weight. Pregnancy and lactation demand 15-25% extra calories. In growing children protein requirement is 2-3 gm/kg/day.

Foot Terminal portion of lower extremity. *f arches* Four arches: internal longitudinal, outer longitudinal, and two transverse arches. *f. athlete's* Fungus infection of interdigital spaces. *f. cleft* A condition where cleft extends between the digits to the metatarsal region, usually due to a missing digit. *f. flat* The inner longitudinal and anterior transverse metatarsal arches are depressed and flat; very often asymptomatic. *f. immersion* Resulting from prolonged immersion of foot in cold water or exposure of foot to extreme cold swampy atmosphere resulting in impaired circulation and anesthesia. *f. madura* Bone hypertrophy and degeneration, frequently followed by suppuration and gangrene, causative agents are—mycetomas. *f. splay* Flat wide foot.

Foot and mouth disease A viral disease of cattle and horses.

Foot board A device that helps to prevent foot drop.

Foot candle An amount of light equivalent to one lumen per square foot.

Foot drop Plantar flexion of foot due to paralysis of muscles in anterior compartment of leg. (lateral popliteal palsy).

Foot plate The flat part of stapes, the bone of middle ear.

Foot print An impression of foot used for identification of infants.

Forage Creating a channel through enlarged prostate by use of an electric cautery.

Foramen A passage; opening; an orifice; a communication between two cavities. *f. apical* Opening at the end of root canal transmitting blood, lymph and nerve supply to dental pulp. *f. condyloid* Opening above the condyle of occipital bone for passage of hypoglossal nerve. *f. epiploic* Opening connecting the peritoneal cavity to lesser sac *SYN* – foramen of Winslow. *f. internal auditory* The opening in the petrous portion of sphenoid bone through which 7th and 8th cranial nerves pass. *f. intervertebral* Opening between adjacent articulated vertebrae for passage of nerves. *f. jugular* Opening at base of skull permitting passage of sigmoid and inferior petrosal sinus and 9th, 10th, and 11th cranial nerves (*see* Figure). *f. magnum* Opening in the occipital bone through which passes the spinal cord. *f. of Monro* Communication between third and lateral ventricles of brain. *f. optic* Opening in the lesser wing of sphenoid bone permitting passage of optic nerve and ophthalmic artery. *f. ovale* Opening between the two atria in fetal heart which often continues into adulthood. *f. rotundum* Opening in greater wing of sphenoid in which maxillary branch of trigeminal nerve passes.

Forbe's disease Type III glycogen storage disease.

Force A push or pull exerted upon an object, measured in newtons. 1 newton is equivalent to 0.225 pound force.

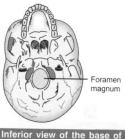

Foramen magnum

Inferior view of the base of the skull, showing the foramen magnum

f. electromotive Energy that causes flow of electricity in a conductor.

Forceps Pincers for holding/extracting. *f. alligator* Toothed forceps with a double clamp. *f. artery* Forceps for holding ends of an artery in order to perform ligation. *f. clamp* Any forcep with automatic lock. *f. dental* Forceps of varying shapes for grasping teeth during extraction. *f. obstetrics* Forceps used to extract the fetal head from pelvis. *f. towel/tissue* Forceps for clipping towels to operation site or grasping delicate tissue (*see* Figure).

Fordyce's disease Enlarged ectopic sebaceous glands in mucosa of mouth and genitals.

Fordyce-Fox disease A disease similar to prickly heat in which itchy follicular papules are present in axilla, areola of breast, labia, etc.

Forensic Pertains to legal.

Forensic dentistry Application of science of dentistry for the purposes of law, e.g., establishing identity.

Forensic medicine Medicine in relation to law, legal aspects of medical ethics and standards.

Foreskin Prepuce; loose skin covering end of penis/clitoris.

Fore waters Mucus discharge from vagina during pregnancy.

Fork turning An elongated instrument that bifurcates at one end, used for testing

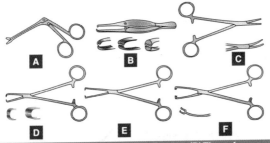

Some types of forceps—(A) Alligator forceps, (B) Tissue forceps, (C) Halsted mosquito forceps (straight and curved), (D) Allis forceps, (E) Schoeder tenaculum forceps, (F) Schoeder vulsellum forceps (with side view of blade)

hearing, bone conduction and vibration.

Formaldehyde A colorless pungent irritant gas formed by oxidation of methyl alcohol, used as disinfectant, preservative in histology and for sterilizing feces, urine, sputum.

Formalin Aqueous solution of 37% formaldehyde.

Formation A structure, shape or figure. *f. reticular* Found in medulla oblongata between the pyramids and floor of the fourth ventricle, supposed to be the activating or arousal system for consciousness.

Forme fruste An aborted or incomplete form of disease arrested before running its course.

Formestane Antiestrogen.

Formic acid A clear pungent acid obtained from oxidation of formaldehyde or wood alcohol, responsible for pain and swelling following stings and bites.

Formication Sensation of insects creeping upon the body.

Formiminoglutamic acid (FI-GLU) A chemical intermediate in the metabolism of histidine to glutamic acid. In folic acid deficiency states FIGLU excretion is increased in urine.

Formoterol Inhaled steroid.

Fornication Sexual intercourse between unmarried partners.

Fornix Anything of arched or vault like shape. *f. conjunc-*

tivae Loose fold connecting palpebral and bulbar conjunctivae. *f. uteri* Anterior and posterior spaces into which upper vagina is divided.

Fosinopril ALE inhibitor.

Forskolin Cardiac stimulant for congestive failure.

Fortification spectrum Appearance of dark patch with zigzag outline in the visual field causing temporary blindness in that portion of eye.

Fossa A shallow depression.

Fourchette Transverse band of mucus membrane at the posterior commissure of vagina.

Fourth cranial nerve Trochlear nerve emerging from dorsal surface of midbrain, supplying superior oblique.

Fovea A pit or cup like depression. e.g., fovea centralis of eye (*see* Figure).

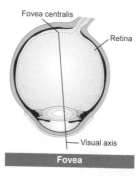

Fovea centralis

Retina

Visual axis

Fovea

Fowler's position Semisitting position with angulation of upper portion of body at 45°-60°; knees may or may not be bent.

Foxglove Common name for plant digitalis purpurea.

Fraction of inspired oxygen (FiO2) The concentration of O_2 in the inspired air.

Fractional testmeal Fractional examination of stomach contents for free and total hydrochloric acid.

Fracture Dissolution in continuity of bone (*see* Figure). *f. avulsion* Tearing of a piece of bone away from the main bone by force of muscular contraction. *f. comminuted* Fracture where bone is broken into many pieces. *f. compound* Fracture where bone fragment protrudes through skin or there is communication between fracture site and exterior. *f. compression* Fracture of vertebra by pressure along long axis of the vertebral column. *f. epiphyseal* Separation of epiphysis from bone, occurs only in young patients. *f. fissured* A narrow split in the bone, the split not extending to other side of bone. *f. gree stick* Fracture when one cortex fractures, the other being intact. *f. hair line* A thin

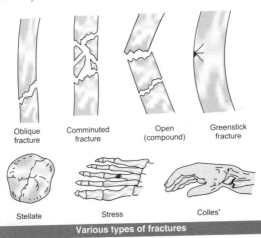

| Oblique fracture | Comminuted fracture | Open (compound) | Greenstick fracture |

| Stellate | Stress | Colles' |

Various types of fractures

narrow incomplete fracture line not extending through the entire bone. *f. impacted* Fracture where one end is wedged into the interior of other. *f. pathologic* Fracture of a weakened bone produced by a force, that would not have fractured a healthy bone. *f. pingpong* Depressed fracture of skull resembling indentation made on pingpong ball by compression. *f. Pott's* Fracture of lower end of fibula with outward displacement of the ankle and foot.

Fragile-X syndrome Mutation in X-chromosome manifesting with mental retardation and greatly enlarged testicles after puberty.

Fragilitas Brittleness as of the hair.

Fragility State of brittleness. *f. erythrocyte* Rupture of RBC in various strengths of salt solution. Normal blood starts hemolyzing at about 0.44% and complete at 0.35%.

Frambesia Infectious disease caused by a spirochete.

Frambesioma Primary lesion of yaws in the form of a protruding nodule.

Franceschetti's syndrome Mandibulofacial dysostosis *SYN*—Treacher-Collin's syndrome.

Francisella tularensis Non-motile, encapsulated, gram –ve organism causing plague.

Fratricide Murder of one's brother or sister.

Freckle Small brownish or yellowish pigmentation of skin.

Freiberg's infarction Osteo-chondritis of head of second metatarsal bone.

Fremitus Vibrating tremors esp. those felt through the chest wall by palpation or auscultation.

French scale A system indicating outer catheter diameters. Each unit of scale is equivalent to 1/3 mm.

Frenkel exercise These exercise involve teaching patient muscle and joint sensation in order to restore the lost co-ordination. Especially useful in cases of tabes dorsalis and other ataxic conditions.

Frenotomy Cutting of the frenum esp. of tongue.

Frenulum linguae A fold of mucus membrane that extends from floor of mouth to the inferior surface of tongue along midline.

Frenzy A state of violent mental agitation or excitement. *f. response* In electrodiagnostic study of spinal reflexes, the time required for a stimulus applied to a motor nerve to travel in the opposite direction up the nerve to the spinal cord and return.

Fretum A constriction.

Freud Sigmund Austrian neurologist and psychoanalyst.

Frey's syndrome A rare condition affecting young children characterized by facial flushing and sweating after eating.

Freudian Freud's theories of unconscious or repressed libido on past experiences or desires as the cause of various neuroses, and cure for which is the restoration of such conditions to consciousness through psychoanalysis.

Friable Easily breakable.

Friction Rubbing, massage.

Friction rub The sound produced by friction of two dry surfaces.

Friedlander's bacillus *Klebsiella pneumonae* causing pneumonia, sinusitis.

Friedrich's ataxia An inherited disease involving degeneration of dorso-lateral columns of spinal cord, kyphoscoliosis and muscular weakness of lower limbs.

Fright Extreme sudden fear.

Frigid Cold, irresponsive to emotions or lack of sexual desire in women.

Frigidity Partial or complete inhibition of sexual excitement.

Frogbelly Flaccid atonic abdomen of children with rickets.

Frog face Facies of chronic sinusitis.

Frohlichs syndrome Obesity, hypogonadism, due to hypothalamic disturbance.

Froin's syndrome High CSF protein content that rapidly coagulates and is yellow caused by spinal canal obstruction.

Fromet's sign Flexion of distal phalanx of thumb when a sheet of paper is held between thumb and index finger, a feature of ulnar nerve palsy.

Frontal lobe 4 main convolutions in front of central sulcus of cerebrum.

Frontal plane Plane parallel with the long axis of body and at right angles to the median sagittal plane.

Frontal sinus A pair of hollow asymmetrical spaces in the frontal bone above the orbits, filled with air and lined by mucus membrane.

Front tap reflex Contraction of gastrocnemius muscles when stretched muscles of extended leg are percussed.

Frost uremic Deposit of urea crystals on skin in uremia patient.

Frostbite Freezing and death of a body part due to cold exposure.

Frottage Orgasm produced by pressing against somebody, massage technique using rubbing.

Frozen section A technique of examining and reporting on pathological tissue cut from a patient while on surgical table, thus deciding future course of action in the theatre itself.

Fructokinase Enzyme that transfers high energy phosphate from a donor to fructose.

Fructose $C_6H_{12}O_6$, fruit sugar, monosachharide akin to glucose.

Fructose intolerance Inability to metabolize fructose in absence of enzyme aldolase thus producing nausea, vomiting, sweating, tremor, hypoglycemia on fructose consumption.

Frustration Disappointment.

Fucose A mucopolysaccharide present in blood group substances and in human milk.

Fucosidosis Hereditary disease with thick skin, heart disease, hyperhydrosis and poor neural growth resulting from improper metabolism of fucose.

Fugitive Inconstant symptoms, transient, wandering.

Fugue A dissociative disorder in which a person acts in normal manner but has complete amnesia for that period of action.

Fulguration Destruction of tissue by high frequency electric sparks.

Full term In obstetric child born between 38-41 weeks of gestation.

Fulminant Coming like flashes of pain, as in tabes dorsalis. Syno fulgurant.

Fumaric acid One of the organic acids in the citric acid cycle.

Fumigation Use of poisonous gases for destroying living organisms like insects, rats, mice, etc; root disinfection.

Functional disease Emotional response to physical disease, taking the form of conversion or hysterical response.

Fundoplication Surgical reduction in size of opening into fundus of stomach, used in treating reflux esophagitis.

Fundoscopy Visual examination of fundus of eye.

Fundus The portion of an organ most remote from its opening (*see* Figure on page 281).

Fungus Plant like organism including yeasts and molds but without chlorophil, hence of having parasitic or saprophytic existence.

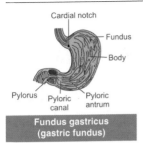

Fundus gastricus (gastric fundus)

Furgemia Presence of fungi in blood.

Fungiform papillae Small rounded eminences on the tongue.

Funicular process That part of tunica vaginalis covering spermatic cord.

Funiculitis Inflammation of spermatic cord.

Funiculopexy Suturing the spermatic cord to tissues in cases of undescended testes.

Funiculus Any small structure resembling cord.

Funnel Conical wide mouthed device for pouring through it with a tubular end.

Funnel chest Sternal depression resembling funnel.

Funny bone Medial epicondyle of humerus.

Fur fur Dandruff scales.

Furor Extreme violent outbursts of anger.

Furosemide Loop diuretic, kaliuretic.

Furrow A groove.

Furuncle A boil.

Furunculoid Resembling boil.

Furunculosis Condition resulting from boil.

Fuscin A dark brown pigment present in pigment epithelium of retina.

Fusiform Spindle shaped, i.e., tapering at both ends.

Fusion Meeting and joining together (*see* Figure below).

Fusobacterium A genus of nonspore forming, nonmotile, non encapsulated gram –ve rods causing gingivitis, and seen in necrotic lesions. *f. waves* Flutter waves in atrial fibrillation.

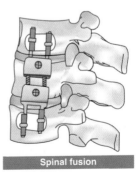

Spinal fusion

G

GABA Gamma amino butyric acid a, neurotransmitter.

Gabapentin An antiepileptic agent.

Gadolinium A rare element used as NMR contrast agent.

Gag An instrument placed between the teeth to keep the mouth open.

Gag reflex Gagging and vomiting resulting from irritation of fauces.

Gail score An indicator for assessing the risk of a woman to develop breast cancer in the next 5 years.

Gait Manner of walking. *g. ataxic* Staggering unsteady gait, e.g., alcoholics. *g. cerebellar* Staggering broad based gait. *g. double step* Gait in which alternate steps are of a different length or at a different rate. *g. equine* High stepping gait of peroneal nerve palsy. *g. festinating* Walking on toes as if pushed from behind. Starts slowly and then accelerates till he holds on to something that stops him e.g., parkinsonism. *g. hemiplegic* The paralyzed limb abducts and makes a circle to come to front to touch the ground. *g. scissor* Gait in which legs cross while walking, e.g. cerebral palsy. *g. slapping* High stepping ataxic gait due to loss of proprioception as in tabes dorsalis. *g. Waddling* Walk resembling that of a duck as in muscular dystrophy.

Galactan A complex carbohydrate that forms galactose on hydrolysis.

Galactase A proteolytic ferment of milk.

Galactocele A tumor caused by occlusion of a milk duct; hydrocele containing milk like fluid.

Galactogogue Agent promoting secretion of milk.

Galactokinase Enzyme transferring high energy phosphate groups from a donor to D-Galactose.

Galactometer Device for measuring specific gravity of milk.

Galactorrhoea Excessive flow of milk, continuation of lactation even without childbirth.

Galactose $C_6H_{12}O_6$ a monosacc-haride, isomer of glucose converted to glycogen in liver.

Galactosemia An autosomal recessive inborn error of metabolism characterized by inability to convert galactose to glucose due to absence of enzyme galactose-1 phosphate uridyl transferase. Symptoms are diarrhoea and vomiting with failure to thrive afterbirth. Infants urine contains high galactose. Intrauterine diagnosis possible from amniocentesis.

Galactosuria Excretion of galactose in urine.

Galeazzi's sign A clinical test for determining presence of congenital hip dislocation in infants and toddlers; with the child lying supine, knees and hips flexed to 90°; dislocation is evidenced if one knee is higher than other.

Galen's veins These veins run through the telachoro-diae formed by the joining of the terminal and choroid veins. They form venacere-bra magna, that empties into straight sinus.

Gallamine triethiodide A drug that inhibits transmis-sion of nerve impulses across myoneural junction of vol-untary muscles. Trade name Flaxedil.

Gallbladder Pear shaped sac on under surface of right lobe of liver holding bile and discharging it into common bile duct through cystic duct during digestion (see Figure).

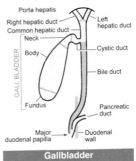

Gallbladder

Gallium Radionucleide of gallium used in bone scan.

Gallon Measure of liquid equivalent to 4.55 liters.

Gallstone Concretion formed in the gallbladder or common bile duct, commonest being cholesterol stone. Excess of cholesterol or decreased bile acid concentration in bile help to precipitate cholesterol leading to stone formation.

Galvanic current Direct electric current from battery.

Galvanometer An instrument for measurement of current.

Galvanoscope An instrument that shows presence and direction of galvanic current.

Gamete A mature male or female reproductive cell.

Gamete intrafallopian transfer (GIFT) The process involves obtaining ova through laparoscope and mating it with sperms and then placing in fallopian tube for completion of fertilization and transfer to uterus.

Gametes The sexually differentiated form of protozoa that when enters mosquito reproduces into sporozoites.

Gametocide Agents that destroy malaria gametocytes.

Gametogenesis Development of gametes.

Gamma benzene hexachloride Scabicidal agent and insecticide.

Gamma globulin Immunoglobulin fraction in plasma containing IgG, IgA, IgD and IgE.

Gamma knife surgery A modality of treatment of brain tumor, where radiation bean is focused on tumor tissue with stereotoxic precison.

Gamma rays Electromagnetic waves of extremely short wave length emitted by radioactive substances having high tissue penetration.

Gammopathy Diseases with high gammaglobulin, e.g., multiple myeloma.

Gamna's disease This is a form of chronic splenomegaly characterised by thickening of the splenic capsule and presence of multiple, small, dense, rust-like densities containing iron. These bodies are known as gamna–gandy bodies.

Gamophobia Neurotic fear of marriage.

Gangliocyte A ganglion cell.

Ganglioma Tumor of lymphatic gland.

Ganglion 1. A mass of nervous tissue composed principally of nerve cell bodies lying outside brain and spinal cord. 2. Cystic tumor developing in a tendon or aponeuroses. *g. cardiac* Tiny ganglion towards which converge the fibers of superficial cardiac plexus, lying on the right side of the ligamentum arteriosum. *g. carotid* Ganglion formed by filamentous threads from the carotid plexus beneath the carotid artery. *g. celiac* One pair of paravertebral or collateral ganglia located near the origin of celiac artery. *g. dorsal root* Ganglia located in dorsal nerve root containing cell bodies of sensory nerves. *g. geniculate* Ganglion on the pars intermedia, the sensory root of facial nerve. *g. jugular* Ganglion located on the root of vagus nerve lying in upper portion of jugular foramen. *g. otic* A small ganglion located in zygomatic fossa below the foramen ovale. *g. sphenopala-tine* Ganglion associated with the great superficial petrosal nerve and maxillary nerve, transmitting both sympathetic and parasympathetic fibers to nasal mucosa, palate, pharynx and orbit. *g. spiral* A long coiled ganglion in the cochlea of ear containing bipolar cells whose peripheral processes terminate in organ of corti. The central processes form the cochlear nerve to terminate in medulla. *g. vestibular* A bipolar ganglion located in the vestibular branch of 8th cranial nerve at the base of internal acoustic meatus. Its incoming fibers arise from macules of utricles and saccules and cristae of ampullae of semicircular canals (*see* Figure).

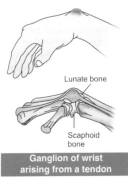

Ganglion of wrist arising from a tendon

Ganglioneuroma A nerve cell tumor containing ganglion cells.

Ganglionic blockade Blockage of neurotransmission in autonomic ganglia by drugs that occupy receptor sites for acetylcholine or stabilize post synaptic membrane against action of acetylcholine liberated in presynaptic nerve endings.

Ganglioside A particular class of glycosphingolipid present in nerve tissue and in the spleen.

Gangrene Necrosis or death of tissue, usually due to deficient blood supply. *g. dry* Aseptic gangrene due to cessation of blood supply, the veins remaining patent. *g. diabetic* Infected gangrene in diabetics. *g. traumatic* Gangrene following extensive injury severing blood supply (*see* Figure below).

Ganser's syndrome A factitious disorder in which

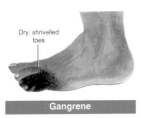

Gangrene

individual mimics symptoms of psychosis.

Gardnerella vaginalis A bacteria causing vaginitis.

Gardner's syndrome Familial polyposis of colon, an autosomal dominant condition with propensity for development of carcinoma.

Gargoylism A congenital condition characterized by dwarfism, kyphosis, and skeletal abnormalities with mental retardation.

Garlic An edible strongly flavoured bulb containing chemical allicin, possessing antithrombotic properties.

Garment (pneumatic-antishock) an inflatable garment used to combat shock, stabilize fracture, promote haemostasis, increase peripheral vascular resistance (*see* Figure).

Garre's disease Chronic sclerosing osteomyelitis.

Gärtner's bacillus It is another name for the bacillus, *Salmonella enteritidis* which is responsible for causing gastroenteritis in man and other animals.

Gartner's duct A vestigial structure representing the persistent mesonephric duct.

Gas mustard Dichlorethyl sulfide, a poisonous gas used in warfare.

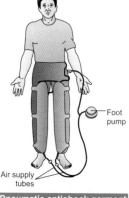

Foot pump

Air supply tubes

Pneumatic antishock garment

Gasoline A distillation product of petroleum often containing toxic additives like tetraethyl lead or tricresyl phosphate.

Gastrectomy Surgical removal of a part or total stomach.

Gastric analysis Analysis of gastric contents to determine quality of secretion, amount of free and combined hydrochloric acid, absence or presence of blood, bile acid, etc. The test is particularly helpful in cases of Zollinger-Ellison syndrome and gastric malignancy.

Gastric digestion Pepsin secreted in stomach hydrolyzes proteins to proteoses and peptones. HCl is essential for activity of pepsin. It also dissolves collagen, splits nucleoproteins, hydrolyzes disaccharides and kills bacteria. Gastric lipase reduces fat to fatty acids and glycerol.

Gastric glands Tubular glands lying in gastric mucosa that contain peptic cells secreting pepsinogen, oxyntic cells secreting HCl and mucus cell lying at the neck of gland secreting cytoprotective gastric mucin.

Gastric inhibitory polypeptide (GIP) A polypeptide in the cells of duodenum and jejunum which inhibits secretion of gastric juice.

Gastric juice Digestive juice of gastric glands containing HCl, pepsin, mucin, small amount of inorganic salts, intrinsic factor. pH is 0.9 to 1.5, total acidity being equivalent to 30 ml of 1/10 N HCl.

Gastric lavage Emptying out of stomach contents to relieve hiccup; before anesthesia for fear of aspiration and in intestinal obstruction, removal of ingested poisons.

Gastric ulcer Ulcer in the stomach.

Gastrin A group of hormones secreted by antral mucosa that circulating via blood stimulate gastric HCl secretion. Gastrins also affect secretory activity of pancreas, small intestine.

Gastrinoma Tumor of gastrin secreting cells causing Zollinger-Ellison syndrome.

Gastritis Inflammation of stomach characterized by epigastric pain, vomiting and dyspepsia. Gastric mucosa may be atrophic or hypertrophic. Dietary indiscretion, excessive indulgence in alcohol, campylobacter are responsible. *g. acute* Manifesting with fever, epigastric pain, vomiting with red angry hyperemic mucosa. *g. hypertrophic SYN* – Menetrier's disease; gastric folds are hypertrophic.

Gastrocnemius Larger superficial muscle in the back of lower leg that helps to plantarflex the foot and flex the knee upon the thigh.

Gastrocolic reflex Peristaltic wave in colon induced by entrance of food into stomach.

Gastroduodenoscopy Visual examination of stomach and duodenum by endoscope.

Gastroenteritis Inflammation of stomach and intestinal tract manifesting with epigastric pain, vomiting, fever and dysentery.

Gastroenterology The branch of medical science dealing with diseases of digestive tract and related structures like esophagus, liver, gallbladder and pancreas.

Gastroepiploic Pertains to stomach and greater omentum.

Gastroesophageal reflux Reflux of acid contents of stomach into lower esophagus due to obesity, hiatus hernia, anticholinergic use, pregnancy, etc.

Gastrografin Diatrizoate meglumine used for radiological examination of G.I. tract.

Gastroileal reflex Physiologic relaxation of ileocecal valve resulting from food in stomach.

Gastrointestinal decompression Removal of gas and fluids from G.I. tract through Ryle's tube.

Gastrojejunostomy Surgical anastomosis between stomach and jejunum.

Gastrolysis Surgical breaking of adhesions between the stomach and adjoining structures.

Gastroptosis Downward displacement of stomach.

Gastrostomy Surgical creation of a stoma in stomach for purpose of introducing food into stomach as in gastroesophageal malignancy.

Gate theory The hypothesis that painful stimuli can be prevented from reaching higher centers for recognition by stimulation of sensory nerves, a key mechanism explaining acupuncture analgesia.

Gatifloxacin A quinolone antibiotic is given once daily.

Gaucher cells Large reticuloendothelial cells with eccentric nucleus seen in Gaucher's disease.

Gaucher's disease A disease due to glycosphingolipid accumulation in RE cells with splenomegaly, bone lesions, skin pigmentation, etc.

Gault's reflex Blinking of eye following a loud noise close to ear, a test helpful in people malingering deafness.

Gauss sign Unusual mobility of uterus in early pregnancy.

Gauze Loosely woven cotton.

Gay's glands Large sebaceous circum anal glands.

Geiger counter Instrument for detecting ionizing radiation.

Geiger reflex Contraction of muscles of lower abdomen on stimulation of inner aspect of thigh in females. It corresponds to cremasteric reflex.

Gel Jelly like semisolid state.

Gelasmus Spasmodic laughter of insane.

Gelatin A protein derivative of collagen, used in X-ray films to suspend silver halide crystals, used in capsule making.

Gelatinase An enzyme present in bacteria, molds, and yeasts that liquefies gelatin.

Gelatinous Having consistency of gelatin.

Gelfoam Absorbable gelatin foam, a hemostatic.

Gemcitabine Anticancer agent.

Gemfibrozil Lipid lowering agent (mainly triglycerides).

Gemifloxacin Quinolone antibiotic given once daily.

Gemination Development of two teeth or two crowns within a single root.

Gemistocyte Swollen astrocyte with eccentric nucleus seen adjacent to areas of infarct/ edema.

Gemmation Cell reproduction by budding.

Gender Sex of an individual.

Gene Basic unit of heredity lying in chromosomes. Their mutation gives rise to new characters. *g. allelic* Pairs of genes located at same site on chromosome pair. *g. dominant* Gene that expresses without assistance from its allele. *g. histocompatible* Gene that controls the specificity of antigenic expression by tissues. *g. recessive* Gene that expresses its effect only when present in both chromosomes.

Gene amplification The duplication of regions of DNA to form multiple copies of a specific portion of the original region.

Gene map A map of the human genome i.e., a map of each cromosome. Man has 100000 genes that determine the amino acid structure of proteins.

General adaptation syndrome Organism's nonspecific response to stress occurring in 3 stages 1. Alarm reaction with pituitary adrenal hyperactivity to face the stress by fight or flight 2. Stage of adaptation when the physical symptoms diminish and 3. Stage of exhaustion when body can no longer respond to stress but manifests with stress related emotional disturbances, cardiovascular problems, etc.

Generation 1. The act of forming a new organism 2. Period of time between birth of parents and birth of their children.

Generator pulse Device producing stimuli intermittently, e.g., cardiac pacemaker.

Generic Distinctive, general.

Genesiology The science of reproduction.

Genesis Act of reproducing, generation, origin of any thing.

Gene splicing In genetic molecular bilogy, the substitution of a portion of a DNA is spliced into the DNA of another gene.

Gene therapy Inserting a normal gene into an organism in order to correct a genetic defect.

Genetic code The information system in living cells that determines the amino acid sequence in polypeptides.

Genetic counselling The application of knowledge of genetics in providing advice to parents to have off springs free of hereditary disease.

Genetic engineering The synthesis, modification or repair of genetic DNA by synthetic means.

Genetics The study of heredity and its variation.

Gene transfer Transfer of gene from one person to another for repair of inherited defect in the recipient.

Geneva convention 1864 declaration in Geneva that the sick and wounded victims of war including persons involved in their care like doctors, nurses, ambulance drivers, stretcher bearers are neutral and would not therefore be target of military action.

Genioplasty Plastic surgery of cheek or chin.

Genitalia Reproductive organs. *g. ambiguous* External genitalia do not clearly conform to that of male or female. (*see* Figure on page 291) *g. female* Labia majora/minora, clitoris, fourchet, vestibular gland, Bartholin's gland, vagina, uterus, two fallopian tubes and two ovaries. *g. male* Penis, two seminal vesicles, two ductus deferens, two testes, two bulbourethral glands.

Genitourinary system Organs and parts concerned with urine formation and excretion and reproductive organs (*see* Figure on page 292).

Genius An individual with exceptional mental or creative capability.

Genome A complete set of chromosomes.

Gentamicin An antibiotic from fungi of genus micromonospora.

Gentian Dried rhizome roots of plant Gentian lutea. *g. violet* A dye derived from coaltar. Widely used as a stain in histology, cytology and bac-

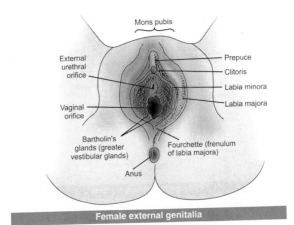

Female external genitalia

teriology. Also is anti-infective and antifungal.

Genu The knee. *g. valgum* Knock knee, a condition in which knees are close to each other and ankles are wide apart (> 5 cm). *g. varum* Bowleg, curving out of the legs. *g. recurvatum* Hyperextension at the knee joint (*see* Figure on page 293).

Genus In biology, taxonomic division between species and family.

Geographic tongue Numerous denuded areas on dorsal surface conforming to geographical pattern.

Gerdy's fibers Superficial transverse ligament of palm.

Geriatrics The study of various aspects of aging including physiology, pathology, economic and social problems.

Gerlach's valve Inconstant valve at the opening of appendix into the cecum.

Germ An organism that causes disease.

Germicidal Agent destructive to germs.

Germinal center A light area of lymphocytopoietic cells that occupies the center of lymphatic nodules, of spleen, tonsils and lymph nodes.

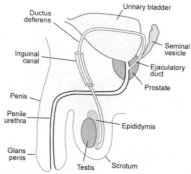

Male genitourinary system

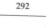

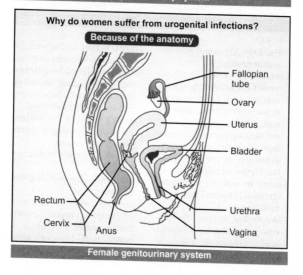

Female genitourinary system

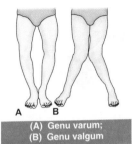

(A) Genu varum;
(B) Genu valgum

Germinal epithelium The epithelium that covers the surface of the genital ridge of an embryo.

Germination Development of impregnated ovum into an embryo or sprouting of spore.

Germinoma Neoplasm arising from germ cells of testes or ovary.

Geroderma Appearance of senility brought about by premature loss of hair, wrinkling of skin, general body atrophy.

Gerontology The study of social, psychological, and biological aspects of aging in humans and the effects of age-related diseases on them.

Gerotophilia Fondness or love for old.

Gerota's capsule The perirenal fascia.

Gerstmann's syndrome Neurological disorder caused by brain lesions near temporal and parietal lobe junction, characterized by inability to write and calculate, inability to distinguish fingers on hand, and left-right side disorientation.

Gestation Time span from conception to birth, usually 259-287 days. *g. ectopic* Fetus develops outside the uterus. *g. interstitial* Tubal gestation in which ovum develops in a portion of fallopian tube. *g. secondary* Gestation in which the ovum becomes dislodged from the original seat of implantation and continues to develop at new site (*see* Figure on page 294).

Gestation assessment Assessment of fetal age and maturity by ultrasound.

Gesture A body movement that assists in expression of thoughts (body language).

Ghon's focus Sharply defined peripheral lesion in X-ray chest with hilar lymphadenitis, a feature of primary kochs.

Ghrelin A 28-amino acid hormone produced by stomach cells and responsible for fat storage and stimulation of hunger.

Giant cell A large cell with several nuclei.

Giant cell tumor 1. A connective tissue tumor of bone marrow

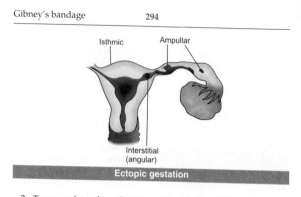

Ectopic gestation

2. Tumor of tendon sheath 3. Epulis 4. chondroblastoma.

Gibney's bandage Used to treat sprain in the ankle or support ankle (*see* Figure).

Gigantism Excessive physical development due to increased growth hormone secretion, late fusion of bones (eunuchoid gigantism)

Giardia A flagellated protozoa inhabiting intestinal mucosa (*see* Figure).

Giardiasis Infestation with *Giardia lamblia*.

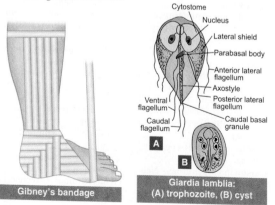

Gibney's bandage

Giardia lamblia: (A) trophozoite, (B) cyst

Gibbus Humped back, commonly due to compression fracture, collapse.

Gibson's murmur Murmur of patent ductus arteriosus.

Giddiness Light headed sensation.

Giemsa's stain A stain for staining blood smears for differential count and detection of parasitic microorganisms.

Gilbert's syndrome Hereditary deficiency of glucuronyl transferase with unconjugated hyperbilirubinemia.

Gilles de la Tourette's syndrome A neurological disorder manifesting with muscular incoordination, ticks and barks.

Gimbernant's ligament The lateral portion of inguinal ligament forming medial portion of femoral ring.

Gingiva The tissue surrounding the neck of tooth in maxilla and mandible. Gingiva has free edge surrounding anatomic crown of tooth, a labial surface and lingual surface (*see* Figure).

Gingivectomy Excision of gingiva in periodontal disease.

Gingivitis Inflammation of gums characterized by redness, swelling and tendency to bleed. *g. necrotizing ulcerative* Ulcerative and necrotic gingivostomatitis, usually by fusiform organisms.

Giralde's organ A remnant of wolffian body at posterior side of testicle.

Girdle Structure that resembles a circular belt or band. *g.*

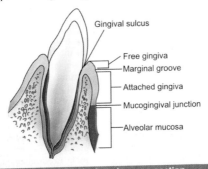

Gingival sulcus

Free gingiva
Marginal groove

Attached gingiva

Mucogingival junction

Alveolar mucosa

Gingiva of an incisor, in cross-section

pelvic Composed of the ileosacral and femoral articulation. *g. shoulder* Two clavicles, scapulae and humeral articulation.

Girdle symptoms Feeling of constriction in the chest, as in tabes dorsalis, or cord compression.

Gitter cell A honey combed cell packed with lipid granules.

Gitalin A cardiac glycoside.

Glabella That portion of frontal bone lying between the superciliary arches just above root of nose.

Glacial Resembling ice.

Gland A secretory organ. *g. acinous* Glands with secreting units in shape of sacs each possessing a narrow lumen. *g. apocrine* Glands in which the secreting cells lose some of their cytoplasmic contents in the form of secretion, e.g., some sweat glands, mammary gland. *g. Bartholin* Numerous glands that open into the vestibule of vagina akin to bulbourethral glands of male. *gs. ceruminous* Glands in external auditory canal, secreting cerumen. *gs. Ebner's* Serous glands of tongue located in the region of valate papillae whose ducts open into the furrows surrounding the papillae. *g. mammary* A compound alveolar gland secreting milk. It has 15-20 lactiferrous ducts each one discharging milk through a separate orifice on the surface of the nipple. The dilatation of these ducts form the milk reservoir during lactation. *g. mixed* 1. Glands having both exocrine and endocrine function, e.g., pancreas 2. Salivary glands secreting mucus and serous secretions. *g. pineal* Tiny conical body lying between two superior quadrigeminal bodies, connected with thalamus. *g. parathyroid* 4 in number of size 6 mm × 4 mm lying at the lower edge of thyroid gland secreting parathormone. *g. prostate* Gland surrounding neck of bladder and upper urethra, consists of a median lobe and two lateral lobes, weighing about 20 gm. Secretes thin opalescent slightly alkaline fluid that forms part of semen. *g. salivary* consist of parotid, submandibular and sublingual glands. *g. sebaceous* A simple or branched alveolar gland secreting sebum, the ducts opening into hair follicle. *gs. of Skene* Two glands at the margin of female urethra, opening into lower urethra on either side.

g. thyroid A ductless gland located in the base of neck; below consists of two lateral lobes connected by isthmus. Histologically consists of large number of closed vesicles called follicles lined with tall columnar cells synthesizing T3 and T4. *gs. Tyson's* Tiny sebaceous glands in the inner surface of perpuce and on the glans penis. *g. Zuckerkandl's* Accessory thyroid gland between genioglosus muscles (*see* Figure).

Glander Contagious disease of horses caused by *Pseudomonas mallei,* transmitted often to man.

Glans The head of the clitoris/penis.

Glanzmann's thrombasthenia Congenital abnormality of platelets with easy bruising, prolonged bleeding time and poor clot retraction.

Glasgow coma scale A scale for evaluating and quantitating the degree of coma by determining the best motor

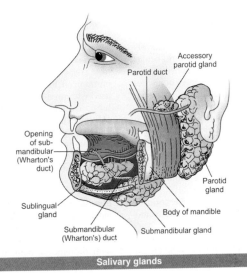

Opening of sub-mandibular (Wharton's duct)

Accessory parotid gland

Parotid duct

Parotid gland

Sublingual gland

Body of mandible

Submandibular (Wharton's) duct

Submandibular gland

Salivary glands

response, verbal and eye opening to standard stimuli. A score of 9 or greater excludes diagnosis of coma. It also has prognostic significance in head injury patients.

Glass photochromatic The glass becoming dark on exposure to light and regaining transparency on being away from light. *g. bifocal* Glasses in which the refractory power of lower portion of glass is for near vision and the upper portion for distant vision.

Glaucoma Raised intraocular pressure which can end in blindness. Narrowing of filtration angle, and sclerosis of canal of Schlemm, ocular diseases are responsible.

Gleet Chronic gonococcal urethritis marked by a transparent mucous discharge.

Glenoid cavity The socket in scapula that receives head of humerus.

Glenoid fossa The fossa of temporal bone that receives the condyle or capitulum of the mandible.

Glia Neuroglia; the connective tissue of the brain and spinal cord.

Gliadin A water insoluble protein present in the gluten of wheat.

Glibenclamide An oral hypoglycaemic agent of the sulphonylurea group used in the treatment of diabetes mellitus.

Glioblastoma A malignant tumor of neurological cells.

Glioma A sarcoma of neurological origin.

Gliomatosis Formation of glioma.

Glipizide Sulphonylurea compound for diabetes.

Globulin Simple protein present in blood. *g. antihemophilic* A clotting component of plasma, deficient in hemophiliacs. *g. gamma* That fraction of globulin responsible for body immunity. *g. antilymphocyte* Globulin from a person who has become immunized to lymphocytes; used as immunosuppressants.

Globus hystericus Sensation of lump in throat in hysterics.

Glomangioma A benign tumor developing from an arteriovenous glomus of skin.

Glomerular disease A group of disorders mostly autoimmune but some secondary (systemic disease, infectious disease, metabolic disease, hypertension, poison, etc) that involve the glomerulus manifesting with proteinuria, hematuria and hypertension.

Glomeruli Cluster of capillary vessels enveloped in Bowman's capsule in cortex of kidney.

Glomerulonephritis A form of nephritis where lesions are confined primarily to glomeruli.

Glomerulopathy Any disease of glomeruli.

Glomerulosclerosis Fibrosis of glomeruli.

Glomoid Similar appearance to glomeruli.

Glomus A small round mass made-up of tiny blood vessels and found in stroma containing many nerve fibers.

Glossina Tsetse flies that transmit trypanosomes, agents of trypanosomiasis.

Glossitis Inflammation of tongue; can be acute, painful or chronic, due to infection or avitaminosis (B complex group).

Glossodynamometer Device for measuring contractile power of tongue muscles.

Glossograph An instrument for measuring tongue's movement during speech.

Glossopharyngeal nerve Ninth cranial nerve carrying taste sensation from posterior third of tongue and distributed to pharynx, meninges, parotids and ears.

Glottis Larynx with the two vocal cords and the intervening space, the rime glottides (*see* Figure).

Glucagon Polypeptide hormone secreted by alfa cells of pancreas that raises blood sugar and relaxes smooth muscles of G.I. tract.

Glucagonoma A malignant tumor of alpha cells of pancreas.

Glucocerebroside A cerebroside with glucose in the

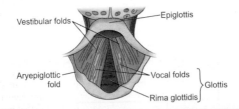

Glottis, comprising the vocal folds (cords) and rima glottidis, seen in a laryngoscopic view of the larynx. The trachea is visible through the rima glottidis

molecule, present in tissues in patients of Gaucher's disease.

Glucocorticoid A class of adrenal hormones that are released in response to stress and effect carbohydrate and protein metabolism.

Glucogenesis Formation of glucose from glycogen.

Glucokinase An enzyme in liver that converts glucose to glucose 6 phosphate.

Gluconeogenesis Formation of glycogen from noncarbohydrate sources like amino or fatty acids.

Glucosamine An amino saccharide present in chitin and mucus.

Glucose Called D-glucose, the primary fuel of human body; in tissue either converted to glycogen, or fat or is oxidized to CO_2 and H_2O (see Figure).

Glucose-6-phosphate dehydrogenase An essential enzyme for pentose-phosphate pathway of glucose metabolism that generates reduced glutathione.

Glucose tolerance test A test performed by giving 1.5 gm/kg wt of glucose to a patient orally in empty stomach and then examining blood samples every ½ hr for 2 hours. The test helps to assess ability of patient to metabolize glucose

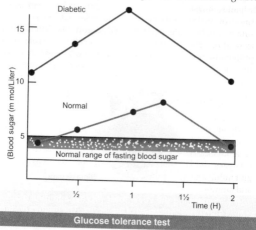

Glucose tolerance test

and is of primary importance in diagnosis of prediabetic states and hyperinsulinemia.

Glucoside A glycoside that upon hydrolysis yields glucose and additional products. e.g., digitalin, present in digitalis.

Glucosuria Abnormal amount of sugar in urine.

Glucoronic acid An acid that possesses detoxifying action.

Glucuronide Combination of glucuronic acid with phenol, alcohol, etc.

Glue ear The accumulation of sticky material in the middle ear resulting in impaired hearing, most common in young school children.

Glue sniffing Solvent abuse

Glutamic acid An amino acid formed during hydrolysis of proteins. It is the only amino acid metabolized by brain.

Glutamic-pyruvic transaminase An enzyme found in the liver. Measurement of serum levels (SGPT) is used in the study and diagnosis of liver diseases.

Glutaminase An enzyme that catalyzes the breakdown of glutamine into glutamic acid and ammonia.

Glutamine The monoamide of aminoglutaric acid, essential for hydrolysis of proteins.

Glutaraldehyde A sterilizing agent effective against all microorganisms.

Glutathione A tripeptide of glutamic acid, cystine and glycine, important for cellular respiration.

Gluten Vegetable albumin, a protein obtained from wheat and other grain.

Gluten free diet Elimination of gluten from the diet by exclusion of all products prepared from wheat, rye, barley and oats.

Gluten induced enteropathy Adult celiac disease manifesting with malabsorption and diarrhea.

Gluburide Sulphonyl urea compound for diabetes mellitus.

Glybenclamide Sulphonyl urea for NIDDM.

Glyceride An ester of glycerin compounded with an acid.

Glycerin $C_3H_8O_3$. A trihydric alcohol present in chemical combination in all fats used extensively as a solvent, preservative and emolient.

Glyceryl The trivalent radical of glycerol. *g. monostearate* An emulsifying agent used in preparing creams and ointments. *g. trinitrate* Nitroglycerin, agent used in angina pectoris.

Glycocholic acid Bile acid present in bile, a conjugate of cholic acid and glycine.

Glycogen Polysaccharide; the storage form of carbohydrate in the body (liver and muscle).

Glycogenase An enzyme in the liver that hydrolyzes glycogen to glucose.

Glycogenesis Formation of glycogen from glucose.

Glycogenolysis Conversion of glycogen to glucose.

Glycogen storage disease Inherited disease with abnormal storage of glycogen in the liver. *gsd type I (von Gierke's disease)* Glucose-6-phosphatase deficiency. *gsd type II* - Lysosomal alfa glucosidase deficiency *gsd type III* - Deficiency of debranching enzymes. *gsd type IV* - (Anderson's disease) brancher enzyme deficiency with hepatic failure. *gsd type V* - (McArdle's disease) Muscle phosphorylase deficiency. *gsd type VI* - Deficiency of liver phosphorylase with growth retardation, hepatomegaly, acidosis and hypoglycemia. *gsd type VII* - Deficiency of muscle phosphofructokinase with weakness and cramping.

Glycolipid Lipid with carbohydrate and nitrogen, but no phosphoric acid; Found in myelin sheath of nerves.

Glyconeogenesis *SYN* – gluconeogenesis

Glycophorin Glycoprotein that spans the bilipid layer of erythrocyte membrane, functioning as a channel for passage of anions in and out of red cells.

Glycopyrrolate An anticholinergic drug used in preanesthetic medication to reduce G.I. and bronchial secretions.

Glycoside A plant product which on hydrolysis yields sugar and additional products.

Glycosphingolipids Carbohydrate containing fatty acid derivatives of ceramide, e.g., cerebrosides, gangliosides and ceramide oligosaccharides. Abnormal accumulation of them in nervous tissue due to deficiency of metabolizing enzymes leads to death.

Glycosuria Presence of glucose in the urine resulting from insulin deficiency, reduced renal threshold, excessive glycogenolysis or adreno pituitary disorders.

Glymidine A drug of the sulphonylurea group used in the treatment of diabetes mellitus.

Gnat Insects smaller than mosquitoes that include black flies, sandflies and midgets.

Gnathion Lowest point on the median line of mandible.

Gnathostoma A genus of nematodes that inhabit alimentary tract of domestic animals and occasionally infest man.

Goblet cells A unicellular gland seen in intestinal and respiratory tract, that secretes mucus by rupture of cell wall.

Godfrey's test Test for identifying tearing of posterior cruciate ligament.

Goiter An enlargement of thyroid gland. *g. adenomatous* Thyroid enlargement due to adenoma. *g. colloid* Thyromegaly with great increase in follicular contents. *g. cystic* Cystic thyromegaly; cyst formation being due to degeneration within an adenoma. *g. diffuse* Diffuse increase in thyroid tissue in contrast to its nodular form as in adenomatous goiter. *g. endemic* Thyromegaly due to iodine deficiency in water in some geographical areas. (*see* Figure) *g. exophthalmic* Grave's disease where antithyroid receptor antibodies play the dominant role with increased TSH and stimulation of thyroid. *g. lingual* Hypertrophied aberrant thyroid tissue forming a mass

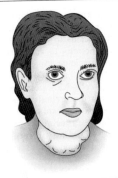

Exophthalmic goiter

on dorsum of tongue posteriorly. *g. toxic* Goiter with excessive production of thyroxine and triodothyronine.

Gold Yellow metal used as alloy (mixed with copper, silver, platinum for dental use (crown, inlays, orthodontics); sodium thiomalate and thioglucose used in rheumatoid arthritis.

Golden hour The initial 60 minutes after a major traumatic injury during which the definitive care and surgical intervention must be given to the patient for counter-acting long-term and irreversible damage to vital organs.

Gold standard A standard with which other tests or procedures are compared.

Golgi apparatus A lamellar membranous structure near the nucleus. In secretory cells it functions to concentrate and package the secretory products.

Golgi cells Multipolar nerve cells in the cerebral cortex and posterior bones of spinal cord.

Golgi corpuscle A sensory nerve ending or receptor found in tendons and apo-neureses.

Goll's tract SYN – fasciculus gracilis, posterior white column of spinal cord.

Gonad A generic term referring to male and female sex glands (testes and ovary).

Gonadal dysgenesis Congenital disorder with failure of ovaries to respond to pituitary gonadotropin stimulation resulting in amenorrhea, failure of sexual maturation and short stature. Webbing of neck, cubitus valgus may be present. Genetic pattern is 45 XO (SYN – Turners' syndrome).

Gonadotrophic Relates to stimulation of gonads.

Gonadotropin *g.s. anterior pituitary* Secreted by anterior pituitary as FSH and LH, called interstitial cell stimulating hormone in male (ICSH) *g. chorionic* Produced by chorionic villi of placenta.

Gonadotropin releasing hormone Produced in hypothalamus, it acts on pituitary to cause release of gonadotropic hormones.

Goniometer Apparatus to measure joint movement and angles.

Gonioscope Device for inspecting the angle of anterior chamber of eye and determining ocular mobility and rotations.

Goniotomy Incision at angle of anterior chamber to promote free flow of aqueous into canals of schleim.

Gonococcus Neisseria gonorrhae, causative organism of gonorrhea.

Gonorrhea Contagious inflammation of genital mucous membrane manifesting with burning micturition, painful induration of penis in males, vaginitis and cervicitis in females. Can cause salpingo oophoritis ending in tubal blockage and sterility in female and chronic prostatitis in male. Can spread to blood to involve principally the joints.

Goodell's sign Softening of the cervix during pregnancy (*see* Figure on page 305).

Goodpasture's syndrome IgA nephropathy with hemoptysis and hemosiderosis.

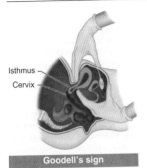

Isthmus
Cervix

Goodell's sign

Good Samaritan law Legal stipulation for protection of those who give first aid in emergency situation.

Goose flesh Transient roughness of skin with contraction of arrector pili muscles, as a reaction to cold or shock.

Gordon's reflex Extension of great toe on pressure to calf muscles, a sign of pyramidal tract disease.

Gorget An instrument grooved to protect soft tissues from injury as pointed instrument is inserted in a body cavity.

Goserelin Gn RH analog.

Gossypol A toxic chemical of cotton seed.

Gouge Instrument for cutting away hard tissue of bone.

Goundou Bilateral hyperostosis of nasal bones.

Gout Hereditary metabolic disease of uric acid metabolism with hyperuricemia and arthropathy. *g. tophaceous* Gout marked by development of tophi (deposits of sodium urate) in the joints, external ear and about the finger nails.

Gower's sign Clinical sign of muscular dystrophy in childhood. Affected children use their arms to push themselves erect by moving their hands up their thighs.

Gower's tract Spinocerebellar tract.

Graafian follicle A mature follicle of ovary which on rupture discharges the ovum. Within the ruptured graffian follicle, the corpus luteum develops that secrets estrogen and progesterone to help in implantation of fertilized ovum (*see* Figure).

A Follicular fluid
B Granulosa cells
C Ovum

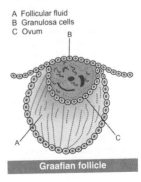

Graafian follicle

Gracile Slender, thin built.

Gracile nucleus Nucleus in medulla oblongata where fasciculus gracilis ends.

Gracilis A long slender muscle on the medial aspect of thigh.

Gradenigo's syndrome Suppurative otitis media with abducens nerve palsy.

Gradient A slope or grade.

Graefe's sign Failure of the upper eyelids to follow a downward movement of the eyeball, a feature of Grave's disease.

Graft Transplanted tissue in a part of body for repair of a defect. *g. allogeneic* Graft from genetically non identical donor of the same species as the recipient. (allograft) *g. cadaver* Grafting tissue taken from cadaver like cornea, bone, heart, lungs, kidney, etc., soon after molecular death. *g. fascicular* Nerve graft with each bundle of nerve stitched separately. *g. full thickness* Graft of entire layer of skin without the subcutaneous fat. *g. homologous* The donor is of same species as the recipient. *g. isologous* Graft in which the donor and recipient are genetically identical, i.e., identical twins. *g. lamellar* Very thin corneal graft used to replace superficial opaque corneal layer. *g. pedicle* A skin graft that is left attached at one end until the free end has begun to receive blood supply from grafted site. *g. sieve* Graft in which a section of skin is removed except for small regularly spaced areas that grow to cover the donor site. *g. Thiersch's* Graft in which only epidermis and small amount of dermis is used.

Graham's law The rate of diffusion of a gas is inversely proportional to the square root of its density.

Gram A unit of weight (mass) of metric system equal to 1000 mg.

Gram's method A method for staining bacteria, a heat fixed blood film is stained with gentian violet, rinsed off and then iodine solution is put and rinsed off and decolorized in 90% ethyl alcohol or acetone. Then the slide is counterstained with carbolfuschsin or safranine. Gram-positive organisms retain violet stain while gram-negative organisms become red.

Grandiose In psychiatry, unrealistic and exaggerated concept of self worth, importance, ability, power and wealth.

Granisetron Antiemetic.

Granular Of the nature of granules, rough.

Granular cast Coarse or fine granules or casts, sometimes yellowish, soluble in acetic acid; seen in inflammatory and degenerative nephropathies (chronic renal failure).

Granulation Formation of granules, often by outgrowth of capillaries *g. arachnoidal* Villus like projections of subarachnoid layer of the meninges that project into the superior sagittal sinus and other venous sinuses of brain. Though these CSF is absorbed into venous systems.

Granule A minute mass in a cell that has an outline but no apparent structure.

Granulocyte A granular leukocyte, i.e. neutrophil, eosinophil and basophil.

Granulocyte colony stimulating factor (G-CSF) a naturally occurring glycoprotein cytokine that stimulates production of neutrophils. It is helpful in cancer chemotherapy and bone marrow transplant.

Granulocyte-Macrophage-colony stimulating factor-(GMCSF) Like G-CSF, this factor stimulates production of macrophages and monocytes in addition to neurophils.

Granulocytopenia Reduction in blood granulocyte count.

Granulocytosis Presence of increased numbers of granulocytes in the peripheral blood film.

Granuloma A granular tumor or growth of lymphoid and epithelioid cell. It occurs in various infectious diseases like leprosy, yaws, syphilis, etc. *g. dental* Granuloma developing at root of a tooth, secondary to pulp infection. It contains chronic inflammatory cells, debris and bacteria. *g. eosinophilic* A form of xanthomatosis with eosinophilia and cystic degeneration of bone. *g. inguinale* Granulomatous ulcerative disease caused by Donovania granulomatis, a gram –ve cocobacillus. *g. Wegener's* A rare disease of unknown etiology characterized by widespread granulomatous lesions of the bronchi, necrotising arteriolitis, and glomerulonephritis.

Granulomatosis The development of multiple granulomas.

Granulopoiesis Formation of blood granulocytes.

Granulosa cell tumor Tumor of ovary secreting estrogens, hence feminizing in nature.

Graphesthesia The ability by which outlines, numbers,

words, symbols, traced or written upon skin are recognized.

Grasp To hold.

Grattage Removal of morbid growth by rubbing with a brush.

Grunt Abnormal sound heard during labored exhalation.

Gravel Coarse sand; concretions in kidneys, made-up of calcium, oxalate, phosphate, uric acid.

Graves' disease Exophthalmic goiter (*see* Figure).

Gravid Pregnant.

Gravitation Force that draws every particle of matter.

Gravity Property of possessing weight. The force of earth's gravitational attraction. *g. specific* Weight of a substance compared with an equal volume of water.

Gray Colour between extremes of black and white.

Gray matter Nervous tissue lying peripherally in brain and somewhat centrally in spinal cord where myelinated fibers do not predominate.

Gray syndrome of the newborn Ashen gray colour, vomiting, cyanosis and flaccidity of newborn when treated with chloramphenicol.

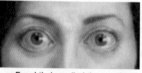

Exophthalmos (bulging eyes)

Graves' disease is a common cause of hyperthyroidism, an over-production of thyroid hormone, which causes enlargement of the thyroid and other symptoms such as exophthalmos, heart intolerance and anxiety

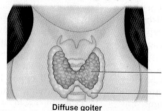

Normal thyroid

Enlarged thyroid

Diffuse goiter

Graves' disease

Grinder's disease Chronic lung disease due to dust inhalation (*SYN*-pneumoconiosis).

Gripes Spasmodic bowel pain, intestinal colic.

Griseofulvin An antifungal antibiotic given orally.

Grits Coarsely ground corn.

Groin Inguinal region, area between thigh and trunk.

Grommet Ventilation tube placed across the tympanic membrane for equalization of pressure in treatment of retracted tympanic membrane secondary to eustachian block/catarrh.

Groove Long narrow channel.

Ground itch Skin inflammation in foot due to invasion by larva of hookworm.

Ground substance The material that occupies the intercellular spaces in fibrous connective tissue, cartilage or bone.

Grouping Classification of individual traits according to shared characteristics. *g. blood* Classification of blood of different individuals according to agglutinating and hemolyzing properties.

Group therapy A form of simultaneous psychotherapy involving many patients by psychotherapist.

Growing pain Pain in the musculoskeletal system in growing children.

Growth The progressive increase in size or development both physical/mental in a living thing.

Growth hormone Anterior pituitary secretion that regulates human growth; *SYN*—somatotropin.

Guaiacol O-methoxyphenol used as antiseptic, germicidel, intestinal antiseptic and expectorant.

Guanabenz A vasodilator.

Guanadrel Adrenergic blocking agent.

Guanase Enzyme that converts guanine into xanthine.

Guanethidine A sympatholytic drug used in hypertension.

Guanidine A protein product.

Guanine $C_5H_5N_5O$. An organic compound of animal and vegetable nucleic acids. Uric acid is its metabolic end product.

Guanosine A nucleoside formed from guanine and ribosome. It is a major constituent of RNA and DNA.

Gubernaculum A structure that guides, a cord like structure linking two structures. *g. dentis* A connective tissue band connecting unerupted tooth with overlying gum. *g.*

testis A fibrous band extending from caudal end of fetal testis through the inguinal canal to scrotal sac; playing no role in descent of testis.

Gudden's law In division of a nerve, degeneration in the proximal portion is towards nerve cell.

Gugeelipid Lipid lowering agent.

Guide wire Wire helpful in positioning and manipulating an intravenous or intraarterial catheter.

Guillain-Barre syndrome Polyneuritis with flaccid muscular palsy following an infectious disease.

Guillotine Instrument for excising tonsils and laryngeal growth.

Guilt Feeling grief for doings what is thought to be wrong.

Guinea pig A small rodent used in laboratory research.

Guinea worm Dracunculus medinensis.

Gum The fleshy tissue covering the alveolar process of jaw.

Gumma Encapsulated granulomatous tumor with central necrosis, characteristic of tertiary syphilis seen in skin, liver, testis, brain and bone.

Gustatory Pertains to sensation of taste.

Gustometry Measurement of sense of acuteness of taste.

Gut The bowel or intestine.

Gutta-percha Purified dried latex of certain trees, used in dentistry for root canal treatment.

Guttering Groove in bone.

Guyon's canal A space at wrist between flexor retinaculum and palmar carpal ligament through which ulnar artery and ulnar nerve enter into the hand (*see* Figure on page 311).

Guyon's sign Ballotment of kidney.

Gymnophobia Abnormal aversion to seeing a naked body.

Gynandroid Individual having hermaphroditic sexual characteristics to be mistaken for a person of opposite sex.

Gynecoid Resembling female.

Gynecology The study of disease of female reproductive organs including breast.

Gynecomastia Abnormally large mammary tissue in male (> 2.5 cm in dm) often secreting milk.

Gypsum Hydrated calcium sulfate, used for plaster, dental casting.

Gyrus Convolution of the cerebral hemispheres (*see* Figure on page 311).

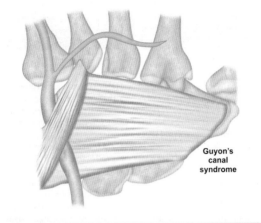

Guyon's canal syndrome

Guyon's canal

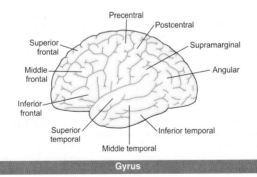

Precentral

Postcentral

Superior frontal

Supramarginal

Middle frontal

Angular

Inferior frontal

Superior temporal

Inferior temporal

Middle temporal

Gyrus

H

HAART therapy *Highly active antiretroviral therapy* involving a combination of various antiretroviral drugs which aim to treat patients of HIV.

Habenula A whip like structure; A stalk attached to pineal body of brain; a narrow band like structure.

Habenular commissure A transverse band of fibers connecting the two habenular areas.

Habenular trigone A depressed triangular area located on the lateral aspect of the posterior third ventricle.

Habilitation The process of education and training persons with disability both physical and mental to improve their ability to function in society.

Habit A motor pattern following frequent repetition or an involuntary act that comes as a reflex action *h. spasm* Involuntary spasmodic muscle contraction; *SYN*-tic

Habituation Act of becoming accustomed to anything from frequent use.

Habitus A physical appearance that indicates a tendency to certain diseases or positioning of internal organs in certain planes.

Hacking cough Recurrent nonproductive cough.

Halsted's operation An operation for inguinal hernia; operation for breast cancer.

Halsted's suture Interrupted suture for intestinal wounds.

Hemogogus A genus of mosquitoes which serves as a vector for yellow fever.

Hailey Hailey disease Benign familial pemphigus.

Hageman factor Blood coagulation factor, helps in kinin synthesis.

Hair A thin keratinized and cornified structure arising from hair follicle. The shaft of hair has 3 layers, the outer cortex containing the pigment melanin. Hair of eyebrow has life of 3-5 months and that of head 2-5 years with continuous turnover (*see* Figure on page 313).

Hair analysis Investigation for chemical composition of

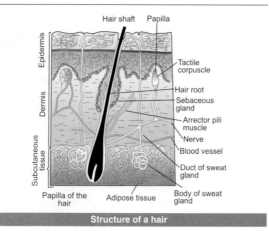

Structure of a hair

hair to exclude toxic chemical intoxication, state of nutrition and monitoring course of certain diseases.

Hair bulb The lower expanded portion of a hair

Hair follicle An invagination of the epidermis that forms a cylindrical depression extending into subepidermal layer. Sebaceous glands and arrectores pili muscles are attached to these hair follicles.

Hair papilla A projection of dermis extending into hair bulb at the bottom of hair follicle. It contains capillaries through which hair receives its nourishment.

Hair transplantation Technique of transferring skin containing hair follicles from one place to another; done to treat alopecia.

Hairy tongue Tongue covered with hair like papilla with threads of aspergillus or candida.

Halazone A chloramine water disinfectant.

Halcinonide A corticosteroid.

Half-life 1. Time required for radioactive substance to reduce to one-half its energy due to metabolism or excretion. 2. Time required for radioactive nuclei undergoing decay to lose half their radioactivity 3. Time taken by body to inactivate half of the administered drug/chemical (biological half-life).

Halfway house A facility to house mental patients who do not need hospitalization but who are not ready for independent living.

Halibut liver oil An oil obtained from liver of halibut fish rich in vit A and vit D.

Halide Compound containing a halogen i.e., bromine, chlorine, fluorine or iodine.

Halitosis Bad breath, offensive breath.

Hallervorden-Spatz disease An inherited progressive degenerative disease beginning in childhood manifesting with rigidity, athetotic movements and mental retardation.

Hallucination A sense of false perception. *h. auditory* Imaginary perceptions of sounds, usually voices. *h. gustatory* Sense of tasting. *h. hypnagogic* Pre-sleep phenomena having the same practical significance as a dream but experienced while consciousness persists. *h. olfactory* Hallucination involving smell. *h. tactile* False sensation of insects creeping under skin. *h. visual* Sensation of seeing objects that are not real.

Hallucinogen Drugs that produce hallucination e.g., LSD.

Hallucinosis The state of having hallucinations.

Hallux The great toe. *h. rigidus* Painful restricted mobility of great toe. *h. valgus* Displacement of great toe toward other toes. *h. varus* Displacement of great toe away from other toes (*see* Figure).

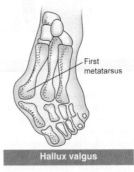

First metatarsus

Hallux valgus

Halo 1. A circle of light surrounding a shining body. 2. A ring surrounding the macula. *h. glaucomatous* Visual perception of rainbow like colors due to glaucoma induced edema of cornea.

Halofantrine Antimalarial agent.

Halogen A substance forming salt like chlorine, iodine, bromine and fluorine which combine with metals to form salt and with hydrogen to form acid.

Haloperidol Antipsychotic agent used in schizophrenia

Haloprogin Halogenated phenolic ether, fungicidal.

Halothane Fluorinated hydrocarbon used as general anesthetic.

Halsted's operation Operation done for radical correction of inguinal hernia.

Halsted's suture Suture placed through the subcuticular fascia that is used for exact skin approximation (*see* Figure).

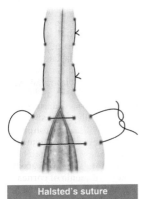

Hamartoma Disorganized self-limited, benign growth of normal tissue; when occur-

ring in blood vessels called haemangioma; common to lungs and kidneys.

Hamate bone The medial bone in the distal row of carpal bones of wrist.

Hammer An instrument with rubber cap to tap muscle, tendon or nerve to initiate reflex response.

Hammer finger Flexion deformity of the distal joint of a finger, caused by avulsion of extensor tendon.

Hamstrings The group of three muscles on the posterior aspect of thigh comprised of semimembranous, semitendinosus and biceps femoris that flex the leg, extend and adduct the thigh.

Ham test Test for diagnosis of paroxysmal nocturnal hemoglobinuria. The red cells lyse in acidic medium.

Hand That part of body attached to forearm at the wrist consisting of 8 carpal bones, 5 metacarpals and 14 phallanges.

Hand-foot-mouth disease Highly infectious coxsackie virus causing painful ulcerative and vesicular lesions of hand and feet.

Handicap Mental or physical impairment preventing or interferring with normal physical and mental activities.

Hand-Schuller-Christian disease A lipid storage disease manifesting with histiocytic granuloma in skull, skin and viscera often with exophthalmos and diabetes insipidus.

Hangman's fracture Fracture dislocation of upper cervical spine due to judicial hanging.

Hang nail Partly detached piece of skin at root or lateral edge of finger or toe nail.

Hangover Headache, depression, fatigue and irritability present some times after consumption of alcohol or CNS depressant.

Hansen bacillus Lepra bacillus

Hansen's disease Synonym for Leprosy.

Haploid Presence of half the number of chromosomes (i.e., 23) as found in ovum and sperm.

Hapten That portion of an antigen determining its immunological specificity.

Haptephobia Aversion to being touched by another person.

Haptoglobin Mucoprotein accepting hemoglobin in plasma on release in hemolytic conditions. Hence haptoglobin is decreased in hemolytic disorders and increased in certain inflammatory conditions.

Hardness Water with less cleansing action due to presence of soluble salts of calcium and magnesium. These compounds precipitate with soap.

Hare lip A cleft in the upper lip due to faulty fusion of median nasal process and the lateral maxillary processes.

Hare lip suture A twisted figure of eight suture used in surgical correction of harelip.

Harlequin fetus Newborn with skin features of ichthyosis with deep red fissures.

Harpoon A device with a hook on the end for obtaining small pieces of tissue.

Harris-Benedict equation Equation for calculating basal body energy expenditure.

Hartman's solution A solution of 0.6 gram NaCl, 0.03 gram KCl, 0.02 gram $CaCl_2$ and 0.31 gram sodium lactate in 100 ml of water used for fluid and electrolyte replacement.

Hartnup disease A disorder of tryptophan metabolism manifesting with pellagra.

Harvey, William British physician who described circulation of blood.

Hashimoto's struma Hashimoto's thyroiditis.

Hashish An extract from flower, stalk and leaves of cannabis sativa, smoked or chewed for its euphoric effect.

Hassal's corpuscle Spherical bodies with central area of degeneration with surrounding flattened cells, seen in thymus gland.

Haunch The hips and buttocks.

Haustra The sacculated pouches of colon, formed because the longitudinal bands are shorter than the gut.

Haversian canal Minute vascular canals in bone transmitting nutrient vessels.

Haversian gland Minute projections from the surface of synovial tissue into the joint space.

Haversian system Architectural unit of bone consisting of haversian canals, with alternate layers of intercellular matrix surrounding it in concentric cylinders.

Hay fever Allergic rhinitis usually caused by airborne pollens, fungal spores.

Head 1. The part of animal body containing brain and organs for vision, hearing, smell and taste. 2. Proximal end of bone.

Headache Acute or chronic pain over the skull not confined to any nerve distribution. *h. cluster* Headache occurring in cluster usually in male soon after falling asleep; akin to migraine. *h. exertional* Headache of short duration, appearing after strenuous physical activity, relieved by rest. *h. histamine* Headache resulting from ingestion of histamine containing foods. *h. post lumbar puncture* Leakage of CSF after lumbar puncture leading to CSF hypotension and headache. *h. tension* Contraction of musculo-tendinous structures of scalp giving rise to a band line compressing around head in situations producing mental strain.

Healing Restoration to normal mental or physical state

Health A state of complete mental, physical and social wellbeing, not being mere absence of disease or infirmity.

Health certificate An official statement signed by a physician attesting to state of health.

Health education Educational program aimed for improving and maintaining good health.

Health hazard Any substance, condition or circumstances not conducive to good health.

Hearing aid An apparatus amplifying sound, worn by persons with impaired hearing.

Heart A hollow muscular 4-chambered contractile pump in the chest cavity, the principal organ of circulating system (*see* Figure on page 318).

Heartburn Indigestion marked by a burning sensation in the oesophagus, often with regurgitation of acid fluid. Pyrosis.

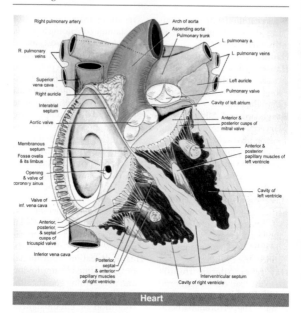

Heart

Heart lung machine A machine that takes over functions of heart and lung during open cardiac surgery (*see* Figure on page 319).

Heat Warmth. A form of energy, which may cause an increase in temperature or a change of state, e.g. the conversion of water into steam. *H. exhaustion* A rapid pulse, anorexia, dizziness, cramps in arms, legs or abdomen and sometimes followed by sudden collapse, caused by loss of body fluids and salts under very hot conditions. *Prickly h.* Miliaria; heat rash. Acute itching caused by blocking of the ducts of the sweat glands following profuse sweating. *H.-stroke* A severe life-threatening condition resulting from prolonged exposure to heat. (*See* Sunstroke).

Hebephrenia A form of schizophrenia characterized by thought disorder and emo-

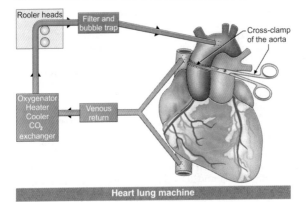

Heart lung machine

tional incongruity. Delusions and hallucinations are common.

Heberden's nodes *W. Heberden, British physician, 1710-1801.* Bony or cartilaginous outgrowths causing deformity of the terminal finger joints in osteoarthritis.

Hebetude Emotional dullness. A common symptom in dementia and schizophrenia.

Hedonism Excessive devotion to pleasure.

Hegar's dilators *A. Hegar, German gynaecologist, 1830-1914.* A series of graduate dilators used to dilate the uterine cervix.

Heimlich maneuver *H.J. Heimlich, American physician, b. 1920.* A technique for removing foreign matter from the trachea of a choking person. Wrap the arms around the person and allow his or her torso to hang forward. Make a fist with one hand and grasp it with the other, then with both hands against the victim's abdomen (above the navel and below the rib cage), forcefully press into the abdomen with a sharp upward thrust. The manoeuvre may be repeated several times if necessary to clear the air passages. If unconscious or prone, turn the victim on to back, kneel astride the torso and with both hands use the manoeuvre as described.

Heinz bodies Inclusions in erythrocytes consisting of damaged aggregated hemoglobin and is associated with some forms of hemolytic anemia.

Heliotherapy Treatment of disease by exposure of the body to sunlight.

Helium *Symbol* He. An inert gas sometimes used in conjunction with oxygen to facilitate respiration in obstructional types of dyspnoea and for decompressing deep-sea divers.

Helix 1. A spiral twist. Used to describe the configuration of certain molecules, e.g. deoxyribonucleic acid (DNA). 2. The outer rim of the auricle of the ear.

HELLP syndrome Life-threatening complication of pregnancy characterized by *hemolysis, elevated liver enzymes, and low platelet* count and considered to be a variant of preeclampsia.

Helminthiasis An infestation with worms.

Hemangioma Common benign tumor of blood vessel; hemangioblastoma occurs in cerebellum, retina and spinal cord; hemangioendothelioma is malignant, hemangio-pericytoma can be benign or malignant usually occurring in kidney, lower extremity or retroperitoneum. *h. cavernous* composed of large dilated blood vessels usually not present at birth. *h.*

capillary the most common type, contain closely packed blood vessels, often present at birth. *h.strawberry* firm red dome shaped.

Hemarthrosis Bleeding into a joint.

Hematemesis Vomiting of blood which may be associated with peptic ulcers, tumors of upper gastrointestinal tract, varices, gastritis, etc.

Hematin Formed from oxidation of free heme of hemoglobin.

Hematochezia Passage of bloody stool.

Hematocrit Red blood cells volume in blood.

Hematoidin A yellow-brown or red pigment formed from hemoglobin under reduced oxygen tension.

Hematoma Localized collection of blood. *h. epidural* blood collected in epidural space due to tear of middle meningeal artery. *h. subdural* blood collected in subdural space due to tearing of venous sinuses; can be acute or chronic.

Hematometra Accumulation of blood in uterus.

Hematuria Passage of blood in urine.

Heme A protoporphyrin with 4 pyrrole groups that binds to oxygen for its carriage to tissues.

Hemianesthesia Anaesthesia (loss of sensation) of one-half of body due to lesion in internal capsule

Hemianopia Partial blindness, in which the patient can see only half of the normal field of vision. It arises from disorders of the optic tract and of the occipital lobe.

Hemiballismus Involuntary chorea-like movements on one side of the body only.

Hemiplegia Paralysis of one-half of body *h. capsular* Lesions of internal capsule producing hemiplegia

Hemisacralization Abnormal development of one half of fifth lumbar vertebra fusing with the sacrum.

Hemispasm Spasm of one side of body or face.

Hemisphere Either half of the cerebrum or cerebellum. *h. dominant* Cerebral hemisphere controlling speech usually the left in 90% right handed persons and 15% of left handed persons.

Hemithorax One-half of the chest.

Hemivertebra Congenital absence or failure of development of half of vertebra.

Hemoagglutination Clumping of RBC.

Hemoagglutinin An agglutinin that clumps RBC.

Hemobilia Blood in bile duct.

Hemochromatosis A congenital disorder of iron metabolism leading to excess iron accumulation in liver, pancreas, and heart. *SYN—* bronze diabetes.

Hemoconcentration A relative or a absolute increase in RBC mass; can be secondary to fluid loss.

Hemocyanin An oxygen carrying blue pigment in the plasma of arthropods and moluscus.

Hemocytoblast The primitive reticuloendothelial stem cell of bone marrow differentiating into various blood components.

Hemocytogenesis Formation of blood cells.

Hemocytology Study of structure and function of blood cells.

Hemodialysis A method of removing poisonous substances, urea, creatinine, etc. from plasma by passing the patient's blood across semipermeable membranes. *SYN—* hemoperfusion.

Hemodialyzer Device used in performing hemodialysis.

Hemodilution Reduction in relative concentration of RBC due to plasma volume expansion.

Hemodynamics Study of blood circulation.

Hemoflagellate Any flagellate protozoan of the blood e.g., trypanosoma, leishmania.

Hemofuscin A brown pigment derived from hemoglobins.

Hemoglobin The iron containing protoporphyrin IX, responsible for carriage of oxygen from lungs to tissues. *h. fetal* Fetal hemoglobin contains 2 alfa and 2 gamma chains in globin unit, constitutes the total Hb in fetus and is replaced by adult Hb after birth. Normal concentration in adults is 2%, level is increased in thalassemia minor. *Hb S* The hemoglobin of sickle cell anemia which polymerizes on exposure to hypoxic conditions, causes hemolysis and organ dysfunction due to vascular occlusion. *Hb M* The iron in HbM is in ferric form and is not able to combine with oxygen (hence called methemoglobin). There is diffuse cyanosis. *Hb A1C* Glycosylated Hb where glucose is attached to terminal amino acid of betaglobin chain. Normal level is $\leq 6\%$. Value above 6% indicates poor blood sugar control.

Hemoglobinemia Presence of free hemoglobin in plasma.

Hemoglobinometer Apparatus for estimating blood Hb.

Hemoglobinuria Presence of hemoglobin in urine.

Hemogram Differential blood count.

Hemolysin Agents destroying blood corpuscles.

Hemolysis Destruction of RBC.

Hemolytic anemia Anemia resulting from haemolysis of red blood cells.

Hemolytic disease of newborn ABO or Rh incompatibility resulting in haemolysis, anemia, jaundice, edema and hepatic enlargement.

Hemolytic uremic syndrome Characterized by microangiopathic hemolytic anemia, acute nephropathy and thrombocytopenia in children usually preceded by upper respiratory illness or G.I. upset.

Hemoperfusion Perfusion of blood through substances, such as activated charcoal or ion exchange resins, to remove toxic material. The blood is not separated from the chemical or solution by semipermeable dialysis membrane unlike hemodialysis.

Hemopericardium Accumulation of blood in the pericardial sac.

Hemoperitoneum Accumulation of blood in peritoneal cavity.

Hemopexin A glycoprotein of beta-globulin that binds to hemin but not hemoglobin.

Hemophilia A sex-linked hereditary disorder of coagulation with prolonged clotting time, repeated hemarthrosis and bleeding from nose or after trivial trauma. There is deficiency of factor VIII.

Hemophilus A genus of bacteria, gram −ve, nonmotile, requiring blood factors X or V for their growth.

Hemopneumopericardium Blood and air in pericardial cavity due to the injury to trachea or mediastinum.

Hemopneumothorax Blood and air in pleural cavity.

Hemopoiesis Formation of blood cells (*see* Figure).

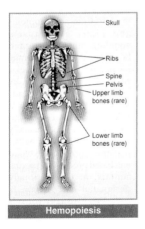

Skull

Ribs

Spine

Pelvis

Upper limb bones (rare)

Lower limb bones (rare)

Hemopoiesis

Hemoptysis Expectoration of blood or coughing up of blood.

Hemorrhage Bleeding, either external or internal. *h. antepartum* Bleeding after 28 weeks of gestation and before onset of labor. *h. accidental* Retroplacental bleeding. *h. postpartum* Bleeding in excess of 500 ml. after childbirth.

Hemorrhagic disease of newborn Bleeding from nose, umbilical stump in newborn due to inadequate prothrombin synthesis (premature fetal liver/poor bacterial flora).

Hemorrhagic fevers A group of diseases due to arthropod-borne viruses like yellow fever, Kyasanur Forest disease.

Hemorrhoid Dilated, tortuous veins in the anorectal region. *h. external* Dilated vein or veins at the junction of anal mucosa with the anal skin. *h. prolapse* Prolapse of internal hemorrhoids through the anus. *h. strangulated* Painful prolapsed hemorrhoids with cessation in their blood supply by pressure from anal sphincter.

Hemorrhoidectomy Removal of hemorrhoids by surgery, ligation or cryo, etc.

Hemosalpinx Bleeding into fallopian tube.

Hemosiderin Iron containing pigment derived from hemoglobin liberated from disintegrated RBC.

Hemosiderosis Deposition of iron in reticuloendothelial cells of liver principally after multiple blood transfusion as in hemoglobinopathy and hemolytic diseases.

Hemostasis Arrest of bleeding.

Hemothorax Blood in the pleural cavity, either due to trauma, tumor of lungs and pleura, connective tissue disease, etc.

Henderson Hasselbalch equation An equation for expression of pH.

Henoch-Schonlein Purpura Allergic purpura with erythema, urticaria accompanied by gastrointestinal and joint symptoms.

Henry's law The weight of a gas dissolved by a given volume of liquid at a constant temperature is directly proportional to the pressure.

Heparin A polysachharide produced by mast cells of liver and basophils, inhibits conversion of prothrombin to thrombin.

Hepatic coma Impaired CNS function due to liver dysfunction. Coma results from increased serum ammonia, false neurotransmitters and middle molecules, the toxic

products of protein metabolism. Common precipitating factors are high protein diet, bleeding into GI tract (varices), infections, electrolyte imbalance, diuretics and drugs. Mousy odor, flapping tremor and EEG changes are characteristic.

Hepatic duct The bile channel from liver that joins with cystic duct to form common bile duct.

Hepatic veins The three veins draining right and left lobes of liver into inferior vena cava.

Hepatitis Inflammation of liver; causative agents include viruses (Hepatitis A, B, C, delta agent), bacteria, alcohol, drugs and autoimmune diseases. Common symptoms and signs are nausea, vomiting, jaundice, fever and hepatomegaly. *h. A* Average incubation period 4 weeks, acute onset, transmitted by feco oral route. Rarely leads to chronic liver diseases. *h. B* Average incubation period 60 days, slow onset, usually progresses to chronic active hepatitis, spread is by blood and blood product and sexual contact. *h. C.* Previously designated non A, non B, acute onset, usually spreads through blood and blood products, mild course. *h. delta* Onset may be acute, usually occurs in those having hepatitis B. Usually self limited. *h. amebic* The liver dysfunction is due to a nonspecific reaction to amebic colitis, not true invasion of ameba into liver. Right subcostal pain, tender hepatomegaly, fever and leukocytosis are present. *h. alcoholic* History of excessive indulgence in alcohol, with tender hepatomegaly, icterus and marked elevation of SGOT and SGPT. *h. fulminant* Rapidly progressive hepatitis with deepening jaundice, liver cell failure and coma.

Hepatitis-associated antigen It was originally applied to hepatitis B surface antigen or Australia antigen. Now other antigens like core antigen (Hbc), 'e' antigen are also identified for diagnosis of hepatitis B infection.

Hepatitis B immunoglobulin Derived from blood plasma of human donors who have high titers of antibodies against hepatitis B.

Hepatitis B vaccine A recombinant vaccine with hepatitis B surface antigen given as 20 μg. Dose-3 doses, to persons at high-risk.

Hepatoblastoma Malignant teratoma of liver.

Hepatogenic Having its origin in the liver.

Hepatogenous Originating in the liver.

Hepatojugular reflex Pressure on the liver or right upper abdomen causes a rise in jugular venous pressure in patients of congestive heart failure.

Hepatolenticular degeneration An autosomal recessive trait with copper deposition in liver, cornea, kidney and brain due to decrease in plasma copper binding protein, the ceruloplasmin.

Hepatology Study of liver.

Hepatoma A primary malignant tumor of liver.

Hepatomegaly An enlargement of liver; may be upward or downward. Commonly due to alcohol, hepatitis, amebiasis, congestive failure, infectious fevers, etc.

Hepatorenal syndrome Kidney dysfunction with uremia secondary to acute or chronic hepatic catastrophe.

Hepatosis Non-inflammatory disease of liver.

Hepatosplenomegaly Enlargement of both liver and spleen; commonly due to enteric fever, malaria, kala-azar, leukemia and lymphoproliferative disorders, cirrhosis, portal hypertension, etc.

Herb A plant with soft stem containing little wood, usually seasonal.

Hereditary Genetic characteristic transmitted from parent to offspring.

Heredofamilial Any disease recurring in family members due to inherited defect or other familial factors.

Hering-Breuer reflex Reflex inhibition of inspiration resulting from stimulation of lung receptors following lung inflation.

Hering's nerve Afferent nerve fibers from carotid sinus passing to brain via glossopharyngeal nerve. A rise in blood pressure stimulates these nerves to reflexly diminish heart rate.

Heritage The genetic and other characteristics transmitted from parents to offsprings.

Hermaphrodite One possessing genital and sexual characteristic of both male and female. The clitoris is usually enlarged to resemble penis of male.

Hermaphroditism Existence of ovarian and testicular tissue in same individual.

Hernia Protrusion of an organ or part of it through a defect in the wall surrounding it. *h. complete* One in which the organ along with its sac has passed completely through the opening. *h. epigastric* Hernia of intestine through an opening in the midline above umbilicus. *h. fascial* Protrusion of muscular tissue through its covering fascia. *h. femoral* Hernia through femoral ring. *h. hiatal* Hernia of fundus of stomach through the esophageal hiatus of diaphragm. *h. incarcerated* Hernia with complete obstruction of herniating bowel segment. *h. inguinal* Herniation of abdominal content (intestine or omentum) through inguinal rings. *h. direct inguinal* The hernial sac protrudes through the external inguinal ring in the region of Hesselbach's triangle. *h. indirect inguinal* The hernial sac protrudes through internal inguinal ring and descends along inguinal canal to protrude in external inguinal ring. *h. labial* Protrusion of a loop of bowel into the labium majus. *h. mesocolic* Herniation between the layers of mesocolon. *h. obturator* Hernia through obturator foramen. *h. retroperitoneal* Hernia into peritoneal sac extending behind the peritoneum into the iliac fossa. *h. Ritcher's* A portion of the wall of the intestinal loop protrudes, the lumen remaining patent. *h. sliding* The herniating organ slides in and out of hernial sac. *h. strangulated* Irreducible hernia where there is complete cut-off blood supply to herniating organ with threatening gangrene. *h. tonsillar* Protrusion of cerebellar tonsils through the foramen magnum, causing often compression of medulla oblongata. *h. transtentorial* Herniation of uncus and part of temporal lobe through tentorium cerebelli (*see* Figure).

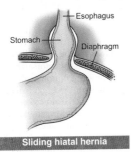

Sliding hiatal hernia

Hernial sac The pouch of peritoneum pushed before the hernia and into which it descends.

Herniated disc Rupture of nucleus pulposus through annulus fibrosus to protrude into spinal canal.

Herniorraphy Surgical repair of hernia.

Herniotomy Surgical correction of irreducible/strangulated hernia by incision over constricting ring.

Heroin An extract of morphine with strong analgesic and addictive potential. Acute intoxication produces euphoria, respiratory depression, hypotension and hypothermia.

Herpangina A coxsackie virus infection with fever, sore throat, and increased salivation. The throat is covered with vesicles.

Herpes Vesiculated eruptions caused by herpes virus. *h. simplex* Thin walled vesicles occurring at mucocutaneous junctions (lips, vagina) or over oral mucous membrane. *h. simplex encephalitis* Caused by herpes simplex virus 'B', predominantly involving temporal lobes and is hemorrhagic. *h. zoster* Caused by varicella zoster virus with inflammation of posterior root ganglia of cranial or spinal nerves. Painful vesicular eruptions, usually unilateral, distributed over few spinal segments or forehead and eye (trigeminal nerve) are characteristic.

Herring bodies Neurosecretory granules in the terminal nerve endings of hypothalamus and hypophyseal tract.

Hertz An unit of frequency equivalent to one cycle per second.

Hesperidin A chemical present in orange and lemon peel that is hemostatic by strengthening the capillaries.

Hesselbach's hernia Hernia passing through cribiform fascia.

Hesselbach's triangle Triangular space bounded by Poupart's ligament below, outer border of rectus sheath and epigastric artery.

Heterogeneous Composed of different kinds of substances.

Heterogenesis Production of offsprings that have different characteristics in alternate generations.

Heterogeusia Perception of an inappropriate quality of taste when food is chewed.

Heterograft Graft from another individual.

Heterolalia The use of meaningless words.

Heterologous 1. Composed of tissue not normal to the part. 2. A tissue, cell or blood obtained from a different individual/species.

Heterometropia Two eyes with different refraction.

Heterophil An antibody reacting with other than specific antigen.

Heterophonia Change of voice occurring esp. at puberty.

Heterophoria Tendency of the eyes to deviate from their normal position for visual alignment due to imbalance or insufficiency of ocular muscles.

Heterosexual One whose sexual orientation is to members of opposite sex.

Heterosmia Perception of inappropriate smell.

Heterotopia Development of normal tissue at an abnormal location or displacement of an organ from its normal location.

Heterotrichosis Growth of different kinds or colors of hairs on the scalp or body.

Heterotroph An organism like man who requires complex organic food for growth and development.

Heterozygote An individual with different alleles for a given characteristic.

Heubner's disease Syphilitic end arteritis in brain.

Hexachlorphene Polychlorinated phenol, antiseptic disinfectant.

Hexokinase An enzyme catalyzing phosphorylation of glucose; present in muscle tissue and yeast.

Hexose Any monosaccharide of formula $C_6H_{12}O_6$.

Hexylresorcinol Anthelmintic agent.

Hiatus An opening. *h. semelunaris* Groove in the external wall of middle meatus of nose into which frontal sinus, maxillary sinus and anterior ethmoidal cells drain.

Hibernation Condition of remaining asleep and immobile for the winter, especially in animals.

Hibernoma A rare multilobular encapsulated tumor containing fetal fat tissue closely resembling fat stored in the foot pads of hibernating animals.

Hiccough Intermittent spasmodic contraction of diaphragm with closure of glottis, causing a short sharp inspiratory cough.

Hick's sign Intermittent painless uterine contraction occurring after third month of pregnancy.

Hidradenoma Adenoma of sweat glands.

Hierarchy In order of importance.

High blood pressure Blood pressure above the normal range for age. Usually 140/90 mmHg if below 50 years and above 160/90 if above 60 years.

High residue diet High fiber/cellulose diet (above 30 gm/day) beneficial for colorectal diseases, diabetes and obesity.

Hilton's law A nerve supplying a muscle also supplies the joint that muscle moves and the skin overlying the insertion of that muscle.

Hilton's line A white line at the junction of skin of the perineum and anal mucosa.

Hilton's sac A pit along the external portion of false vocal cord.

Hilum (*SYN* – hilus) 1. The root of lungs at the level of 4th and 5th dorsal vertebra. 2. Depression or recess at exit or entrance of a duct into a gland or nerves and vessels into an organ.

Hind gut The caudal portion of entodermal tube giving rise to ileum, colon and rectum.

Hinge joint A joint permitting only flexion and extension in a single axis.

Hip Upper part of thigh formed by femur, ilium, ischeum and pubis.

Hip joint The ball and socket articulation between head of femur and acetabulum.

Hippocampal commissure A thin sheet of fibers passing transversely under posterior portion of corpus callosum.

Hippocampal formation Olfactory structures including hippocampus, dentate gyrus, supracallosal gyrus, diagonal band of Broca and hippocampal commisure.

Hippocampus major Elevation of floor of inferior horn of lateral ventricle.

Hippocampus minor Small elevation on the medial wall of lateral ventricle formed by end of calcarine fissure.

Hippocrates Greek physician who first established the scientific basis of medical practice; hence known as father of medicine.

Hippocratic facies The appearance of face at the time of impending death.

Hippocratic oath The oath Hippocrates exacted from his students which reads like "I will follow that system of regimen which, according to my ability and judgment, I consider for the benefit of my patients, and abstain from whatever is deleterious and mischievous. I will give no deadly medicine to anyone if asked nor suggest any such counsel, and in like manner I will not give to a woman a pessary for abortion. With purity and holiness I will pass my life and practise my art, into whatever houses I enter, I will go into them for the benefit of the sick, and I will abstain from every voluntary act of mischief and corruption, and further from seduction of females or males, of free men and slaves. Whatever in connection with my professional practice, or not in connection with it, I see or hear in the life of men, which ought not to be spoken of abroad, I will not divulge, as reckoning that all such should be kept secret. "While I continue to keep this oath unviolated, may it be granted to me to enjoy life and the practice of this art, respected by all men in all times. But should I trespass and violate this Oath, may the reverse be my lot".

Hippuric acid Endogenous acid formed in the human body from combination of benzoic acid and glycine and excreted by kidneys.

Hippus Rhythmical and rapid dilatation and contraction of pupil.

Hirschberg's reflex Adduction of foot when sole at base of great toe is stimulated.

Hirschsprung's disease A dynamic megacolon due to failure of development of myenteric plexus in the rectosigmoid area of colon.

Hirsutism Excessive hair growth in women.

Hirudicide Any substance that destroys leeches.

His bundle Atrioventricular bundle arising in AV node and ending in the ventricles.

Histamine A derivative of histidine that is secreted by mast cells and is responsible for triple response.

Histamine blocking agents H_1 receptor blocking agents are antiallergic and H_2 receptor blockers reduce gastric acid production.

Histamine headache Headache after taking histamine containing foods.

Histidine An amino acid obtained by hydrolysis from tissue proteins.

Histiocyte A phagocytic cell with ameboid activity, present in most connective tissues.

Histiocytosis Abnormal presence of histiocytes in the blood.

Histiocystosis-X A granulomatous destructive disease.

Histochemistry Light and electron microscopy and special chemical tests and stains done to study chemistry of cells and tissues.

Histocompatibility The ability of cells to survive without any immunological influence or interference; important in blood transfusion and tissue transplantation.

Histocompatibility antigens A number of antigens expressed by all nucleated cells which are controlled by genes located in major histocompatibility gene complex (mhc) in chromosome 6.

Histogenesis Origin and development of tissue.

Histoid Resembling one of the tissues.

Histology Study of microscopic structure of cells and tissues.

Histone A class of simple proteins present in cell chromatin.

Histonomy The law governing development and structure of tissues.

Histoplasmosis A systemic fungal infection with histoplasma capsulatum, manifesting as fever, anemia, splenomegaly, leukopenia and pulmonary infiltrations.

Histotomy Cutting of thin sections of tissue for microscopic study.

Histozyme A renal enzyme that converts hippuric acid into benzoic acid and glycine.

Histrionic Theatrical, dramatic.

Hives Eruption of itchy wheals due to allergy; local or systemic.

Hoarseness A rough quality of voice due to simple chronic laryngitis, vocal cord palsy, or infiltration of vocal cords.

Hobnail liver Liver with an irregular surface, usually cirrhosis.

Hodgkin's disease A lymphoproliferative disease with painless lymphadenopathy, hepatosplenomegaly, and often relapsing fever. Reed-Sternberg's giant cells in lymph node biopsy are characteristic.

Hoffman's sign Flicking the terminal phalanx of finger causes reflex flexion of other fingers of same hand in pyramidal damage.

Holistic medicine Comprehensive and total care of a patient, taking into account his physical, mental, social, economic and spiritual needs.

Holodiastolic Covering entire diastole i.e., closure of aortic valve to closure of mitral valve.

Holoendemic A disease affecting almost all population in a given area. In malaria epidemiology, spleen index rate of $\geq 5\%$ in children under 10 implies the disease to be holoendemic.

Holography A method of producing 3 dimensional pictures. The picture obtained is called hologram.

Holoprosencephaly Deficiency in fore brain with CSF accumulation due to trisomy of 13, 14, 15, or 18 chromosomes.

Holorachischisis Complete spina bifida.

Holosystolic Related to entire period of systole.

Holter monitor An ECG recording system capable of recording ECG for 24 hours, particularly useful for recording arrhythmias, and silent ischemia.

Homan's sign Pain in the calf on passive dorsiflexion of great toe, an evidence of deep vein thrombosis.

Homatropine Anti-muscarinic agent used to dilate pupil.

Homeopathy A system of medicine developed by Hahnemann based on the theory "like cures likely", i.e., large doses of a drug that produces symptoms of disease in healthy people will cure the same symptoms in small doses.

Homeostasis. State of equilibrium of internal environment of the body.

Homicide Murder.

Homoblastic Developing from a single type of tissue.

Homocystine A homologue of cystine formed during catabolism of methionine.

Homocystinuria An inherited metabolic disease due to absence of an enzyme essential in the metabolism of homocystine. Clinical features include marfanoid features, mental retardation, subluxation of lens, etc.

Homogeneous Uniform in structure, composition or nature.

Homogenesis Reproduction by same process in succeeding generations.

H1 and H2 receptor blockers Agents that block H$_1$ and H$_2$ receptors e.g., terphenadrine and ranitidine respectively.

Homologue Similar in position, origin and structure.

Homonymous In ophthalmology pertains to corresponding vertical halves of visual field.

Hookworm An intestinal blood sucking nematode ancylostoma duodenale and necator Americanus.

Hormone A chemical substance produced in body subserving specific function *h.*

adrenocorticotropic (ACTH) 39 amino acid peptides secreted by adrenal cortex. *h. follicle stimulating* (FSH) secreted by anterior pituitary causing growth and maturation of ovarian follicle. *h. gonadotropin releasing* (GnRH) hypothalamic hormone causing FSH, LH release. *h. growth* secreted by anterior pituitary affecting metabolism and thus control of skeletal and visceral growth. *h. luteinizing* (LH) anterior pituitary hormone causing ovulation and secretion of progesterone. *h. melanocyte stimulating* secreted by anterior pituitary causing skin pigmentation *h. parathyroid* secreted by parathyroid glands promoting release of calcium from bone by stimulation of osteoclasts and increases gut calcium absorption.

Horn Cutaneous outgrowth composed chiefly of keratin. *horn anterior* Gray substance in anterior portion of spinal cord SYN-ventral horn. *horn dorsal* Posterior projection of gray matter in spinal cord. *horn of Ammon* Hippocampus.

Horner's syndrome Myosis, ptosis, enopthalmos and loss of sweating over affected side of face due to paralysis of cervical sympathetic trunk.

Horse power A unit of power equals to 33.000 foot pounds per minute or 745.7 watts.

Horse-shoe shaped kidney A congenital renal abnormality in which both the kidneys are united at their lower poles.

Hospice Palliative and supportive care services for terminally ill.

Hospital Institution for treatment of sick and injured.

Hospitalization Admission of a patient into hospital.

Host 1. The organism which nourishes the parasite. 2. The individual receiving the graft in transplantation program. *host definitive* The final host in which parasite has sexual maturity and sexual union for reproduction. *host intermediate* Host in which parasite undergoes sexual development.

Hostility Manifestations of anger, animosity or antagonism directed towards oneself or others. It may be a symptom of depression.

Hotline A continuously functioning telephone connection.

Hot water bag A rubber or plastic bag for application of dry heat or keeping moist applications warm.

Hour-glass contraction Excessive contraction of an organ at its center resembling hour-glass e.g., in malignancy of stomach or gastric ulcer.

House maid's knee Patellar bursitis in house maid due to prolonged kneeling.

House physician An intern or resident responsible for patient care under direction of a senior staff.

Houston's valves Crescent shaped folds of mucous membrane in the rectum.

Howell-Jolly bodies Spherical granules in the erythrocytes seen in asplenia, thalassemia, leukemia, etc.

Howship's lacunae Grooves or pits occupied by osteoclasts during bone resorption.

Hubbard tank Tank of suitable size and shape for active and passive underwater exercises.

Huguier's canal Canal in the base of skull through which chorda tympani nerve exits from brain

Huhner's test Aspiration of vagina within an hour of coitus to test for sperm motility in investigation of infertility.

Hum Soft continuous sound.

Human immunodeficiency virus. (See AIDS).

Human insulin Insulin prepared by recombinant DNA technology using *E. coli.*

Human placental lactogen Placental secretion that helps to prepare the breast for milk secretion.

Humerus Bone of upper arm that articulates with scapula above and radius, ulna below (*see* Figure).

Humidity Moisture in the atmosphere.

Humor Any fluid or semifluid substance in the body. *h. aqueous* The secretion of cilliary body occupying anterior and posterior chambers of eye. It is absorbed to venous system through canal of Schlemm. *h. vitreous* The transparent jelly like substance occupying the space between lens and retina.

Humpback Curvature of spine or kyphosis.

Hunchback Kyphosis with prominent rounded deformity of back.

Hunger A desire to eat with dull pain in epigastrium. Appetite in contrast is pleasant sensation of seeking food to eat to enjoy it.

Hunter's canal Adductor canal.

Hunter's disease Mucopolysaccharidosis II.

Hunterian chancre Indurated syphilitic chancre.

Huntington chorea Inherited disease of CNS manifesting with chorea, progressive dementia.

Hurler's syndrome A form of mucopolysaccharidosis with skeletal abnormality, cloudy

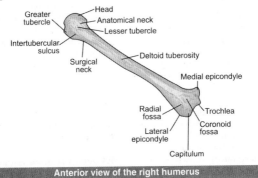

Greater tubercle — Head — Anatomical neck — Lesser tubercle — Intertubercular sulcus — Surgical neck — Deltoid tuberosity — Medial epicondyle — Radial fossa — Trochlea — Lateral epicondyle — Coronoid fossa — Capitulum

Anterior view of the right humerus

cornea, and often mental deficiency.

Hürthle cells Eosinophilic staining cells of thyroid gland.

Hutchinson Sir British surgeon.

H.'s pupil Widely dilated pupil in CNS disease.

H.'s teeth A feature of congenital syphilis in which the lateral incisors are peg shaped and the central incisors are notched.

H.'s triad In congenital syphilis this diagnostic triad consists of deafness, interstitial keratitis and Hutchinson's teeth.

Hyaline It refers to any alteration within cell or in the extracellular space, which gives a homogeneous, glassy, pink appearance in histologic sections stained with hematoxylin and eosin.

Hyaline Bluish-white glassy translucent cartilage, e.g. semilunar cartilage of knee, thyroid cartilage.

Hyaline cartilage Smooth, pearly true cartilage covering articular surface of bone.

Hyaline casts Pale, transparent casts with homogeneous rounded ends seen in urine in nephropathy.

Hyaline membrane disease A respiratory disease of newborn with poor gas transfer.

Hyalinization The development of an albuminoid mass in a cell or tissue.

Hyalinosis Waxy or hyaline degeneration.

Hyalitis Inflammation of vitreous humor; can be asteroid, punctate and suppurative.

Hyalogen A protein substance in vitreous humor and cartilage.

Hyaloid artery A fetal artery supplying nutrition to the lens. It disappears afterbirth.

Hyaloid canal Lymph channel in vitreous extending from optic disk to posterior capsule of lens; contains hyaloid artery in fetus.

Hyaloid membrane Membrane that envelops the vitreous humor.

Hyaluronic acid An acid mucopolysaccharide forming the ground substance of connective tissue; functioning as a binding and protective agent.

Hyaluronidase An enzyme that depolymerizes hyaluronic acid, thereby increases permeability of connective tissues.

Hybrid The offspring of parent that are of different species.

Hybridization Production of hybrids by cross-matching.

Hybridoma It is the cell produced by fusion of an antibody producing cell and a multiple myeloma cell. The hybrid cell thus formed can be a source of continuous monoclonal antibodies.

Hydantoin A colorless base, glycolyl urea.

Hydatid A cyst formed in internal organs, commonly lungs or liver by developing larva of *E. granulosus*.

Hydatid disease The disease produced by the cysts of larval stage of echinococcus (*see* Figure).

Hydatidiform mole Degenerative process of chorionic villi with formation of multiple cysts within uterus (*see* Figure).

Hydatid of Morgagni Cyst like remnant of mullerian

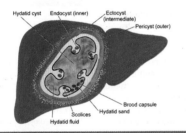

Hydatid disease

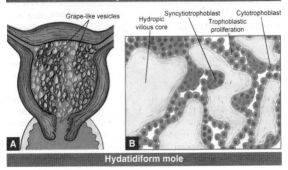

Hydatidiform mole

duct that is attached to fallopian tube.

Hydradenitis Inflammation of sweat glands.

Hydradenoma Tumor of sweat gland.

Hydragogue Drug promoting watery evacuation of bowel like sodium sulphate or magnesium sulphate.

Hydralazine Antihypertensive acting through vasomotor center in CNS.

Hydramnios An excess of liquor amnii around the developing fetus.

Hydranencephaly Hydrocephalus due to congenital absence of cerebral hemispheres.

Hydrarthrosis Serous effusion into a joint cavity.

Hydraulics The science of fluids.

Hydriatrics Application of water for treatment *SYN* hydrotherapy.

Hydrocarbon Compound made of only hydrogen and carbon.

Hydrocele Fluid accumulation in tunica vaginalis testes or in any sac like cavity (*see* Figure). *h. cervical* Hydrocele of neck resulting from accumulation of fluid in persistent cervical duct or cleft. *h. congenital* Hydrocele present since birth resulting in failure of tunica

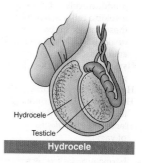

Hydrocele

Testicle

Hydrocele

vaginalis to close. *h. encysted* Hydrocele in the processus vaginalis with closure of its abdominal and scrotal ends.

Hydrocephalus Increased content of CSF within the ventricles resulting from decreased absorption of CSF, its increased production or blockage to its circulation resulting from developmental anomalies, infection, injury or tumor. *h. communicating* Hydrocephalus in which normal communication between 4th ventricle and subarachnoid space is maintained. *h. normal pressure* Hydro-cephalus with normal CSF pressure and without demonstrable block, to CSF circulation.

Hydrochloric acid Produced by oxyntic cells of gastric

glands, serves to convert pepsinogen into pepsin, dissolves and disintegrates nucleoproteins, precipitates caseinogen, hydrolyzes sucrose, inhibits bacterial multiplication, etc.

Hydrochlorothiazide Diuretic.

Hydrocodone Opioid alkaloid, analgesic and hypnotic.

Hydrocolpos Retention cyst of vagina.

Hydrocortisone Corticosteroid hormone produced by adrenal gland.

Hydroflumethazide A diuretic.

Hydrogen A colorless, odorless and tasteless gas with atomic weight of 1. Three isotopes of hydrogen, e.g. protium, deuterium and tritium have (appx) atomic weights of 1,2, 3 respectively.

Hydrogenase An enzyme that catalyzes reduction by molecular hydrogen.

Hydrogenation Addition of hydrogen to convert unsaturated fat to solid fat.

Hydrogen donor In oxidation-reduction reactions a substance that gives up hydrogen to another substance.

Hydrogen ion The positively charged hydrogen particle.

Hydrogen ion concentration The pH value is the negative logarithm of H. ion concentration of a solution, expressed in gram ions (moles) per liter. A solution with pH of 1 is ten times more acid than one with pH of 2 and 100 times more acid than one with pH of 3. A pH above 7 means alkalinity. The blood pH is around 7.35.

Hydrogen peroxide H_2O_2 colorless greasy liquid with irritating odor and acrid taste, decomposes easily liberating oxygen in presence of light. 3% solution is a mild antiseptic, germicide and cleansing agent. Used commercially as a bleaching agent.

Hydrogen sulfide H_2S. A poisonous, gas with pungent odor of rotten egg.

Hydrolase An enzyme causing hydrolysis.

Hydrolysis Combination of water with salt to produce acid and base or a chemical decomposition in which a substance is split into simpler compounds by addition or the taking up of the elements of water.

Hydrometer An instrument that measures density of liquid.

Hydromorphone An analgesic, opium derivative.

Hydromyelia Distention of central canal of spinal cord with fluid.

Hydromyelocele Protrusion of spinal CSF sac through spina bifida.

Hydromyoma Cystic uterine fibroid.

Hydronephrosis Collection of fluid in renal pelvicalicyeal system usually due to obstruction to urine flow, ultimately causing atrophy of renal parenchyma (*see* Figure).

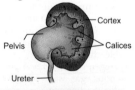

Hydronephrosis

Hydropericarditis Inflammatory condition of the pericardium along with the accumulation of serous fluid inside the pericardial sac.

Hydroperitoneum Also known as ascites in which there is accumulation of serous fluid inside the peritoneal cavity.

Hydrophobia Morbid fear for water, synonym for rabies in which attempt to drink water causes spasm of pharynx due to CNS irritation.

Hydrophilic ointment Topical ointment that absorbs water and hence is emollient.

Hydropneumatosis Liquid and gas in tissues producing combined edema and emphysema.

Hydropneumopericardium Fluid and gas in pericardial cavity.

Hydropneumothorax Gas and fluid in pleural sac.

Hydrops Edema. *h. endolymphaticus* Edema of labyrinth.

Hydropyonephrosis Dilatation of renal pelvis with pus and urine.

Hydroquinone A depigmenting agent.

Hydrorrhoea Production of profuse watery discharge from any part or organ of the body, e.g. Hydrorrhoea gravidarum refers to discharge of watery fluid from the vagina during the third trimester of pregnancy.

Hydrostatic densitometry An underwater weighing technique for determination of body components, usually percentage of fat.

Hydrostatic test A test to know if the dead infant has breathed prior to death. If the infants lungs float in water, breathing had been established prior to death.

Hydrotherapy Scientific application of water in treatment of diseases for following therapeutic objectives. Brief hot tub and shower baths relieve fatigue, cold bath to constrict blood vessels, to reduce tissue edema after injury. Hot bath dilates blood vessels, encourages perspiration.

Hydrothorax Accumulation of noninflammatory fluid within thorax.

Hydroureter Distension of ureter due to obstruction.

Hydroxocobalamin A chemical with activity similar to B_{12}.

Hydroxyapatite Calcium phosphate in combination with calcium carbonate present in the bones; when it combines with fluorine, it becomes decay resistant fluoroapatite.

Hydroxybenzene Phenol.

Hydroxybutyric acid A component of ketone body produced by abnormal metabolism of fat in diabetic ketosis.

Hydroxychloroquin Antimalarial agent.

Hydroxyproline An amino acid found in collagen.

Hydroxypropyl methyl cellulose A substance used to increase viscosity of solutions.

Hydroxystilbamidine isethionate Antiprotozoal antimonial. *5 hydroxy tryptamine* Serotonin.

Hydroxyurea Cytotoxic agent used in leukemia.

Hydroxyzine An antihistamine.

Hygiene Study of methods and means of preserving health.

Hygroma A sac containing fluid. *h. cystic* A rapidly growing cystic swelling in neck of lymphatic origin.

Hygrometer Instrument for measuring moisture in air.

Hymen A fold of mucous membrane that partially covers the entrance to vagina. *h. annular* Hymen with ring shaped opening in the center. *h. biforis* Hymen with two parallel openings with a thick septum in between. *h. cribiform* Hymen with many small openings. *h. denticulatus* Hymen opening has serrated edges.

Hymenolepsis A genus of tapeworm. *h. nana* Dwarf tapeworm, average length 1". capable of completing lifecycle within one host.

Hymenology Science of the membranes and their diseases.

Hymenoptera An order of insects that includes ants, bees, hornets and wasps.

Hymenorrhaphy Plastic surgery of hymen to restore it to preruptured state.

Hyoglossus Muscle arising from hyoid bone and inserted into dorsum of tongue. It draws sides down and retracts the tongue.

Hyoid bone Horse-shoe shaped bone lying at the base of tongue (*see* Figure).

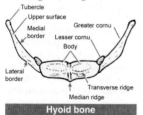

Hyoid bone

Hyopharyngeus Middle pharyngeal constrictor.

Hyoscine hydrobromide Belladona alkaloid having atropine like effect.

Hyper Prefix meaning excessive, beyond.

Hyperacidity Excess of acid in stomach.

Hyperactivity Excessive activity of an organ or entire organism.

Hyperacusis Abnormal sensitivity to sound, e.g., in hysteria.

Hyperalgia Excessive sensitivity to pain.

Hyperalimentation IV infusion of hypertonic solution that contains sufficient amino acids, electrolytes and glucose to sustain life and achieve normal growth and development.

Hyperammonemia Excess of ammonia in blood, e.g., cirrhosis can be congenital either due to deficiency of carbamyl phosphate synthetase or ornithine transcarbamylase that metabolize ammonia.

Hyperamylasemia Increased blood amylase.

Hyperbaric oxygen Oxygen on increased pressure to treat gas gangrene, air embolism, decompression sickness, CO poisoning, nonhealing ulcers, etc.

Hyperbetalipoproteinemia Excessive amount of betalipoprotein in blood.

Hyperbilirubinemia Excessive amount of bilirubin in blood.

Hypercalcemia Excessive amount of calcium in the blood (12.2 mg%) either idiopathic, or secondary to malignancy, prolonged recumbency, vit D intoxication, etc.

Hypercalciuria Excessive excretion of calcium in urine.

Hypercapnia Excess CO_2 in blood.

Hyperchloremia Increased chloride content of blood e.g., hyperchloremic acidosis.

Hyperchlorhydria Excess secretion of HCl in stomach.

Hypercholesterolemia Excessive ($\geq$250 mg%) cholesterol in blood; often familial, but usually dietary.

Hyperchromatic Overpigmented.

Hyperchromatopsia Defect of vision in which all objects appear colored.

Hypercorticism Excessive production of adrenocortical hormones.

Hypercyesis Presence of more than one fetus in uterus.

Hyperdontia Presence of more than normal number of teeth.

Hyperemesis Excessive vomiting.

Hyperemesis gravidarum Nausea and vomiting during pregnancy threatening dehydration, and acidosis.

Hyperemia Vascular congestion; can be active as in increased blood flow or passive due to venous stasis.

Hypereosinophilic syndrome Idiopathic persistent hyper- eosinophilia often with CNS and cardiac involvement.

Hyperesthesia Increased sensitivity to sensory stimuli especially pain and touch.

Hyperextension Excessive degree of extension movement in a joint, a feature of collagen disorder.

Hyperferremia Increased iron content of blood.

Hyperfibrinogenemia Increased blood fibrinogen, often threatening spontaneous coagulation.

Hyperglycemia Increased blood sugar as in diabetics.

Hyperglycinemia Accumulation of amino acid glycine in blood manifesting with mental and growth retardation.

Hypergnosia Distorted or exaggerated perception.

Hypergonadism Excessive secretion of sex hormones.

Hyperhidrosis Unusually high sweating, often due to fever, drugs, anxiety.

Hyperhydration Excess amount of water in the body.

Hyperinsulinism Excess of insulin in the body causing hypoglycemia that manifests with hunger, sweating, weakness, convulsion and often coma.

Hyperkalemia Serum potassium exceeding 5 mEq/lit.

Hyperkeratosis Thickening of horny layer of epidermis often due to vitamin A deficiency.

Hyperkinesia Increased muscular movement and physical activity. In children often due to brain dysfunction and phenobarbitone.

Hyperlipemia Excessive quantity of fat in the blood.

Hyperlipoproteinemia Increased lipoprotein content in blood due to increased synthesis or decreased breakdown.

Hypermelanosis Increased melanin content of skin either in epidermis (melanoderma) in which the coloration is brown, or in the dermis in which skin color is blue or slate grey. Conditions responsible for hypermelanosis are ACTH producing tumors, Wilson's disease, biliary cirrhosis, chronic renal failure, etc.

Hypermenorrhea Abnormal increase in duration or amount of menstrual blood loss.

Hypermetabolism Increased metabolic rate seen in hyperthyroidism, fever, following trauma and surgery.

Hypermetria Unusual range of movement as in cerebellar disease.

Hypermetropia Far-sightedness, i.e., the parallel rays fall behind the macula.

Hypermimia Making great number of gestures while speaking.

Hypermnesia Great ability to remember or memorize minute details as in mania or in conditions of temporal lobe stimulation.

Hypermobility Increased range of joint movement due to lax surrounding structures as in Ehlers-Danlos syndrome, Marafan's syndrome.

Hypermorph Large limb length causing high standing height in comparison to sitting height.

Hypernatremia Excess sodium content of blood (150 mEq/lit).

Hypernephroma Renal cell carcinoma.

Hypernormal Abnormal.

Hyperosmia Abnormal sensitivity to odors.

Hyperosmolarity Increased osmolarity of blood (300 mOsms/lit.)

Hyperostosis Abnormal and excessive growth of osseous tissue. *h. frontalis interna* Multiple osteomas arising from frontal bone internally into nasal sinuses. *h. infantile cortical* Excessive subperiosteal bone growth in the mandible or clavicles.

Hyperoxaluria Increased oxalic acid excretion in urine. *h. enteric* Caused by disease or surgical removal of ileum. *h. primary* Defective oxalate metabolism causing oxlate calculi in urinary system.

Hyperparathyroidism Increased parathormone secretion, causing osteitis fibrosa cystica, bone pain, renal stone and fracture.

Hyperpathia Hypersensitivity to sensory stimuli.

Hyperphasia Abnormal desire to talk.

Hyperphenylalaninemia Increased phenylalanine in blood.

Hyperphonia Explosive speech in stammerers.

Hyperphoria Tendency of one eye to turn upward.

Hyperphosphatasemia Raised alkaline phosphatase in blood either due to biliary obstruction or bone destruction.

Hyperphosphatemia Increased blood phosphorus content.

Hyperphosphaturia Increased amount of phosphates in urine.

Hyperphrenia Excessive mental ability as in mania.

Hyperpituitarism Overactivity of pituitary, commonly the anterior lobe producing gigantism/ acromegaly.

Hyperplasia Excessive growth of normal cells with normal tissue architecture.

Hyperploidy Condition having one extra chromosome, e.g., Down syndrome (trisomy 21).

Hyperpnea Increased rate and depth of breathing.

Hyperpraxia Excessive activity and restlessness.

Hyperprolactinemia Amenorrhea, galactorrhea produced by increased serum prolactin due to hypothalamic pituitary dysfunction.

Hyperprolinemia Excess blood proline level due to inherited metabolic defect.

Hyperproteinemia Excess of protein in plasma, as in multiple myeloma.

Hyperproteinuria Protein excretion in urine exceeding 150 mg/24 hours.

Hyperptyalism Excess salivary secretion.

Hyperpyrexia Body temperature exceeding 106°F. (41.1°C). *h. malignant* Hyperpyrexia occurring with inhalant anesthetics and muscle relaxants.

Hyperreflexia Increased tendon reflexes.

Hyperresonance Increased resonance to percussion especially over cavity, bullae, pneumothorax and emphysematous lung tissue.

Hypersensibility Hypersensitivity to a foreign protein or drug.

Hypersomnia Prolonged sleepiness, usually pathological, i.e. narcalepsy.

Hypersplenism Enlarged spleen with enhanced removal

of blood components from circulation.

Hypersthenia Abnormal strength or excessive tension of the entire body or part of it.

Hypersthenuria Passage of abnormally concentrated urine.

Hypersusceptibility Unusual susceptibility to a disease, pathological process, parasite or chemicals.

Hypertelorism Abnormal width between two paired organs, usually the eyes.

Hypertension Blood pressure considered abnormally high for an age. *h. essential* Hypertension without apparent cause. *h. malignant* Severe hypertension with diastolic pressure exceeding 130-140 mmHg with papilledema. *h. portal* Increased portal vein pressure caused by obstruction to portal flow as in cirrhosis, portal vein thrombosis/compression and Budd-Chhiari syndrome. *h. renal* Hypertension secondary to renal artery occlusion leading to hyperreninemia.

Hyperthecosis Hyperplasia of theca interna of ovary often leading to amenorrhea and hirsutism.

Hyperthelia Presence of more than 2 nipples.

Hyperthermia Unusual high fever; a treatment modality by which foreign protein is introduced into body to raise body temperature.

Hyperthrombinemia Increased thrombin concentration in blood.

Hyperthyroidism Over production of thyroxine by thyroid gland with tachycardia, tremor, anxiety, weight loss, increased appetite.

Hypertonia Increased vascular/muscle tone.

Hypertonic Having higher osmotic pressure or having greater than normal tension.

Hypertrichosis Excess growth of hair due to endocrine disease.

Hypertrophy Nontumorous enlargement of an organ or structure due to increase in size or number of cells. *h. concentric* The walls of the organ become symmetrically thick without increase in size of cavity. *h. eccentric* Regional hypertrophy with dilatation. *h. pseudomuscular* An inherited disease affecting boys where the muscles commonly of calf, thigh, buttocks enlarge due to deposition of fat and fibrous tissue. The involved muscles are weak and atrophied with waddling gait and increased spinal curvature.

Hyperuricemia Increased serum uric acid (8 mg%).

Hypervascular Excess vascularity.

Hyperventilation Increased rates and depths of inspiration and expiration.

Hyperviscosity Excess adhesiveness or stickiness property of fluid, commonly blood.

Hypervitaminosis Excessive vitamin content of body tissues, commonly involves fat soluble vitamins like A, D, E and K; usually secondary to excess ingestion.

Hypervolemia Abnormal increase in volume of circulating blood.

Hypesthesia Lessened sensibility to touch.

Hyphema Bleeding into anterior chamber of eye.

Hypnagogic Induced by sleep; inducing sleep; in psychiatry relates to hallucinations and dreams just before loss of consciousness.

Hypnodontics The application of controlled suggestions and hypnosis to practice of surgery.

Hypnology Scientific study of sleep.

Hypnosis A subconscious condition in which the patient responds to suggestions made by the hypnotist, useful for treatment of phobias, anxiety and chronic pain disorder.

Hypnotics Drugs that cause insensitivity to pain by inducing hypnosis.

Hypnotism An induced sleep like state during which the patient is peculiarly susceptible to the suggestions of the hypnotist.

Hypoacusis Decreased sensitivity to sound stimuli.

Hypoalbuminemia Decreased plasma albumin manifesting with edema, usually due to malnutrition or cirrhosis.

Hypoaldosteronism Decreased plasma aldosterone with hypotension and hyperkalemia.

Hypoalimentation Insufficient nourishment.

Hypobaric Decreased atmospheric pressure.

Hypocalcemia Decreased plasma calcium manifesting with stridor and tetany.

Hypocalciuria Decreased calcium excretion in urine.

Hypocarbia Decreased CO_2 in blood.

Hypocapnea Decreased CO_2 in blood.

Hypocellularity Decreased cell population in any tissue.

Hypochloremia Decreased chloride content in blood.

Hypochlorhydria Decreased HCl secretion in stomach often indicative of malignancy of stomach.

Hypochlorous acid HClO, used as disinfectant/bleaching agent.

Hypochondriac Abnormal and excessive fear of disease.

Hypochondrium Part of the abdomen below the lower ribs.

Hypochromasia Lack of hemoglobin in RBC *SYN*—hypochromia.

Hypocomplementemia Decreased complement concentration in blood.

Hypocorticism Decreased cortical hormone.

Hypodermic Inserted under the skin.

Hypodontia Absence or poor tooth development.

Hypofunction Decreased function.

Hypogammaglobulinemia Decreased gammaglobulin concentration in blood leading to frequent infections; can be congenital or acquired (AIDS).

Hypogastrium Region below the umbilicus, between the right and left inguinal regions.

Hypogeusia Blunting of taste sensation.

Hypoglossal Situated below the tongue.

Hypoglossal nerve 12th cranial nerve originating in medulla and supplying intrinsic and extrinsic muscles of tongue.

Hypoglottis Under surface of tongue.

Hypoglycemia Decreased blood glucose below 50 mg% manifesting as tremor, sweating, weakness, etc.

Hypoglycemic agents Sulphonylurea compounds causing a decrease in blood sugar.

Hypoglycemic shock Shock produced by hypoglycemia induced by insulin injection to treat schizophrenia.

Hypokalemia Decreased blood potassium ($\geq$ 3mEq/l) manifesting with weakness, paralysis and hypotension.

Hypokinesia Decreased motor activity.

Hypolipidemic Reducing lipid concentration.

Hypomagnesemia Decreased plasma magnesium with neuromuscular excitability.

Hypomelanosis Decreased melanin in epidermis, e.g. vitiligo, burn.

Hypomenorrhea Decreased menstrual flow.

Hypomorph Individual with disproportionately short legs.

Hyponatremia Decreased blood sodium concentration. (< 130 mEq/L).

Hypoparathyroidism Insufficient parathormone production with hypocalcemia and tetany.

Hypopharynx Lowermost portion of pharynx leading to esophagus and larynx.

Hypophonia Weak voice.

Hypophoria Tendency of one visual axis to fall below the other.

Hypophosphatasia Decreased alkaline phosphatase in serum, usually an inherited metabolic disease manifesting with rickets, osteomalacia, poor dentition, etc.

Hypophosphatemia Decreased plasma phosphate concentration.

Hypophyseal Pertains to hypophysis or pituitary.

Hypophysectomy Excision of hypophysis.

Hypophysis The pituitary gland occupying sella turcica.

Hypophysitis Inflammation of pituitary body.

Hypopituitarism Diminished pituitary hormone secretion secondary to pituitary destruction by tumor, infarction, compression resulting in secondary dysfunction of thyroid, adrenal, testis/ovary and growth disturbance in children.

Hypoproteinemia Decreased plasma protein.

Hypopyon Pus in anterior chamber usually secondary to corneal ulcer.

Hypospadius Abnormal urethral opening, either in the under surface of glans, penile shaft or in perineum.

Hypostasis Diminished blood flow or circulation.

Hyposthenia Weakness, subnormal strength.

Hyposthenuria Secretion of low specific gravity urine.

Hypotension Abnormally low blood pressure.

Hypothalamus The portion of diencephalon comprising the ventral wall of third ventricle and adjacent structures responsible for regulation of body temperature, sugar and fat metabolism, and secretion of releasing and inhibiting hormones. It is the principal center for integration of sympathetic and parasympathetic activities (*see* Figure on page 350).

Hypothenar The fleshy prominence at the base of little finger along inner side of palm.

Hypothermia Subnormal (below 96°F) body temperature, induced for open heart

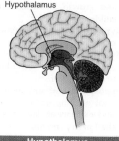

Hypothalamus

Hypothalamus

surgery and neurological procedures.

Hypothesis An assumption not proved by experiment or observation.

Hypothrombinemia Deficiency of thrombin in blood.

Hypothyroidism Deficiency of thyroid hormones causing thick coarse hair, dry thick inelastic skin, hoarse voice, obesity, depressed muscular activity, slow pulse and hypercholesterolemia. Mental retardation and growth failure may occur in children (cretinism).

Hypotonia Loss of muscle or arterial tone.

Hypotrichosis Sparse hair.

Hypotrophy Degeneration and atrophy of tissues.

Hypotympanum The part of middle ear below the level of tympanic membrane.

Hypoventilation Reduced rate and depth of breathing.

Hypovitaminosis Condition arising from lack of vitamins.

Hypovolemia Diminished circulating blood volume.

Hypoxanthine A purine derivative formed during protein decomposition to form urea and uric acid.

Hypoxemia Insufficient oxygen content of blood.

Hypoxia Decreased O_2 concentration in inspired air.

Hypsarrhythmia An abnormal EEG pattern in which there is persistent generalized slowing and very high voltage discharge; characteristic of infantile epilepsy.

Hypsiloid U or Y shaped.

Hypsiloid ligament Iliofemoral ligament.

Hypsokinesis Tendency to fall backwards when standing as seen in Parkinson's disease.

Hypsophobia Fear of being at great heights.

Hysterectomy Surgical removal of uterus either by abdominal or vaginal route. It can be subtotal, total or radical. In radical hysterectomy (Wertheim's operation) uterus, tubes, ovaries, adjacent lymphnodes and part of vagina are removed; usually done in stage I and II cancer cervix.

Hysteresis Failure of the manifestation of an effect to keep up with its cause.

Hysteria A conversion disorder in which patient transforms longstanding mental conflict into somatic symptoms. There is no organic disease to account for the symptoms. Patient is amnesic for the period of illness as the primary consciousness reasserts itself.

Hysteric chorea A form of hysteria with choreiform movements.

Hysterography Recording of frequency and intensity of uterine contractions.

Hysterogram X-ray of uterus.

Hysteroid Resembling hysteria.

Hysteromania Nymphomania.

Hysterometry Measurement of size of uterus.

Hysteromyemectomy Excision of uterine fibroid.

Hystero-oophorectomy Excision of uterus and ovaries.

Hysteropia Hysteric visual defect.

Hysterorrhexis Rupture of pregnant uterus.

Hysterosalpingectomy Excision of uterus and tubes.

Hysterosalpingography X-ray visualization of uterus and the tubes by introduction of contrast media.

Hystero salpingostomy Anastomosis of uterus with the remaining healthy portion of fallopian tube after excision of diseased part.

Hysteroscope Instrument for examination of inside of uterus.

Hysterotomy Incision of uterus as in evacuation of mole, dead fetus or cesarian section.

Hysterotrachelectomy Amputation of uterine cervix.

Hysterotrachelorrhaphy Repair of torn cervix.

I

Iatrogenic Adverse body effect induced by drug, procedure or the doctor.

Ibuprofen A nonsteroidal anti-inflammatory agent.

Ice Solid form of water at temperature of 0°C or below.

Icebag A water tight bag to hold ice for cold sponging over bruised or sprained area.

Ichnogram A footprint taken while standing.

Ichor Fetid discharge from an ulcer.

Ichthammol A reddish brown viscous fluid acting as an antiseptic, often used in ear-dressing and skin applications.

Ichthyosis Condition in which skin is dry, scaly resembling fish skin. Ichthyosis vulgaris is hereditary.

Ichthyotoxin Any toxin present in fish.

Ictal Pertains to acute attack of epilepsy or stroke.

Icteric Pertains to jaundice.

Icteroid Resembling jaundice.

Icterus Yellow pigmentation of sclera, mucous membrane and skin due to excess bile salts in blood.

Id. In psychiatry one of the three divisions of psyche, the other two being ego and super ego. The id is the obscure, inaccessible part of our personality that serves as a repository of instinctual drives continually striving for expression.

Idarubicin Anthracycline antinerplastic antibiotic.

Idea A mental image, concept. *i. compulsive* A persistent obsessional thought. *i. dominant* Idea that controls one's thought and action. *i. fixed* Idea dominating one's mind and not amenable to change irrespective of evidence to contrary. *i. of reference* An impression that the conversations or actions of others have reference to oneself.

Ideal A goal regarded as a standard of perfection.

Ideation The process of thinking or formation of ideas.

It is quick in mania but slow in depression, and dementias.

Identical Exactly alike.

Identification 1. The process of determining the sameness of a thing or person with that described or known to exist 2. A defense mechanism operating unconsciously, by which a person patterns himself after some other person. This plays a major role in personality development. *i. dental* The use of dental charts, radiographs or records to establish a person's identity. *i. palm and soles* Prints of palm and sole used for one's identification.

Identity The physical and mental characteristic by which an individual is known and recognized.

Ideology A philosophy, the science of ideas and thoughts.

Ideomotor Muscular automatic movement regulated by a dominant idea.

Idiocy Severe mental deficiency due to defective mental development, the cause of which may be genetic, vascular or birth asphyxia.

Idioglossia Inability to articulate properly so that the language is not comprehensible.

Idiogram Graphic representation of chromosome karyotype.

Idiopathic A disease without recognizable cause.

Idiopathic pulmonary fibrosis A form of interstitial lung disease with diffuse fibrosis and rapid deterioration.

Idiophrenic Pertaining to or originating in the mind alone.

Idiosyncrasy A peculiar or individual reaction to an idea, action, drug, food or some other substance. Special characteristic by which one person differs from another or reacts differently from another.

Idiot Person with severe mental deficiency.

Idiotropic In psychology turning inward mentally and emotionally, i.e. introvert who is satisfied with his own emotions and is content to live apart from social contacts.

Idiotype In immunology, the specific Fab region of the immunoglobulin to which the specific antigen binds.

Idioventricular A heart rhythm arising from conduction tissue or ventricular muscle without any influence from sinus node.

Idoxuridine Antiviral agent; used for herpes infection of eye in the form of ointment 2%.

Ifosfamide Anticancer drug.

IgA Principally present in exocrine secretions like milk, saliva, intestinal secretions and tear. Hence it protects against mucosal invasion by pathogenic organism. **IgE** is secreted by mast cells and is responsible for allergy, asthma, eczema, etc. **IgG** is the principal immuno-globulin and is the major antibody against bacteria, viruses and fungi. **IgM** is formed during early period of antigenic stimulation or infection.

Ileal bypass A method of treating obesity whereby absorption of nutrients from intestine is decreased from anastomosis of one portion of upper small intestine to another portion down below.

Ileal conduit Method of diverting the urinary flow by transplanting the ureters into an isolated segment of ileum opening into the abdominal wall.

Ileitis Inflammation of ileum. *i. regional* A nonspecific chronic granulomatous lesion involving terminal ileum giving rise to pain, weight loss, intestinal obstruction and often fistula formation.

Ileocecal valve A muscular ring at the terminal ileum that regulates passage of food from small intestine to large intestine and prevents re-entry of food back into small intestine.

Ileocecostomy Surgical formation of an opening between ileum and cecum.

Ileocolostomy Anastomosis between the ileum and colon.

Ileoileostomy Surgical formation of an opening between two parts of ileum.

Ileorrhaphy Surgical repair of ileum.

Ileostomy Surgical opening of ileum through external abdominal wall.

Ileum Lower 3/5 of small intestine from jejunum to ileocecal valve. Average length 15-31 feet.

Ileus A form of intestinal obstruction due to intestinal muscle paralysis, spasm or obstruction in intestinal lumen, e.g., meconium ileus of newborn.

Iliac crest Upper free margin of hip bone or ileum.

Iliac fascia Transversalis fascia over the anterior surface of iliopsoas muscle.

Iliac region Inguinal region on either side of hypogastrium.

Iliac spine One of the four spines of ilium namely the anterior and posterior inferior spines, and the anterior and posterior superior spines.

Iliotibial band A thick wide fascial layer from the iliac crest to knee joint.

Ilizarov method A method of bone lengthening by distraction using external fixators.

Illness Sickness, ailment.

Illumination Lighting up of a part for examination or of an object under microscope. *i. darkfield* A method used to observe spirochetes or colloid particles in which the central or axial light rays are stopped and the object is illuminated by light rays coming from sides.

Illusion Inaccurate perception, misinterpretation of sensory impressions; when an illusion becomes fixed, it is called delusion.

Image A mental picture representing real object or the picture of an object produced by lens or mirror.

Image intensifier Device that increases brightness of an image and permits discrimination of much smaller objects in the image.

Imagery The calling up of events or mental pictures pertaining to sound, smell, taste, etc.

Imagination Formation of mental images of things, persons or situations.

Imaging Production of image of an object by X-ray, ultrasound, magnetic resonance, etc.

Imbalance Loss of balance usually between opposing body forces. *i. autonomic* Sympathetic- parasympathetic imbalance. *i. vasomotor* Excessive vasoconstriction or dilatation.

Imatinib Anticancer agent for CML.

Imbecile Severe mental deficiency.

Imbed In histology, to surround with a firm substance such as paraffin or colloidium.

Imbibition The absorption of fluid by a solid.

Imbricated Overlapping as tiles.

Imidazole An organic compound with heterocyclic ring as in histamine and histidine.

Imipenem An antibiotic, beta-lactamase resistant.

Imipramine A tricyclic antidepressant, also used in migraine and enuresis.

Immature Not fully developed or mature.

Immedicable Incurable.

Immersion Placing body or object under water or fluid; in microscopy the act of immersing the objective (lens) in oil.

Immersion foot A form of cold injury due to dampness and cold.

Immiscible Which cannot be mixed, e.g. oil and water.

Immobilization To make a part or limb immovable by splint, traction, plaster cast.

Immune Protected from or resistant to disease due to development of antibodies.

Immune reaction Reaction of host cells to antigenic stimulation.

Immune response The response of body to substances that are foreign or are interpreted as foreign. Immune response can be cell mediated, humoral or nonspecific.

Immunifacient Making immune.

Immunity State of being protected against disease either by previous infection or by vaccine. *i. acquired* Immunity due to active or passive immunization. *i. cell mediated* The T-cells interact with antigen with a delayed response as seen in graft rejection or infection with tuberculosis, leprosy. *i. natural* Immunity conferred by natural inherent factors like race, species. *i. passive* Immunity due to transplacental trans-

fer of maternal antibodies, antibodies secreted in milk or injection of hyperimmune specific sera.

Immunization The process of rendering a person immune by active (toxoid, inactivated, killed organisms) or passive process.

Immunoassay Assay of concentration of a substance by using the reaction of an antigen with specific antibody.

Immunobiology Study of immune phenomena in biological systems.

Immunochemistry The chemistry of antigen, antibodies and their relation to each other.

Immunocompetence Being capable of developing antibody response stimulated by an antigen.

Immunocompromised Unable to have adequate immunological response because of genetic defect of T and B-cells, immunosuppressive drugs or AIDS virus infection.

Immunodiagnosis Use of specific immune response in diagnosing medical conditions.

Immunodiffusion A test method in which antigen and antibody are placed in a gel where they diffuse towards each other and when they meet a precipitate is formed.

Immunoelectrophoresis A method of investigating the amount and character of antibodies and immunoproteins present in body fluids.

Immunofluorescence The use of fluorescein stained or fluorescein labeled antibodies to locate antigen in tissues. The sample is examined in fluorescent microscope.

Immunogen A substance that stimulates formation of antibody.

Immunogenetics The study of genetics by use of immune responses.

Immunogenic Capable of inducing immunity.

Immunogenicity The capability to stimulate antibody formation.

Immunoglobulin Proteins capable of acting with antigens; can be IgG, IgA, IgM, IgD and IgM.

Immunology Study of immunity to disease.

Immunopathology Study of tissue alterations resulting from immune or allergic reactions.

Immunoselection Selective survival of cell populations due to their having least amount of cell surface antigenicity.

Immunostimulant Agent capable of stimulating antibody production.

Immunosuppressant Agent suppressing body immune response, usually employed in treatment of autoimmune diseases.

Immunosurveillance The immune system's recognition and destruction of newly developed abnormal cells arising from mutations. This process eliminates some cancer cells.

Immunotherapy Modalities to enhance immunity.

Impaction Condition of being tightly wedged into a part e.g., tooth impaction, impaction of feces in bowel (*see* Figure).

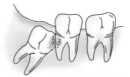

Impaction of the third molar

Impairment Any loss or abnormality of psychological, physiological or anatomical structure or function.

Impalpable Not perceptible to touch.

Impedance Resistance met by alternating current while

passing through a conductor.
i. acoustic Resistance to the
passage of sound waves.

Imperative Obligatory,
involuntary.

Imperception Lack of perception, inability to form a mental picture.

Imperforate Without an opening. In imperforate hymen the menstrual blood accumulates behind to cause hematocolpus. In imperforate anus the infant has absolute constipation.

Impervious Difficult to be penetrated.

Impetigo Inflammatory skin disease marked by formation of pustules which rupture with crust formation, may occur in crops, are contagious. *i. herpetiformis* A rare pustular eruption of unknown etiology that occurs especially during pregnancy and in association with hypocalcemia.

Implant To graft, to insert. *i. dental* Prosthetic device; endosseous, subperiosteal, mucosal or endodontic (*see* Figure).

Implosion A violent collapse inward; opp. (explosion).

Impotency Inability of male to achieve erection, can be anatomic (defect in the genitalia), atonic (paralysis of

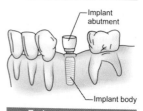

Endosseous implant

nervi erigentis), functional or vasculogenic.

Impotent Inability to copulate and procreate.

Impregnate Saturate, to make pregnant.

Impression A hollow or depression on surface; effect produced upon mind by external stimuli, the imprint of dental arch.

Impression material Materials appropriate for dental impression work, like plaster of paris, zinc oxide paste, reversible colloids.

Impression tray A tray to carry impression material to mouth and hold it in opposition to jaw/teeth.

Impulse An incitement of mind; in physiology passage of stimulating/inhibitory wave across muscle or nerve.

Impulsion Idea to do something or commit some act suddenly imposed upon the subject that tortures him until the accomplishment of that act.

Inaction Decrease response or failure of response to a stimulus.

Inactivate To make inactive or to cause loss of activity.

Inadequacy Insufficiency, incompetence.

Inanimate Dull, lifeless.

Inanition Physical debility due to lack of food.

Inapparent Not noticeable.

Inarticulate Without joints, unable to express oneself intelligibly.

Inassimilable Not capable of being utilized by body.

Incarcerated Confined, constricted, constriction as in hernia.

Incarnation To grow in (e.g., toe nails); the process of being converted to flesh.

Inception The beginning, ingestion.

Incest Coitus between close relatives.

Incidence The frequency of occurrence of any event or condition over a period of time in a specified population.

Incident A happening, event or occurrence, falling or striking ray of light.

Incipient Beginning, coming into existence.

Incise To cut, as with a sharp instrument.

Incisor One of the cutting teeth, that which cuts.

Incisura Indentation at edge of any structure, e.g. stomach incisura at distal end of lesser curvature.

Incitant The stimulus that sets off a reaction, disease.

Inclination Leaning from normal or from a vertical as in case of tooth, vertebra or pelvis.

Inclinometer Device for measuring ocular diameter from vertical and horizontal lines.

Inclusion Being included or enclosed.

Inclusion bodies Bodies present in the nucleus of cytoplasm of certain cells, e.g. Negri bodies.

Inclusion conjunctivitis *Chlamydia trachomatis* infection of the conjunctiva.

Incoercible Uncontrollable, not able to be held in check.

Incoherent Not coherent or understandable.

Incombustible Unfit for burning.

Incompatible Not being in harmony.

Incompetence Inadequacy in function of a part or organ or commonly a valve (ileocecal, mitral, aortic, pulmonary, venous, etc.).

Incompetent One legally unable to execute; incapable.

Incompetent palatal syndrome Distortion of speech (whinolalia) due to ineffective function of soft palate.

Incontinence Inability to retain urine, feces because of sphincter laxity.

Incontinence stress (urinary) Leaking of urine during coughing, sneezing, laughing, lifting, etc.

Incontinence urge Involuntary loss of urine after a strong feeling of the need to urinate.

Incoordination Inability to produce harmonious, rhythmic muscular movement.

Incorporation Combining two substances to produce a homogeneous mass.

Increment Something added or gained; an addition in number, size or extent.

Incrustation Formation of crusts or scabs.

Incubation Interval between exposure to an infection and appearance of first symptoms; in bacteriology period of culture.

Incubator 1. Enclosed crib in which temperature and humidity are controlled for nursing premature babies 2. Apparatus for maintaining bacterial culture.

Incus The middle of the three ossicles in middle ear (*see* Figure).

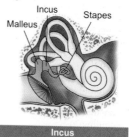

Incus

Indecision Inability to make-up one's mind.

Indentation A depression or hollow.

Index case In hereditary disease, the initial patient whose condition led to investigation of the disease.

Index The forefinger, the ratio of the measurement of a given substance with that of a fixed standard. *i. cardiac* Cardiac output expressed as liters/min divided by body surface area in m². *i. cephalic* Skull breadth to length multiplied by 100. *i. cerebral* Ratio of greatest transverse to anteroposterior diameter of skull. *i. pelvic* Ratio of pelvic conjugate and transverse diameters. *i. therapeutic* The maximum tolerable dose of a drug divided by minimum curable dose.

Indicator In chemical analysis, a substance that can be used to determine pH.

Indifferent Not responsive to normal stimuli, apathetic, neutral.

Indigenous Native to a country or region.

Indigestion Imperfect digestion manifesting as nausea, vomiting heart burn, belching, etc.

Indium A rare metallic element, its isotope ^{113}I used in scanning.

Indocyanine green A dye used in testing hepatic and renal excretory function.

Indole A solid crystalline substance found in feces, a bacterial decomposition product of tryptophan.

Indolent Inactive, sluggish.

Indolent ulcer Ulcer slow in healing.

Indomethacin Antiprostaglandin agent with anti-inflammatory, analgesic and antipyretic properties.

Induction The process of facilitating labor with oxytoxic drugs.

Inductor Any substance that will cause cells exposed to it to differentiate into an organized tissue.

Induration The act of heardening.

Inebriant Any intoxicant; making drunk.

Inebriation State of intoxication.

Inelastic Not elastic.

Inert Not active; in chemistry not able to react with other chemicals.

Inertia 1. Sluggishness, lack of activity 2. In physics tendency of body to remain in its state uptill acted upon by external force. *i. uterine* Absence of uterine contractions.

Infant From time of birth to one year of age. *i. preterm* Born prior to 37 weeks of gestation. *i. post term* Born after 42 weeks of gestation. *i. term* Born between 38-41 weeks of gestation.

Infanticide The killing of a child during the first year of its life.

Infantile Concerning an infant; childish. *i. paralysis* poliomyelitis.

Infantilism Persistence of the characters of childhood into adult life, marked by underdevelopment of the reproductive organs, and often short stature.

Infarct Area of necrosis consequent to cessation of blood supply.

Infarction Formation of an infarct.

Infection Tissue invasion with pathogenic agent that produce injurious effect. *i. acute* Infection appearing suddenly. *i. chronic* Infection having protracted course. *i. concurrent* Existence of two or more infections at the same time. *i. cross* Transfer of one disease from one hospitalized patient to another. *i. droplet* Infection acquired through microorganisms disbursed to air via breath or nasobronchial secretion. *i. pyogenic* Infection by pusforming organisms. *i. lowgrade* Mild inflammation without pus formation.

Infectious disease Disease caused by an infecting agent, not necessarily contagious.

Infertility Biological inability of a female to become pregnant during an year or more of unprotected intercourse. *i. primary* present in a woman who has never conceived. *i. secondary* present in a woman who has previously conceived, even if the pregnancy did not reach the term.

Infiltration The process of passing into or through a substance or space.

Infinity Space, time and quantity without limits.

Infirmary A small hospital, a place for care of sick.

Inflammation Tissue reaction to injury with vasodilatation, exudation, leukocyte migration followed by healing. *i. acute* Rapid onset and short course. *i. catarrhal* Inflammation of mucous membrane with excessive mucous secretion. *i. exudative* Inflammation with extreme vasodilatation, and large accumulation of blood cells. *i. granulomatous* Inflammation with excessive granular tissue production as in tuberculosis, syphilis and systemic fungal infections.

Inflation Distention of a part by air, gas or fluid.

Inflator Device used to force air into an organ.

Inflection An inward bending; change of tone or pitch of the voice.

Influenza A viral acute contagious upper respiratory infection.

Influenza virus vaccine Vaccine containing inactivated influenza virus A and B; given every year with different strains of A and B.

Infolding Process of enclosing within a fold.

Informed consent Competent and voluntary permission for a medical test, procedure or medication.

Infra Prefix meaning below, under, beneath.

Infrared rays Invisible heat rays beyond the red end of spectrum, of 7500-150,000 AU used for local application of heat and pain relief.

Infracotyloid Beneath the cotyloid cavity of the acetabulum of hip.

Infraction An incomplete fracture of bone.

Infradentale The bony point between the mandibular central incisors.

Infundibulum 1. Funnel shaped passage or structure. 2. Tube connecting the frontal sinus with middle nasal meatus. 3. Stalk of pituitary gland. 4. Peritoneal end of fallopian tube. 5. Upper end of cochlear canal.

Infusion Liquid substance introduced into body vein.

Infusion pump A pump that aids in regulated infusion into artery or vein.

Ingestion Intake of food or the process by which cells take foreign particles.

Ingravescent Becoming more severe.

Ingredient Any unit or part of a complex compound or mixture.

Ingrowing Growing inward.

Ingrown nail Growth of nail edge deep into soft tissues causing pain and inflammation.

Inguinal Pertains to region of groin.

Inguinal canal The canal ½" long, providing passage for spermatic cord in the male and round ligament of uterus in the female. A potential source of weakness; may serve as site of inguinal hernia and undescended testis (see Figure on page 364).

Inguinal glands Lymph nodes of groin draining from lower limb and perineum.

Inguinal ligament *SYN*— Poupart's ligament. Fibrous band extending from anterior superior iliac spine to pubic tubercle.

Inguinal region The iliac region on either side of pubes.

Inguinal ring Interior and exterior openings of inguinal canal, termed as internal and external inguinal rings.

Inhalation The act of drawing in the breath, vapor or gas into the lungs.

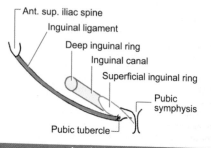

Inguinal canal

Inhalation therapy Administration of medicine, water vapor and gases (O_2, CO_2, NO_2).

Inhaler Device for administering medicines by inhalation.

Inherent Natural *SYN*—innate, intrinsic.

Inheritance Something hereditary, acquired through eggs and sperms.

Inhibin A testicular hormone that inhibits LH secretion by pituitary.

Inhibition 1. Restraint of a function. 2. In physiology slowing or stopping the function of an organ. *i. competitive* Inhibition by competing with cell receptors. *i. psychic* Arrest of an impulse, thought, action or speech.

Inhibitor That which inhibits.

Inhomogeneity Lack of uniform quality or consistency.

Iniencephalus Congenitally deformed fetus in which brain substance protrudes through a fissure in the occiput.

Inion External occipital protruberance.

Iniopagus Twins fused at the occiput.

Initials. Beginning or commencement.

Initis Inflammation of fibrous tissue.

Inject To introduce.

Injection Forcing a fluid into body via vessel or skin. *i. epidural* Injection of anesthetic agent into epidural - space. *i. hypodermic* Injection of substance beneath the skin. *i. alveolar* dental infiltration of anesthetic agent. *i. intramuscular* Injection directly into muscles, e.g., thigh, deltoid, glutei. *i. intra-articular*

Injection into joint space. *i. z. track* An injection technique, the needle taking a Z track to make the injected fluid difficult to track back (*see* Figure).

Injectors Instruments used for injection of fluids.

Injury Damage or trauma to some body part. *i. steering wheel* Automobile accidents where victims lung and heart are contused by pressure of steering wheel.

Inlay A solid filling made to the precise shape of a cavity of a tooth and cemented into it.

Innate Something natural, belonging from birth.

Innervation Nerve supply, distribution and function of nervous system. *i. collateral*

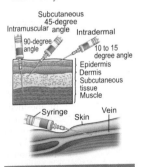

Subcutaneous
45-degree
Intramuscular angle   Intradermal
90-degree
angle   10 to 15
                    degree angle
                    Epidermis
                    Dermis
                    Subcutaneous
                    tissue
                    Muscle
Syringe   Skin   Vein

Intramuscular, subcutaneous, intradermal and intravenous injections

Outgrowth of nerves from adjacent nerves, once the original nerve supply is damaged. *i. reciprocal* An innervation mechanism by which if flexors are stimulated, the extensors are inhibited.

Innocent Harmless, benign, clinically unimportant.

Innocuous Harmless, benign, without serious effects.

Innominate artery The artery arising on right side from aortic arch and dividing into right subclavian and right common carotid.

Innominate Nameless.

Innominate bone The hip bone composed of ilium, ischium and pubis.

Innominate vein Formed by union of internal jugular and subclavian veins.

Inoculate To inject microorganism, serum or toxic materials into body.

Inoculation The process of being inoculated.

Inoculum Substance introduced by inoculation.

Inocyte Fibroblast.

Inogenesis Formation of fibrous tissue.

Inoperable Unsuitable for surgery.

Inopexia Tendency of blood to coagulate spontaneously.

Inorganic compound A chemical compound without carbon.

Inosemia An excessive amount of fibrin in the blood.

Inositis Inflammation of fibrous tissue.

Inositol A sugar like crystalline substance, a part of vitamin B complex group.

Inotropes An agent capable of altering the force or energy of muscular contractions inside the body of the living organism after administration.

Inotropic Augmenting force of muscular contraction.

Inpatient Hospitalized patient.

Inquest Investigation into circumstances, manner and cause of health.

Insalubrious Not healthy.

Insanitary Not conducive to health.

Insanity Severe mental derangement.

Insatiable Unable to be appeared or satisfied.

Inscription A prescription slip with name of the drug and its doses.

Insect bites and stings The venom of stinging insect, may be more toxic than that of poisonous snake but fortunately the quantity injected is small.

Insecta A class of phylum Arthropoda characterized by three distinct body divisions like head, thorax and abdomen, two pairs of wings and three pairs of jointed legs.

Insecticide An agent destructive to insects.

Insectifuge Insect repellant.

Insecurity Feeling of helplessness, apprehension.

Insemination Fertilization of ovum, semen discharge into vagina during coitus.

Insenescence Process of growing old.

Insensible Without feeling or perception.

Insertion 1. Placement or implanting of some thing into another. 2. Distal end of muscle attachment through which it moves a part.

Insidious Used to denote the onset of a disease so silently without patient's awareness.

Insight Self-understanding; absence of awareness.

Insipid Lacking in spirit, without taste.

In situ In position, localized, without invasion.

Insolation Heat stroke.

Insoluble Unable to be dissolved.

Insomnia Lack of sleep.

Inspect To examine visually.

Inspection Visual examination.

Inspersion Sprinkling with powder or a fluid.

Inspiration Indrawing of air into lungs.

Inspissate To thicken by evaporation or absorption of fluid.

Insterscapular reflex Scapular muscular contraction following percussion between the scapula.

Instillation Slowly pouring or dropping a liquid into body cavity.

Instinct The inherited tendency for the members of a specific species to react to certain environmental conditions and stimuli in a particular way.

Instruction Directions or command.

Instrumentation The use of instruments.

Insufficiency Inadequacy of function. *i. adrenal* Decreased adrenal function. *i. aortic* Imperfect closure of aortic leaflets with back flow. *i. cardiac* Poor cardiac pump function. *i. coronary* Diminished blood flow through coronary vessels. *i. hepatic* Hepatic insufficiency with cholemia. *i. mitral* Inefficient mitral valve closure with backflow of blood into left atrium during ventricular systole. *i. respiratory* Hypoxemia and hypercarbia due to poor pulmonary function.

Insufflate The act of blowing into or pumping air into a cavity/lung as in infants.

Insufflation Introduction of a gas or a powdered drug into a cavity.

Insula Triangular area of the cerebral cortex lying in the floor of the lateral fissure.

Insulator That which insulates.

Insulin Hormone secreted by the beta cells of islets of Langerhans of pancreas. *i. human* Synthesized by recombinant DNA technology using *E. coli. i. monocomponent* Highly purified insulin containing impurity 10 parts per million. *i. isophane (NPH)* Intermediate acting insulin with 18-28 hours of action.

Insulin lipodystrophy Atrophy or hypertrophy of skin fat at the insulin injection site.

Insulin pump A battery driven pump delivering insulin subcutaneously into abdominal wall according to preset program.

Insulin shock Hypoglycemic shock due to overdose of insulin.

Insulinase An enzyme that inactivates insulin.

Insulinemia Excess of blood insulin.

Insulinogenesis Production of insulin by the pancreas.

Insulinogenic Pertains to production of insulin.

Insulinoid Resembling or having properties of insulin.

Insulinoma Insulin producing tumor of pancreas.

Intake Things taken up like food and liquids.

Integration The bringing together of various parts or functions for harmonious working.

Integrator Device for measuring body surfaces.

Integument A covering, the skin.

Integumentary system The skin and its appendages.

Intellect The mind, conscious brain function.

Intelligence quotient A standard score that places an individual in reference to the scores of others within the same age group. This is determined through the subject's answers to arbitrary chosen questions.

Intelligence test A test designed to determine the intelligence of an individual.

Intelligence The ability to think, the capacity to comprehend.

Intemporance Lack of moderation, excess in use of anything.

Intensity The degree or extent of activity, strength, force.

Intensive Related to or marked by intensity.

Intensive care unit A special unit of hospital that provides constant monitoring and intensive care medicine to the patients with most serious diseases and injuries.

Intention Goal or purpose, a natural process of healing.

Intention tremor Occurrence of tremor on attempted coordinated movements.

Intercadence A supernumerary pulse wave between two regular beats.

Intercalated ducts Short narrow ducts that lie between secretory ducts and the terminal alveoli in the parotid and submandibular glands and in the pancreas.

Intercalated Inserted between.

Intercilium The space between the eyebrows.

Intercostal Between the ribs.

Intercostal muscles, external Outer layer of muscles between the ribs, originating from the lower margin of rib and inserted to the upper margin of next rib below; act to draw adjacent ribs together thereby increasing volume of thorax.

Intercostal muscles, internal Lie beneath external intercostal and function in the same way.

Intercourse Sexual union; social interaction between individuals or groups.

Intercurrent Intervening.

Interdent A specially designed knife used for removing interdental tissue.

Interdentium The space between contiguous teeth.

Interface In computers, a device that enables two normally noncompatible circuits or parts to function together.

Interference Clashing.

Interferon A protein formed by leucocytes and plasma cells in response to viral or other foreign nucleic acids, used in treatment of hepatitis B and C, hairy cell leukemia.

Interferon i Can be IFN-alfa, IFN-alfa 2b, IFN-beta, IFN-gamma and IFN-gamma 1b.

Intergemmal Between taste buds.

Interglobular spaces Gaps in dentin due to failure of calcification.

Intergluteal Between the two buttocks.

Interictal Between the two seizure attacks.

Interleukin I Substance from monocytes and macrophages responsible for acute phase response.

Interleukin II A lymphokine that stimulates growth of T-lymphocytes, often used in treatment of metastatic renal cancer.

Interleukin 15 variety of interleukins have been discovered, IL-3 stimulates haematopoitic and lymphoid stem cells, IL-4 regulates IgE and eosinophil mediated reactions, IL-5 stimulates growth and differentiation of eosinophils; IL-6 and IL-7 are differential factors for B-cells, IL-8 is a chemotactic and activator for neutrophils, IL-9 is a growth factor for T-cells, IL-10 inhibits cytokine production by T-cells, IL-11 stimulates megakaryocytes, IL-12 stimulates production of IFN- gamma, IL-13 inhibits inflammatory cytokine production, and IL-15 promotes NK-cell proliferation.

Intermarriage Marriage between persons of two distinct populations.

Intermediary Situated between two bodies; occurring between two periods of time.

Intermediary metabolism The series of intermediate products formed during process of digestion and excretion.

Intermedin A substance secreted by pituitary controlling pigmentation of skin in lower animals.

Intermenstrual Between menstrual periods.

Intermission Interval between two paroxysm of disease.

Intermittent Coming and going.

Intermittent fever Fever in which there is complete absence of symptoms between paroxysms.

Intermittent positive pressure breathing Assisted breathing in patients of respiratory failure, myasthenia gravis.

Intermural Between the walls or sides of an organ.

Internal bleeding Hemorrhage especially from G.I. tract.

Internal ear The cochlea, semicircular canals, vestibule.

Internal injury Any injury not visible from outside.

Internal secretion Secretion of ductless glands.

Internalization The unconscious mental mechanism in which the values and standards of society and one's parents are taken as one's own.

Internatal Between the buttocks.

International classification of diseases A classification code devised by WHO, helpful for international comparison.

International unit Internationally accepted amount of substances like vitamins, hormones, vaccines, etc.

Interneuron A neuron situated in between neurons.

Internist Physician specializing in internal medicine.

Internuncial Acting as a connecting medium.

Interocclusal Between the occlusal surfaces or cusps of opposite teeth.

Interoceptive Sensations arising within body itself, not those arising from outside the body.

Interoceptor A receptor activated by stimuli within the body.

Interoinferior Inward and downward position.

Interparietal Between the parietal bones; between the parietal lobes of cerebrum, between walls.

Interpersonal Concerning the relations and interactions between persons.

Interphase The resting stage of a cell between divisions.

Interpolation 1. In surgery transfer of tissue from one site to another. 2. In statistics the calculation of an intermediate value from the observed values.

Interposition The state of being interposed or inserted between.

Interpretation Analysis, significance.

Interradicular Between the roots of teeth.

Intersection Site where one structure crosses another or joins similar structure.

Intersex A person having both male and female sex characteristics but genetically either male or female.

Interspinal Between the two spinous processes of the spine.

Interstitial cells of testes Cells of leyding in seminiferous tubules producing testosterone.

Interstitial cystitis Idiopathic inflammation of bladder.

Interstitial fluid Fluid that surrounds cells.

Interstitial lung disease A large group of diseases, chronic non- infectious in nature that hamper oxygen transfer from alveoli to the capillaries.

Interstitial tissue Intercellular connective tissue.

Interstitium Space or gap in a structure or an organ.

Intertransverse Joining the transverse processes of vertebrae.

Intertriginous Having similarity with intertrigo.

Intertrigo Superficial dermatitis of the skin folds.

Intertrochanteric Between greater and lesser trachanter of femur.

Intertrochanteric line Ridge between greater and lesser trochanter of femur.

Intervaginal Between the sheaths.

Interval Space, time or period between two objects or happenings. *i. AV* Interval between beginning of atrial systole and ventricular systole. *i. cardio-arterial* Time between apex beat and radial pulse. *i. isometric* Time between onset of ventricular systole and opening of semilunar (aortic-pulmonary) valves. *i. lucid* Brief remission of symptoms in head injury and psychosis. *i. PR* Period between onset of P wave and beginning of QRS complex. Normalless than 0.2 sec. *i. QR* Period between onset of Q wave and peak of R wave. *i. QRS* - QRS duration from beginning of Q wave to end of S wave. Normal 0.12 sec. *i. QT* Interval between beginning of Q wave and end of T wave.

Intervention Taking appropriate action.

Intervertebral disc A broad and flat disk of fibrocartilage between the bodies of vertebra.

Intervillous Between the villi.

Intestinal bypass Surgical short circuiting of small intestine to produce controlled malabsorption to treat massive obesity.

Intestinal flora Bacteria present in intestine that synthesize vitamins.

Intestinal gas H_2, methane, CO_2, H_2S and methyl mercaptan produced in GI tract during digestive process.

Intestinal juice Secretion of small intestine containing a number of enzymes like maltase, lipase, peptidase, sucrase, etc.

Intestinal obstruction Blockage of intestinal lumen due to stricture, worms, fibrous band, foreign body, stone, fecolith, etc. producing absolute constipation, abdominal distension, dehydration and pain.

Intestinal perforation Soiling of peritoneal cavity with intestinal content; commonly a complication of enteric fever, tuberculosis or prolonged intestinal obstruction.

Intestinal putrefaction The putrefying effect of intestinal bacteria producing indole, skatole, paracresol, phenol, phenylpropionic acid, phenyl acetic acid, and gases.

Intestinal reflex Intestinal contraction and relaxation above the portion of bowel that is stimulated.

Intestinal tubes Plastic or rubber tubes placed in intestinal tract through nose or mouth to suck gas, fluids or solids.

Intestine The alimentary canal extending from pylorus to anus. The small intestine is 7 meter long and the large intestine 1.5 meter. Cecum is the beginning of large intestine and appendix (3-4" long) is attached to it. The duodenum is 8-10" long; jejunum 9 feet and ileum 14 feet. In the wall of the small intestine are Brunners glands, crypts of Lieberkuhn and Peyers's patches.

Intolerance Unable to bear pain, effects of a drug or other substance.

Intorsion Rotation of eye inward.

Intoxication State of being intoxicated with alcohol, drugs and chemicals.

Intra-aortic balloon counterpulsation Placement of an inflatable balloon in aortic root to lower/decrease systolic work of LV and to promote coronary blood flow; useful in treating shock. The balloon is inflated with helium during diastole and deflated during systole.

Intra-atrial Within the atrium.

Intracardiac Within the heart.

Intracisternal Within cistern of brain.

Intradural Enclosed by dura mater.

Intragastric balloon Placement of inflatable balloon in stomach to treat obesity.

Intralocular Within the cavity of any structure.

Intramedullary Within the medulla oblongata of brain; within bone marrow; within the spinal cord substance.

Intramural Within the walls of a hollow organ or cavity.

Intraosseous infusion Technique performed in the emergency treatment of a child in which blood, medications, or fluids are injected into the bone marrow rather than a vein (*see* Figure).

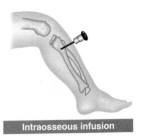

Intraosseous infusion

Intrapartum Occurring during childbirth.

Intraperitoneal Inside the peritoneal cavity.

Intrauterine Within the uterus.

Intrauterine contraceptive device Copper or other metallic device placed within uterus to prevent conception (*see* Figure on page 374).

Intrauterine growth retardation Occurs when the unborn baby is at or below the 10% of his/her gestational age (*see* Figure on page 374).

Intravasation Entry into blood vessels.

Intravenous Into a vein.

Intravenous infusion Injection of colloid or crystalloid solutions into a vein to treat hypovolemia, or maintenance.

Intravenous infusion pump A device to provide constant but adjustable rate of flow of IV solutions.

Intravesical Within urinary bladder.

Intravitreous Within the vitreous of eye.

Intrinsic Belonging to or embedded in, essential nature of a thing.

Intrinsic factor Substance present in the gastric juice that facilitates absorption of vit B_{12}.

Intrinsic muscles Muscles having their origin and insertion

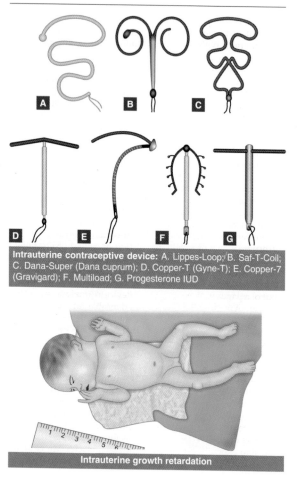

Intrauterine contraceptive device: A. Lippes-Loop; B. Saf-T-Coil; C. Dana-Super (Dana cuprum); D. Copper-T (Gyne-T); E. Copper-7 (Gravigard); F. Multiload; G. Progesterone IUD

Intrauterine growth retardation

entirely within a structure, e.g., intrinsic muscles of eye, tongue and larynx.

Introducer Device for controlling, directing and placing intubation tube within trachea, blood vessels or heart.

Introitus Entrance into a canal or cavity.

Introjection In psychoanalysis, identification of self with another, the victim assuming the supposed feelings of the other personality.

Intromission An insertion or placing of one part into another.

Introns The noncoding region between the coding regions (exons) of the DNA in gene.

Introspection Looking within one's mind.

Introversion Preoccupation with one's self; turning inside out of a part.

Introvert A personality characterized by withdrawal from reality, fantasy formation, as in schizophrenia.

Intubation To insert a tube, e.g. into larynx.

Intuition Knowing something spontaneously in advance.

Intumescence Swelling-up or enlarging.

Intussusception Invagination; slipping of one part of intestine into another part below (*see* Figure).

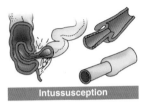

Intussusception

Intussusceptum The inner segment of intestine in intussusception.

Intussuscipiens That portion of intestine that receives the intussusceptum.

Inuction Ointment rubbed into skin for medicinal effect.

Inulase Enzyme that converts inulin to levulose.

Inulin A polysaccharide found in plants yielding levulose on hydrolysis. Used in study of renal function (GFR).

In utero Within uterus.

Invaginate To insert one part of a structure within a part of same structure; to ensheath.

Invalid A sick person confined to bed or wheelchair.

Invasion Entrance of microorganisms into body and their distribution into tissues.

Invasive Tending to spread, e.g. malignant growth.

Invasive procedure Procedure in which the body cavity is entered that could interfere with bodily function.

Inverse square law Law stating that the intensity of radiation or light at any distance is inversely proportional to the square of the distance between the irradiated surface and a point source.

Inversion Reversal of normal relationship; turning inside out. *i. uterine* Uterus is turned inside out with internal surface protruding at vagina, a serious complication of placental delivery and causes of post-partum bleeding.

Invert sugar A mixture of levulose and dextrose, formed by inversion of sucrose by the enzyme invertase.

Invertase A sugar-splitting enzyme found in GI tract.

Invertebrate Those species without a backbone.

Investment A covering or sheath.

Inveterate Chronic, firmly seated habit.

In vitro Outside the living body, e.g. tests done in laboratory involving isolated tissue or cell preparation.

In vivo Within the living body or organism.

Involucrum The covering of newly formed bone enveloping the sequestrum in infected bone.

Involuntary Independent, not depending upon volition.

Involution Turning inward, reduction in size of uterus following delivery, the retrogressive change in vital processes after their functions have been fulfilled.

Involutional melancholia Depression visiting men and women between 50-65 years and 40-55 years of age.

Iodameba A genus of ameba seen in GI tract.

Iodide A compound of iodine, e.g. pot iodide.

Iodine A nonmetallic halogen giving violet vapour on melting. Total body content is 50 mg, one-third of it being present in thyroid. Daily requirement is 100-150 µg. *i. protein bound* That iodine bound to plasma protein. *i. radioactive* Isotopes of iodine ^{131}I or ^{125}I, used for thyroid uptake studies, hepatic studies or in treatment of hyperthyroidism and thyroid cancer.

Iodine tincture Preparation of iodine in alcohol and water.

Iodipamide meglumine Agent used for gallbladder X-ray.

Iodism Condition resulting from excess and prolonged use of iodine.

Iodized salt Salt containing 100 mg of sodium or potassium iodide per gram.

Iododerma Dermatitis due to iodine.

Iodoform A compound formed by action of iodine on acetone in the presence of an alkali. Used topically for mild antibacterial action.

Iodohippurate sodium A radio-active dye used in renal studies.

Iodophilia Unusual pronounced affinity of polymorphs for iodine in some infections and anemia.

Iodophor Iodine in a solubilizing agent, e.g., povidone iodine.

Iodoquinol Antiamebic agent, can cause subacute myelooptic neuropathy.

Iodotherapy Use of iodine medication.

Ion A particle carrying an electric charge. Ions carrying positive charge aggregate near cathode and those with negative charge near anode.

Ion exchange resins Resins that bind to some ions, e.g., cholestyramine.

Ionium A natural radioactive ion of thorium.

Ionization Dissociation of acids, bases and salts into their constituent ions.

Ionometer A device to measure amount of radiation and intensity of rays.

Iontophoresis Introduction of various ions into the skin by means of electricity.

Iopanoic acid Radio-opaque dye used for gallbladder studies.

Iophendylate Radio-opaque dye used in myelography.

Iothalamate meglumine Radioopaque material for angiography.

Ipatropium bromide An anticholinergic given by inhalation in bronchial asthma.

Ipecac Dried roots of plant ipecacuanha, source of emetine.

Ipodate calcium Radioopaque material for X-ray studies of gallbladder.

Iproniazid Antitubercular drugs.

Ipsilateral On the same side.

Iridalgia Pain in the iris.

Iridauxesis Increase in thickness of iris as in glaucoma.

Iridectome Instrument for cutting iris in iridectomy.

Iridectomy Surgical removal of a portion of iris as in glaucoma, corneal scar.

Irideremia Partial or total congenital absence of iris.

Irides Pleural of iris.

Iridium A white hard metallic element.

Iridoavulsion Tearing away of iris.

Irido capsulitis Inflammation of iris and capsule of lens.

Iridocele Protrusion of a portion of iris through a defect in cornea.

Iridocoloboma Congenital defect or fissure in iris.

Iridocyclectomy Surgical removal of iris and ciliary body.

Iridodialysis Separation of outer margin of iris from its ciliary attachment.

Iridodonesis Tremulousness of iris seen in aphakic eye or subluxated lens.

Iridokinesis Contraction and expansion movement of iris.

Iridorrhexis Rupture of or tearing of the iris from its attachment.

Iridotasis Stretching of the iris in the treatment of glaucoma.

Iridotomy Incision of iris for making a new aperture.

Iris The organ between lens and cornea. *i. bombe* Bulging of iris forwards with annular posterior synechia (*see* Figure).

Iritis Inflammation of the iris, with photophobia, lacrimation, irregular pupil, dull-muddy looking iris. *i. plastic* Iritis with fibrinous exudate.

Iron A metallic element existing as Ferrous (Fe^{++}) and Ferric (Fe^{+++}) forms, essential part of hemoglobin

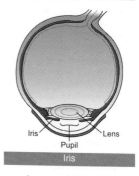

Iris   Lens

Pupil

Iris

and myoglobin. Adult requirement of iron is 0.5-1 mg per day; manganese, copper and cobalt are necessary for proper utilization of iron.

Iron-dextran Injectable form of iron.

Iron storage disease Hemo-chro-matosis.

Irradiation Therapeutic application of X-ray, radium as in malignancy.

Irrational Contrary to what is reasonable or logical.

Irreducible Not capable of being reduced or made smaller.

Irrelevance Unrelated to, in appropriate.

Irreversible Impossible to reverse.

Irrigation Cleansing with fluids.

Irrigator Device used to flush or irrigate.

Irritability Excitability; impatience.

Irritations Reaction to what is irritating.

Ischemia Lack of blood supply.

Ischiocavernosus An erectile muscle extending from ischium to penis or clitoris.

Ischiococcygeus Coccygeus muscle forming posterior portion of levator ani.

Ischiorectal abscess Collection of pus in ischiorectal fossa.

Ischiorectal fossa Pararectal fat filled fossa bounded laterally by obturator internus and ischial tuberosity, posteriorly by gluteus maximus and medially by levator ani.

Island A structure detached from surrounding structures or a tiny, isolated mass of one kind of cells within another type.

Ismelin Guanethidine sulphate.

Isoagglutination Agglutination of red blood cells by agglutinin from blood of another person.

Isoagglutinin Antibody in the serum that agglutinates RBC of same species.

Isoantigen A substance present in certain individuals that stimulates production of antibody in other members SYN—alloantigen.

Isobucaine hydrochloride A local anesthetic agent.

Isochromatic Having the same color.

Isochromosomes A chromosome with arms that are morphologically identical and contain the same genetic loci.

Isochronal Taking place at regular intervals or in uniform time.

Isochronia The correspondence of events with respect to time, rate or frequency.

Isocoria Equality in size of both pupils.

Isocytosis Cells of equal size.

Isodontic Having teeth of equal size.

Isoelectric Having equal electric potentials.

Isoelectric period The time or point when no electric energy is produced.

Isoenzyme A form of an enzyme.

Isoetharine hydrochloride A sympathomimetic agent, used as bronchodilator.

Isoflurophate An anticholinesterage drug used to treat glaucoma and atony of intestinal and vesical smooth muscles.

Isogamete A cell which on fusion with a similar cell reproduces.

Isogamy Reproduction resulting from conjugation of isogametes or identical cells.

Isohemaglutin Blood group antibody normally present in blood that causes clumping of incompatible blood.

Isoimmunization Immunization of an individual against the blood of another individual of same species.

Isolation Limitation of movement and social contact of patients suffering from or a known carrier of communicable disease.

Isoleucine An essential amino acid.

Isomer Substances having same molecular formula but different chemical and physical properties, e.g. dextrose is an isomer of levulose.

Isomerase Any enzyme that catalyzes isomerization of its substrate.

Isomerism Compounds with equal number of atoms but with different atomic arrangements.

Isomerization Conversion of a substance to its isomer.

Isometric contraction Contraction without change in muscle length i.e., tension development without any mechanical work.

Isoniazid Antitubercular agent, bacteriocidal, can cause peripheral neuritis.

Iso-osmotic Having the same total concentration of osmotically active molecules.

Isophoria Equal tension of vertical muscles of each eye with visual lines in the same horizontal plane.

Isoprenaline Beta-adrenergic agonist.

Isopropamide iodide A synthetic antimuscarinic drug with actions similar to belladona.

Isopropyl alcohol C_3H_8O, an alcohol used in medical preparations for external use, antifreeze, cosmetics, and as a solvent.

Isoproterenol A sympathomimetic, used in bronchial asthma.

Isosexual Concerning or characteristic of same sex.

Isosorbide dinitrate Antianginal drug.

Isospora A genus of sporozoa, e.g. *I-Hominis*, a nonpathogenic protozoa inhabiting small intestine.

Isosthenuria Passage of urine having constant specific gravity; a sign of advanced renal disease.

Isotherapy Treatment of a disease by the same causative agent.

Isotonic Having same osmotic pressure.

Isotonic exercise Contraction of a muscle during which the force of resistance to the movement remains constant throughout the range of motion.

Isotonic solution A solution with osmotic pressure same as that of another solution with which it is compared.

Isotope Elements with nearly identical chemical properties but different atomic weights and electric charges.

Isotretionin A retinoid used in acne.

Isotropic Possessing similar qualities in every direction; having equal refraction.

Isoxsuprine hydrochloride A vasodilator and smooth muscle relaxant.

Isradipine A calcium channel blocking agent, antihypertensive.

Issue Offspring.

Isthmoplegia Paralysis of fauces.

Isthmus A narrow passage connecting two cavities, a narrow structure connecting two larger parts, a constriction between two larger parts.

Isuprel hydrochloride Isoproterenol hydrochloride.

Itch Irritation of skin inducing desire to scratch. *i. barber's* Fungus infection of beard area. *i. dhobie* Fungus infection of groin and perineum. *i. ground* Itching in feet due to penetration by hookworm larva. *i. swimmer's* Dermatitis due to swimming in water containing larvae form of schistosomes.

Itraconazole Antifungal agent.

Ivy method A method for estimation of bleeding time

Ivy poisoning Poison ivy dermatitis.

Ixodes A genus of ticks.

J

Jacket A bandage usually applied to the trunk to immobilize the spine or correct deformities. *J. Minerva* a plaster of Paris jacket used for fracture cervical spine. *j. porcelain* Crown restoration with procelain. *j. Sayre's* Plaster of Paris jacket to support spinal deformity.

Jackscrew A threaded screw used for expanding the dental arch.

Jacksonian epilepsy Focal epilepsy with spasm confined to a group of muscles.

Jackson's syndrome Unilateral muscular and structural paralysis which are innervated by tenth, eleventh, and twelfth cranial nerves.

Jacobson Danish anatomist. *j's cartilage* Cartilage lying along anterior inferior border of nasal septum. *j's nerve* Tympanic nerve.

Jacquemier's sign Blue or purple color of vagina in early pregnancy.

Jactitation Restless to and fro movement of body.

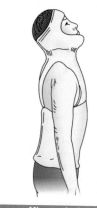

Minerva jacket

Jaegers test types A reading test type for near vision.

Jamais vu Feeling of being placed in a strange environment or unfamiliarity; a feature of temporal lobe epilepsy.

James fiber Preexcitation of ventricles by fibers connecting atria to ventricle or distal. His bundle, bypassing AV node.

Janeway lesion Small painless red blue macular lesions in palms and soles in bacterial endocarditis.

Jargon Speech or writing that includes unfamiliar terms or abbreviations.

Jarvi's snare Snare for removing growth in nasal cavity.

Jaundice Yellow coloration of skin, conjunctiva and mucous membranes due to hyperbilirubinemia. *j. acholuric* Jaundice with clear urine i.e., unconjugated hyperbilirubinemia of hemolysis. *j. cholestatic* Conjugated hyperbilirubinemia due to stasis of bile excretion, either intrahepatic or extrahepatic. *j. hemolytic* Jaundice due to hemolysis. *j. hepatocellular* Jaundice due to hepatitis. *j. obstructive* Conjugated hyperbilirubinemia with itching due to bile duct stricture, compression or luminal obstruction.

Jaw Maxilla and mandible bearing teeth and forming the framework of mouth. *j. cleft* Lack of fusion of the right and left mandible into a single bone. *j. crackling* Noise of normal or diseased temperomandibular joint during movement of jaw. *j. dislocation* The jaw is pushed downward and forward,

occurring due to trauma, following yawning, hearty laugh or chewing large chunks of food. *j. winking* Voluntary movement of lower face causing unilateral contraction of orbicularis oculi, seen during the process of recovery from Bell's palsy.

Jejunitis Inflammation of jejunum.

Jejunocolostomy Anastomosis of colon with jejunum.

Jejunoileitis Inflammation of jejunum and ileum as in Crohn's disease.

Jejunorrhaphy Surgical repair of jejunum.

Jejunostomy Making a surgical opening into jejunum.

Jejunotomy Making surgical incision into jejunum.

Jejunum The second portion of small intestine next to duodenum, about 8 feet in length, making about 2/5 of small intestine.

Jelly A thick semisolid gelatinous substance. *j. Wharton's* Soft gelatinous connective tissue that constitutes the matrix of umbilical cord.

Jendrassik's maneuver Facilitation of deep tendon reflexes of lower extremity by hooking the fingers of both hands by the patient and trying to pull them apart.

Jenner, Edward British physician who invented cowpox vaccine for immunization against smallpox.

Jenner's stain Eosin methylene blue stain.

Jerk Sudden muscular movement, often as a reflex from tapping of the tendon. *j. ankle* Contraction of soleus-gastrocnemius by tapping tendoachiles. *j. biceps* Contraction of biceps following tapping of biceps tendon at elbow. *j. jerk* Tapping of mandible when jaw is half open. Vigorous mouth closure indicates bilateral supranuclear cerebral lesions. *j. knee* Striking the patellar tendon causes contraction of quadriceps with extension of knee.

Jessner's solution Combination of resorcinol, lactic acid, and salicylic acid that acts as a peeling agent.

Jogger's heel Irritation of fibrofatty tissue of heel in joggers.

Joint An articulation, between two bones. Joints are grouped according to motion: ball and socket (enarthrosis), hinge (ginglymus); condyloid, pivot (trochoid), gliding (arthrodial) and saddle joint. Joints can move in four ways 1. gliding, in which one bony surface glides on another without angular or rotatory movement. 2. angular 3. circumduction and 4. rotation. Angular movement when occurs forwards or backwards is called flexion and extension and away from the body abduction and towards median plain of body adduction. *j. ball and socket* Rounded end of one bone fits into cavity of another. *j. Charcot's* Denervated joint with increased range of movement as in syringomyelia and tabes dorsalis. *j. condyloid* Joint permitting all forms of angular movements except axial rotation. *j. hinge* Joint having only forward and backward motion. *j. pivot* Joint permitting rotation. *j. saddle* Joint in which the opposing surfaces are reciprocally concavoconvex.

Joint capsule The sac like covering enclosing the articulating ends of bones in a diarthrodial joint. It consists of an outer fibrous layer and inner synovial layer.

Jones criteria USA physician who devised the major and minor criteria for diagnosis of acute rheumatic fever. The major criteria include 1. fleeting polyarthritis 2. chorea, 3. erythema marginatum and 4. subcutaneous nodules.

Joule Work done in one second by current of one ampere against a resistance of one ohm.

Jugular Pertains to throat.

Jugular foramen Opening formed by jugular notches of the occipital and temporal bones.

Jugular ganglion Nodes of vagus root and glossopharyngeal nerve in jugular foramen.

Jugular process Projection of occipital bone towards the temporal bone.

Jugular vein 1. *External* lies superficial to sternocleido mastoid and joins subclavian vein. 2. *Internal* is direct continuation of transverse sinus and joins subclavian vein to form innominate vein. The vein is more prominent during expiration. The height of pulsating blood column in internal jugular gives an indication of right atrial pressure.

Junction The place of union of two parts.

Jurisprudence The scientific study or application of the principles of law and justice. *j. medical* The application of the principles of law as they relate to the practice of medicine.

Jury-mast Apparatus for support of head in diseases of spine.

Juster's reflex Finger extension instead of flexion when palm of the hand is irritated.

Juvenile Youth or childhood.

Juxta Close proximity.

Juxtaglomerular apparatus The myoepithelioid cell structure cuffing afferent renal arteriole concerned with production of renin.

Juxtaglomerular cells Myoepithelioid cells resembling those of carotid body in juxtaglomerular apparatus.

Juxtangina Inflamed condition of pharyngeal muscles.

Juxtaposition Positioned side by side.

K

Kader's operation Surgical formation of gastric fistula with the feeding tube inserted through a valve like flap.

Kakidrosis Unpleasant odor of the sweat.

Kakosmia Perception of bad odor that does not exist.

Kakotrophy Malnutrition.

Kala-azar Protozoal tropical disease caused by *Leishmania donovani* manifesting with fever, lymphadenopathy and hepatosplenomegaly with darkening of skin.

Kalimeter Device for determining alkalinity of a substance.

Kalium A mineral (potassium).

Kaliuresis Excretion of potassium in urine.

Kallikrein An enzyme, when activated is a potent vasodilator.

Kanamycin Aminoglycoside antibiotic, used in tuberculosis.

Kanner syndrome Infantile autism.

Kaolin Clay powder containing hydrated aluminium silicate used as adsorbent in diarrhea.

Kaolinosis Pneumoconiosis caused by inhalation of kaolin particles.

Kaposi Hungarian physician.

Kaposi's disease Xeroderma pigmentosum.

Kaposi sarcoma AIDS associated sarcoma of skin.

Kaposi's varicelliform eruption Herpes or vaccinia infection in presence of pre-existing eczema.

Karaya gum Plant product, used as adhesive and bulk laxative.

Karman catheter Catheter used in performing suction curettage of uterus.

Karnofsky's index A tool used in studying chronic illnesses and cancers to clinically estimate the physical state, performance, and prognosis of a patient after a therapeutic procedure.

Kartagener's syndrome Hereditary syndrome consisting of bronchiectasis, sinusitis and transposition of viscera.

Karyocyte Nucleated red blood cell, normoblast.

Karyolysis Destruction of cell nucleus.

Karyopyknosis Shrinkage of nucleus of a cell with condensation of chromatin.

Karyorrhexis Fragmentation of chromatin in nuclear lysis.

Karyosome Irregular clumps of nondividing chromatin in cell nucleus.

Karyotype A photomicrograph of a single cell in the metaphase to show chromosomes in descending order of size (*see* Figure).

Kasabach-Merritt syndrome Capillary hemangioma associated with thrombocytopenic purpura.

Kata (Cata) Prefix meaning down, wrongly, back, against.

Kawasaki disease Mucocutaneous lymphnode syndrome;

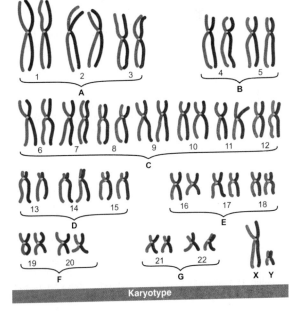

Karyotype

children are the prime victims and run a risk of coronary arteritis with infarction.

Kayser-Fleischer ring The green-ring around the cornea due to deposition of copper in Descemet's membrane in Wilson's disease.

Kegel exercise An exercise for strengthening the pubococcygeal levator ani muscles in control of urinary and fecal incontinence.

Keith-Wagener-Barker classification A classification of hypertensive changes of retina. Grade I-moderate narrowing of retinal arterioles Grade II-retinal hemorrhages Grade III-cotton wool exudates and grade IV-papilledema.

Kell blood group One of the human blood groups, composed of three forms of antigens.

Keloid Hypertrophied, raised, firm, thick scar following trauma or surgical incision.

Kelvin scale Temperature scale in which absolute zero is equal to minus 273° on Celsius scale.

Kemadrin Procyclidine hydrochloride, used in Parkinsonism for anticholinergic effect.

Kenalog Triamcinolone hydrochloride.

Kenny treatment Physical therapy for treating poliomyelitis consisting of application of hot moist packs, early muscle education.

Kenophobia Fear of empty spaces.

Kent's bundle Accessory conduction pathway joining atria with ventricles as in WPW syndrome.

Kerasin A cerebroside.

Keratectomy Excision of a portion of cornea.

Keratin A tough protein substance in hair, nail, horny tissue, produced by keratinocytes.

Keratinization The process of keratin formation within keratinocytes and its progress upward through the layers of epidermis to the surface stratum corneum.

Keratinocyte Cell synthesizing keratin.

Keratitic precipitates Inflammatory cells in anterior chamber that stick to inner endothelial surface of cornea.

Keratitis Inflammation of cornea.

Keratoacanthoma A papular keratin filled lesion resembling squamous cell carcinoma but subsiding spontaneously.

Keratocele Herniation or protrusion of Descemet's membrane through a weakened or absent corneal stroma as a result of corneal ulcer or corneal trauma.

Kerato-conjunctivitis Inflammation of cornea and conjunctiva.

Keratoconus Conical protrusion of center of cornea without inflammation (*see* Figure).

Keratoderma blenorrhagica Prominent hyperkeratotic scaling lesions of palms, soles associated with Reiter's syndrome.

Keratodermia Hypertrophy of stratum corneum of palms and soles of feet.

Keratoiritis Inflammation of cornea and iris.

Keratoma A callosity, a horny growth.

Keratomalacia Softening of cornea as in childhood vit A deficiency.

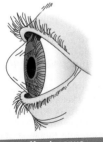

Keratoconus

Keratometer An instrument for measuring curvature of cornea.

Keratometry Measurements of cornea.

Keratomileusis Plastic surgery of cornea in which a portion of cornea is removed, frozen, its curvature is reshaped and then reattached in its place.

Keratonosis Any noninflammatory disease or deformity of horny layer of skin.

Keratonyxis Surgical puncture of cornea.

Keratopathy band Calcium deposit in superficial layer of cornea and Bowman's capsule, occurring in hypercalcemia or chronic intraocular inflammation.

Keratoplasty Plastic surgery of cornea. *k. optic* Replacement of corneal scar with healthy donor corneal tissue. *k. refractive* Treatment of myopia or hypermetropia by reshaping corneal curvature either by multiple incision or as in keratomileusis.

Keratoprotein The protein of hair, nail and epidermis.

Keratorrhexis Rupture of cornea.

Keratoscope Instrument for examination of cornea.

Keratosis Any condition of skin with excessive horny

growth. *k. actinic* A horny keratotic premalignant lesion due to prolonged exposure to sunlight. *k. follicularis SYN* – Darier's disease, characterized by verrucous papular growths that colaesce into plaques affecting face, neck, axillae and scalp. *k. pilaris* Chronic inflammation of unknown etiology involving hair follicle.

Keratotome A knife for corneal incision.

Keratotomy Incision of cornea. *k. radial* Very shallow, bloodless, hairline incisions are made in outer portion of cornea thereby allowing it to flatten; a treatment modality for axial myopia up to 5 diopters (*see* Figure).

Keraunophobia Morbid fear of thundering and lightening.

Kerion A lesion secondary to tinea capitis.

Kerley lines Thickening of inter alveolar septa due to pulmonary edema. See—lines kerley.

Kernicterus Bilirubin infiltration of basal ganglia and other areas of brain and spinal cord occurring in erythroblastosis fetalis of newborns when unconjugated hyperbilirubinemia touches 25 mg% or above.

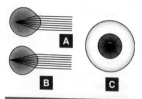

Radial keratotomy. (A) Presurgery, the myopic eye focusing in front of the retina, (B) postsurgery, the corneal flattening causing the light to focus on the retina, (C) anterior view of the eye, showing the lines of incision

Kernig's sign Reflex spasm and pain in hamstrings when attempting to extend the knee after flexion of hip; a sign of meningitis.

Kerosene A flammable liquid fuel distilled from petroleum. Fumes of it can cause pneumonitis.

Ketamine A nonbarbiturate analgesic-hypnotic substance used IM/IV.

Ketanserine 5 HT antagonist.

Keto acid Any organic acid containing ketone (CO) radical.

Ketoacidosis Acidosis due to excess of ketone bodies.

Keto aciduria Presence of ketoacids in urine.

Ketoconazole Systemic antifungal agent.

Ketogenic diet Diet insufficient in calories to produce mild ketosis helpful in some cases of childhood epilepsy.

Ketohexose A nonsaccharide consisting of a six-carbon chain and containing a ketone group in addition to alcohol group (e.g., fructose).

Ketone A substance containing carbonyl group (C=O) attached to two carbon atoms. e.g., acetone. The ketones are end-products of fat metabolism.

Ketone bodies A group of compounds produced during oxidation of fatty acids and include acetone, beta hydroxy butyric acid and acetoacetic acid.

Ketonemia Presence of ketone bodies in blood in excess quantity.

Ketone threshold Level of ketones in blood above which they appear in urine.

Ketonuria Presence of ketone bodies in urine.

Ketoprofen NSAID group of drug.

Ketorolac Non-opioid analgesic.

Ketotifea Mast cell stabilize to.

Ketose A carbohydrate containing the ketones.

Ketosis The accumulation in the body of the ketones causing acidosis commonly occurring in starvation, high fat diet, pregnancy, uncontrolled diabetes mellitus, following ether anesthesia. They impart a fruity odor to the breath.

17 ketosteroid One of a group of neutral steroids having a ketone group in 17th position, principally produced by adrenal cortex and gonads. They are androsterone, dehydroisoandrosterone, corticosterone, compound E, 11 hydroxy isoandrosterone.

Ketotifen Mast cell stabilizer used in asthma.

Kidney Paired retroperitoneal structures, one on each side of spinal column, wt - 4-6 OZ, size 4" long, 2-3" broad. The kidneys in the newborn are about 3 times as large in proportion to body weight as in the adult. The outer cortex contains the glomeruli, 1 million in number. The inner medulla contains the pyramids 8-18 in number made-up of collecting tubules being penetrated by cortical substance. Known as columns of Bellini; kidneys are instrumental to the formation of urine in which in 95% water and 5% solids (urea, uric acid, cretinine, hippuric acid, sodium and potassium); conversion of vit D into active form and secretion of renin and erythropoietin. *k. artificial* Haemodialysis device that removes wastes like that of kidney. *k. contracted* The small kidneys characteristic of chronic glomerulonephritis or interstitial nephritis. *k. fatty* Kidney with fatty infiltration causing degeneration of renal substance. *k. flee bitten* Arteriosclerotic kidney. *k. floating* Displaceable and movable kidney due to weak fascial support. *k. granular* Kidney of chronic nephritis where it is small, and of fibrous hard granular texture. *k. horse shoe* Congenital malformation where the upper or lower poles of both kidneys united by a fibrous isthmus. *k. polycystic* Kidney with multiple cysts, congenital in origin, can be adult onset type or infantile type. *k. sacculated* A condition in which renal parenchyma is absorbed leaving behind the distended capsule. *k. sponge* Multiple small cysts in the renal parenchyma. *k. wandering* Hypermobile kidney (*see* Figure on page 392).

Kidney failure Diminished function of the kidneys. This may be acute and temporary or may progress to complete loss of renal function.

Kidney stone Calculus present in renal parenchyma, calyx or renal pelvis, composed principally of calcium, urate, oxalate, phosphates and carbonates, ranging from small granular masses to 5 cm or more in diameter. Most common in patients of hyperparathyroidism, oxaluria, gout and chronic pyelonephritis.

Kiesselbach's plexus A rich network of capillaries on the anteroinferior part of nasal septum; the most common site of bleeding in epistaxis.

Kilocycle One thousand cycles as in electricity.

Kilogram One thousand gram.

Kilohertz One thousand cycles as in electricity.

Kilometer 1000 meters, 3281 feet or 0.61 mile.

Kilowatt A unit of electrical energy equivalent to 1000 watts.

Kimmelstiel-Wilson syndrome Nodular glomerulosclerosis in longstanding diabetes mellitus with hypertension, edema, retinal lesions, and proteinuria.

Kinanesthesia Inability to perceive extent of movement or direction resulting in ataxia.

Kinase An enzyme that catalyzes the transfer of phosphate from ATP to an acceptor.

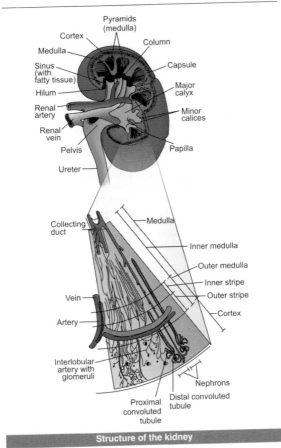

Structure of the kidney

Kinematograph Device for viewing photographs of objects in motion.

Kineplasty A form of amputation enabling the muscles of stump to impart motion to artificial limb.

Kinescope Device for conducting refraction of eye.

Kinesiatrics Treatment involving active and passive movements.

Kinesics Systematic study of the body and use of its static and dynamic position as a means of communication.

Kinesiology The study of muscles and body movement.

Kinesthesia Ability to perceive extent, direction and weight of movement.

Kinetic Pertaining to or consisting of motion.

Kinetosis Any disorder caused by motion, such as sea sickness.

Kinin A general term for a group of polypeptides capable of causing smooth muscle contraction, hypotension, hyperpermeability of capillaris and pain.

Kininogen Precursor of kinin.

Kinky hair disease Congenital autosomal recessive syndrome consisting of short, sparse kinky hair, poor physical and mental development, associated with degenerative changes of cerebral gray matter.

Kinomometer Device for measuring degree of motion in a joint.

Kinship The descendants from a common ancestor.

Kiotome Device for amputation of uvula.

Kisch's reflex Closure of an eye from stimulation of auditory meatus.

Kite apparatus Apparatus for reeducation of weak muscles and prevention of contractures around forearm, wrist and fingers.

Klebsiella Short mump gram-negative bacilli, encapsulated, nonspore forming frequently causing respiratory infection. *k. pneumoniae* A species causing pneumonia. *k. rhinoscleromatis* Species causing rhinoscleroma, a destructive granuloma of nose and pharynx.

Klepto To steal.

Kleptolagnia Sexual gratification obtained from stealing.

Kleptomania Impulsive stealing, the motive not being for substantial gain, stolen without prior planning or assistance from others. Stealing provides gratification and mental relaxation.

Kleptomaniac A psychopathic personality suffering from impulsive stealing.

Kleptophobia Morbid fear of stealing.

Klieg eye Conjunctivitis, lacrimation and photophobia from exposure to intense lights as used in making television, film shooting.

Klinefelter's syndrome XXY chromosomal disorder of male manifesting with gynecomastia, tall height, subnormal intelligence, small firm testes (*see* Figure).

Klippel's disease Pseudoparalysis due to generalized arthritis.

Klippel-Feil syndrome Congenital anomaly characterized by short wide neck, low hair line, reduction in number of cervical vertebra often with features of upper cervical myelopathy.

Klumpke's paralysis Atrophic paralysis of forearm usually due to birth trauma with stretching, avulsion of brachial plexus.

Kluver-Bucy syndrome Behavioral syndrome usually following bilateral temporal lobectomy, manifesting with hypersexuality, rage, memory deficit, hyperreligiosity, hyperphagia, failure of visual recognition, etc.

Knapp's forceps Forceps with roller like blades for expressing trachomatous granulations on the palpebral conjunctiva.

Kneading A form of massage consisting of grasping, wringing, lifting, rolling, pressing.

Knee Femerotibial articulation covered anteriorly with patella. *k. internal derangement* Pertains to a knee with injury to collateral/cruciate ligaments, the menisci, fracture of tibial spine. *k. housemaid* Bursitis of bursa anterior to patella due to prolonged

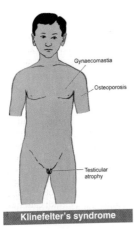

Gynaecomastia

Osteoporosis

Testicular atrophy

Klinefelter's syndrome

kneeling. *k. knock* Outward bending of legs allowing the knees to touch each other *SYN* – genu valgum. *k. locked* Inability to extend the leg due to torn semilunar cartilage.

Knee cap Patella.

Knee chest position Position in which patient is on knees with thighs straight, head and upper part of chest resting on table and arms crossed in front of head. Employed for sigmoidoscopic examination of colon and rectum, repositioning of retroverted uterus or displaced ovary.

Knee jerk reflex Contraction of quadriceps on tapping ligamentum patellae, while the leg hangs loosely with knee at right angle. The reflex arc is via L_3, L_4 Pyramidal tract lesions exaggerate knee jerk and it is absent in lesions of peripheral nerves and anterior horn cells of involved spinal segments.

Knemometry A precise method of determining the length of a limb.

Knob A mass or nodule.

Knot 1. In surgery, the intertwining of the ends of a suture, ligature, bandage so that the ends will not slip or get loose. 2. An intertwining of a cord or cord like structure to form a knob or lump.

Knuckle Prominence of the dorsal aspect of any of the phallangeal joints.

Kocher's reflex Contraction of abdominal muscles following moderate compression of testicle.

Koebner phenomenon Appearance of skin lesion as a result of nonspecific trauma.

Kohler's disease Aseptic necrosis of navicular bone of wrist.

Koilocyte An abnormal cell of squamous epithelium of the cervix, a forerunner of cervical intraepithelial neoplasia.

Koilonychia Dystrophy of finger nails, thinning spooning as in iron deficiency anemia.

Koniology Science of dust and its effect.

Koniometer Device for estimating amount of dust in air.

Koplik's spots Small red spots with blue white centers on the oral mucosa opposite the molars, a diagnostic sign of measles.

Korotkoff's sounds Sounds heard in auscultation of blood pressure.

Korsakoff's syndrome Personality characterized by psychosis, polyneuritis, disorientation, delirium, confabulation, a feature of chronic alcoholism.

Krabbe's disease Globoid cell leukodystrophy due to collection of galactocerebrocides in the tissues. Clinically manifesting with seizure, deafness, blindness, and mental retardation.

Kraurosis Atrophy and dryness of skin and mucous membrane—esp. of vulva, malignant degeneration may occur.

Krause's glands Accessory lacrimal glands opening into fornix of eye.

Krause's valves Fold of mucous membrane of the lacrimal sac at the junction of lacrimal duct.

Krause's end bulbs Encapsulated nerve endings present in skin.

Kreb's cycle The chain reaction cycle involving oxidation of pyruvic acid and production of ATP.

Krukenberg's tumor A malignant tumor of ovary, usually bilateral and frequently secondary to malignancy of G.I. tract (through peritoneal seedling).

Krypton A gaseous element in the atmosphere.

Kufs' disease Adult form of cerebral sphingolipidosis with dementia, retinitis pigmentosa, blindness and myoclonic jerks.

Kugelberg-Welander disease Juvenile spinal muscular atrophy.

Kummell's disease Spondylitis following compression fracture of vertebra.

Kupffer's cells Fixed phagocytic cells lining hepatic sinusoids.

Kuru A progressively fatal encephalopathy probably of slow virus infection spreading by practice of cannibalism.

Kussmaul's breathing Very deep and gasping respiration in acidosis.

Kussmaul's disease Periarteritis nodosa.

Kwashiorkor A severe protein deficiency syndrome in children manifesting with lethargy, dry brittle hair, growth failure, subcutaneous edema, skin changes and hepatomegaly.

Kyasanur forest disease Tick born encephalitides of South India.

Kymograph 1. A device for recording movements of a stylus on a moving drum, thus helpful to record respiratory movements, muscle contractions. 2. A radiographic device for recording the range of motion of involuntary movements of the heart or diaphragm.

Kymoscope Device for measuring variations in blood flow and pressure.

Kyphoscoliosis Forward bending of spine along with increased lateral curvature.

Kyphosis Excessive curvature of spine with convexity backwards. May be congenital or secondary to compression fracture, malignancy *SYN*— hump back.

L

LA 50 The total body surface size of a burn that will kill 50% of victims, used for statistical analysis of mortality figures in burn patients.

Labelling The process or procedure followed in using chemical or radioactive labels as an aid in reaching a diagnosis or for experimental study.

Labetalol Both alpha and beta-blockers used in hypertension.

Labile Unstable, emotions that are easily changeable.

Labioplasty Plastic surgery of labium majus or minus.

Labium A lip shaped structure, a fleshy margin or fold.

Labor The onset of forceful uterine contraction to expel the fetus; divided into three phases, first: from onset of contraction till full dilatation of cervix, second: from full dilatation till delivery of fetus and third: delivery of placenta. *l. arrested* Failure of progression of labor. *l. dry* Premature rupture of membranes with escape of liquor. *l. false* Uterine contractions that do not progress. *l. induced* Labor precipitated by drugs, (oxytocics) or artificial rupture of membrane. *l. obstructed* Arrest in progress of labor due to cephalopelvic disproportion, contraction ring, abnormal fetal position, etc. *l. precipitate* Rapidly progressing labor threatening fetal and maternal injury. *l. prolonged* Extended duration of labor as first phase exceeding 20 hours in nullipara, 14 hours in multipara or cervical dilatation less than 1.2 cm/hr in nullipara and 1.5 cm in multipara.

Labrum Lip like structure. *l. acetabulare* Triangular rim of fibrocartilage, base of which is fixed to acetabular margin, deepening its cavity. *l. glenoidale* A triangular rim of fibrocartilage, the base of which is fixed to circumference of glenoid cavity of scapula.

Labyrinth Any thing twisted or of spiral shape. *l. membranous* A closed system of communicating sacs in the internal ear, containing endolymph and surrounded by perilymph. *l. osseous* The bony cavities in petrous part of temporal bone housing the membranous labyrinth and connected to middle ear by fenestra vestibuli and fenestra cochleae. *l. vestibularis* The portion of membranous labyrinth comprising sacculus, utriculus and their connections and the three semicircular canals (*see* Figure).

Labyrinthectomy Partial or complete surgical destruction of labyrinth as in Menier's disease; Techniques employed include injection of absolute alcohol, diathermy, ultrasound, cryosurgery or avulsion of lateral semicircular

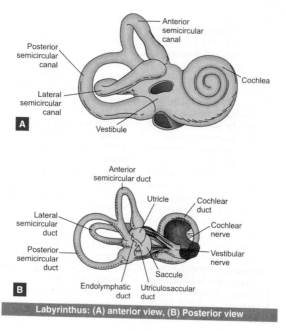

Labyrinthus: (A) anterior view, (B) Posterior view

canal/transtympanic avulsion of utricle.

Labyrinthitis Inflammation of inner ear; can be circumscribed, serous or suppurative.

Laceration Tearing of tissues with ragged irregular margins and surrounding contusion. *l. first degree obstetric* Laceration of perineum involving the fourchette, vaginal mucosa, and skin but not underlying fascia and muscle. *l. second degree obstetric* Involves underlying fascia and muscle but does not extend to anal sphincter. *l. third degree obstetric* Laceration extends to involve anal sphincter. *l. fourth degree obstetric* Laceration involves anal sphincter and rectum with rectovaginal fistula.

Lacrimation Production of tears, weeping.

Lactalbumin Proteins in milk that are not precipitated with ammonium sulfate. β. *lactamase* Bacterial enzyme that hydrolyzes the β lactam bond antibiotics like penicillin and cephalosporins leading to loss of antibiotic activity.

Lactate dehydrogenase An enzyme catalysing reaction of lactate to pyruvate with liberation of NADH and H⁺, helping hereby in anaerobic glycolysis. The enzyme is a tetramer consisting of 2 types of chains, the alfa is predominant in heart muscle and beta in skeletal muscle.

Lactic acid A product of anaerobic glycolysis in muscles and by milk-souring bacteria.

Lactiferrous Capable of producing, transporting or secreting milk.

Lactobacillus Gram-positive, anaerobic nonspore forming bacilli producing D or L lactic acid in the milk.

Lactoferrin Iron binding protein of milk.

Lactogen Agent stimulating lactation, like prolactin; human placental lactogen is a polypeptide hormone structurally related to human growth hormone and prolactin secreted by placenta. It is essential in maintenance of growth of fetus.

Lactoglobulin A milk protein with a concentration of 3 gm per liter in cow's milk, second only to casein among milk proteins.

Lactose The principal sugar of milk hydrolyzed by β galactosidase to glucose and galactose. Those deficient in this enzyme have discomfort on drinking milk.

Lactose synthetase Enzyme helping in synthesis of lactose, found in mammary glands.

Lactosuria Presence of lactose in the urine.

Lactulose A synthetic disaccharide that is not hydrolyzed or absorbed but broken down by clonic bacteria with formation of organic acids. It reduces ammonia level of blood and acts as purgative.

Lacune A space or cavity between cells or structures. *l. cerebral* Hypertensive lipohyalunosis causing minor infarction with lacune formation within cerebral hemisphere (lacunar syndrome). *l. Howship's* Bony pits occupied by osteoclasts.

Lag Slowness to act or react, the interval between an expected action or reaction and its occurrence. *l. anaphase* A retarded movement of chromosome during mitosis. *l. eyelid* Failure of upper eyelid to descend promptly while looking down as in Grave's disease. *l. globe* While looking upward, upper eyelid pulls faster than the eyeball is raised, thus exposing the sclera above the iris. *l. jet* Altered biological rhythms like sleep, satiety, hunger, after rapid jet transport.

Lagophthalmos Inability to close the eyelids completely as in facial palsy.

Lambda The 11th letter of Greek alphabet; the junction of sagittal and lambdoid sutures.

Lamella Thin plate, layer or sheet as of compact bone.

Lamina A plate or thin sheet of material. *l. dental* A flat band of epithelial cells that develops in the embryos along which develop the tooth germs giving rise to primary and secondary dentition. *l. of Rexed* Lamination of cells in spinal gray matter marked 1 to 9, arranged in dorsoventral direction and lamina 10 situated centrally. *l. terminalis* A membrane formed in the developing embryo remaining to adulthood as a thin layer of gray matter extending from superior surface of optic chiasma to rostrum of corpus callosum (*see* Figures).

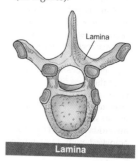

Lamina

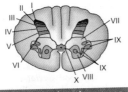

Rexed's laminae in a cross section of the spinal cord at approximately the level of the seventh cervical vertebra (C7)

Laminated Arranged in layers.

Laminotomy Division or partial removal of vertebral lamina.

Lamotrigine Antiepileptic.

Lamp A device producing light artificially. *l. Eldridge Green* Color vision testing device using spectral filters. *l. Finsen* Carbon arc lamp utilized for treating lupus vulgaris. *l. kromayer* Mercury quartz ultraviolet lamp for treatment of skin ulcers. *l. Wood's* Lamp producing ultraviolet rays at 365 nm giving characteristic fluorescence of some fungi. Infected hairs have bright green fluorescence; *T. versicolor* has gold fluorescence.

Lancet A small surgical blade, used for making small drainage incisions (*see* Figure).

Lancinating Sudden sharp transient pain as if tearing into pieces.

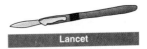

Lancet

Landsteiner's classification A classification of blood groups into A, B, AB, and O on the basis of presence of antigens A and B on red blood cells.

Langers lines The structural orientation of fibrous tissues of skin. Incisions made parallel to them produce less scar.

Lanolin A waxy fatty secretion of sebaceous glands of the sheep deposited on wool fibers, used as an ointment base.

Lansoprazole Proton pump inhibitor, used in peptic ulcer.

Lanugo The fine downy hairs devoid of medulla, covering fetus.

Laparoscope An endoscope devised for examination of abdomino-pelvic organs.

Laparotomy Surgical incision of abdominal wall for access to abdominal organs.

Laplace's law Pressure within a tube is inversely proportional to its radius.

Larva Motile developing stage of worms, maggots, caterpillars. l. fillariform: Infective larva of nematodes.

Larva migrans Migratory phase of the cycle of helminth in an abnormal host/

site with random wandering. *l.m cutaneous* Linear eruption caused by hookworm larva. *l.m visceral* Disorder of visceral larval migration from normal i.e., intestine to liver, heart, lungs, trachea, mouth and back to intestine so that the larva migrate in random with ultimate encapsulation in aberrant site.

Larvicide Medication effective against larval form.

Larviparous Deposition of hatched larvae than eggs.

Laryngectomy Excision of a part or total larynx.

Laryngismus stridulus Brief nocturnal attack of laryngo spasm.

Laryngitis Inflammation of lining of larynx, may be catarrhal, chronic hyperplastic (often precancerous), chronic nonspecific, diphtheritic, membranous (diphtheria, streptococci, pseudomonas).

Laryngocele An air containing pouch, usually bilateral in wind instrument players and glass blowers.

Laryngomalacia A flaccid supraglottic larynx in babies causing inspiratory stridor but with spontaneous cure.

Laryngoplasty Reconstruction of larynx to improve airway as in bilateral abductor palsy.

Laryngoscopy Inspection of interior of larynx. *l. fiberoptic* Indirect (mirror) laryngoscopy.

Laryngospasm Spasm of glottic sphincter produced by foreign material, blood, secretion getting access to laryngeal inlet.

Laryngostomy Making an opening into subglottic larynx for relief of upper airway obstruction.

Laryngotracheobronchitis Inflammation of larynx, trachea and bronchi often producing critical respiratory embarrassment in small children chiefly due to subglottic swelling and tenacious secretion usually of viral origin.

Larynx The musculocartilaginous structure continuous with trachea below and inferior of pharynx above, formed by 9 cartilages and 8 muscles, acting as the organ of voice (*see* Figure on page 405).

Laser Light amplification by stimulated emission of radiation. *l. carbondioxide* Used to remove lesions of skin or other superficial organs. *l. argon* Its blue green light causes coagulation of bleeding sites in surgery. *l. neodymium Yag* Laser used for capsulotomy, vitrectomy (*see* Figure on page 405).

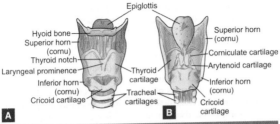

Larynx: (A) anterior view, (B) posterior view

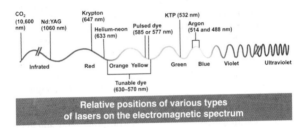

**Relative positions of various types
of lasers on the electromagnetic spectrum**

Latency The period between stimulation application and onset of response.

Latent Existing but not apparent, dormant.

Lateral On the side of body.

Lateralization The tendency to perform an act predominantly on left or right side of the body.

Lathyrism Spastic paraplegia with sensory impairment due to consumption of khesari dal containing fungus *Lathyrus sativatus*.

Laurence-Moon-Biedl syndrome An autosomal recessive disorder affecting specially males and characterized by obesity, polydactyly, mental retardation, sub-normal development of genitals, and retinitis pigmentosa.

Lauric acid A fatty acid found in neutral fat like butter.

Lavage The washing out of hollow organ, e.g. gastric, peritoneal, intestinal.

Law An accepted and tested phenomena. *l. Collin's* After removal of a tumor in infancy or childhood if metastasis or recurrence does not develop within period equal to age of patient plus 9 months then risk of such development is small. *l. Courvoisier's* Obstruction of common bile duct by a gallstone rarely causes dilatation of gallbladder. *l. Faget's* Lack of correlation between body temperature and heart rate in yellow fever. *l. Flatav's* The longer ascending and descending tracts of spinal cord tend to be displaced peripherally by shorter axons arriving or terminating at that level. *l. Graham's* The rate of diffusion of a gas is inversely proportional to the square root of its density. *l. Laplace* The transmural pressure in a free sphere or cylinder is directly proportional to the circumferential tension in the wall; inversely proportional to the radius. *l. Ohm's* Voltage across a resistor is equal to current ×-resistance. *l. Starling's* The force of contraction in cardiac muscle is equivalent to fiber length at beginning of contraction. *l. Teevan's* Fractures of bones occur in lines of extension and in the line of compression.

Laxative Agent promoting or stimulating bowel movement.

Lean body mass Body weight without fat content.

LE cell A nutrophil containing phagocytosed nucleus of another neutrophil; seen in SLE.

Lecithin A fatty substance like phospholipids found in blood, bile, brain, egg yolk, nerves and other animal tissues.

Lecithin-Sphyngomyelin ratio This ratio in amniotic fluid indicates fetal maturity. Level more than 1 occurs in full-term. Low level in associated with hyaline membrane disease in newborn.

Leflunomide Used in rheumatoid arthritis.

Legionella *L pneumophila,* a non-motile gram -ve rod present in air conditioning system causing pneumonia.

Leiomyoma A low mitotic benign tumor of smooth muscle cell. Can be seen on skin (dermatomyoma) uterus, seminal vesicles, blood vessels (angiomyoma) (*see* Figure on page 407).

Leiomyosarcoma Malignant tumor of smooth muscle cells.

Leishmaniasis Infectious disease caused by flagellate

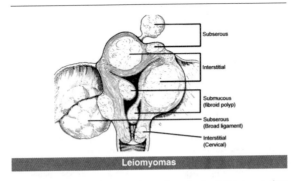

Leiomyomas

protozoan parasites and transmitted to man by sandflies.

Leishmanoid Facial cutaneous lesion containing leishmania.

Lemniscus A ribbon, band, bundle of axons. *l. lateral* Longitudinal tract of auditory system terminating in inferior colliculus and medial geniculate body. *l. medial* Myelinated tract emerging from nucleus gracilis and cuneatus and crossing over to opposite side in medulla and terminating in ventrobasal thalamic nucleus. *l. trigeminal* A large band of myelinated axons originating from principal trigeminal nucleus and crossing over to opposite side in pons to join medial lemniscus.

Length *l. cranial* Skull length between glabella and inion.

l. crown heel Fetal or infant length from crown to heel. *l. foot* Toe to heel length for estimation of age of fetus. *l. sitting* Distance between vertex and coccyx.

Lens 1. Transparent biconvex disk lying between iris and vitreous. 2. A medium with refractile surfaces. *l. contact* Resin lens fitting directly on cornea. *l. photo chromatic* Lens that darkens on exposure to ultraviolet light, used in sunglasses.

Lentiasis Bilateral symmetrical hypertrophy of bones of face and cranium of unknown cause.

Lentiform Shaped like a lentil or lens of eye.

Lentigo A small brown macule resulting from increased number of melanocyte at dermo-epidermal junction, Pleural - Lentigines.

Lentigomelanosis Irregular brownish black localized pigmentation produced by senile lentigo.

Leopold's Maneuver A method to determine position, presentation, and engagement of fetus (*see* Figure).

Lepothrix A superficial corynebacterium infection of axillary or pubic hair in which nodules form on hair.

Leprosy Chronic mycobacterial disease of skin and peripheral nerves caused by *mycobacterium leprae;* can be divided into borderline, borderline lepromatous, lepromatous, border line tuberculoid and tuberculoid types. *l. borderline* Affects persons with moderate degree of cell mediated immunity, can upgrade to tuberculoid or downgrade to lepromatous pole. *l. lepromatous* Diffuse bilaterally symmetrical lesions in persons with poor cell mediated immunity. Bacilli are plenty and well disseminated. *l. lucio* A diffuse non-nodular variant of lepromatous leprosy. *l. tuberculoid* Few hyposthetic macules, enlarged cutaneous nerves, well developed cellular immunity and few bacteria.

Leptocyte A thinner erythrocyte, appearing hypochromic, seen in iron deficiency anemia, thalassemia, etc.

Leptodactyly Unusual slenderness of fingers.

Leptomeninges Pia-arachnoid membranes together.

Leptophonia A weak thin quality of voice.

Leptoscope An optical instrument used to measure thickness of a thin film.

Leptospira A genus of coiled ectopic spirochete.

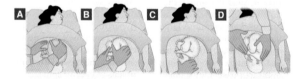

Leopold's Maneuver

Leptospira icterohemorrhagica A febrile illness caused by leptospira manifesting with hemolysis, jaundice, anemia, bleeding tendency.

Lergotrile Ergot alkaloid.

Lesbian Female homosexual.

Lesch-Nyhan syndrome It is X-linked recessive genetic disease characterized by the deficiency of the enzyme hypoxanthine – guanine phosphoribosyl transferase (HPRT). It is associated with symptoms of severe gout, poor muscle control, mental retardation, self mutilating behaviour (e.g. Lip and finger biting), failure to thrive, choreoathetosis, etc.

Lesion A pathological alteration in structure or function of an organ.

Lethal Deadly, capable of causing death.

Lethargy A state of excessive fatigue, diminished physical and mental activity.

Lithotomy position Common position for surgical procedures and medical examinations involving the pelvis and the lower abdomen and a common position for child birth in western nations. The patient lies on back, thighs flexed on abdomen and abducted.

Letrozole Aromatase inhibitor.

Letterer-Siwe disease Granulomatous destructive disease.

Leucine An essential amino acid.

Leucovorin A calcium salt of folinic acid that counteracts toxic effects of folic acid antagonists.

Leukapheresis Selective removal of leukocytes by hemopheresis, useful in treatment of blast crisis or to obtain leukocyte donation.

Leukemia Malignant proliferation of leukocytes and their bone marrow precursors with organ infiltration. Principal types are: acute myeloid, acute lymphoblastic, chronic myeloid, chronic lymphocytic. Acute myeloid has six subtypes- M_1 to M_6. that includes monocytic, myelomonocytic, promyelocytic and erythroleukemia. *l. aleukemic* Peripheral blood picture is normal but there is pancytopenia. Bone marrow puncture yields the excess blast cells. *l. basophilic* Marked increase in basophils of blood and marrow, a variant of chronic myeloid leukemia. *l. eosinophilic* Peripheral eosinophilia with increased blasts in marrow.

Leukemid A nonspecific cutaneous lesion containing infiltration of leukemic cells.

Leukemoid Resembling leukemia with appearance of immature leukocytes in peripheral blood and leukocytosis. Seen in some infectious diseases.

Leukoblastosis Any malignant disorder of white cells including leukemia and lymphoma.

Leukocyte Nucleated cells of blood and marrow excluding erythrocyte precursors (*see* Figure).

Leukocytoblast The earliest recognizable leukocyte precursor.

Leukocytoma Tumorous accumulation of leukocytes including chloroma, granulocytic leukemia and lymphoma.

Leukocytosis Increased number of leukocytes in blood may be lymphocytic, neutrophilic, eosinophilic. It can be seen in newborn, often physiological after exercise, terminal (before death) and toxic (severe infection).

Leukocytotaxis Migration of leukocytes to the site of inflammation and injury.

Leukocytotoxin Any substance that selectively damages leukocytes.

Leukoderma Lack of normal skin pigmentation.

Leukodystrophy Myelin degeneration in white matter of brain and spinal cord consequent to inherited disorders of lipid metabolism.

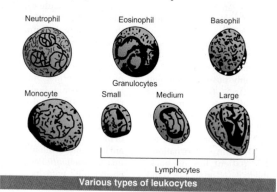

Neutrophil   Eosinophil   Basophil

Granulocytes

Monocyte   Small   Medium   Large

Lymphocytes

Various types of leukocytes

Leukoencephalitis Encephalitis predominantly involving cerebral white matter.

Leukoencephalopathy Any disease of cerebral white matter; may be hemorrhagic, necrotizing.

Leukoerythroblastosis Presence in the blood of numerous normoblasts together with precursors of granulocyte series.

Leukokoria White reflex of pupil as in retinopathy or any pathological condition posterior to crystalline lens.

Leukoma Dense white scar of cornea.

Leukopedesis Migration of lymphocytes through walls of blood vessels.

Leukopenia Abnormal decrease in number of blood leukocytes. ($\leq 4000/\mathrm{cmm}$).

Leukoplakia Epithelial hyperplasia with keratosis of mucous membrane appearing as white patch. It chiefly affects gums, lips, cheeks, tongue, larynx, urinary bladder and female genitalia.

Leukopoiesis Formation, growth and maturation of leukocytes.

Leukopsin The colourless product of bleaching of rhodopsin.

Leukorrhea Abnormal white nonbloody discharge from vagina.

Leukotactic Capable of attracting leukocytes.

Leukotaxis Active ameboid, unidirectional movement of leukocytes towards an attractant.

Leukotomy Trans orbital frontal lobotomy.

Leukotrienes Mediators of inflammation derived from arachidonic acid. Leukotriene $C_4 D_4 E_4$ play roles in anaphylaxis (slow reacting substance) and B_4 is a chemoattractant and aggregator of neutrophils.

Leuprolide Gonadotropin releasing hormone analog for prostatic carcinoma.

Levallorphan tartarate A narcotic antagonist for treatment of respiratory depression caused by narcotics.

Levamisole The l-form tetramisole, used for treatment of roundworm, hookworm, strongyloides. Also used as an immunopotentiator.

Levarterenol Norepinephrine.

Levator A muscle that raises up the part into which it is inserted.

Levobunolol Antiglaucone drug.

Levocardia Visceral situs inversus with a normally positioned left sided heart. Such a heart often has aortic arch and valvular malformations.

Levodopa 3-hydroxyl-L-tyrosine, administered orally in parkinsonism and heart failure.

Levonorgestrel Progesteron for emergency contraception.

Levorotatory Capable of rotating the plane of polarized light counter-clockwise.

Levorphanol Narcotic analgesic similar to morphine.

Levothyroxine L thyroxine; yellow crystalline powder for oral supplement in hypothyroid cases.

Levoxadrol L-isomer of dioxadiol, used as local anesthetic and smooth muscle relaxant.

Levulinic acid 4 oxopentanoic acid, source of aminolevulinic acid which is an intermediate in biosynthesis of porphyrins.

Levulose Levorotatory glucose.

Lhermitte's sign Also sometimes known as the Barber Chair phenomenon. There is a production of electrical sensation which runs down the back, arms and legs when the person flexes his head. It is usually present in lesions of dorsal columns of the cervical cord, e.g. multiples sclerosis, Behçet's disease, vitamin B_{12} deficiency, etc. It may persist for a few days or weeks and then disappear on its own without treatment.

Libido Sexual desire or appetite.

Lichen A tree moss, localized thickening, shining itchy skin lesion due to continuous friction or rubbing.

Lidocaine A local anesthetic applied as sprays, creams to skin and mucous membrane.

Lidoflazine A coronary vasodilator.

Lie The relation of longaxis of fetus to that of mother; can be longitudinal, transverse or oblique.

Linorenal Pertaining to spleen and kidney.

Life The time span between birth and death.

Ligament 1. Any band of fibrous tissue connecting bones. 2. Any membranous fold sheet or cord like structure that holds an organ in position. *l. broad, of uterus* Fibrous sheets of peritoneum extending from uterus to lateral pelvic wall. *l. cruciate of knee* One anterior and one posterior crossing each other like *x* that prevent rotation in knee joint. *l. deltoid* The medial reinforcing ligament of ankle. *l. falciform* A sickle shaped ligament composed of two layers of peritoneum attaching liver to anterior abdominal wall. *l. inguinal* Rolled inferior margin of external oblique aponeurosis extending from anterior superior iliac spine of ileum to pubic tubercle. *SYN*—Poupart's ligament. *l. lacunar* A triangular band extending horizontally from the inguinal ligament to iliopectineal line of pubis. *l. ovarian* A cordlike bundle of fibers between the folds of broad ligament joining ovary to uterus. *l. pectineal* A strong aponeurotic band extending from pectineal line of pubis to the lacunar ligament. *l. round of liver* Remnant of umbilical vein extending from umbilicus to anterior border of liver *SYN* – ligamentum teres hepatis. *l. round of uterus* A fibromuscular cord extending from either side of uterus to labium majus passing through inguinal canal (*see* Figure).

Ligand Any of the molecules or ions, identical or different that bind to same central entity by multiple coordination bonds. e.g., O_2 and N_2 attaching to same iron molecule contained in Hb.

Ligate To tightly tie a thread to compress a vessel, pedicle of a tumor.

Ligation The action to ligate. *l. tubal* Both fallopian tubes are tied and cut or crushed for purpose of sterilization.

Ligator Surgical instrument facilitating ligation, superficial or deep.

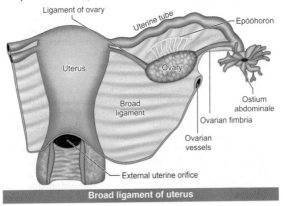

Broad ligament of uterus

Ligature A suture tied around a vessel or tube in order to obliterate the lumen. Ligature can be grassline, double, interlocking and continuous type.

Light Electromagnetic radiation of 400-700 nm.

Lightening The descent of fetus deeper into pelvis.

Lignocaine A local anesthetic.

Limbic system The parts of brain including hippocampus, amygdala, dentate gyrus, cingulate gyrus responsible for emotion, arousal, behavior and motor autonomic functions.

Lincomycin An antibiotic obtained from Streptomyces.

Lindane Gamma benzene hexachloride, used in pediculosis.

Line A connection between two points or a boundary between two areas. *l. Beau's* Superficial transverse depressions in the nail plates appearing after an illness. *l. Camper's* Line drawn from base of anterior nasal spine to upper end of tragus of ear. *l. Chamberlain's* A line drawn in lateral X-ray of skull from posterior end of hard-palate to the posterior margin of foramen magnum. In normal individual the odontoid process should not lie above this line. *l. Kerley's* Thin linear soft tissue densities seen in X-ray chest representing thick interlobular septa. Kerley B lines are located in costophrenic area. A lines are located centrally and C lines are tiny lace like densities in hilum. They are all seen with interstitial pulmonary edema and with pulmonary fibrosis. *l. Nelaton's* A line drawn from anterior superior iliac spine to ischial tuberosity, passing above greater trochanter of femur in a normal person. *l. pectinate* An uneven horizontal line formed by the continuity between the anal valves and bases of rectal columns 2 cm. above the anal opening. The line represents ectoentodermal junction. *l. Schoemaker's* The line joining greater trochanter of femur and anterior superior iliac spine passes normally above umbilicus. *l. simian* A transpalmar crease more common to those with Down's syndrome. *l. white of Frankel* Line of increased radiodensity in the metaphysis at the provisional zone of calcification; a sign of scurvy.

Linea A long thin mark, ridge, crease or line. *l. alba* Midline tendinous band extending from xiphoid process to symphysis pubis, formed by aponeurosis of external oblique, internal oblique and transversalis muscles. *l. nigra* Pigmented linea alba of pregnancy.

Lineage The direct descendants of an individual.

Linear Having the properties of a line.

Lingula A narrow band of white matter in brainstem connecting nucleus gracilis to inferior cerebellar peduncle, tongue shaped lobule of superior vermix of cerebellum.

Lingulectomy Surgical resection of lingula of left upper lobe.

Liniment An oily medicinal liquid applied to skin by friction as an counter irritant.

Linin Fine thread like achromatic substance of the cell nucleus that interconnects the chromatin granules.

Lining In dentistry, the coating applied to the walls of a tooth cavity to protect the pulp from irritation by restorative filling e.g., zinc oxide, eugenol, zinc phosphate and calcium hydroxide.

Linitis Inflammation of cellular tissue of stomach. *l plastica* Extensive thickening of stomach wall due to infiltration by scirrhous carcinoma.

Linkage 1. The force that holds together the atoms in a chemical compound. 2. The relationship existing between two or more genes in the same chromosome.

Linoleic acid An essential fatty acid, precursor of prostaglandin.

Linseed The oil acts as a demulcent and laxative.

Lip Any projecting labrum, fleshy parts surrounding mouth opening. *l. cleft* Notch, furrow or open space in upper lip developmental in origin.

Lipase Enzyme that catalyzes hydrolysis of fat.

Lipectomy Excision of subcutaneous adipose tissue.

Lipemia Increased turbidity of plasma due to increased lipids.

Lipid Any natural compound soluble in apolar but insoluble in polar solvents. Lipids contain fatty acids, one chain alcohols, steroids or sphyngolipids.

Lipid A The endotoxic component of lipopolysaccharide consisting of glucosamine disaccharide.

Lipidosis Disease state with abnormal lipid storage by RE cells e.g., metachromatic leukodystrophy (sulfatide); Niemann-Pick disease (sphingomyelin), gangliosidosis, cerebral lipidosis.

Lipoadenoma A tumor with mixture of glandular and fat tissue e.g., parathyroid adenoma.

Lipoatrophy Atrophy of subcutaneous tissue at sites of insulin injection.

Lipoblast A polyhedral cell with small lipid droplets which becomes a fat cell.

Lipoblastomatosis A benign lobulated tumor of fetal fat cell, may be localized or diffuse.

Lipodermatosclerosis A brawny pigmented fibrosis of the skin and subcutaneous tissue of lower leg resulting from venous stasis.

Lipodystrophy A condition due to abnormal fat metabolism.

Lipofuscin A brown pigment, partially soluble in fat, occurring in nerve and muscle cells.

Lipogranulomatosis A rare metabolic disorder in which ceramides and gangliosides accumulate as a result of ceramidase deficiency.

Lipohyalin Lipid material sometimes seen in hyalinized beta cells of pancreatic islets of Langerhans in diabetes.

Lipoma A benign growth of mature adipose tissue cells.

Lipomatosis Presence of multiple or diffuse lipomas. *l. dolorosa* Presence of multiple painful lipomas.

Lipophilic Fat soluble.

Lipophore A pigmented cell whose color is caused by lipochrome pigment.

Lipopolysaccharide Any substance made-up partly from lipid and partly from polysaccharide e.g., bacterial cell wall which is highly antigenic.

Lipoprotein Compounds of lipid and protein. *l. high density* Contains 50% protein, 25% phospholipid, 20% cholesterol, and 5% fat, originate both in liver and intestine, function in cholesterol transport, have longer half-life and are cardioprotective. *l. low density* Contains more of cholesterol and lipids and little triglyceride high blood level is atherogenic. *l. very low density* Density 1.006 mg/ml. Contains 50% fat, 25% cholesterol and 20% phospholipid.

Lipoprotein lipase The enzyme that catalyzes hydrolysis of fat into fatty acids and glycerol. VLDL is hydrolyzed in this way. The enzyme lies bound to capillary wall by glycosaminoglycan.

Liposarcoma Malignant tumor of adipose tissue common to

soft tissue and retroperitoneum. It can be well differentiated, myxoid (embryonal), round cell, pleomorphic or mixed.

Liposis Diffuse fatty infiltration of body tissues. *SYN* – adiposis.

Liposome A small vesicular structure which forms spontaneously when phospholipids are placed in water.

Liposuction A method of subcutaneous fat removal.

Lipoteichoic acid The teichoic acid found in bacterial membranes.

Lipotropin Any hormone that causes release of fatty acids from fat. β *lipotropin* A single chain polypeptide hormone with 91 amino acids, functions as a prohormone for endorphins, encephalins and MSH. γ *lipotropin* Single chain polypeptide hormone with 58 amino acids, physiologic property unknown.

Lipoxygenase An oxidising enzyme for linoleate group.

Lippes loop A type of intrauterine contraceptive device.

Lipping A bony spur.

Liquefaction Becoming liquid, often due to hydrolysis.

Liquor The fluid secreted by choroid plexus of ventricles, ovarian follicles.

Lisch nodule A hamortoma of iris, seen in neurofibromatosis.

Listeria Small gram-positive aerobic rods, e.g., L. monocytogenes causing meningitis, septicemia, abscess.

Listerosis Infection with listeria organisms.

Lithiasis Formation of stones; renal, biliary, conjunctival.

Lithium A silvery, soft element, the carbonate form used for manic depressive disorder.

Lithocholic acid Bile acid, found conjugated with taurine and glycine.

Lithogenesis Formation of calculi.

Litholysis Fragmentation or dissolution of stones.

Litholyte An instrument designed to administer stone dissolving agents directly inside bladder.

Lithopedion A retained calcified fetus.

Lithotomy An incision into a duct or organ for removing stone.

Lithotony Formation of bladder fistula for stone removal.

Lithotripsy Breaking up of gall/urinary stones by shock waves, delivered directly or extra corporeally.

Lithotrite Surgical instrument designed to crush or fragment stones and help their removal.

Litmus A natural pigment from lichens whose principle is azolitmin. It is used as pH indicator being red at pH and blue at pH 8.3.

Litter A stretcher for transporting the invalid.

Livedo A discoloration, skin erythema that follows a reticular pattern of the cutaneous vascular network. *l. reticularis* Circulatory disorder of unknown origin causing constant bluish discoloration on large areas of extremity.

Liver Largest glandular organ in the body weighing 1200-1600 gm (1/40 of body wt), located in right upper quadrant below right dome of diaphragm; major functions are secretion of bile, synthesis of plasma proteins, fibrinogen, prothrombin; detoxification, metabolism of carbohydrate, fat and protein and storage of glycogen. *l. amyloid* Large pale gray waxy looking liver due to deposition of amyloid. Amyloid deposits appear as an amorphous eosinophilic substance, in the space of Disse, between hepatocyte and sinusoidal endothelial cells. *l. cirrhotic biliary* Deeply bile stained nodular liver caused by autoimmune damage to small bile ducts (primary biliary cirrhosis) or obstruction to bile outflow. *l. cirrhotic* Scarred nodular liver, post-hepatitis, alcoholic. *l. Indian childhood cirrhosis* Enlarged firm liver with a leafy edge. *l. fatty* Yellow soft greasy liver with increased cytoplasmic fat within hepatocytes. *l. nutmeg* Liver affected by chronic vascular congestion as in CHF. *l. polycystic* Liver with multiple congenital cysts, often associated with polycystic kidney, usually asymptomatic (*see* Figure).

Lividity A black and blue discoloration of skin such as caused by contusion.

Loa A genus of filarial nematode transmitted by blood sucking flies.

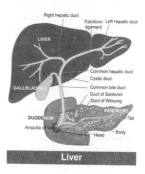

Liver

Loa-loa The thread like eye worm of Africa causing blindness and calabar swelling. The microfilarae with nuclei extending right up to tail are found only during day.

Lobe 1. A fairly well defined portion of an organ or gland bounded by structural borders such as fissures, sulci or septa 2. Projecting fibro fatty lobule of human ear. 3. One of the main divisions of crown, formed from distinct point of calcification. *l. azygos* An occasional small triangular lobe on the mediastinal surface at the apex of the right lung. *l. caudate* A small lobe of liver situated posteriorly between the inferior vena cava and fissure for ligamentum venosum. *l. frontal* The portion of each cerebral hemisphere bounded behind by central and below by lateral sulci. *l. limbic* Cingulate and parahippocampal gyri, as well as underlying hippocampal formation, and dentate gyrus, the oldest portions of cerebral cortex. *l. occipital* Most posterior portion of each cerebral hemispheres, bounded anteriorly by parietooccipital sulcus and the line joining it to the preoccipital notch.

l. olfactory A general term usually denoting olfactory bulb, tract, trigone plus anterior perforated substance. *l. parietal* Upper central portion of each cerebral hemispheres between the frontal and occipital lobes and above the temporal lobes, separated from frontal lobe by central sulcus. *l. median of prostate* The portion of prostate between ejaculatory ducts and urethra, forming the superior part of posterior surface of prostate, only becomes obvious when enlarged and enlargement causes bladder neck obstruction. *l. flocculonodular* Oldest division of cerebellum made up of the midline nodules and two stalk like flocculi located in the posterior and ventral surface of cerebellum. It is functionally related to vestibular nerve and nuclei. *l. piriform* A portion of the anterior and ventromedial face of temporal lobe composed of the terminal extensions of the lateral olfactory striae, the uncus and the anterior part of parahippocampal gyrus. *l. pyramidal of thyroid gland* An inconstant, narrow cone-shaped lobe of thyroid, arising from upper border of isthmus, often attached to hyoid bone by a fibrous band. *l. Riedel's* A tongue shaped mass of tissue often extending downward from right lobe of liver. *l. quadrate* A small lobe on inferior surface of liver between gallbladder and ligamentum teres. *l. temporal* A long lobe on outer side and inferolateral surface of cerebral hemispheres bounded above by lateral sulcus (*see* Figure).

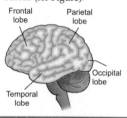

Frontal lobe
Parietal lobe
Occipital lobe
Temporal lobe

Lobes of the cerebrum

Lobeline Ganglionic stimulant.

Lobotomy Incision of a lobe. *l. prefrontal* A psychosurgical procedure with division of fibers connecting prefrontal and frontal lobes with thalamus. Also called prefrontal leukotomy.

Lobulated Consisting of or divided into lobules.

Lobule A small lobe.

Lochia Discharge from uterus following childbirth.

l. alba Light colored uterine discharge consisting of leukocytes. *l. rubra* Bloody uterine discharge immediately after delivery.

Lochiometra A condition in which lochia is retained inside the uterine cavity.

Lockjaw Trismus, a symptom of tetanus.

Loculation 1. A tissue or structure having numerous small cavities. 2. formation of small cavities.

Loculus A small cavity.

Locus A place or spot, as the specific site occupied by a gene in the chromosome. *l. ceruleus* A bluish gray area in the floor of fourth ventricle. *l. histocompatibility* One of the genes located within major histocompatibility complex that specifies transplantation antigens or immune response functions. *l. operator* A regulator locus that governs the transcription of adjacent structural genes of the operon and is the binding site of a repressor protein molecule.

Loeffler's syndrome Disorder lasting less than a month, characterized by transient infiltrates in lungs, low fever and eosinophilia.

Loeffler's disease Also called eosinophilic endomyocardial disease with eosinophilic coronary arteritis, congestive cardiac failure, eosinophilia and multiple systemic emboli.

Logorrhea Excessive uncontrolled speech, i.e., logomania.

Loin The part of back and sides of body between the ribs and the pelvis.

Lomustine Antineoplastic agent.

Loop A bend in a cord or cord like structure, the arched dermal ridges in dermatoglyphics. *l. Lippe's* S-shaped intrauterine contraceptive device. *l.Meyer's* The portion of geniculocalcarine radiation that loops around inferior horn of lateral ventricle. *l. of recurrent laryngeal nerve* The arching of recurrent laryngeal nerves after their origin from vagus in the chest. The left one hooks below the arch of aorta behind attachment of ligamentum arterisoum and then up the left side of trachea while the right one hooks around first part of subclavian artery.

Loperamide A meperidine congener, intestinal smooth muscle relaxant.

Lophophorine An extreme toxic alkaloid found in cactus.

Loraadine H$_1$ receptors blocker, antiallergic.

Lophotrichous Bacteria possessing multiple flagella at one pole only.

Lorazepam A benzodiazepine anxiolytic.

Lorbamate A cyclopropane carbamate ester used as muscle relaxant.

Lorcainide Antiarrhythmic agent, for ventricular tachycardia.

Lordosis Abnormally increased forward curvature of lumbar spine. Also called sway back or saddle back. *l. compensatory* Lordosis secondary to pelvic obliquity/deformity (*see* Figure).

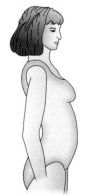

Abnormally increased curvature of the lower spine characteristic of lordosis

Larnoxican Analgesic, anti inflammatory.

Losartan Angiotensin receptor blocker used in hypertension.

Loss *l. dissociated sensory* Pain and temperature severely lost with preservation of touch as in syringomyelia or central cord tumors. *l. hearing* 1. Sensory neural due to ageing or autoimmune 2. Conductive due to disease of middle ear or external ear.

Lotion Medicated liquids for external application or cosmetic liquid preparations e.g., benzyl benzoate, l. calamine, (calamine, zinc oxide, glycerin, bentonite, calcium hydroxide).

Loudness The intensity of noise or sound.

Loupe Small magnifying lens.

Louse Small flat bodied parasitic insect. e.g., body louse, crab louse, head louse, pubic louse).

Lovastatin Ester of methyl butanoic acid, given orally for increased LDL and cholesterol.

Lowe's syndrome Oculocerebrorenal syndrome.

Loxapine A tricyclic antipsychotic agent with tranquillizing properties.

Loxotomy Surgical amputation by means of an oblique incision.

Lozenge A tablet, often diamond shaped, containing medication in a flavoured and sweetened base.

Lubb - dupp First and second heart sound auscultatory appearance.

Lubricant Agent used to reduce friction.

Lucid Easily understood, clear, able to think properly.

Luciferase An enzyme which catalyzes the transfer of an electron from luciferin to oxygen with emission of light. (bioluminescence of fire flies, glow worms and bacterial fungi).

Luetic Syphilitic.

Lumbago Pain in lumbar region.

Lumbar Pertaining to loins (*see* Figure).

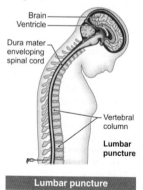

Brain
Ventricle
Dura mater enveloping spinal cord
Vertebral column
Lumbar puncture

Lumbar puncture

Lumbarization Fusion between the transverse processes of the lowest lumbar and adjacent sacral vertebra.

Lumbosacral Pertaining to lumbar portion of spine and the sacrum.

Lumbrical Resembling an earth worm, lumbrical muscles of hand.

Lumbricoid Earthworm like appearance.

Lumefantrine An antimalarial.

Lumen The cavity within tubular structure; the SI unit of luminous flux.

Luminescence Emission of infrared, visible light or ultraviolet by matter from any cause except incandesence.

Luminiferous Capable of transmitting light.

Lumiracoxib Anti-inflammatory, analgesic.

Lumpectomy Localized excision of breast lump.

Lunate Moon or crescent shaped, semilunar.

Lunacy Major mental illness.

Lung Paired organ of respiration in the chest enveloped by pleura. Subserving the function of oxygen uptake and CO_2 elimination. *l. farmer's* Extrinsic allergic alveolitis occurring in farmers due to inhalation of moldy hay manifesting with cough, dyspnea and fever. Repeated exposures lead to pulmonary fibrosis. *l. honey comb* Small multiple areas of radiolucency with intervening borders of soft tissue density as seen in interstitial pulmonary fibrosis. *l. post perfusion* A condition of atelectasis, pulmonary arterio-venous shunting and consolidation following cardiopulmonary bypass. *l. uremic* Pulmonary edema with butterfly appearance of lung in X-ray due to circulatory overload and uremic dysfunction of L.V.

Lupoma A small granulomatous nodule characteristic of lupus vulgaris.

Lupus Resembling wolf. *l. discoid* A disease confined to skin, marked by scaly rash usually in butterfly pattern over nose and cheeks, sometimes extending to scalp but no visceral involvement. *l. pernio* Sarcoid lesions of the hands and face, especially the ears and nose resembling frost bite. *l. vulgaris* Redbrown nodular skin lesions of face in tuberculosis. *l. systemic* Chronic autoimmune disease marked by an erythematous rash on face and other areas exposed to sunlight with vasculitis involving kidneys, brain and arthritis. Antinuclear antibodies to double stranded DNA and native DNA nucleohistone are diagnostic. *l. drug induced* Similar to systemic lupus induced by drugs like procainamide and hydralazine but without renal and brain involvement.

Luteal Relating to corpus luteum of ovary.

Luteinization Transformation of granulosa cells into lutein cells in the ovary. Other cells may undergo luteinization including theca cells, celomic cells and cervical cells.

Lutembacher'ssyndrome Congenital cardiac abnormality with ASD and mitral stenosis.

Luteoid Acting like progesterone.

Luteolysis Involution or destruction of corpus luteum.

Luteoma Growth of lutein cells of ovary during third trimester with regression after parturition, often may secrete androgens.

Luteotropic Promoting development, maturation or hormonal secretion of corpus luteum.

Lutetium Element No 71, isotopes used in nuclear medicine.

Lutheran blood group Antigens of red blood cells, specified by lugene that react with antibodies designated as anti-Lu^a and anti-Lu^b, first detected in serum of an individual who had received many transfusions and who developed antibodies against erythrocyte of a donor named Lutheran.

Lux A unit of illumination, equal to one lumen per square meter.

Luxation Dislocation.

Lye Sodium potassium hydroxide.

Lying-in Confinement of a woman during childbirth.

Lyme disease A spirochetal disease transmitted by ticks characterized by erythema chronicum migrans, fever, myalgia, lymphadenopathy, arthritis, pericarditis, myocarditis, and CNS involvement.

Lymph A transparent or slightly opalescent fluid containing lymphocytes, which flows through lymph channels and enters finally into venous system via thoracic ducts (*see* Figure on page 425).

Lymphaden Lymph node.

Lymphadenectasia Enlargement of lymph nodes with excessive lymph.

Lymphadenectomy Surgical excision of lymph nodes.

Lymphadenitis Inflammation of lymph nodes.

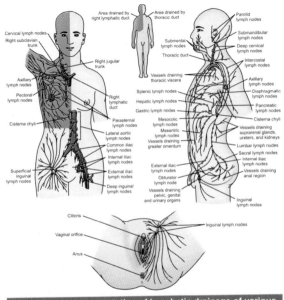

Diagrammatic representation of lymphatic drainage of various parts of the body

Lymphadenography X-ray examination of lymph nodes.

Lymphadenoma A tumor made of lymphoid tissue.

Lymphadenomatosis Presence of numerous enlarged lymphnodes.

Lymphadenopathy A diseased state of lymph nodes.

Lymphadenosis Generalized enlargement of lymph glands and lymphatic tissue, may be benign (e.g., infectious mononucleosis) or malignant.

Lymphagogue An agent that increases formation and flow of lymph.

Lymphangiectasia Abnormal dilatation of lymphatic vessels. *l. intestinal* Dilatation of intestinal lymphatic with subsequent protein losing enteropathy, steatorrhea and diarrhea. It may be congenital due to hypoplasia of thoracic duct or acquired due to inflammation or malignancy of lymphatics. Small intestinal biopsy is diagnostic with dilated lacteals in intestinal villi.

Lymphangiectasis Dilatation of lymph vessels.

Lymphangioendothelioma A tumor composed of small masses of endothelial cells and aggregation of tubular structures thought to be lymphatic vessels.

Lymphangiography X-ray visualization of lymphatic vessels after injection of contrast medium.

Lymphangioleiomyomatosis A proliferation of lymphatic and smooth muscle cells typically affecting lung and lymph node, a lesion of women in reproductive age, with honey combing and respiratory insufficiency.

Lymphangioma A benign growth composed exclusively of lymph vessels lined by a single layer of endothelial cells. The lesion is often congenital, can be subtyped into capillary, cavernous and cystic. The latter two are most frequent in cervical, mediastinal and retroperitoneal regions of infants (hygroma); capillary lymphangioma is difficult to identify from hemangioma.

Lymphangiosarcoma Malignant tumor of lymphatic tissue, mainly associated with chronic lymph stasis usually secondary to radical mastectomy.

Lymphangitis Inflammation of lymphatic vessels. *l. carcinomatosa* Growth of carcinoma in lymphatics or lymphatic obstruction by carcinoma.

Lymphedema Chronic unilateral or bilateral swelling of extremities caused by obstruction of lymph vessels or disease of lymph nodes, usually congenital, **type I** : autosomal dominant, associated intestinal protein loss and pleural effusion (Millroy's disease). **type II:** slowly progressive form with onset around puberty. *l. praecox* Lymphedema occurring in girls approaching puberty.

Lymph node A rounded body consisting of accumulations of lymphatic tissue found in the course of lymphatic vessels (*see* Figure on page 427).

Lymphoblast An immature cell, the precursor of lymphocyte, also known as lymphocytoblast/immunoblast.

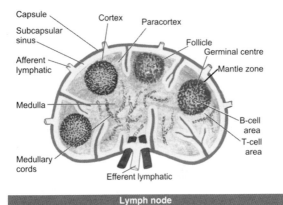

Capsule
Cortex
Paracortex
Subcapsular sinus
Follicle
Germinal centre
Afferent lymphatic
Mantle zone
Medulla
B-cell area
T-cell area
Medullary cords
Efferent lymphatic

Lymph node

Lymphoblastoma A form of malignant lymphoma, composed mainly of lymphoblasts.

Lymphocyte A white blood cell derived from lymphoid tissue constituting 25-33% of white blood cells in peripheral blood. It has a round nucleus with well condensed chromatin, no nucleolus, and agranular cytoplasm staining pale blue. *l. B* Derived from bone marrow, involved in humoral immunity. They recognize antigens irrespective of MCH molecule and transform to plasma cells to secrete antibodies on antigenic stimulation. They are thymus independent. *l. T.* Thymus derived lymphocyte, that has been exposed to antigen on an antigen presenting cell. They play large role in cellular immunity. Can be helper cells, killer cells, suppressor cells or null cells.

Lymphocytoma A tumor of low grade malignancy arising in a lymph node, composed mainly of mature lymphocyte.

Lymphocytopenia Marked reduction in number of circulating lymphocytes.

Lymphocytosis Greater than normal number of lymphocytes in peripheral blood. *l. acute infectious* An acute benign infectious disease of obscure etiology in children with headache, upper respiratory symptoms, and lymphocytosis.

Lymphocytotoxin A complement fixing antilymphocyte antibody.

Lymphoepithelioma A malignant tumor derived from epithelium around tonsils and nasopharynx containing abundant lymphoid tissue.

Lymphogranuloma venereum A chlamydial infection marked by appearance of transient ulcer on the genitalia, and enlargement of lymph node in the groin. Can lead to urethral and rectal strictures, rectovaginal fistula.

Lymphokine A hormone like factor produced by sensitized lymphocytes when they come in contact with antigen to which they were sensitized, acts as an intercellular messenger to regulate immunologic and inflammatory responses.

Lymphokinesis 1. Circulation of lymph through lymphatic vessels and nodes 2. Movements of endolymph in the membranous labyrinth of the internal ear.

Lymphoma Malignant disease of lymphoreticular system. *l. Burkitt's* Malignant lymphoma involving extranodal sites like jaw, orbit, abdominal viscera, and ovaries, the most common childhood tumor of tropical Africa. Possibly caused by EB virus and linked to falciparum malaria. *l. histiocytic* Lymphoma composed of histiocytes (poorly differentiated lymphocytic lymphomas). *l. lymphocytic* A malignant lymphoma composed of lymphocytes. The pattern may be nodulas or diffuse, and the cells may be poorly differentiated, well-differentiated. *l. prolymphocytic* The cells are larger and have less condensed nuclear chromatin. *l. sclerosing* A lymphoma with prominent stromal component. *l. signet ring cell* Cells with a large cytoplasmic vacuole of immunoglobulin which displaces the nucleus to periphery. *l. stem cell* Composed of large basket like cells.

Lymphopoietin A soluble factor required for maturation of lymphocytes.

Lymphorrhea Flow of lymph from ruptured lymph channel.

Lymphotaxis The induction of lymphocyte movement.

Lymphotoxin Substance destructive to lymphocytes.

Lymphotrophic Attracted to lymphatic system.

Lynestrenol A semisynthetic progestin.

Lyon hypothesis Inactivation of one X chromosome in female during embryogenesis forming the barr body.

Lyophilic Dispersing or dissolving easily because of affinity for solvent.

Lyophobic Difficult to disperse because of poor affinity for solvent.

Lyophilize To separate a solid from solution by rapid freezing and dehydration under vacuum.

Lypressin Vasopressin with lysine in place of arginine in position 8. An antidiuretic and vasopressor.

Lysergic acid diethylamide A hallucinogen, can induce chromosomal changes.

Lysin Any substance capable of causing lysis.

Lysine One of the twenty amino acids. It is an essential amino acid deficient in plant proteins.

Lysis 1. Destruction of cell by specific lysin 2. gradual recovery from an acute disease.

Lysochrome A lipid soluble pigment that is suitable for staining fat.

Lysogen An antigen that stimulates the formation of specific lysin.

Lysogeny A form of viral parasitism in which viral DNA becomes incorporated in a (bacterial) cell genome, without destroying the cell, thereby permitting transmission of virus to subsequent bacterial generations.

Lysokinase An activator agent of fibrinolytic system.

Lysolecithin A lecithin without unsaturated fatty acid residue. It is strongly hemolytic, a good detergent.

Lysosome A membrane limited cytoplasmic organelle containing hydrolytic enzymes capable of breaking down most of the constituents of living matter.

Lysozyme An antibacterial enzyme present in tear, sweat, saliva and nasal secretion.

M

Macerate 1. To soften a solid or tissue by soaking the tissue in enzyme/acid. 2. The autolysis of fetal tissue after fetal death.

Machine A device for accomplishing a specific objective. *m. heart - lung* A combination of pump and oxygenator to affect extracorporeal circulation and oxygenation of blood during open heart surgery. *m. Holtz* A machine for developing high voltage static electricity by multiplication of an induced charge. *m. panoramic rotating* An X-ray machine capable of radiographing all the teeth and surrounding structures by using a reciprocating motion of the tube and extraoral film.

Macroamylase A form of amylase that occurs as a complex joined to a serum globulin.

Macrocyte Red blood cell 2 micron larger than normal RBC, also called megalocyte.

Macrocytosis A condition in which red blood cells are larger than normal, e.g., Vit. B_{12} and folic acid deficiency.

Macroencephaly Malformation and increase in size and weight of brain due to proliferation of glia with small ventricles and mental retardation.

Macrogamete The female gamete, larger egg fusing with microgamete, leading to zygote formation.

Macrogametocyte The mother cell producing macrogamete.

Macroglia The astrocyte and oligodendrocyte, the two neuroglial elements of ectodermal origin.

Macroglobulin Plasma globulin with molecular weight of 1000000, increased in multiple myeloma, cirrhosis, collagen disorders.

Macroglobulinemia Plasma cell myeloma, a disorder with excessive production of IgM with anemia and bleeding; also called Waldenstrom's macroglobulinemia.

Macroglossia Enlarged tongue.

Macrogyria Congenital malformation in which the cerebral gyri are large due to few sulci.

Macrolides A group of antibiotics having molecules made-up of large ring lactones e.g., erythromycin

Macromelia Enlarged limbs.

Macromolecule Any molecule composed of several monomers.

Macrophage A large mononuclear cell that ingests degenerated cells, widely distributed in body but greatest accumulation in spleen where they remove senescent RBC. In brain and spinal cord known as microglia and in the blood as monocyte. *m. alveolar* A cell that moves on the alveolar surface of lung engulfing airborne particles reaching the alveoli.

Macropsia Condition of seeing objects larger than their actual size.

Macroscopic Visible with naked eye.

Macrostomia Abnormally large mouth.

Macrotia Abnormally large ears.

Macula A small area differing in appearance from surrounding structure. *m. densa* That portion of distal convoluted tubule of the kidney in contact with the wall of afferent arteriole just before the latter enters the glomerulus. It contains cells that are tall and narrow, secreting renin. *m. retinae* A small yellow oval depression on the retina 2 disc diameter lateral and slightly below the optic disc containing fovea centralis. *m. sacculi* The oval neuroepithelial sensory area in the medial wall of the saccule that houses the terminal filaments of vestibular nerve.

Macule A nonelevated discolored lesion on the skin.

Maculoerythematous Both red and spotted.

Maculopapular Spotted and elevated.

Maculopathy Any disease of macula of retina.

Mad Suffering from mental disorder, rabid, angry.

Maddox rod Multiple parallel cylindrical rods of glass fused side to side and shaped into a trial lens used for testing of squint and fusion.

Madelong deformity Subluxation of distal radioulnar joint secondary to abnormal growth and curvature of distal radius.

Madarosis Loss of eye lashes.

Maduramycosis A chronic disease affecting feet with draining sinuses discharging yellow to black granules.

Madurella A genus of fungi causing maduramycosis.

Maffucci's syndrome A combination of multiple cutaneous hemangiomas and dyschondroplasia.

Magaldrate Hydroxy magnesium aluminate, an antacid.

Maggot A legless soft bodied larva of various insects, common housefly, developing in dead organic matter.

Magma 1. A paste like preparation of any organic matter. 2. Finely divided material suspended in a small quantity of water.

Magnesia Magnesium oxide, it neutralizes acids to give soluble magnesium salts.

Magnesium Element number 12, the silvery white metal, one of the principal cations governing electrochemical properties of living system. *m. carbonate* $MgCO_3$, insoluble in water, used as laxative and antacid. *m. citrate* Used as laxative. *m. hydroxide* Insoluble in water, used as laxative and antacid. *m. oxide* also called magnesia (see above). *m. sulphate* $MgSO_4$. Effective cathartic, antiarrhythmic and antiepileptic, useful in certain poisonings.

Magnetic resonance imaging A technique of soft tissue imaging using radiofrequency pulse, best for evaluating musculoskeletal system, spine, brain and joints.

Magnetism 1. The properties of mutual attraction, or repulsion produced by magnet or electric current. 2. Study of magnet and their properties. 3. The force exhibited by a magnetic field.

Magneton A unit of measure of the magnetic movement of an atomic or subatomic particle.

Magnification An enlargement of an object by an optical element or instrument.

Maim To disable, mutilate, cripple by injury.

Main Hand. *m. d' accoucheur* The characteristic position of hand produced by tetany. *m. en griffe* Permanent extension of metacarpophallangeal joints.

Mainlining Term used by drug addicts denoting IV injection of heroin or other drugs.

Majocchis' disease Annular telangiectatic purpura.

Majority The age at which a person becomes legally entitled to full civil rights of an adult. It is 18 in UK, 21 in India, USA, Canada and 20 in Japan.

Makeshift Denoting a shunt from a large variceal collateral vessel to a systemic vein when a standard shunt cannot be employed. Employed for portal hypertension.

Mal A disease.

Mala The cheek bone, cheek.

Malabsorption Impaired or incomplete absorption of nutrients by the intestine. *m. lactose* Lactase deficiency, mostly inherited, commonly manifesting in adults, with pain and diarrhoea after lactose ingestion. Unabsorbed lactose is converted to butyric and lactic acid by colonic bacteria, that causes pain. Lactose being hyperosmolar draws fluid to add to stool volume. *m. syndrome* Manifests with pallor, potbelly, bleeding tendency, weakness due to malabsorption of nutrients, caused by any disease.

Malachite green Green crystalline substance used as a pH indicator.

Malacia Softening of tissues. *m. cordis* Morbid softening of heart.

Malady Illness.

Malaise A vague general discomfort or feeling ill.

Malakoplakia. The formation of soft, fungus like growths on the mucous membrane of a hollow organ, esp. urinary bladder.

Malalignment 1. Incorrectly aligned fractured parts. 2. Displacement or abnormal position of tooth.

Malar Relating to cheek or cheek bone.

Malaria An infectious disease caused by any of the four plasmodia, transmitted by mosquitoes of the genus *Anopheles*, manifesting with chill and fever, anemia, splenomegaly. *m. falciparum* Caused by *plasmodium falciparum,* the parasite develops within small vessels of internal organs frequently blocking them. Fever paroxysm often occurs daily and is often continuous. Patient can have cerebral, gastrointestinal, renal and pulmonary complications. Also known as malignant tertian. *m. malarae* Caused by *plasmodium malarae,* Fever paroxysm occurs on every third day. *m. quotidian* A form in which paroxysms occur daily, can be caused by combination of *plasmodium vivax* and falciparum or two generations of falciparum. *m. relapsing* A type in which exoerythrocytic cycle persists in liver with relapse e.g., in vivax and ovale infection. *m. vivax* Caused by plasmodium vivax or ovale, the fever paroxysm occurring every other day (*see* Figure on page 434).

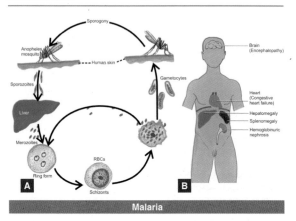

Malaria

Malassizia furfur Fungus that causes tinea versicolor.

Malate Salt of malic acid.

Malathion Insecticide.

Male Sex of an individual containing organs that produce spermatozoa, with one X-and one Y-chromosome.

Malformation A defect or deformity. *m. Klippel-Feil* Short webbed neck due to malformation of cervical vertebrae. *m. Mondini* Congenital deafness due to hypoplasia of latter part of cochlea.

Malfunction Abnormal or inadequate function.

Malic acid An intermediate in carbohydrate metabolism, present in unripe apples, cherries, tomatoes, etc.

Malignant Denoting any disease resistant to treatment, and of fatal nature. In case of tumor it denotes uncontrollable undifferentiated growth and dissemination.

Malinger To pretend to be ill, for personal gains.

Malingerer Who pretends to be sick.

Malleable Pliable, capable of being made into small sheets.

Malleation A spasmodic movement.

Malleolar Relating to one or both prominences on either side of ankle.

Malleolus One of the two projections on either side of ankle.

Malleus The club shaped and most lateral of the three

auditory ossicles involved in sound transmission across middle ear. It is attached to tympanic membrane and articulates with incus.

Mallory-Weiss syndrome Laceration of lower esophagus with hematemesis following severe retching and vomiting.

Malnutrition Faulty nutrition due to inadequate diet, metabolic abnormality, wrong proportions of items, etc.

Malocclusion Abnormal contact of opposing teeth.

Malonic acid It competitively inhibits the oxidation of succinate to fumarate.

Malonyl-Coenzyme A Formed from acetyl COA, helpful in fatty acid biosynthesis.

Malpighian body Renal corpuscle.

Malpractice Improper, unskillful, or negligent treatment of an individual by a medical man.

Malrotation Developmental failure of rotation in the normal direction and to normal degree, most common to digestive tract.

Malt Grain, especially barley, containing dextrin, maltose, glucose and some enzymes.

Maltase Digestive enzyme promoting conversion of maltose to glucose.

Maltose $C_{12}H_{22}O_{11}$; a sugar formed by action of a digestive enzyme on starch.

Malunion Faulty union of fractured bones.

Mamma Breast, rudimentary in male and but containing milk producing glands in female (*see* Figure).

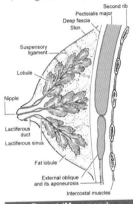

Breast (Mammary)

Mammal Vertebrates that nourish their offspring with milk.

Mammilities Inflammation of the nipples.

Mammilliplasty Plastic surgery of the nipples and the areola.

Mammitis Also known as mastitis. This is the infection or inflammation of the breast tissue which occurs commonly among breast-feeding women.

Mammoplasty Plastic surgery of breast; can be augmentative (increase in size by implants) or reductive.

Mammary Relating to breast.

Mammila Nipple, nipple like protruberance.

Mammilate Having nipple like structures.

Mammiloplasty Reparative surgery of nipple.

Mammogram X-ray of mammary gland.

Mammography A soft tissue X-ray technique for visualization of female breast; used to detect nonpalpable lesions and identify palpable lesions.

Mammotrophic Promoting development, and growth of mammary glands.

Mandelate Salt of mandelic acid.

Mandelic acid Urinary antibacterial agent.

Mandible The horse shoe shaped bone of lower jaw in mammals. Articulating with skull at temperomandibular joint and housing the lower teeth (*see* Figure).

Mandibullectomy Removal of lower jaw.

Maneuver A skillful movement. *m. Bracht's* In obstetrics, maneuver used in breech extraction whereby breech is allowed to deliver spontaneously up to umbilicus and then the fetal body is held anteriorly toward mother's abdomen to facilitate delivery of vertex. *m. credes* A method of expressing the placenta

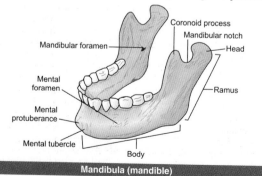

Mandibula (mandible)

in which body of uterus is vigorously squeezed inorder to produce placental separation. *m. Hallpikes* a test for benign positional vertigo. *m. Heimlich* method of dislodging food and other material from the throat. *m. Pinard* Method of fetal extraction in frank breech presentation; two fingers are passed along fetal thigh to push it away from midline and flex the leg, the foot then easily grasped and brought down and out. *m. Prague* A procedure used in breech delivery in which the finger is hooked over shoulder of fetus to exert traction and allow engagement of the head. *m. Scanzoni's* Rotation of fetal head with mid forceps from posterior to anterior position. *m. valsalva* 1. Forced expiration against closed glottis to increase pressure within lungs. 2. Forced expiration with mouth closed and nose pinched to open up auditory tubes (*see* Figure).

Manganese Element no. 25, an essential micronutrient.

Manganous Bivalent salts of manganese.

Mange Scabies.

Mania Emotional disorder characterized by excitement, hyperactivity and garrulousness.

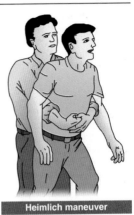

Heimlich maneuver

Maniac Emotionally disturbed individual with violent behavior.

Manifestation Display of characteristic signs and symptoms of a disease. *m. neurotic* The use of various defense mechanisms like conversion, dissociation, depression in an attempt to resolve emotional conflicts. *m. psychotic* Loss of contact with reality, personality disintegration.

Manikin An anatomic model of human body for practice of certain manipulations as those of obstetrics and dentistry.

Manipulation Treatment by skillful use of hand in reducing dislocation or changing the fetal position.

Manna The dried sugary exudate of ash tree, rarely used as a laxative.

Mannerism Distinctive characteristic or behavioral trait.

Mannitol An alcohol, $C_6H_{14}O_6$, derived from fructose, used in preparation of dietetic sweets and as an osmotic diuretic.

Manometer An instrument for measuring pressure of liquid and gases.

Mansonia A genus of mosquitoes transmitting filaria.

Manubrium A structure that resembles a handle but when used alone refers to manubrium sterni (*see* Figure).

Manus The hand.

Mantle A covering.

Mantoux test An intradermal test to know exposure to tuberculous protein. Induction less than 5 mm is negative, 5-10 mm in doubtful and more than 10 mm is positive.

Maple syrup urine disease An autosomal recessive disorder marked by deficient oxidative decarboxylation of alpha keto acids; the urine has characteristic Maple syrup odor and the symptoms soon afterbirth are hypoglycemia, hypotonia, convulsion etc. Also known as branched chain ketonuria.

Mapping In genetics, locating the position and order of gene loci on a chromosome

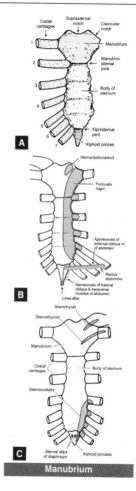

Manubrium

by analyzing the frequency of recombination between the loci.

Maprotiline Tricyclic antidepressant.

Marasmus Protein calorie malnutrition in young children with progressive wasting, wizened face, shrunken eyeballs but alerted mind.

Marble bone disease Abnormally calcified bone with spotted appearance in X-ray.

Marcus Gunn's pehnomenon Closing of the eyes when mouth is closed and exaggerated opening of the eyes when mouth is opened. *SYN* – Jaw winking syndrome.

Marfan's syndrome Autosomal dominant trait with defective formation of elastic fibers marked by abnormally long slender extremities, spidery fingers, high arched palate, lax joints, aortic regurgitation, MVP and dislocation of lens.

Margin The edge or border of a structure or organ. *m. of safety* A measure of drug safety based on the dose required to produce an effective, therapeutic response in most individuals versus the dose required to produce toxic effects in few individuals. It is similar to but not same as therapeutic index.

Margination Adhesion of leukocytes to the interior of capillary wall during early stages of inflammation.

Marijuana The dried, chopped leaves, flowers and stems of the common hemp plant *canabis sativa*, smoked or eaten to induce euphoria.

Marie Strumpel disease Ankylosing spondylitis.

Mark A blemish, a spot. *m. port wine* Congenital discoloration of skin, usually on the face varying from pink to purple.

Marker 1. A characteristic factor by which a cell or molecule can be identified or a disease can be recognized. 2. A general term for any trait that helps to throw light on the genetic nature of a disorder.

Maroteaux Lamy syndrome.

Marmot Ticks that transmit rocky mountain spotted fever.

Maroteaux-Lamy syndrome A form of mucopolysaccharidosis characterized by dwarfism, chest deformity, knock knee, stiff joints, cloudy cornea, short hands and fingers, inherited as autosomal recessive and there is excessive dermatan sulphate excretion in urine.

Marrow The meshy material filling the medullary cavities of bones. *m. red* Marrow in the cancellous or spongy bones of sternum, ribs, iliac crest, vertebrae and ends of long bones. Concerned with formation of blood. *m. yellow* The fatty marrow in center of long bones.

Marsupialization Surgical procedure for eradication of cyst in which the sac is incised, and its edges are stitched to the edges of external incision e.g., pilonidal cyst.

Masculine Relating to characteristics of male sex.

Mask 1. A covering for the face and nose to prevent spread of infection. 2. An expressionless appearance of face, e.g. Parkinson facies. 3. A metal frame covered with gauze placed over face for giving inhalation anesthesia. 4. To cover metal parts of a denture with an opaque material. *m. BLB* An oxygen mask used at high altitudes, having a combination of inspiratory and expiratory valves in a rebreathing bag. *m. Venturi* Mask that develops a constant concentration of oxygen, using the Venturi Principle of entrainment of air to dilute the flow of pure oxygen.

Masking 1. The introduction of noise in one ear for the purpose of excluding that ear from a hearing test given to the other ear. 2. The opaque material placed over the metal or any other part of a dental prosthesis.

Masochism 1. A form of sexual perversion where satisfaction is dependent upon physical torture. 2. The infliction of physical or psychological pain upon oneself to relieve guilt.

Masochist 1. The passive partner in practice of masochism. 2. One who for psychological purposes exposes himself unnecessarily to sufferings.

Mass A collection of tissue; in pharmacology, a soft pasty mixture of drugs suitable for rolling into pills.

Massage Rubbing body parts for therapeutic goals. *m. Cardiac* Rhythmic manual compression of heart either by thoracotomy (open cardiac massage) or by pressure applied to sternum (closed cardiac massage). *m. carotid sinus* Massage of carotid sinus at the angle of jaw for treatment of SVT or identification of tachycardia. *m. prostatic* Massage of prostate through rectum to express its secretions into prostatic urethra (examination for gonococci).

Masseter Muscle of lower jaw used for chewing.

Masseur A person trained in or who practises the art of massage.

Mastectomy Surgical excision of breast. *m. extended radical* Mastectomy that includes removal of chest muscles, axillary lymph nodes and the internal mammary chain of lymph nodes. *m. Halstead radical* Removal of breast, chest muscles and lymph nodes of axilla. *m. modified radical* Removal of breast and axillary lymph nodes without removal of pectoralis muscle. *m. total* Removal of breast only.

Masticate To chew.

Mastication The process of chewing.

Mastigophora The subphylum of protozoa that includes leishmania and trypanosomas; organisms with one or more flagella and a single nucleus.

Mastitis Inflammation of the breast.

Mastochondroma A benign breast tumor composed chiefly of cartilaginous tissue.

Mastocytogenesis The formation of mast cells.

Mastocytoma A nodule resembling a tumor, composed chiefly of mast cells.

Mastocytosis Disorder characterized by yellow, brown macules and papules on skin due to skin infiltration by mast cells.

Mastodynia Pain in the breast.

Mastoid 1. Resembling a breast or nipple in shape. 2 The downward projection of the temporal bone located behind the ear.

Mastoidectomy Removal of mastoid air cells indicated for persistent or recurrent mastoiditis not controlled by antibiotics. *m. conservative* The operation does not interfere with sound conducting system of middle ear. *m. modified radical* The pars tensa of tympanic membrane and attached handle of malleolus are spared. *m. radical* Done by transmeatal or transmastoid routes with tympanectomy and excision of all diseased tissue of middle ear and mastoid leaving intact the posterosuperior bony canal wall to facilitate subsequent tympanoplasty.

Mastoiditis Inflammation of mastoid process of temporal bone.

Mastomenia Vicarious menstruation from breast.

Mastoptosis Dropping or pendulous breasts.

Mastoplastia Hypertrophy or enlargement of the breast.

Masturbation Self-manipulation of genitals to achieve sexual gratification.

Materia Latin for substance or matter.

Materia alba White cheese like deposit along gum line.

Material The substance from which something is made or composed. *m. impression* Substances used for taking impressions like plaster of paris, hydrocolloid compounds.

Maternal Relating to mother.

Maternity Pertaining to pregnancy, the state of being pregnant.

Mating The union of male and female for reproduction.

Matrilineal Relating to inheritance of traits through the maternal line rather than the paternal.

Maturation 1. The process of becoming mature. 2. A stage of cell division in which chromosome is halved.

Mature Complete in natural development, the reproductive cell which has undergone meiosis.

Matrix 1. The intercellular substance in a tissue. 2. The mold for dental restoration in the form of thin steel or plastic strip surrounding tooth. *m. bone* The ground substance of bony tissue which is composed of protein and mucopolysaccharide. As the bone matures, the content of collagen fibers and bone salt increases. *m. cartilaginous* A basic, homogeneous basophil substance of embryonic skeletal tissue in the center of which articular cartilage develops. *m. mesangial* A mesh in the space between the renal glomerular loops, formed from material similar to that of capillary basement membrane. The phagocytic mesangial cells are dispersed in this matrix. The matrix is permeable to substances of higher molecular weight which aggregate to form deposits.

Matron The chief nursing officer in a hospital.

Mattress ripple Mattress containing transverse inflatable tubes linked in a series to pump so that alternate tube is inflated. Thus, the area of compression between skin and mattress changes that prevents formation of decubitus ulcer/bedsore.

Maxilla The upper jaw bone supporting upper teeth and taking part in the formation of orbit, nasal cavity, and hard palate (*see* Figure).

Maximum 1. The greatest quantity, value or degree. 2. The height of a fever or any acute state. *m. glucose transport* The maximum rate at which kidneys can reabsorb glucose (300 mg/min). *m. tubular (Tm)*. The maximum ability of renal tubules either to excrete or secrete a substance.

Maze An intricate labyrinth of walled pathways frequently used to study the learning process in laboratory animals.

Mazindol A CNS stimulating agent with properties similar to amphetamine, hence used as anorexogenic agent.

Mcburney's sign A sign of acute appendicitis, characterized by tenderness over the Mcburney's point, located in right lower quadrant, during palpation.

Meal Food. *m. Boyden* Meal used to test the evacuation time of gallbladder; it consists of flour, egg yolks, and milk mixed with sugar. *m. test* Bland food given before analysis of gastric secretion.

Mean An average of a set of values. *m. arithmetic* The ratio of the sum of the terms in a statistical series to their number. *m. geometric* A value indicating the central tendency of a statistical series of 'n' terms, equal to the positive 'n'th root of their products. *m. harmonic* For a given set of values, the reciprocal of the mean of the reciprocals of the individual values.

Measles Highly contagious disease caused by paramyxo

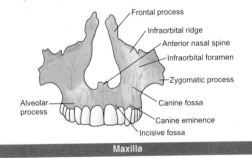

Maxilla

virus occurring in young children with fever, coryza, Koplik spots, erythematous maculopapular rash spreading from head to trunk to limbs, often complicated by meningitis, carditis.

Measure 1. The dimensions, quantity, capacity like length, area, volume, etc. 2. The act of determining such dimensions, quantity or capacity. 3. A device used for measuring like graduated glass, tape.

Measurement The act of measuring. *m. skin fold* Skin fold measurement by caliper for assessing body fat percentage.

Meatometer Apparatus for measuring urinary meatus.

Meatoplasty Reconstructive surgery usually of external auditory meatus.

Meatorraphy Enlarging the urethral meatus by suturing the urethral membrane to glans penis.

Meatotomy An incision of a meatus to increase its diameter.

Meatus An opening to a canal, or passage in the body. *m. external acoustic* S shaped canal of external ear, up to tympanic membrane lined by skin which continues on to the tympanic membrane. *m. internal acoustic* A short canal above the anterior part of jugular foramen in the petrous part of temporal bone transmitting facial, intermediate, and vestibulocochlear nerves and the labyrinthine vessels.

Mebendazole A benzimidazole given for hookworm, round worm, trichuriasis and enterobiasis.

Mebeverine A smooth muscle relaxant used for gastrointestinal motility disorder like IBS.

Mebutamate Orally acting hypotensive agent.

Mecamylamine An orally acting ganglion blocking agent rarely used to treat severe hypertension.

Mechanics The branch of physics concerned with the interaction of force and matter.

Mechanism 1. An aggregation of parts that interact in order to perform a specific or common function. 2. The means by which an effect is obtained *m. cough* A mechanism for expulsion of foreign material from respiratory tract, consisting of short inspiration, closure of glottis, forced expiration with opening of glottis with a air flow rate of 3000 - 4000 ml/sec. *m. counter current* Mechanism essential to the production of an osmotically concentrated urine; it involves two basic processes, counter current multiplication in loop of Henle and countercurrent exchange in vasa recta. *m. defense* A psychic structure, usually unconscious, which serves as a protection against awareness of conflicts or anxiety.

Mechlorethamine Alkylating agent used in treatment of lymphomas.

Meclizine Drug used in treatment and prevention of motion sickness.

Meclocycline A topically applied antibiotic closely related to chlortetracycline.

Mecloqualone A compound with hypnotic and sedative properties.

Mecobalamine Neuroprotective agent, congener of methyl cabalamime.

Mecometer Instrument used to measure newborn infant.

Meconism Opium addiction or opium poisoning.

Meconium The odorless, sticky, greenish-black semisolid intestinal content of fetus. It is replaced by feces within 2 days of birth.

Medallion A circumscribed red, scaly patch, characteristic of pityriasis rosea.

Medazepam A week tranquilizer, anxiolytic agent.

Medial 1. Towards the midline. 2. Relating to tunica media or middle layer.

Median In statistics denoting the middle value in a distribution i.e., the point in a series at which half of the plotted values are on one side and half on the other.

Mediastinitis Inflammation of mediastinum.

Mediastinography X-ray visualization of mediastinum by injection of NO_2.

Mediastinoscope An endoscope to visualize superior mediastinum, introduced through a small suprasternal incision.

Mediastinum 1. The central space in chest bounded anteriorly by sternum, posteriorly by vertebral column and laterally by pleural sacs. 2. Any septum or partition between two parts of an organ. *m. anterior* That portion of lower mediastinum located in front of heart behind the sternum. It contains thymus gland, few lymph nodes and loose areolar tissue. *m. lower* The part of mediastinum below the plane of manubriosternal joint in front and lower border of 4th thoracic vertebra behind. It is divided into anterior, middle and posterior. *m. middle*

It contains the heart, pericardium and the emerging great vessels. *m. posterior* It contains esophagus, thoracic duct, thoracic aorta, vagus and lymph nodes *m. superior* It lies above the pane of manubriosternal articulation and contains aortic arch and its branches, superior vena cava, brachiocephalic veins, left recurrent laryngeal nerve, thoracic duct, thymus, vagus nerve and some lymph nodes (*see* Figure).

Medicament A remedy, healing agent.

Medicate To treat disease with medicine, to impregnate with a medicinal substance.

Medicated Treated medically, permeated with a medicinal substance.

Medicine A drug: The art and science dealing with the maintenance and restoration of health. *m. adolescent* The branch of medicine dealing with care and treatment of individuals from onset of

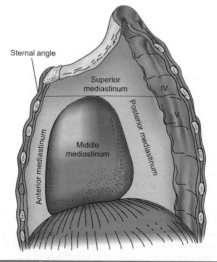

Sternal angle

Superior mediastinum

IV

V

Posterior mediastinum

Anterior mediastinum

Middle mediastinum

Subdivisions of the mediastinum

puberty to the age of 19. *m. aviation* A specialized branch of medicine dealing with physiologic, pathologic, psychologic conditions which occur in fliers, and people transported in air. It helps in selection of aircraft personnel, air transport of sick and wounded. *m. behavioral* The applications of the principles of learning and learning theory to treat those disorders caused at least in part by psychologic factors as if they were behavioral. Specific techniques are applied to reverse the expressions of maladaptive functioning whether purely psychologic as in phobias or partly physiologic as in faulty patterns of learned autonomic nervous system response leading to cardiovascular disease. *m. clinical* The study and practice of medicine at bedside, as opposed to theoretical and laboratory investigations. *m. community* Medicine dealing with community health care and their solution as a whole rather than individual health problem e.g., preventive medicine, public health services. *m. family* Medical speciality dealing with first patient contact, long-term care, and a broad responsibility to all members of the family irrespective of age. *m. folk* Treatment of disease at home with remedies and techniques passed from generation to generation. *m. emergency* A branch of medicine that specializes in providing immediate diagnosis and treatment of those who are acutely or often suddenly ill or severely injured. *m. environmental* The study of environmental aspects related to health and their modification for better health. *m. experimental* Study of disease process and various therapies in animal models. *m. forensic* The application of medical knowledge and skill to the solution of problems encountered in administration of justice. *m. geriatric* Medicine dealing with diagnosis, treatment and prevention of disease in elderly. *m. holistic* An approach to health care based on theory that health is the result of harmony between body, mind and spirits and that stress of any kind including physical, psychological and social pressure is inimical to health. *m. internal* The branch of medicine which deals with the diagnosis and nonsurgical treatment of diseases. *m. nuclear* Application of nuclear energy in the diagnosis and treatment of disease e.g., use of radioisotopes. *m. occupational* A branch of medicine dealing with prevention of disease and injury among people at work. It has two functions: to ensure suitability of an individual for particular work and to identify and control health and safety hazards in the work. *m. oral* The study and treatment of diseases of soft tissues of mouth. *m. perinatal* A specialized branch of medicine dealing with the mangement of mother and fetus during pregnancy and the infant immediately after delivery. *m. physical and rehabilitation* The branch of medicine concerned with use of physical agents and modalities including electricity light, heat, sound, mechanical devices and physical activity, in the diagnosis, treatment and prevention of disease. *m. space* A special branch of aviation medicine which deals with the stresses imposed on man by projection through and beyond the earth's atmosphere, flight in interplanetary space and return to earth. Such stresses include the agravic state, exposure to radiation and isolation. *m. tropical* The medical speciality concerned with diseases and disorders contracted in tropic or which exhibit unique characteristics in tropical countries.

Medico A medical student, a combining form meaning medical.

Medicolegal Pertaining to a matter that involves both medicine and law.

Medionecrosis Necrosis of middle layer (tunica media) of an artery.

Meditation (transcendental) (TM) An exercise of contemptation that induces a temporary hypometabolic state, a sense of wellbeing , and a feeling of complete relaxation; this hypometabolic state is associated with change in physiologic function including a reduction in oxygen consumption, a decrease in cardiac output and altered EEG activity.

Medium 1. A material in which a substance, an impulse, or information is transported. 2. A material in which interaction takes place. 3. Culture medium. *m. contrast* In radiology, a substance of different radio-opacity from that of the organ or tissue studied, to allow X-ray demonstration of contour or lumen. When the substance is more radiopaque than tissue is positive contrast, e.g. barium sulphate, iodine, when the substance is less radio-opaque than tissue— negative contrast e.g., air. *m. Neal and Nicolle* A saline rabbit's blood medium suitable for culture of *Leishmania donovani*.

Medlars (Medical Literature Analysis and Retrieval System). A computerized system of online databases containing citations of world's biomedical literature available through a network of centers at medical schools, hospitals. Govt organizations which are connected by telephone to central library's computers. Any data required can be retrieved; only available in advanced countries like USA.

Medroxyprogesterone A progesterone widely used as contraceptive and to treat precocious puberty in female, functional uterine bleeding, dysmenorrhea, endometriosis, threatened and habitual abortion and to suppress post-partum lactation.

Medulla The innermost or middle part of an organ. *m.*

oblongata The caudal portion of brainstem that extends between pons and most rostral part of cervical spinal cord. Its upper posterior part forms the floor of fourth ventricle. It contains central nuclei of glossopharyngeal, vagus, accessory and hypoglossal nerves and regulates life sustaining cardiovascular and respiratory reflexes (*see* Figure).

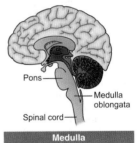

Pons

Medulla oblongata

Spinal cord

Medulla

Medullated Having a myelin sheath, having a medulla.

Medulloblast An undifferentiated cell of embryonic neural tube. It is rounded, poor in cytoplasm without processes found in middle layer of neural tube and is derived from germinal cells of inner ependymal layer.

Medulloblastoma A rapidly growing malignant brain

tumor composed of poorly differentiated small preneuroglial cells that tend to form pseudorosettes. Common to children, arising from cerebellar vermis and floor of fourth ventricle.

Medulloepithelioma A tumor of eye, primarily of children, characterized by formation of multilayered sheets of undifferentiated cells resembling primitive medullary epithelium of optic vesicle. The malignant form resembles retinoblastoma.

Mefenamic acid An agent with analgesic, anti-inflammatory and antipyretic properties.

Mefexamide A CNS stimulant, used to treat fatigue and depression.

Mefloquine Antimalarial agent, schizonticide.

Mefruside A diuretic with use similar to chlorthiazide.

Megabecquerel A unit of activity in radionuclide equal to 10^6 becquerel. Symbol - MBq.

Megacolon Abnormally large colon, either segmental or total, manifesting with constipation.

Megadyne Unit of force equal to 1 million dynes.

Mega electron volt (MeV) One million electron volts.

Megaesophagus Abnormal enlargement of lower esophagus.

Megakaryoblast A primitive cell of megakaryocyte series with a large oval or kidney shaped nucleus and scanty cytoplasm. It develops into a promegakaryocyte and finally then to megakaryocyte.

Megakaryocyte A giant cell with usually multilobed nucleus, (up to $100\,\mu$) the precursor of platelets.

Megaloblast Large nucleated erythrocyte precursor seen in bone marrow in vit B_{12} and folic acid deficiency.

Megaloblastoid Having some features resembling megaloblastic maturation. An erythrocyte precursor is said to be megaloblastoid when nuclear chromatin condensation is in clumps but with a prominent parachromatin, i.e., open, transparent, unstained cleft are prominent in the nucleus and the contours of nucleus are irregular.

Megalomania A psychopathologic condition in which the individual has unfounded conviction of his great importance and power.

Megaloureter Abnormally dilated ureter in absence of obstruction.

Megavitamin A vitamin dose far in excess of daily recommended dose.

Megavolt A unit of electromotive force equal to one million volts.

Megavoltage Electromotive force in the range of 2-10 MeV. used in radiotherapy.

Megestrol acetate A synthetic progestin used as antineoplastic agent in palliation of metastatic endometrial cancer.

Meglitinide Antidiabetic agent.

Meglumine A substance used in the preparation of radio-opaque compounds.

Meig's syndrome Polyserositis associated with ovarian fibroma.

Meiosis The reduction cell division during maturation of sex cells in which two nuclear cell divisions occur in quick succession thus forming four gametes each containing half the number of chromosomes.

Meissner's corpuscle End-organ for touch present in epidermis.

Meissner's plexus Autonomic plexus in submucosa of alimentary tract regulating intestinal secretions.

Melalgia Pain in the lower extremity.

Melancholia A condition characterized by severe depression as manifested by loss of pleasure in all activities, early morning awakening, anorexia and feeling of guilt. *m. involutional* A major depression occurring in the involutional period, i.e., 40-55 years in female and 50-65 years in males. Its characteristic triad of symptoms are delusions of guilt or poverty, obsession with death, and delusional fixation on gastrointestinal functioning all within a setting of depression and agitation.

Melanic Having a dark colour.

Melanin The natural pigment of hair and skin formed by oxidation of tyrosine via dopa and dopaquinone to a complex polymeric material.

Melanoameloblastoma Benign tumor of anterior maxilla, usually occurring in infants.

Melanoblast A derivative of neural crest which differentiates in an embryo into a melanocyte.

Melanocyte A cell capable of forming melanin, mature pigment cell.

Melanoma Any benign or malignant melanocytic tumor. *m. acral lentiginous* A malignant melanoma occurring on palms, soles, nail beds and characterized by a lentiginous growth of atypical melanocytes in the epidermis, elongated rete ridges and acanthosis. *m. lentigo maligna* An irregularly shaped, flat patch with various shades of brown, blue, red, white and tan, typically occurring in sun exposed skin and old people. *m. malignant* Malignant tumor of melanin producing cells commonly in the skin, uveal tract of eye, oral mucosa, vagina, lung, meninges. Metastasis are typically widespread at unusual sites like heart and small bowel. Tumor can be nodular, i.e., spreading vertically and rapidly exhibiting deep dark brown discoloration or may be superficial spreading type with irregular borders.

Melanophore A pigment cell carrying melanin.

Melanosis Abnormal deposits of dark pigment in various organs.

Melanosome A single melanin containing organelle that has finished synthesizing melanin.

Melarsoprol A trivalent arsenic containing antiprotozoal drug for trypanosomiasis.

Melasma Cloasma affecting cheeks, forehead and lips (*see* Figure).

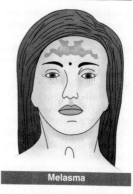

Melasma

Melatonin A hormone believed to be secreted by pineal gland. It has action opposite to that of MSH. It stimulates aggregation of melanosomes in melanophores, thus lightening the skin.

Melena Black tarry stool due to GI bleed. *m. spuria* Melena in breast-fed babies where blood originates from fissures in mother's nipple.

Meleney's ulcer Incision of an operative site which typically appears after one to two weeks after surgery.

Melioidosis An infectious disease primarily affecting rodents. Caused by *Pseudomonas pseudomallei*, often transmitted to man via open wounds, manifesting with fever, pneumonia and metastatic abscess formation.

Melitis Inflammation of cheek.

Mellitum Any pharmaceutical preparation having honey as excipient.

Mellitus Latin for honeyed.

Melomelia A condition of unequal conjoined twins in which both normal limbs and rudimentary accessory limbs are present.

Melphalen A phenylalanine analogue of nitrogen mustard, an antineoplastic agent for multiple myeloma.

Membrane A thin sheet of tissue that covers a surface, envelops a part, lines a cavity, divides a space or connects two structures. *m. alveolocapillary* The blood air barrier in the lungs consisting of alveolar epithelium, basal lamina and capillary endothelium. *m. basement* A thin transparent noncellular layer under the epithelium of mucous membranes and secreting glands. *m. basilar of cochlear duct* Membrane extending from the osseous spiral lamina to the basilar crest of cochlea, forming the floor of the cochlear duct and supporting the spiral organ of corti. *m. Bowman's* One of the five layers forming the cornea, consisting of fine inter woven fibrils. *m. Brusch's* Basal lamina of choroid in contact with the pigmented layer of retina. *m. cell* A delicate structure about 90Å thick that encloses a cell. Composed of mucopolysaccharides and lipids, regulates the movement of substances in and out of cell. *m. cricothyroid* A broad thin membrane originating from upper border of cricoid cartilage and extending to the vocal process of arytenoid cartilage and to the thyroid cartilage. *m. Descemet's* One of the five layers of cornea covering the posterior surface of substantia propria, also called posterior limiting membrane and is extremely thin, elastic, transparent and homogeneous. *m. diphtheritic* Yellowish-gray leathery exudate on the mucous membrane of upper respiratory tract seen in diphtheria. *m. dialysis* A semipermeable cellulose membrane separating blood from dialysate in hemodialysis. *m. external limiting* The third of ten layers of retina, it has the form of chicken wire. *m s fetal* Extraembryonic membranes concerned with respiration, excretion, nutrition, and protection of embryo. They include amnion, chorion, allantois, yolk sac, decidua and placenta. *m. hyaline* Like the eosinophilic homogeneous, transparent membrane lining the alveoli in premature infants afflicted with hyaline membrane disease. *m. internal limiting* The last of ten layers of retina forming the inner limit of retina and outer limit of vitreous. *m. mucous* Membrane lining tubular structures and consisting of epithelium, basement membrane, lamina propria and lamina muscularis. *m. perineal* The inferior layer of the fascia of urogenital diaphragm. *m. tympanic (TM)* The membrane separating the external ear from the middle ear cavity, kept tense by tensor tympani. The displacement of tympanic membrane (vibration) during ordinary conversation is only that of the diameter of molecule of hydrogen.

Memory 1. To remember; the persistence of the effects of experience on the behavior of living organism which includes learning, retaining, recalling and recognizing. 2. That portion of computer in which instructions and data are stored. *m. iconic* The hypothesized first stage of visual memory formation in which a faint copy of visual input persists very briefly allowing a longer interval for extraction of information. *m. immunologic* The capacity of immune system to mount a vigorous and sustained response to a subsequent exposure to a particular antigen than was mounted to initial exposure. This memory is retained by a subpopulation of T lymphocytes (memory cells). *m. kinesthetic* Memory of movement rather than event. *m. long term* The hypothesized substage of memory process in which information is stored in a relatively permanent way for the rest of life. *m. retrograde* The memory for events prior to a trauma or other incident that has affected one's memory. *m. short term* A hypothesized substage of memory process not exceeding 25 minutes per event.

Menacme The height of menstrual activity in a woman life.

Menadiol sodium diphosphate A synthetic derivative of menadione.

Menadione (Vit. K₃) Methyl naphthoquinone, parent

substance of various forms of vitamin K.

Menadione sodium bisulfite The water soluble form of menadione, used in the treatment of hemorrhage consequent to hypoprothrombinemic states.

Menaquinone Any of the several substituted menadiones with Vitamin K activity.

Menarche Appearance of first menstrual period.

Mendel's laws Laws that explain transmission of hereditary characteristics, first studied in garden peas.

Menetrier's disease/syndrome A disease of unknown etiology characterized by large gastric rugae, and pseudopolyps which may be associated with ulcer like symptoms, bleeding or idiopathic hypoproteinemia, *SYN*—Hypertrophic gastritis.

Meniere's disease/syndrome Paroxysmal labyrinthine vertigo with deafness and tinnitus, due to unexplained increase in endolymphatic pressure.

Meninges The three membranes that cover the brain and spinal cord; consisting of dense fibrous outer dura mater, thin innermost pia mater and trabeculated middle arachnoid mater. The last two are grouped as leptomeninges (*see* Figure).

Meningitis Inflammation of meninges; can be cerebral, spinal or cerebrospinal. Pachymeningitis involves dura mater while leptomeningitis involves pia arachnoid but the latter is more common.

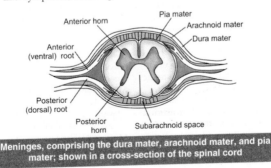

Meninges, comprising the dura mater, arachnoid mater, and pia mater; shown in a cross-section of the spinal cord *m. mollarets* Acute meningitis with CSF pleocytosis and presence of abundant large endothelial cells in CSF; rapid spontaneous remission. *m. tuberculous* Occurs due to hematogenous spread or rupture of cortical tuberculoma into CSF. Subacute onset with chronic course, often with encephalomyelopathy, cerebral arteritis, subarachnoid adhesions.

Meningioma Tumor of meninges, especially from dura where arachnoid villi are numerous. Usually benign, producing symptoms due to compression or bone erosion, can undergo sarcomatous changes.

Meningiomatosis Presence of multiple meningiomas.

Meningism A group of symptoms and signs suggesting meningitis but without identifiable pathologic lesion of meninges. Occurs in children suffering from febrile infections like pneumonia, tonsillitis, systemic viral infection.

Meningocele A congenital sac like skin covered protrusion of meninges through a defect in skull or vertebral column. Common to mid occipital area or lumbosacral area.

Meningococcemia Presence of meningococci in blood, often associated with petechial rash, cardiovascular collapse and meningitis/(Waterhouse-Fredrichson syndrome), chronic persistent meningococcemia may be associated with lowgrade fever, rash and arthritis.

Meningocyte A mesenchymal epithelial cell of subarachnoid space.

Meningoencephalitis Inflammation of brain and meninges. *m. primary amebic* Caused by *Naegleria* or *Acanthamoeba*, infection travelling via cribiform plate with fatal course in a week. *m. trypanosomal* Subacute or chronic meningoencephalitis predominantly involving the base of brain caused by trypanosoma gambiensae or rhodesiense. Producing sleeping sickness and dementia.

Meningoencephalomyelitis Combination of meningitis, encephalitis and myelitis.

Meningoencephalomyelopathy Any disease involving brain, meninges and spinal cord.

Meningoencephalomyeloradiculoneuritis Inflammation of brain, spinal cord, meninges, nerve roots and peripheral nerves.

Meningoencephalopathy A diffuse disorder of function of brain and meninges; commonly relates to toxic and metabolic encephalopathies.

Meningomyelitis Inflammation of spinal cord and its covering membranes.

Meningomyelocele A protrusion of spinal cord and associated meninges through a developmental defect in spinal canal.

Meningovascular Concerning meninges and adjacent blood vessels.

Meniscectomy Surgical removal of semilunar cartilage especially of knee. *m. arthroscopic* Removal of a part of damaged meniscus through arthroscope.

Meniscus A crescent shaped structure; one of the fibrocartilaginous discs of knee joint . *m. lateral* A nearly circular crescent shaped fibrocartilage attached to lateral articular surface of upper end of tibia. *m. medial* A crescent shaped fibrocartilage attached to medial surface of upper end of tibia.

Menolipsis The temporary cessation of menstruation.

Menometrorrhagia Abnormal bleeding during or between menstrual periods.

Menopause The normal physiologic cessation of menstruation commonly between 45-50 years of age. Frequent symptoms include hot flushes, headache, vulvar dyscomfort, painful sexual intercourse and mental depression. *m. artificial* Cessation of menopause by irradiation or surgical removal of ovaries. *m. premature* Early menopause, idiopathic or secondary to pituitary disease, systemic illness.

Menorrhagia Excessive or prolonged menstruation, *SYN* – hypermenorrhea.

Menoschesis Suppression of menses.

Menostasis Amenorrhea.

Menses Periodic bloody discharge from uterus, called menstruation.

Menstrual Relating to menses.

Menstruation The periodic discharge from uterus of a non-clotting bloody fluid at 4-5 weeks interval. *m. anovulatory* Menstruation not preceded by ovulation. *m. vicarious* Bleeding from sites other than uterus occurring at the time of normal menstruation (*see* Figure on page 458).

Mensual Monthly.

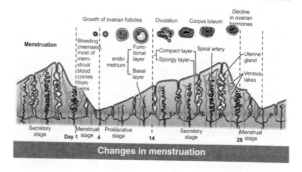

Changes in menstruation

Mensuration Measurement by immediate comparison.

Mental 1. Relating to mind 2. relating to chin.

Mentation Mental activity.

Menthol Peppermint camphor, an organic compound derived from pippermint oil or prepared synthetically. It provides a sensation of coolness in mucosal membranes by stimulation of cold receptors.

Mentoanterior In a face presentation, having the fetal chin pointing anteriorly in relation to maternal pelvis.

Mentoplasty Plastic operation on chin.

Mentoposterior In face presentation, having fetal chin pointing posteriorly in relation to maternal pelvis.

Mentotransverse In face presentation, having the fetal chin pointing laterally in relation to maternal pelvis.

Mentum The anterior prominence of mandible produced by mental protruberance; the chin.

Mepacrine An anthelmintic for tapeworm and giardiasis, also an antimalarial agent.

Meperidine A synthetic narcotic analgesic, with spasmolytic properties and high addiction potential.

Mephenesin An agent used for skeletal muscle relaxation.

Mephenoxalone A skeletal muscle relaxant, also has mild anxiolytic properties.

Mephentermine An adrenergic agent used as a nasal decongestant or in certain hypotensive states to augment vascular tone.

Mephenytoin Anticonvulsant agent for focal, Jacksonian,

grandmal and psychomotor seizure.

Mephobarbitol Long acting barbiturate with anxiolytic and anticonvulsant properties.

Mepivacaine An analogue of lidocaine for local anesthesia, peripheral nerve block or epidural block.

Meprednisone A synthetic glucocorticoid used to treat corticosteroid responsive diseases, allergic conditions.

Meprylcaine A local anesthetic for infiltration and nerve block anesthesia.

Mepyramine malleate An antiallergic.

Meralein sodium A water soluble topically applied antibacterial agent.

Meralgia Pain in the thigh, **m. Paresthetica** is troublesome tingling, pricking or numbness in lateral aspect of thigh due to compression of lateral femoral cutaneous nerve while it passes beneath or through the inguinal ligament just medial to anterior superior iliac spine.

Meralluride A mercurial salt of succinamic acid used as a parenterally administered diuretic.

Merbromin Topically used antibacterial and antiseptic Synmercurochrome.

Mercaptan Any substance containing the radical -SH bound

to carbon, analogous to alcohol and phenols but containing sulfur instead of oxygen. Used in dentistry as an elastic impression compoud.

Mercaptoethanol Most commonly used reagents containing thiol group.

Mercaptoethylamine A component of coenzyme A, used in treatment of radiation sickness and chronic leukemia.

2-Mercaptoimidazole A thiourea group of antithyroid drug, five times more potent than methylthiouracil.

Mercaptomerin sodium A mercurial diuretic given SC/IM.

Mercaptopurine 6-Purinethol, A hypoxanthine and adenine analogue used as antineoplastic agent for its growth inhibitory effect on DNA synthesis.

Mercapturic acid An S-aryl-N acetyl cysteine found in the urine after ingestion of aromatic halogen compounds.

Mercurialism Poisoning by mercury or its compounds.

Mercuric Bivalent mercury.

Mercurous Monovalent mercury.

Mercury A heavy, silvery poisonous metallic element liquid at room temperature, atomic No. 80, used in thermometer.

Mercury197 (^{197}Hg) A radioactive mercury isotope used in brain tumor localization and in the study of renal function.

Meridian A line surrounding a spherical body passing through both poles or half of such circle containing both poles.

Merocrine Denoting secretory cells that remain intact during discharge of secretory products as those in the salivary glands.

Merocyte An incompletely isolated cell found in the vicinity of the yolk of a fertilized ovum during segmentation. Its nucleus is generally derived from accessory spermatozoa.

Meropenem Highly potent antibiotic.

Merotomy Cutting into parts.

Merozoite The product of asexual schizogony of a protozoan in the body of host; in malaria merozoites are liberated from rupture of RBC to invade fresh RBC or form gametocyte, the sexual form in man, infective to mosquito.

Merogony The development of only a portion of an egg. If the egg contains only male pronucleus, the development is called andromerogony and if only female pronucleus gynomerogony.

Merology Study of rudimentary tissue.

Meromycin One of the two proteins – heavy meromycin and light meromycin formed by enzymatic digestion of muscle protein mycin.

Merphalon A racemic mixture of melphalan and medphalan; antineoplastic drug.

Mersalyl sodium A mercurial diuretic given parenterally.

Mesangium The framework of glomerulus which arises from vascular pole and extends into intercapillary spaces. It contains matrix and mesangial cells which are phagocytic in nature.

Mescaline A hallucinogenic alkaloid.

Mesencephalon The embryonic midbrain; the second cephalic dilatation of neural tube that develops into corpora quadrigemina, the cerebral peduncles and aqueduct of sylvius.

Mesenchyme Embryonic connective tissue consisting of an aggregation of cells in close contact by means of long processes thus forming a loose network. (stellate cells).

Mesenchymoma A rare benign or malignant tumor consisting of two or more clearly identifiable mesenchymal elements in addition to fibrous tissue.

Mesentery A double layer of peritoneum attaching various organs to body wall and conveying to them their blood vessels and nerves; commonly referred to peritoneal fold attaching small intestine to the posterior body wall (*see* Figure).

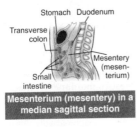

Mesenterium (mesentery) in a median sagittal section

Mesial Situated in, near, or towards the midline or apex of dental arch.

Mesna Uroepithelial protector.

Mesoappendix A triangular fold of peritoneum around the vermiform appendix, attaching the latter to posterior surface of the mesentery of the ileum. The artery to appendix runs along the free margin of this fold.

Mesocardium The double layer mesoderm attaching the embryonic heart to the wall of pericardial cavity.

Mesocephalic Denoting a skull having cephalic index between 75-80; intermediate between dolichocephalic and brachy cephalic.

Mesocolon The double layer of peritoneum attaching colon to posterior abdominal wall. Only the transverse colon and sigmoid colon have actual mesentery.

Mesocolopexy Surgical procedure in which the mesocolon is fixed or resuspended to prevent ptosis or torsion of transverse colon.

Mesocoloplication A surgical procedure of folding back the mesocolon on itself and stitching in place in order to restrict mobility of transverse colon.

Mesocord An umbilical cord, a segment of which is bound to placenta by an accessory fold.

Mesocortex The cerebral cortex of the cingulate and retrosplenial gyri that does not pass through a six layered developmental stage.

Mesoderm The middle of primary germ layers, in between outer ectoderm and inner entoderm. From this layer are derived the majority of skeletal system, the circulatory system, the musculature, the excretory system and most of the reproductive system in vertebrates.

Mesoduodenum A part of the primitive midline dorsal mesentery in relation to embryonic duodenum.

Mesoepididymis A fold of tunica vaginalis that connects the testis to the epididymis.

Mesogastrium That part of primitive dorsal mesentery which is related to developing stomach and becomes greater omentum.

Mesomorph A person having a body build with prominent musculature and heavy bony structure.

Mesonephroma Rare ovarian tumor believed to be formed from displaced mesonephric tissue.

Mesonephros An intermediate excretory organ of the embryo, it is replaced by permanent metanephros (kidney). While its ductal system is retained in male as epididymis and deferent duct and in female as tubules of epoöphoron. Also known as wolffian body.

Mesorchium A thick fold of peritoneum which connects the developing testis to the mesonephric fold in embryo. It contains testicular vessels and nerves.

Meso-ovarium It is that part of the broad ligament which encloses the ovary. It lies between the mesosalpinx and the mesometrium.

Mesosalpinx Part of the broad ligament investing the fallopian tube. It represents the upper free part of the broad ligament which is above its attachment to the uterus.

Mesorectum A short peritoneal fold investing the upper part of rectum and connecting it to sacrum.

Mesoridazine Antipsychotic agent.

Mesosalpinx The upper free portion of broad ligament investing the fallopian tube.

Mesosigmoidopexy Attaching the sigmoid mesocolon to anterior abdominal wall to prevent sigmoid volvulus or rectal prolapse.

Mesotendon The connective tissue fold of synovial membrane extending from a tendon to the wall of its synovial tendon sheath.

Mesothelioma A benign or malignant tumor arising from the mesothelial lining of one of the coelomic cavities, commonly pleura or peritoneum, consisting of epithelial and spindle cell elements.

Mesovarium A short thick peritoneal fold that attaches ovary to posterior layer of broad ligament and permits passage of blood vessels and nerves to ovary.

Messenger 1. The RNA that carries the information coded in DNA sequence to the site of protein biosynthesis where it specifies the order of amino-acid residues. 2. The mediator of an effect.

Mesterolone Anabolic and rogen.

Mestranol An estrogen used in preparation of oral contraceptive.

Mesurpine HCl A vasodilator and smooth muscle relaxant.

Meta Prefix means 1. changed in form, or position transformed, 2. after, behind, following 3. next to.

Metabiosis The dependence of an organism upon the preexistence of another for its development.

Metabolism A general term applied to chemical processes taking place in the living tissues for maintenance of life. *m. acid-base* The processes influencing hydrogen ion concentration in the body. *m. aerobic* Metabolic activity dependent upon oxygen. *m. intermediary* The chemical changes associated with the synthesis of cellular components from food materials and their degradation.

Metabolite A substance taking part in or produced by metabolic activity.

Metabutethamine Used in dentistry as a local anesthetic for nerve block/infiltration anesthesia.

Metacarpus The five bones of hand between the carpus and the phallanges (*see* Figure).

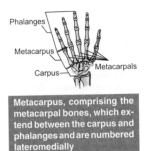

Phalanges

Metacarpus

Carpus

Metacarpals

Metacarpus, comprising the metacarpal bones, which extend between the carpus and phalanges and are numbered lateromedially

Metacentric Pertaining to chromosome with centromere in the middle.

Metachromasia 1. The property by which some cells stain in a colour different from the dye with which they are stained 2. The property through which a single dye stains different tissues in different colours.

Metachromatic Term applied to cells and dyes exhibiting metachromasia.

Metacercaria The encysted stage of a digenetic trematode which occurs in the tissues or on the surface of intermediate host such as snail. This stage is usually infective or is the transfer stage to definitive host.

Metacresol A local antiseptic.

Metacryptozoite A member of a second or subsequent generation of the extra erythrocytic, tissue dwelling malarial parasite; it develops from sporozoites.

Metacyesis Extrauterine pregnancy.

Meta female A female with 3 X chromosomes (trisomy X) usually short statured, mentally retarded and obese.

Metagonimus A genus of small flukes which may infect man upon eating fish containing the larvae.

Metakinesis The separation of two chromatids of a chromosome during the anaphase of mitosis.

Metal Any of the several chemical elements that share a group of characteristic properties, are good conductors of electricity, malleable and liberate cations. *m. heavy* Any metal 5 times or more heavier than water. *m. noble* Metal that cannot be oxidized by heat nor can be easily dissolved, e.g., gold, silver, platinum. *m. rare earth* Any metal with atomic no. 57 through 71.

Metaldehyde A polymer of acetaldehyde formerly used as an antiseptic.

Metalloenzyme An enzyme having a metal ion as an integral part of its active form, e.g., cytochrome (Fe^{2+}, Fe^{3+}). Cytochrome oxidase (Cu^{2+}, Cu^2) or alcohol dehydrogenase (Zn^{2+}).

Metalloprotein A protein with metal ion bound to it. Many enzymes are metalloproteins.

Metamale A male with one X chromosome but 2 Y chromosomes; usually tall, lean, often having tendency towards aggressive behavior.

Metamorphopsia Distortion of visual image as in parietal lobe disease, retinal lesion or intoxication.

Metamorphosis A change in form or structure as in the development of certain insects from larva to adult.

Metamyelocyte An immature granulocyte, an early stage of granulocyte derived from myelocyte with kidney shaped nucleus and finely granulated cytoplasm containing azurophilic granules.

Metanephrine One of the catabolic products of epinephrine excreted in urine.

Metanephros The permanent kidney in the human fetus,

formed caudal to mesonephros close to termination of cloaca. It is composed of metanephric duct (primitive ureter) and the metanephrogenic tissue.

Metaphase The second stage of cell division by mitosis during which the chromatids are aligned along the equatorial plate of cell and attached by spindle fibers to centromere.

Metaphysis The line of junction of epiphysis with diaphysis (shaft).

Metaplasia The abnormal transformation from one differentiated adult tissue to another type adult tissue within a given organ (*see* Figure).

Metaproterenol A potent beta-adrenergic stimulant used as bronchodilator.

Metarhodopsin An intermediate formed in retina from degradation of lumirhodopsin. It is unstable and degrades to scotopsin and transretinene.

Metarminol A compound with vasopressor activity used to treat acute hypotension.

Metastasis Transfer of a disease from its primary site to a distant location either by blood, lymphatic channel, CSF flow, etc (*see* Figure on page 466).

Metatarsus The anterior portion of foot between the toes and the instep. Composed of 5 cylindrical bones (*see* Figure on page 466).

Metathalamus That portion of thalamus composed of medial and lateral geniculate bodies.

Metathrombin A thrombin-antithrombin complex formed during clotting and is inactive.

Metaxalone Orally administered smooth muscle relaxant.

Metazoa A subkingdom of animals comprising all multicellular organisms having specialized cells producing a different type of tissue.

Metazoonosis A type of zoonosis requiring both a vertebrate

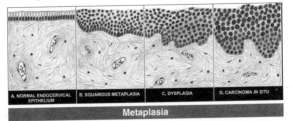

A, NORMAL ENDOCERVICAL EPITHELIUM   B, SQUAMOUS METAPLASIA   C, DYSPLASIA   D, CARCINOMA *IN SITU*

Metaplasia

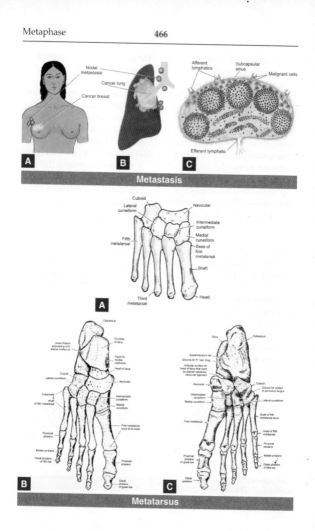

Metastasis

Metatarsus

and an invertebrate host stage in the lifecycle of causative organism.

Metencephalon The more rostral part of brain in embryo that develops into cerebellum and pons.

Meteorism Distention of intestine with gas.

Meter (m) Measure of length equal to 39.37 inches or 100 cm.

Met formin A structural analogue of phenformin, hypoglycemic agent.

Methacholine A derivative of acetyl choline with only muscarinic effect.

Methacycline A semisynthetic antibiotic of tetracyclic group given orally.

Methadone A synthetic narcotic analgesic with morphine like effect. It is used in opium withdrawal and as a maintenance treatment in heroin addicts.

Methallenestril A synthetic nonsteroidal estrogenic agent.

Methamphetamine A sympathomimetic amine similar to amphetamine; used as a CNS stimulant.

Methandriol Anabolic steroid.

Methandrostenolone A compound of methyl testosterone with anabolic and androgenic properties.

Methane CH_4. Marsh gas, the simplest hydrocarbon.

Methanol Methyl alcohol, prepared synthetically or from distillation of wood. Toxic and causes blindness when drunk.

Methantheline bromide An anticholinergic agent used to suppress gastric motility and secretion.

Methapyrilene Antihistaminic of medium potency and short duration; used as fumarate or hydrochloride.

Methaqualone A sedative and hypnotic, chronic use can lead to psychologic and physical dependence.

Metharbital A barbiturate used as anticonvulsant for grandmal, petitmal and myoclonic seizures.

Methazolamide An agent inhibiting carbonic anhydrase, hence used in glaucoma; given orally.

Methemalbumin A complex of plasma albumin with heme released from hemoglobin when there is intravascular hemolysis.

Methemoglobin A derivative of hemoglobin with oxidized iron, hence incapable of carrying oxygen.

Methemoglobinemia Methemoglobin greater than 1% of total hemoglobin in blood; therefore causing cyanosis.

Methenamine $C_6H_{12}N_4$ Used in treatment of infections of urinary tract because of its slow hydrolysis to formaldehyde. Hippurate and mandelate salts are in use.

Methetoin An analog of phenytoin used as oral anticonvulsant.

Methicillin sodium A semisynthetic derivative of penicillin given IM. in infections resistant to penicillin G.

Methimazole Potent, widely used antithyroid drug. It acts by interfering with incorporation of iodine.

Methiodal sodium Iodine containing contrast for urinary tract.

Methionine One of the essential amino acids, the main biologic donor of methyl groups for protein synthesis.

Methisazone A synthetic antiviral agent, not in use.

Methixene hydrochloride Anticholinergic agent used orally in gastrointestinal hypermotility and spasm.

Methocarbamol A muscle relaxant, given orally, IM and SC.

Method A set form or mode of procedure, a systemic way of performing an examination, test or operation.

Methohexital sodium Short acting barbiturate used IV like pentothal sodium.

Methotrexate A potent folic acid antagonist used as cytotoxic agent and immunosuppressant.

Methotrimeprazine A phenothiazine with potent analgesic properties used in obstetric analgesia, and as a preanesthetic medication.

Methoxamine An adrenergic vasopressor, often used in supraventricular tachycardia.

Methoxsalen A psoralen compound used in association with ultraviolet exposure to enhance repigmentation in vitiligo. It is also used to precipitate a phototoxic response in the treatment of psoriasis.

Methoxychlor An insecticide used to control mosquito larva and flies.

Methoxyflurane A colorless nonexplosive liquid used as a slow anesthetic.

Methoxyphenamine An adrenergic agent used as bronchodilator.

Methoxypromazine A phenothiazine tranquilizer.

Methscopolamine A quaternary derivative of scopolamine with anticholinergic actions; used as gastrointestinal sedative.

Methsuximide An anticonvulsant for petitmal and psychomotor epilepsy.

Methyclothiazide A thiazide antihypertensive diuretic.

Methylal Dimethoxymethane, anesthetic and hypnotic agent.

Methylchloride A refrigerant, used in spray form for local anesthesia, also same property by m. iodide. *m. methacrylate* An acrylic resin for dental use. *m. salicylate* An antipyretic, analgesic, used in pain killing ointments.

Methyl orange Used as an indicator with a pH range of 3.2-4.4 (yellow at 3.2 and pink at 4.4).

Methyl red Used as an indicator, red at 4.4 and yellow at 6.

Methylate To combine with methyl alcohol or the methyl radical.

Methyl benzenethonium chloride A topical anti-infective agent.

Methylcellulose A bulk forming cellulose derivative with laxative properties. Used for constipation, as appetite suppressant in management of obesity, and in ophthalmic solutions/ointment.

Methyl cholanthrene One of the carcinogenic polycyclic hydrocarbons of coaltar.

Methyldopa Sympathetic activity inhibitor used in treatment of hypertension.

Methylene blue Methyl thionine chloride, an aniline dye formerly used as urinary antiseptic; now used in treatment of methemoglobinemia, as an antidote for cyanide poisoning, as a staining agent for basophilic and metachromatic substances.

Methylene dioxyamphetamine (MDA) A hallucinogen commonly referred as the love drug.

Methylene green A synthetic metachromatic dye used to distinguish mast cell granules.

Methylergonovine maleate An oxytocic agent used to induce uterine contraction to reduce postpartum hemorrhage.

Methyl glucamine ditrizoate An organic compound used as a contrast medium in the making of X-ray transparencies.

Methyl malonic aciduria Elevation of methyl malonic acid in blood with excessive excretion in urine. Caused due to congenital enzymatic deficiency or B_{12} deficiency.

Methyl malony CoA Formed from propionyl CoA, helpful for utilization of fatty acids.

Methyl methacrylate Acrylic resin used to make denture bases, artificial teeth, crowns and restorations.

Methyl phenidate Mild psychomotor stimulant, used to treat hyperkinetic children, and narcolepsy.

Methyl prednisolone Methylated analog of prednisolone given orally as immunosuppressant.

Methyl salicylate A colorless oily liquid with strong odor used in perfumes and as counter irritants.

Methyl testosterone Orally given androgenic steroidal agent as a replacement therapy for androgen deficiency states.

Methyl tetrahydrofolic acid An intermediate subserving as a donor of methyl group to homocystine to form methionine.

Methyl violet Dye for staining amyloid.

Methyprylon A compound with sedative and hypnotic properties.

Methysergide A serotonin receptor antagonist used as vasoconstrictor in migraine.

Metitepine 5 HT antagonist.

Metmyoglobin Oxidized (Fe^{3+}) myoglobin.

Metocurine A derivative of tubocurarine which is more potent and longer acting.

Metolazone A diuretic acting on proximal and distal tubules.

Metoprolol A beta-adrenergic antagonist used in treatment of hypertension and angina pectoris.

Metorchis A genus of flukes in animals, occasionally transmitted to man.

Metrectomy Hysterectomy.

Metrifonate A drug effective against bladder flukes (*Schistostoma hematobium*).

Metritis Inflammation of uterus.

Metrizamide A nonionic radiographic contrast agent.

Metrizoate sodium A contrast medium for coronary angiography.

Metrizoic acid A compound used as contrast medium in diagnostic procedures.

Metrodynamometer Instrument used to measure the strength of uterine contractions.

Metronidazole A nitroimidazole compound used for treatment of amebiasis, trichomoniasis, anaerobic infections.

Metropathia hemorrhagica Excessive prolonged bleeding from uterus associated with cyst formation in the endometrium.

Metyrapone An inhibitor of adrenocortical steroid C-11 beta-hydroxylation, administered orally or IV as a diagnostic test to determine the capability of pituitary to increase production of corticotropin.

Mevalonic acid A product of methyl valeric acid produced in the pathway of biosynthesis of sterols.

Mevinolin HMG CoA reductase inhibitor used as lipid lowering agent.

Mexiletine Antiarrhythmic drug.

Micelle 1. A submicroscopic unit of a protoplasm. 2. A molecular aggregate as that of a colloid often formed by action of detergents on a hydrocarbon in water.

Miconazole Antifungal, topically used 2%.

Micrencephaly A condition in which the brain is abnormally small and underdeveloped.

Micro One millionth (10^{-6}); very small, minute.

Microabscess A small abscess usually less than a mm, often multiple. *m. of Munro* One of the characteristic lesions of psoriasis consisting of focal accumulation of polymorphonuclear leukocytes in the upper layer of epidermis. *m. Pautrier's* Focal collection of atypical T lymphocytes in the epidermis in mycosis fungoides.

Microadenoma A small (≤ 10 mm diameter) non-malignant glandular tumor, as associated with Cushing's disease.

Microaerophil An anaerobe that can tolerate low O_2 tension.

Microaerosol A suspension in the air of minute particles of 1-10 μ.

Microalbuminuria Excretion in urine of less than 100 μgm per minute of albumin.

Microanalysis Analysis using small amounts of material than classical methods of chemical analysis that involves weighing precipitated material.

Microaneurysm An aneurysmal dilatation affecting small arteries, arterioles and capillaries; a feature of diabetes mellitus, thrombotic thrombocytopenic purpura. Diabetic microaneurysms of retina with exudates and hemorrhages constitute characteristic features of diabetic retinopathy.

Microangiopathy A disease process affecting small blood vessels. *m. diabetic* Thickening of capillary basement membrane, in the retina, kidney, heart with microaneurysm formation.

Microbe A microorganism, a one-celled plant.

Microbiology Branch of science concerned with microorganisms subdivided into virology, bacteriology, mycology, protozoology and phycology.

Microcurie A unit of activity of radionuclides equal to 10^{-6} curie, $3.7 \geq 10^4$ becquerels.

Microcyte A small red blood cell at least 2 μ smaller than normal, as seen in iron deficiency.

Microcytosis Condition in which RBCs are abnormally small.

Microfilaria A prelarval or embryonic form of filarial worms.

Microgamete The smaller male element in the conjugation of cells of unequal size.

Microgametocyte The mother cell that produces microgametes.

Microgamy Conjugation between two young cells in certain protozoans.

Microglia The smallest neuroglial cell, the macrophage of brain and spinal cord that remove cellular debris in CNS.

Micrognathia Abnormal smallness of jaw, especially the lower jaw producing bird like profile.

Microgram Unit of weight equivalent to 10^{-6} gram.

Micrometer 1. One millionth of a meter. 2. An instrument containing a microscope for accurate linear measurement of very small units of length.

Micronutrient Any essential dietary constituent like vitamins and minerals required by body in small quantities.

Microorganism Any single celled organism.

Microphonics Electrical potentials generated in the cochlea by passage of sound waves.

Micropipette A pipette calibrated for accurate delivery of very small quantities less than 0.5 ml.

Micropore A submicroscopic break in the membrane of a protozoan cell or microbe through which exchange of materials, pinocytosis occur.

Microprobe An ultrafine probe used for exploration and fixation of tissues in microsurgical procedures.

Micropsia Perception of objects as smaller in comparison to their actual size. It occurs in retinal detachment, temporal lobe epilepsy, delirium and drug intoxication.

Microradiograph A recorded image obtained by microradiography, used in high resolution imaging of thin objects like tissue sections.

Microscope An optical instrument used for viewing magnified images of small objects. *m. electron* A microscope that uses electrons rather than visible light to irradiate clear magnified images; capable of magnifying objects having dimensions smaller than wavelength of light. *m. laser* A microscope in which laser beam is focussed on microscopic field, causing it to vaporize; the emitted radiation is analyzed by a microspectrophotometer. *m. operating* A microscope used in operating room for magnifying the surgical field. *m. phase contrast* A microscope that makes use of the relationship between two paths of light 1. light that enters microscope objective through the specimen and 2. light that enters objective after being diffracted by the specimens; all points of divergence between these two paths of light reveal a specimen or object whose lack of contrast would make it invisible under other types of illumination. *m. polarizing* A microscope especially equipped to polarized light and to examine the alterations of polarized light by the specimen, useful in identification of crystals. *m. electron scanning* A microscope where specimen is examined point by point by an electron beam and an image is formed on television screen from the secondary electrons given off the surface. *m. ultraviolet* A microscope whose energy source is electromagnetic radiation with a wavelength of 180-400 nm. *m. X-ray* A microscope which uses a beam of X-ray instead of light with the image usually being recorded on photographic film.

Microscopic Extremely small.

Microscopy The study of objects using a microscope.

Microsecond One millionth of a second.

Microsection A thin slice of tissue prepared for examination under a microscope.

Microsome A fragment of endoplasmic reticulum with associated ribosomes.

Microspectrography Study of composition of an object, especially of cellular constituents using a spectroscope. That makes a photographic record of the spectrum.

Microspectrophotometer An instrument used to measure the absorption, reflection or emission of light by objects under a microscope, especially used for spectral analysis of individual cells.

Microstomia Disproportionately small oral orifice.

Microtia Abnormally small auricle or pina.

Microtome A mechanical device used for preparing histologic sections for microscopic examinations; can be m. freezing or m. rotary.

Microtomography A technique for rotating a small sample in an electron microscope through 90°, processing the data by computer and displaying three dimensional images.

Microtonometer An instrument for measuring the partial pressure of gases in minute quantities of material.

Microtubule A small, hollow, cylindrical structure found in the cell cytoplasm. During cell division they increase greatly in number to form the mitotic spindle, play an important role in intracellular movements and in maintaining shape of the cell.

Microvilli Submicroscopic finger like projections on the surface of cell membrane which greatly increase the surface area.

Microvolt One millionth of a volt, 10^{-6} volt.

Microwave Any electromagnetic radiation having a very short wavelength between 1 mm and 30 cm. wavelength 1 mm are in infrared region and that beyond 30 cm. are radio waves. Sources of emission include radar, cathode ray tubes, induction furnaces, and electrotherapy devices. Microwave exposure can cause cataract.

Micturition The act of urination.

Midazolam A benzodiazepine.

Midbrain The part of brain developing from embryonic mesencephalon, divided into three parts; tectum (quadrigeminal plate), tegmentum (cephalic continuation of pontine tegmentum) and the crus cerebri.

Middle lobe syndrome A form of chronic atelectasis marked by collapse of middle lobe of the lung resulting from compression of bronchus by enlarged lymph nodes/ tumor. Symptoms include chronic cough and recurrent respiratory infections. *SYN*— Brock's syndrome.

Midfoot The middle portion of foot consisting of navicular, cuboid and cuneiform bones.

Midgut 1. The small intestine comprising jejunum and ileum. 2. The middle segment of embryonic intestine, precursor of stomach to transverse colon.

Midpelvis The area of pelvis extending from the posterior inferior aspect of symphysis in a line through ischial spines to sacrum intersecting it at S_2 or S_3 vertebra.

Midwife A woman who attends women during delivery.

Midwifery Practical obstetrics.

Mifepristone Progestine antagonist.

Miglitol Alphaglucosidase inhibitor for diabetes.

Migraine A recurrent hemicranial intense headache associated with nausea, vomiting and visual disturbances. *m. abdominal* Episodic abdominal pain, nausea, vomiting in migraine sufferers. *m. complicated* An attack of migraine accompanied by prolonged aphasia, hemiplegia, hemianopia, epilepsy, etc. *m. hemiplegic* Migraine in which recurrent attacks of hemiplegia occur. *m. ophthalmoplegic* Oculomotor palsy occurring during an attack of migraine. *migraine equivalent* Symptoms produced by migraine like mechanism but without an associated headache e.g., transient partial loss of vision.

Mikulicz's disease Benign bilateral swelling of the lacrimal and salivary glands associated with dryness of mouth and reduced, lacrimation, identical to Sjögren's syndrome.

Mikulicz's drain A procedure used in emergency medicine as a last resort to control bleeding while all the other methods fail.

Mikulicz's syndrome Painless bilateral enlargement of salivary and lacrimal glands with dryness of mouth and decreased lacrimation as in sarcoidosis.

Miliaria Skin eruption due to retention of sweat in sweat follicles. *SYN*—sweat fever, summer eruption; can be m. papulasa, profunda, rubra and even pustular types.

Miliary Of the size of a millet (2 mm diameter).

Milieu Environment, surroundings.

Milium A minute whitish or yellowish papule on the skin caused by retention of fatty material (sebum) or densely packed keratin.

Milk The secretion of mammary glands. *m. witch's* A few drops of milk expressed from newborn's nipple during first few days of life.

Milk alkali syndrome Hypercalcemia without hypercalciuria or hypophosphaturia induced by prolonged ingestion of large quantity of milk and soluble alkali as in therapy of peptic ulcer.

Milking A manual or mechanical technique for removing fluid from body part.

Milkman's syndrome Osteoporosis with multiple fractures as seen in postmenopausal women.

Milk teeth Deciduous teeth.

Millard-Gubler syndrome Paralysis of facial muscles on one side and extremities on opposite side by brainstem lesions.

Millicurie A measure of radioactivity; one thousandth of a curie.

Milliequivalent A quantity equal to 10^{-3} of the equivalent weight of an element or compound.

Milligram One thousandth of a gram.

Milligray A unit of absorbed dose in the field of ionizing radiation equal to 10^{-3} gray.

Millimeter One thousandth of a meter.

Millimicrogram One billionth of a gram, biller called a nano gram.

Milliosmole One thousandth of an osmole; the osmotic pressure exerted by the concentration of a substance in solution; expressed as milligrams per kilogram divided by atomic weight for an ionized substance or divided by molecular weight for nonionized solute. Normal plasma osmolality is 280-300 mOsm/kg.

Millirad A unit of absorbed dose of ionizing radiation equivalent to 10^{-3} rad, 10^{-5} gray.

Millirem A unit of radiation dose equivalent to 10^{-3} rem 10^{-5} joule/kg, 10^{-5} silvert.

Milliroentgen A unit of ionization exposure equal to 10^{-3} roentgen; $2.58 \geq 10^{-7}$ coulomb/kg.

Milrinone Sympathomimetic, cardiac stimulant.

Milroy's disease Familial and congenital swelling of subcutaneous tissues usually confined to extremities with large accumulation of lymph.

Mimesis State in which one disease presents the symptoms of another.

Mimetic Of or relating to mimesis.

Mimicry The imitation of one species by another in an adaptation tending to improve its chances of survival.

Minaserine 5HT antagonist, antidepressant.

Mind The organized total of psychological processes and

contents that allow the individual to respond to external and internal stimuli in an integrated and dynamic way, relating response of present to both past and future of the individual. The principal processes of mind are perceiving, learning, thinking, remembering, feeling and behaving with intelligence.

Mineral Any naturally occurring homogeneous inorganic substance, having a characteristic crystalline structure and chemical composition.

Mineral corticoid One of the steroids in the adrenal cortex that act principally on renal retention of sodium and excretion of potassium e.g., aldosterone.

Mineralization The conversion of organic material to inorganic material.

Minim A unit of fluid measure; about a drop or 1/60th of a dram.

Minimal brain dysfunction syndrome A complex of symptoms that involve impairment of some or all of the following functions: language, perception, memory, concentration, and motor functions.

Minimal change disease A form of nephrotic syndrome in which minimal or no glomerular abnormalities are noted by light microscopy but fusion of foot processes of podocytes in electron microscopy.

Minocycline A semisynthetic antibiotic of tetracycline group used for acne.

Minoxidil Vasodilator; used for alopecia locally as 2% solution.

Miopus Unequal conjoined twins united at head in such fashion that face of one member is rudimentary.

Miosis Marked constriction of pupils, can be spastic or paralytic.

Miotic Any agent causing miosis.

Miracidium A free swimming ciliated larva of a trematode that penetrates a small intermediate host where it develops into a sporocyst.

Mirror A polished surface that forms optical images by reflection. *m. head* A concave mirror worn on a headband or spectacle frame used for focussing a beam of light. *m. laryngeal* A circular plane mirror used to examine the interior of larynx and hypopharynx.

Mirtazapine Antidepressant.

Miscarriage Spontaneous abortion.

Miscarry To give birth to a nonviable fetus.

Misce Mix, a direction given in pharmacy.

Miscible Capable of being mixed.

Misdiagnosis Wrong diagnosis.

Misogyny Hatred of women.

Misophobia Abnormal fear of contamination.

Mistura Mixture; used in pharmacy.

Mite Any of various minute arachnids that are often parasitic on man and animals; they may infest food and propagate disease.

Mithramycin An antineoplastic antibiotic given IV in testicular malignancy and hypercalcemia.

Miticide An agent for killing mite.

Mitigate To make or become milder.

Mitochondria A double membrane cytoplasmic organelle, self reproducing, present in cell cytoplasm of all living cells; responsible for energy production (ATP), Each cell has several hundreds of mitochondria, each of 15.00 Å length.

Mitogen Agent promoting cell mitosis and lymphocyte transformation.

Mitogenesis The induction of mitosis in a cell.

Mitomycin A group of antibiotic substances produced by species of streptomyces and differentiated as mitomycin A, B, and C. Mitomycin C inhibits cell division by blocking the cross linking of DNA strands; hence used as antineoplastic agent in lymphomas and solid tumors.

Mitosis Multiplication or division of a cell that results in formation of two daughter cells normally receiving the same chromosome and DNA as that of original cell (*see* Figure on page 479).

Mitoxantrone Antineoplastic agent.

Mitotane Antineoplastic agent.

Mitral Left atrioventricular valve.

Mitralization Straightening of left cardiac border due to enlarged left atrial appendage and pulmonary artery in mitral stenosis.

Mittelschmerz Intermenstrual pain specially at the time of ovulation.

Mixture 1. An aggregation of two or more substances that are not chemically combined. 2. A pharmaceutical preparation consisting of an insoluble substance suspended in a liquid by viscid material such as sugar, glycerol etc.

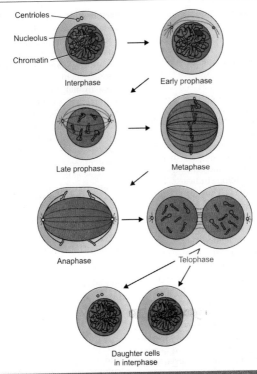

Mitosis shown as occurring in a cell of a hypothetical animal with a diploid chromosome number of six (haploid number three); one pair of chromosomes is short, one pair is long and hooked, and one pair is long and knobbed

Mizolastine Anti allergic agent.

M. mode A motion B mode tracing of ultrasound to visualize moving structures.

Mnemonic The use or devising of techniques to facilitate memory.

MNS blood groups A system of erythrocyte antigen determined by the allelic genes, MN and S; the grouping is primarily used to solve identification problems such as disputed paternity and genetic linkage, population studies.

Mobility The capacity for movement. *m. electrophoretic* The velocity at which ions of a substance migrate in an electric field.

Mobilization A process or an operation whereby an object or a substance is freed or made mobile. *m. stapes* The transmeatal operative mobilization of the stapes as ankylosed in otosclerosis, thereby restoring hearing loss.

Mobius sign Convergence weakness of eyes occurring in exophthalmic goiter.

Mobius syndrome A congenital disorder characterized by bilateral paralysis of both external recti and hypotrophy of facial musculature due to agenesis of ganglion cells in the brainstem of occulomotor and facial nerve nuclei.

Moclobemide Antidepressant.

Modality 1. Any of the several forms of therapy. 2. Any of the main forms of sensation.

Modafinil Wakefullness promoting agent.

Mode In statistics, the value occurring most often.

Modiolus The central pillar or column of bone around which the spiral canals of cochlea turn.

Modulation The changes that take place in response to changes in the environment.

Moiety One of two, more or less equal parts. One of two or more main components, such as the groups of atoms in a complex molecule.

Molality The amount of substance of a solute divided by mass of the solvent; expressed in mole per kg.

Molar Any of the most posterior teeth in jaw.

Molarity The concentration of a substance expressed in moles per liter.

Mold 1. Any fungus having a cottony appearance, usually growing on decaying material. 2. A receptacle for shaping any cast material. 3. to shape.

Molding 1. The process of shaping. 2. The changes in shape of the fetal head as it passes through the birth canal (*see* Figure on page 481).

Fetal head molding

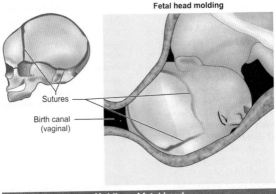

Sutures

Birth canal
(vaginal)

Molding of fetal head

Mole 1. Intrauterine mass.
2. Pigmented cellular nevus;
circumscribed pigmented
growth on skin. 3. Gram
molecule. *m. carneous* A spontaneous abortion in which
the ovum is surrounded by
a capsule of clotted blood.
m. hydatidiform A developmental anomaly of placenta
consisting of a nonmalignant
mass of clear vesicles resembling bunch of grapes formed
from cystic swellings of chorionic villi. The moles may
cause uterine enlargement
disproportionate to period of
gestation (*see* Figure).

Molecular Relating to or consisting of molecules.

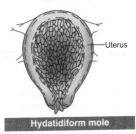

Uterus

Hydatidiform mole

Molecular weight The sum of
the atomic weights of all the
atoms making up a molecule.

Molecule The smallest unit of
a substance which can exist
in a free state and still retain
the chemical properties of the
substance.

Molindone Antipsychotic agent.

Molluscum A skin disease marked by the presence of soft rounded tumors. *m. contagiosum* An infectious disease of skin marked by small wart like lesions containing a substance resembling curd, usually of viral etiology.

Molt To cast off.

Molybdenum Element No. 42, a silvery white hard metal required for many animal enzyme function.

Moment of death That point in time when an individual is declared dead. This determination is based on criteria which are defined by law and which differ according to situation. For autopsy and burial purposes, criteria include the clinical judgement that respiration and circulation have ceased and rigor mortis has started. For organ transplantation brain death is employed even though functional circulatory and respiratory activities may persist.

Momentum The product of mass and velocity of a body, an index of quantity of motion.

Mometasone A steroid for topical use.

Momism The state of being excessively dependent on or subordinate to one's mother.

Monoamine oxidase inhibitors A group of drugs for treatment of depression.

Monarthritis Arthritis of single joint.

Monday disease The return of symptoms after a weekend away from work, as in the case of an allergic reaction to a substance encountered while at work.

Mondor's disease Inflammation of the subcutaneous veins of the chest and breast, usually extending from epigastric region to the axilla and occurring in both sexes.

Mongolism Down syndrome due to trisomy 21.

Mongoloid Having characteristics or resembling mongolism.

Monilethrix Beaded hair, an anomalous condition in which the hair shaft exhibits nodosities or points of thickening alternating with normal or constricted areas.

Monilia A genus of molds or fungi, commonly known as fruit molds, now called candida.

Moniliasis Infection with any fungus of genus *Monilia*.

Moniliform Having the shape of a necklace.

Monitor 1. To keep close watch over. 2. An apparatus used to record or display data.

m. apnea An alarm system for alarming attendants to the occurrence of apnea commonly in a premature infant. *m. cardiac* Continuous display of cardiac rhythm in a screen to detect irregularities in the heart rhythm. *m. electronic fetal* An electronic instrument monitoring fetal heart rate and patterns of uterine contraction.

Monkey rhesus Macaca mulatta widely distributed in India and China; easily raised in captivity, hence amply used in medical and biological research.

Monoamine Compound containing only one amine group. *m. oxidase* An enzyme that catalyzes the oxidation of a wide variety of physiologic amines into aldehydes and ammonia. It is important for catabolism of epinephrine and tyramine.

Monobenzene The monobenzyl ether of hydroquinone used as ointment to cause hypopigmentation in the treatment of hyperpigmentation.

Monoblast An immature cell of monocytic series, 18-22 μ in diameter, having many nucleoli, formed primarily in spleen and lymphoid tissue.

Monochromatic Having one colour.

Monoclonal antibody A group of antibodies of high purity made by hybridoma technology, used for identification of infectious organisms and hormones.

Monocrotic Forming a smooth single crest on the downward line of a curve, e.g. pulse.

Monocular Relating to, having, or used by one eye.

Monocyte A large mononucleated white blood cell 15-25 μ with a round kidney shaped or lobulated nucleus and gray-blue cytoplasm. It is the largest cell in blood film and on leaving blood it becomes macrophage.

Monocytosis Abnormal increase in number of monocytes in blood.

Monograph A detailed written account of one particular subject or a small area of a special field of learning.

Monohybrid A cross between parents that differ in one character.

Monoiodotyrosine (MIT) An amino acid formed by iodination of tyrosine at C_3, the first step in production of thyroxin.

Monokine A hormone like factor produced by activation of monocytes; acts as an intercellular messenger to regulate immunologic and inflammatory responses.

Monomania Pathologic preoccupation with only one idea.

Monomer A single unit or molecule which can polymerize with similar units to form a chain or polymer.

Monomorphic Having but one shape, unchangeable in size and form.

Mononeuritis Inflammation or degeneration of a single nerve trunk or some of its branches. *m. multiplex* Neuritis involving single nerves at several distant sites, usually vascular origin (PAN).

Mononuclear Unicellular.

Mononucleosis EB virus infection marked by fever, sore throat, splenomegaly, lymphadenopathy and peripheral atypical lymphocytosis. *SYN*—kissing disease; similar symptoms also occur in post- transfusion patients.

Monophasia Disorder in which the individual's vocabulary is limited to a single word or sentence.

Monoplegia Paralysis of one limb.

Monorchid An individual with only one testis.

Monosaccharide A carbohydrate which cannot be further broken down, simple sugar.

Mono sodium glutamate (MSG) The sodium salt of glutamic acid with one sodium ion per molecule used as a food flavoring agent, causative agent for chinese restaurant syndrome.

Monosome A chromosome without its homologous chromosome.

Monosomy Condition in which one chromosome of a pair of homologous chromosomes is missing.

Monoxide An oxide containing only one oxygen atom.

Monozygotic Denoting identical twins, or twins formed by division into two of the embryo derived from a single fertilized egg.

Mons In anatomy, a slight prominence, or elevation. *m. pubis* The fleshy prominence formed by a pad of fatty tissue over the symphysis pubis in female.

Monster A congenitally severely deformed individual.

Montelukast Leukotriene antogonist for asthma.

Montgomery strap A band of adhesive tape featuring a lace-up design, used to secure dressings that must be changed frequently (*see* Figure on page 485).

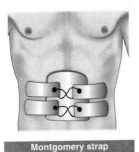

Montgomery strap

Mood A prevailing emotional state of mind.

Moraxella Short, aerobic, gram- negative bacteria.

Morbid Diseased, pathologic, pertaining to or affected by disease.

Morbidity The condition of being diseased; within a given population, the number of sick persons or cases of disease recorded as of a stated point in time or over a stated period. Thus, morbidity can be expressed as the number of new cases arising (incidence) or the number of cases existing whether old or new (prevalence).

Morbilliform Resembling the skin eruption of measles.

Morbus Latin for disease.

Morgan (m) The unit of map distance on a chromosome.

Morgue A place where dead bodies are kept pending identification, autopsy or burial/cremation.

Moribund Dying; Close to death.

Moro reflex An infantile reflex where striking infant's bed abduction and extension of arms.

Morphea A circumscribed form of scleroderma presenting as a central atrophic lesion with a pigmented border occurring chiefly on the chest, face or neck.

Morphine The principal alkaloid of opium; white, crystaline, insoluble in water, alcohol and ether; potent narcotic analgesic, can cause respiratory depression. Repeated use causes physical dependence and addiction. Used as morphine sulfate or tartarate.

Morphogenesis The embryonic differentiation of cells leading to formation of characteristic structure or form of the organism or its parts.

Morphologic Relating to structure or form of organism.

Morphology 1. The study of configuration or structure of living organism. 2. The form or structure of an organism.

Morquio's syndrome A form of mucopolysaccharidosis characterized by dwarfism, knock knee, pectus carinatum, flat vertebra, corneal clouding, deformed wrist and hands. There is excess excretion of keratin sulfate in urine and the disease is autosomal recessive, also called mucopolysaccharidosis IV.

Morrhuate sodium The oily salt used as sclerosing agent and is injected into veins.

Mortal Subject to death, deadly.

Mortality The quality of being mortal. The death rate. *m. neonatal* Death during first month or four weeks of life. *m. perinatal* The combined mortality from stillbirths and deaths in first week of life.

Mortar A small receptacle in which substances are crushed or pulverized with a pestle.

Mortification Gangrene or necrosis, death of a part.

Mortuary A funeral home where bodies of deceased are prepared for cremation *SYN*—morgue.

Morula A cluster of cleaving blastomeres resulting from early division of zygote; a stage in the development of the embryo prior to the blastula.

Morulus The lesion characteristic of yaws, resembling a mulberry or raspberry.

Mosaic 1. In genetics an individual whose cells consist of at least two geno typically distinct populations that arose after fertilization through somatic mutation or somatic nondisjunction.

Mosapride GI prokinetic agent.

Mosquito Blood sucking winged insects of family culicidae, responsible for transmission of malaria, dengue etc.

Mother surrogate One who replaces an individual's mother in emotional feelings. A mother who bears offspring of another.

Motile Having capacity to move spontaneously.

Motion sickness A condition marked by nausea, dizziness, and often vomiting and headache, induced by some movement as in travel by aeroplane, train, bus or ship.

Motilin A gastrointestinal peptide of 22 amino acids located in enterochromaffin cells, chiefly of duodenum and upper jejunum that stimulates gastric and colonic motility.

Motility The capacity for spontaneous movement. *m. segmental* Regularly spaced ring like contractions of small intestine.

Motivation An incentive to act or the reason for an attitude;

an inner state of a person that serves to arouse, maintain and guide behavior towards a goal.

Motor 1. Carrying or transmitting an impulse to a peripheral effector organ of the nervous system, either to elicit a response or to inhibit it. 2. Producing movement.

Mottling 1. A condition marked by spotty coloration. 2. Macular lesions of varying shades and hues.

Moulage The making of a mold of a bodily structure, especially for identification, prosthetics and teaching models.

Mount To prepare slides of tissues for microscopic examination.

Mounting A dental laboratory procedure in which a maxillary or mandibular cast is attached to an articulator.

Mouse pleural A round soft tissue density seen in chest X-ray representing a fibrin body in the pleural space.

Mouth The body opening through which one takes food. *m. tapir* The characteristic pouting appearance of lips seen in facioscapulo humoral muscular dystrophy.

Mouth trench Necrotizing ulcerative gingivitis.

Mouthwash A solution for rinsing the mouth, having antibacterial, astringent or deodorant properties.

Movement 1. Change of place or position. 2. The act of defecation. *m. ameboid* Locomotion of cells like leukocytes or amebas resulting from protoplasmic streaming into pseudopodia. *m. brownian* Erratic motion of microscopic particles suspended in a liquid or gas resulting from collision with molecules in the suspending medium. *m. dystonic* Slow and often bizarre involuntary movement with alteration of posture. *m. conjugate* (of eyes) Movement of both eyes in one direction. *m. involuntary* Involuntary contraction of one or more muscle groups producing movement of a limb or body part e.g. tremor, chorea, athetosis, tics, myoclonus, dystonia and hemiballismus.

Moxa A small mass of combustible material placed near the skin and ignited to produce counter irritation.

Moxalactam A cephalosporin group antibiotic.

Moxibustion Counter irritation by means of a moxa.

Moxifloxacin A quinolone antibiotic.

Muciferous Secreting or producing mucus.

Mucilage In pharmacology, a thick viscous liquid, a water solution of the mucilaginous principles of certain vegetable substances.

Mucin A substance secreted by mucous membranes containing mucopolysaccharide which raises the viscosity of medium around it.

Mucinase Any of several enzymes that breakdown the mucin or glycosaminoglycan.

Mucinosis An abnormal accumulation of mucopolysaccharides in the skin.

Mucocele 1. An intrasinus cyst arising from mucosal lining. 2. An enlarged cavity containing mucus. 3. Mucus polyp.

Mucoclasis The surgical removal or destruction of the inner lining of any hollow organ.

Mucocyte An amorphous extracellular basophillic metachromatic mass averaging 100μ found in white matter of normal and abnormal brains; probably artifactual, derived from precipitation of myelin during tissue fixation.

Mucocutaneous lymph node syndrome (Kawasaki disease) Condition affecting mainly infants and young children; marked by fever, conjunctivitis, reddening of oral cavity and lips, cervical lymphadenopathy, peeling of hands and feet. Coronary arteritis with infarction is a complication and aneurysms in coronary circulation may occur.

Mucoenteritis Inflammation of intestinal mucous membrane.

Mucoid Resembling mucus.

Mucolipidosis Any inborn error of metobolism that has characteristics of both mucopolysaccharidosis and sphyngolipidosis. 4 distinct types of disease known and are autosomal recessive.

Mucopolysaccharidase Enzyme that catalyzes hydrolysis of polysaccharides.

Mucopolysaccharide Polysaccharide that forms chemical bonds with water. It is thick, gelatinous and forms intercellular ground substance. It is found in mucous secretions and synovial fluid. *SYN*—Glycosaminoglycan.

Mucopolysaccharidosis (MPS) A group of inherited disorders with accumulation of mucopolysaccharides in reticuloendothelial system, intimal smooth muscle cells and fibroblasts within body; manifesting with coarse facies, mental retardation, corneal clouding, skeletal dysplasia, joint stiffness, etc. *MPS IH* is known as Hurler syndrome. It is due to deficiency of the enzyme alpha-L-iduronidase with accumulation of heparan sulphate and dermatan sulphate. *MPS IS* Scheie's syndrome. It is a variant of *MPS IH* but without mental retardation. *MPS IHS* It is intermediate between MPSIH and MPSIS. *MPS II* Hunter syndrome. It is due to deficiency of L-iduronosulphate sulphatase. Unlike *MPS IH* there is no corneal clouding. *MPS III* Sanfilippo syndrome. Corneal clouding is absent and skeletal growth is normal. *MPS IV* Morquio's syndrome The deficient enzyme is N-acetyl galactosamine-6-sulphatase. Distinguishing features, are dwarfism, kyphoscoliosis, cardiac lesions and joint hypermobility. *MPS VI* Maroteaux-Lamy syndrome. Deficient enzyme is N-acetyl galactosamine-4-sulphatase. Clinically it is similar to *MPS IH* but there is no mental retardation. *MPS VII* The deficient enzyme is beta-glucoronidase.

Mucoprotein A complex of protein and mucopolysac-charide. *m Tamm-Horsfall* It is secreted in renal tubules (not from plasma) and is contained in most urinary casts.

Mucor A genus of fungi seen on dead or decaying matter; often causes infection of external ear, skin and respiratory passage.

Mucosa A mucous membrane with epithelial lining, basement membrane, and often lamina propria. It may contain goblet cells, may be keratinized and the covering epithelium may be stratified squamous, columnar or pseudostratified columnar depending upon location.

Mucositis Inflammation of mucous membrane.

Mucoviscidosis *SYN*—cystic fibrosis.

Mucus A viscid secretion containing mucin, leukocytes, epithelial cells, etc. secreted by mucous membrane.

Multi Prefix indicating many or much.

Multigravida A woman who has been pregnant two or more times. *SYN*—*multipara.*

Multiple endocrine neoplasia (MEN) An inherited disease involving hyperplasia/malignancy of multiple endocrine glands. **MEN I** *SYN*—*Wermer's Syndrome* Tumors of parathyroids, pancreatic islets and adrenal cortex.

MEN II Pheochromocytoma, parathyroid hyperplasia, medullary carcinoma thyroid.

Multiple personality Condition in which the subject may develop more than one personality.

Multiple sclerosis (MS) An autoimmune demyelinating disorder due to decrease in suppressor T lymphocyte function, manifesting with visual loss, gait disorder, motor dysfunction and bladder bowel disturbance. Multiple sites of involvement in brain and spinal cord common.

Mummification Drying and shrivelling of body; mortification producing a dry hard mass.

Mumps A febrile viral disease characterized by inflammation of salivary and parotid glands.

Munchausen syndrome A psychiatric disorder in which patient feigns illness by self-mutilation.

Mupirocin Broad spectrum topical antibacterial.

Muramidase *SYN*—lysozyme. An enzyme richly present in leukocytes. Level increased in leukemias.

Murmur A soft blowing or rasping sound heard during cardiac auscultation; pro-duced due to excess blood flow through normal valves or normal flow through diseased valves. *m. Austin Flint* A mid or late mitral diastolic murmur heard in aortic regurgitation due to partial closure of mitral valve due to aortic regurgitant jet. *m. Carey Coomb* Diastolic murmur of mitral valvulitis in rheumatic fever. *m. Durozeiz* Systolic and diastolic murmurs heard over femoral artery in aortic insufficiency. *m. Graham Steell's* Early diastolic murmur of pulmonary insufficiency in pulmonary hypertension.

Murphy's sign Pain and catch in right hypochondrium to pressure during deep inspiration in acute cholecystitis.

Musca domestica The common house fly transmitting cholera, typhoid, amebic/bacillary dysentery, and other diseases.

Muscae volitantes Black floaters in visual field due to vitreous opacities.

Muscarine A toxic poison found in fungi.

Muscle Contractile tissue of mesodermal origin with properties like irritability, conductivity, and elasticity. Can be smooth, striated and cardiac. Smooth muscles (involuntary muscle) are found to line GI tract, bronchi, urinary and genital ducts, gallbladder, urinary bladder. The cells are fusiform or spindle-shaped with one central nucleus. Striated (skeletal) muscles are under conscious control. The muscle fibers are grouped into bundles called fasciculi and each cell or fiber has multiple nuclei. Denervation causes complete paralysis of striated muscle but not of cardiac or smooth muscle (*see* Figure).

Muscle cramp Painful contraction of muscle, idiopathic or due to electrolyte imbalance.

Mushbite Making a dental impression by asking the patient to bite into a soft wax.

Mushroom Umbrella-shaped fungus growing on decaying material.

Musset's sign Nodding movement of head synchronous with ventricular contraction as in gross aortic incompetence.

Mussitation The muttering of delirium or moving of the lips without production of sound.

Mustard Powder of mustard seeds used as counter-irritant, rubefacient, emetic, stimulant, and condiment.

Mutagen Any agent that causes gene mutation, e.g. ionizing radiation.

Mutant A variant of genetic structure.

Mutase Enzyme that accelerates oxidation-reduction reactions.

Mutation Change in genetic structure; can be natural or induced by drugs, chemicals and radiation.

Mutilation Destruction, maiming.

Mutism Unable to speak. *m. akinetic* Condition in which patient can neither speak nor can move body parts.

Myalgia Pain in the muscles often with tenderness.

Myasis Infestation with larva of flies or maggots.

Myasthenia Weakness of muscles. *m. gravis* An autoimmune disease with extreme muscle weakness due to presence of acetyl choline receptor antibodies.

Mycetes The fungi.

Mycetoma A suppurative condition due to actinomycetes and fungi.

Mycobacterium A genus of acid fast organism causing leprosy and tuberculosis. They are Gram-positive, nonsporeforming and nonmotile rods. *m. atypical* Forms of mycobacteria causing mild but resistant form of tuberculosis in man. They are *M. avium-intracellulare, M. kansasii, M. chelonei, M. marinum, M. xenopi*, etc.

Mycology Science of fungi.

Mycoplasma Organisms in between bacteria and viruses, responsible for atypical pneumonia, urethritis; common forms are – *M. hominis, M. orale, M. salivarium*.

Mycosis fungoides A malignant disease of RE system of skin, with intense itching and lymph node and internal organ involvement.

Mydriasis Dilatation of pupils.

Mydriatic Drug/agent causing pupillary dilatation, e.g. atropine, belladona.

Myelencephalon The embryonic hindbrain giving rise to medulla oblongata.

Myelin The complex lipid-protein sheath around axons in nervous system.

Myelinosis Fatty degeneration during which myelin is produced.

Myelitis Inflammation of spinal cord.

Myeloblast Immature white cell precursor of marrow from which develop myelocytes and eventually granulocytes.

Myelocele Protrusion of spinal cord through a defect in spinal arch—usually spina bifida.

Myelocyte A leukocyte precursor in bone marrow.

Myelofibrosis A condition where bone marrow is replaced by fibrous tissue.

Myelogram 1. X-ray of spinal canal after injection of radiopaque material into spinal subarachnoid space. 2. Differential count of bone marrow cells.

Myelolysis Dissolution of myelin.

Myeloma A tumor originating from marrow element. *m. multiple* A plasma cell tumor with multiple lytic bone lesions and increased paraprotein in blood and urine (*see* Figure).

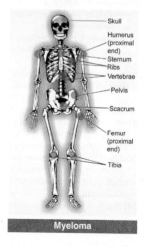

Skull
Humerus (proximal end)
Sternum
Ribs
Vertebrae
Pelvis
Scacrum
Femur (proximal end)
Tibia

Myeloma

Myelomalacia Abnormal softening of spinal cord.

Myelomeningocele A condition where spinal cord along with meningeal covering protrudes through the spinal defect. (*see* Figure)

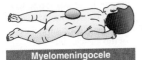

Myelomeningocele

Myelopathy Any pathological condition of spinal cord.

Myelopoiesis Development of bone marrow.

Myeloproliferative Concerning proliferation of bone marrow elements.

Myenteric reflex Intestinal contraction above and relaxation below the point of stimulatioin.

Myerson's sign Inability to stop blinking on tapping the forehead as in Parkinson's disease.

Myoblast Embryonic cell developing into muscle fiber.

Myocardial infarction Death of myocardium usually due to coronary thrombosis or spasm (*see* Figure).

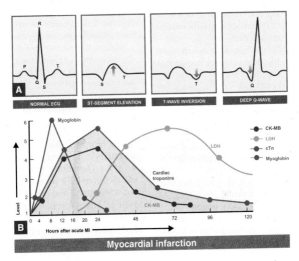

Myocardial infarction

Myocarditis Inflammation of myocardium, mostly viral, due to coxsackie group of viruses.

Myocyte A muscle cell.

Myodynamometer Device for determining muscle strength.

Myoepithelial cells Spindle-shaped contractile cells found between glandular elements and basement membrane of sweat, mammary and salivary glands.

Myoepithelium Tissue containing contractile epithelial cells.

Myofilament Electron microscopic picture of muscle showing thick *myosin* and thin *actin* filaments, essential for muscle contraction.

Myoglobin The respiratory pigment in muscle tissue that serves as oxygen carrier.

Myograph Instrument for graphic recording of muscle contraction.

Myoma A tumor containing muscle tissue.

Myonectomy Removal of myomatous tumor, generally of uterus.

Myometrium The muscular layer of uterus.

Myopathy Any disease or abnormal condition of striated muscle; may be an acquired or hereditary.

Myope One suffering from myopia or short sightedness.

Myopia Short sightedness, the parallel rays passing through optical axis are focussed in front of retina. Can be axial (elongation of eyeball), curvature or lenticular types. Corrected by use of minus lens.

Myoplasm The contractile part of the muscle cell.

Myorrhaphy Suture of a muscle wound.

Myosin The contractile protein of myofibrils constituting about 65% of muscle proteins. Myosinogen is the precursor of myosin.

Myositis Inflammation of striated muscle. *m. ossificans* Calcification and osteoblastic invasion of muscle hematoma, commonly after supracondylar fracture of elbow.

Myotonia Tonic spasm of a muscle. *m. congenita* SYN – Thomsen's disease. A hereditary disease with tonic spasm of muscle induced by voluntary movements. *m. dystrophica* Hereditary disease characterized by myotonia, muscle atrophy and cataract.

Myringa The tympanic membrane.

Myringitis Inflammation of tympanic membrane.

Myringoplasty Plastic surgery of tympanic membrane usually for closure of perforation.

Myringotomy Incision of tympanic membrane as to relieve pain in acute otitis media (*see* Figure).

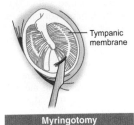

Tympanic membrane

Myringotomy

Mythophobia Abnormal fear of making an incorrect statement.

Myxedema A condition resulting from hypofunction of thyroid; commonly autoimmune or due to iodine lack, dyshormonogenesis.

Myxoma Tumor composed of mucous connective tissue similar to that present in embryo or umbilical cord. It is soft, gray, lobulated, translucent and incompletely encapsulated.

Myxovirus Family of viruses, the common member being influenza virus.

Nabothian cyst Retention cysts of the nabothian glands in the cervical canal, usually associated with ectropion.

Nabumetone Anti-inflammatory pain killer.

Nadolol A betablocker, used in hypertension.

Nadroparin Factor Xa inhibitor anticoagulant.

Naegele German obstetrician (1777-1851). *n. obliquity* Anterior parietal presentation of fetal head in labor. *n. pelvis* An obliquely contracted pelvis. *n. rule* The method of counting expected date of delivery by counting 90 days backwards from LMP and adding 7 days to that date.

Nafarelin GnRH analog.

Nafcillin A semisynthetic penicillinase resistant penicillin.

Nafoxidin Antiestrogen.

Nail A modified epidermal structure forming flat plate on dorsal aspect of terminal phallanx. *n. intermedullary* Surgical rod inserted into the intermedullary canal to fix the fracture. *n. Smith-Peterson* A three flanged nail used to fix fracture neck of femur. *n. spoon* Nail with depressed centre and raised borders, feature of iron deficiency *SYN*—koilonychia. *n. fold* The groove in the cutaneous tissue surrounding the nail except at its free edge (*see* Figure).

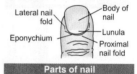

Lateral nail fold — Body of nail — Lunula — Eponychium — Proximal nail fold

Parts of nail

Naked Exposed to view; without cloth.

Nalbuphine Opioid receptor antagonist.

Nalidixic acid Urinary antibiotic; also used for gastrointestinal infections.

Nalorphine Narcotic antagonist.

Naloxone Narcotic antagonist.

Naltrexone Narcotic antagonist.

Nandrolone decanoate Anabolic steroid.

Nanism Dwarflike body build.

Nano 10^{-9} or one billionth part.

Nap Short sleep.

Nape Back of neck.

Naphazoline hydrochloride Topical vasoconstrictor, ingredient of nasal and eye drops.

Naphthalene A coaltar derivative, used as antimoth agent.

Naproxen Anti-inflammatory pain killer.

Narcissism Sexual pleasure sought by observing one's own naked body; self-admiration.

Narcoanalysis A form of psychotherapy where the subconscious is exposed after light anesthesia.

Narcolepsy Recurrent attacks of uncontrollable desire to sleep but easily awakenable.

Narcotic An agent that in moderate doses relieves pain but in higher doses causes coma and respiratory paralysis.

Narcotism State of stupor induced by a narcotic.

Nasal feeding Feeding through a tube passing through nose.

Nasal index The greater width of nasal aperture in relation to a line from the lower edge of nasal aperture to the nasion.

Nasal obstruction Blockage of nasal passage.

Nasal reflex Inducible sneezing from irritation of nasal mucosa.

Nascent Just born, beginning; substance being set free from a compound.

Nasion The point where sagittal plane intersects frontonasal suture (root of nose).

Nasmyth's membrane Epithelial membrane that envelops the enamel of a tooth after birth.

Nasogastric tube Tube inserted through nose into the stomach for feeding or stomach wash.

Nasomental reflex Percussion on side of nose causing contraction of mentalis muscle with elevation of lower lip and wrinkling of skin of the chin.

Nasopharyngitis Inflammation of nasopharynx.

Nasopharynx Part of pharynx situated above the level of soft palate.

Natal Relating to birth.

Natality See birth rate.

Natamycin Topical antibiotic.

Nateglinide Antidiabetic.

Nates Gluteal region *SYN*—buttocks.

Native Born with, inherent.

Natriuresis Excess excretion of sodium in urine.

Natural killer cells Large T-lymphocytes that bind to cells infected with viruses and kill them and often kill tumor cells; the most natural defence against tumor/viral infection.

Naturopathy A therapeutic system that employs natural forces as light, heat, air and water to cure ailments rather than drugs.

Nausea Unpleasant epigastric sensation preceding vomiting. *n. gravidarum* Morning sickness of pregnancy.

Nauseant Provoking nausea.

Navel The depressed scar in the center of abdomen; *SYN*—umbilicus.

Navicular Shaped like a boat.

Near point Closest point of near vision with maximum accommodation. It is 3" at 2 year and recedes to 40" at 60 years.

Nearsighted Only able to see clearly the near objects; *SYN*—myopia, corrected by concave lens.

Nebivolol A betablocker for hypertension.

Nebula Very thin scar on cornea.

Nebulizer An apparatus for producing fine spray or mist.

Necator A genus of nematode hookworms, includes *N. americanus.*

Neck That part of body lying between shoulders and the head. *n. femoral* The thick compact portion of femur joining head with the shaft. *n. of mandible* The narrow area below the articular condyle where are attached the lateral pterygoid muscle and the articular capsule. *n. surgical of humerus* The narrowed portion of humerus below the tuberosity; more prone for fracture. *n. wry SYN*—torticollis; muscle contraction involving sternocleidomastoid, the neck rotated to opposite side.

Necklace of Casal Ring of pigmented reddened skin around the neck in pellagra.

Necrobiosis Degeneration and swelling of collagen in the dermis, common to diabetics.

Necromimesis A delusion in which one believes to be dead.

Necrophilia Sexual intercourse with dead; abnormal interest in corpses.

Necrosis Death of tissue following cut-off in blood supply, physical or chemical injury, infection, etc. *n. coagulation* Necrosis where the necrosed area is converted to a homogeneous mass.

Necrotizing Causing necrosis.

Needle holder Forceps used for holding surgical needle.

Nefopam Pain killer.

Negativism Behavioral disorder in which patient does opposite to suggested action or does not do it at all, a sign of dementia.

Negri bodies Aggregations in nerve cells as in rabies.

Neisseria Gram-negative bacteria, lie in pairs, e.g. *N. gonorrhea, N. meningitidis, N. sicca* and *N. catarrhalis* (last two cause respiratory infection and often endocarditis).

Nelfinavir Anti-HIV agent.

Nelton's line Line from anterior superior iliac spine to tuberosity of ischium.

Nematoda Spindle shaped or rounded worms.

Neocerebellum The posterior lobe of cerebellum that develops last and is concerned with integrations of voluntary movements.

Neodymium A silvery rare earth metal used in LASER.

Neogenesis Regeneration of tissue.

Neologism A new work or phrase or a new meaning put to an old work/phrase; a feature of mental diseases.

Neomycin An aminoglycoside antibiotic isolated from streptomyces, toxic to kidney and eighth cranial nerve but effective against many gram +ve and –ve bacteria, particularly resistant tubercle bacilli.

Neon A rare inert gas.

Neonate First six weeks after birth.

Neonatology The study dealing with the development and diseases of newborn.

Neoplasia The development of neoplasms.

Neoplasm A tumor or new growth. *n. benign* Growth having a definite capsule and noninfiltrating. *n. malignant* Growth that lacks a capsule, infiltrates surrounding structures or has distant metastasis, or recurs after surgery.

Neostigmine Cholinergic drug used for myasthenia; bromide and methyl sulfate salts are used.

Neostriatum Caudate nucleus and putamen together.

Neothalamus The lateral and dorsomedial parts of thalamus.

Nephrectomy Removal of kidneys.

Nephritis Inflammation of kidneys involving glomeruli, tubules and interstitial tissue singly or combinedly, can be acute/chronic; interstitial, salt losing.

Nephritogenic Causing nephritis.

Nephrocalcinosis Deposit of calcium in renal tubules.

Nephroid Resembling kidney.

Nephrolithiasis Presence of stones in kidneys.

Nephrology Study of structure and function of kidneys and diseases related to them.

Nephromere The intermediate mesoderm of embryo from which kidney develops.

Nephropathy Any diseased condition of kidney including inflammatory, degenerative, arteriosclerotic lesions. e.g. analgesic nephropathy, hypokalemic nephropathy, membranous nephropathy, etc.

Nephroptosis Downward displacement of kidney.

Nephrosclerosis Arteriosclerosis of kidney vessels resulting in ischaemic atrophy and fibrosis of kidney.

Nephrosis Non inflammatory degenerative disease of kidney e.g., lipoid nephrosis manifesting as nephrotic syndrome.

Nephrotic syndrome A symptom complex with leakage of protein in urine due to damage to capillary wall of glomeruli.

Nephrotomography Tomography of kidney after injection of radiopaque dye to opacify the kidneys.

Nerve Bundles of nerve fibers connecting CNS or spinal cord with various parts of body. *n. adrenergic* Sympathetic nerves that liberate noradrenaline at the neuroeffector synapse. *n. afferent* Any nerve that transmits impulses from periphery towards centre. *n. cholinergic* Parasympathetic nerve liberating acetylcholine for impulse transmission. *n. efferent* Nerves that transmit impulses from center towards periphery. *n. mixed* Nerve contains both motor (efferent) and sensory (afferent) fibers. *n. secretory* Nerve that stimulates secretion from glands. *n. spinal* 31 pairs of peripheral nerves, 8 cervical, 12 thoracic, 5 lumbar, 5 sacral, 1 coccygeal.

Nerve gas Materials used in chemical warfare; get absorbed through skin to cause paralysis, apnea and often death.

Nerve growth factor A protein necessary for growth and maintenance of certain nerves.

Nesiblastoma Islet tumor of pancreas.

Netilmicin Amino glycoside antibiotic.

Neural crest A band of cells along the neural tube of embryo from which cells forming cranial, spinal and autonomic ganglia arise.

Neural fold One of two longitudinal elevations of the neural plate of embryo that unite to form the neural tube.

Neural plate A thickened band of ectoderm along the dorsal surface of an embryo.

Neural tube Tube formed from fusion of neural folds.

Neural tube defect Defective closure of neural tube during embryogenesis leading to defects like spina bifida, anencephaly, meningocele, meningomyelocele.

Neuralgia Sharp pain along the course of nerve. *n. glossopharyngeal* Severe pain in the back of throat, tonsils and middle ear along the distribution of glossopharyngeal nerve. *n. trigeminal* Neuralgia involving the gasserian ganglion or one or more branches of trigeminal nerve.

Neurasthenia Psychiatric illness with unexplained chronic fatigue and lassitude.

Neurilemma The peripheral covering of nerve fiber around myelin sheath that contributes to regeneration of damaged nerve fiber.

Neurilimmoma Firm encapsulated tumor of peripheral nerve.

Neurinoma A peripheral glioma arising from endoneurium.

Neuritis Inflammation of nerve; inflammatory or degenerative.

Neuroablation The act of destroying nerve tissue by surgery, cautery, injection of sclerosing agents, lasers or cryotherapy.

Neuroblastoma A malignant tumor of neuroblasts in children giving rise to cells of sympathetic nervous system; especially adrenal medulla.

Neurocirculatory asthenia Functional circulatory and nervous disturbance with precordial pain and fatigue.

Neurodermatitis Cutaneous inflammation with itching mostly due to emotional disturbances.

Neuroepithelium Specialized epithelial structure forming the gustatory cells, olfactory cells, hair cells of inner ear, rods and cones of retina.

Neurofibril Tiny fibrils in the cytoplasm of nerve cell body.

Neurofibroma Tumor of connective tissue around nerve.

Neurogenesis Growth and development of nerve tissues.

Neurogenic Originating from nervous tissue or happening due to nervous dysfunction.

Neuroglia Supporting tissue of nervous system, includes astrocytes, microglia, Schwann cells, satellite cells, ependyma etc. All except microglia are of ectodermal origin.

Neurohypophysis Posterior lobe of pituitary secreting oxytocin and vasopressin.

Neuroleptic Synonymous with antipsychotic.

Neurology The study dealing with nervous system and diseases related to it.

Neurolysis Stretching of a nerve to relieve tension; release of a nerve from fibrous tissue.

Neuromatosis Multiple tumors of nerve tissue.

Neuromyasthenia Muscular weakness consequent to emotional disorder.

Neuron A nerve cell; consisting of cell body and its processes i.e., axons and dendrites. *n. afferent* Neurone conducting impulses to the brain and spinal cord. *n. associative* Neurone coordinating impulses between sensory and motor neurons. *n. efferent* Neurones conducting impulses away from brain and spinal cord. *n. lower motor* Neurone with cell body in anterior gray column. *n. upper motor* Neurone with cell body in motor cortex. *n. preganglionic* Neurone of autonomic nervous system whose cell body lies in central nervous system and axon terminates in peripheral ganglia. *n. postganglionic* Neurone whose cell body lies in an autonomic ganglion and its axon terminates in effector organ (*see* Figure).

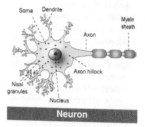

Neuron

Neuronitis Inflammation of nerve cell.

Neuropathy Any disease of nerves. *n. entrapment* Nerve inflammation secondary to entrapment in a closed constricting space e.g., median nerve in carpal tunnel of wrist. *n. hypertrophic* Inflammation with thickening of nerves as in Refsum disease.

Neurophysin Proteins that bind oxytocin and ADH, secreted by posterior pituitary.

Neuropraxia Trauma to a nerve followed by loss of conduction even though anatomical integrity is maintained.

Neuroradiology Branch of medical science utilizing radiography for diagnosis of neurological diseases.

Neurosis A minor mental disease where person's insight is maintained. *n. anxiety* Neurosis where vague anxiety or apprehension interferes with effective functioning. *n. obsessional* Neurosis where obsession dominates.

Neurosyphilis Syphilis affecting the nervous system. *n. meningovascular* The meninges and the cerebral blood vessels are affected the most with ischemia, infarction, hydrocephalus.

Neurotensin Tridecapeptide from hypophysis stimulating pituitary.

Neurotic Person suffering from neurosis.

Neurotmesis Nerve injury with complete loss of function in absence of anatomical disruption.

Neurotransmitter Chemical substance released by stimulation of presynaptic neurone that excites or inhibits target cell, e.g. acetyl choline, dopamine, norepinephrine.

Neutral Neither alkaline nor acidic, indifferent.

Neutralization The process of counteracting the effects of any harmful agent/substance.

Neutral point A pH of 7.0 which is neither acid nor alkaline.

Neutral red An indicator dye.

Neutron Electrically neutral particle equal in mass to proton.

Neutrophil A leukocyte staining easily with neutral dyes.

Nevirapine Anti-HIV agent.

Nevus Congenitally discolored localized area of skin; vascular skin tumor due to hyperplastic blood vessels. *n. junctional* Nevus in the basal layer of epidermis appearing as a non-hairy pigmented area, with high malignancy potential.

Niacin Nicotinic acid used for pellagra.

Niche A depression or recess on a smooth surface e.g., ulcer niche.

Nicergoline Cerebral activator.

Nicking Compression of retinal vein at the site crossed by artery.

Niclosamide Anthelmintic.

Nicorandil Vasodilator for angina.

Nicotinamide adenine diphosphate (NADP) An enzyme that accepts electrons.

Nicotine Alkaloid of tobacco, a vasoconstrictor, stimulant and addictive agent.

Nidus Focus of infection, nest like structure.

Niemann-Pick disease A disturbance of sphingolipid metabolism characterized by hepatosplenomegaly, lymphadenopathy and mental deterioration.

Nifedipine Calcium channel blocker.

Nightblindness (nyctalopia) Inability to see in dark due to deficient rhodopsin or its slow regeneration after exposure to light, a feature of retinal pigmentary degeneration or vitamin A deficiency.

Nightmare A bad dream accompanied by fear.

Night sweat Profuse sweating during night sleep e.g., diabetes, with hypoglycemia due to excess insulin, chronic debilitating diseases (tuberculosis), rickets.

Nigrostrial Bundle of nerve fiber connecting corpus striatum with substantia nigra.

Nikethamide Respiratory and CNS stimulant.

Nikolsky's sign Spreading of a pemphigus bleb by application of mild pressure due to easy epidermal separation.

Nimesulide Analgesic antiinflammatory agent.

Nimodipine Calcium channel blocker.

Nipple The conical protuberance at center of breast containing erectile tissue and pierced by milk ducts.

Niridazole Anthelmintic used for guinea worm and schistosomiasis.

Nissl bodies Chromophil granules in cell bodies and dendrites of neurones composed of RNA.

Nit Egg of louse or any parasitic insect.

Nitazoxamide Anti-amoebic agent.

Nitrate Salt of nitric acid.

Nitrazepam Benzodiazepine, anxiolytic.

Nitrendipine Calcium channel blocker.

Nitric oxide A potent vasodilator, released from vascular endothelium, synthesized from arginine.

Nitrite Salt of nitrous acid, an antispasmodic and smooth muscle dilator.

Nitroblue tetrazolium test A test of ability of leukocytes to transform nitroblue tetrazolium from a colorless state to deep blue, a test of leukocyte bacterial killing ability.

Nitrofurantoin Urinary antibacterial agent.

Nitrofurazone Topically used antibacterial agent.

Nitrogen mustards Anti-lymphoid agents used in treating lymphosarcoma, rheumatoid arthritis, leukemia, nephritis. Agents in this group are cyclophosphamide, mechlor ethamine, melphalan and chlorambucil.

Nitrogen balance The difference between the amount of nitrogen ingested and excreted per day.

Nitroglycerin Any nitrate of glycerol used for vasodilatation in angina pectoris as 2% ointment or tablets; be kept in tinted glass (not plastic) container without cotton plug.

Nitromersol Topically used mercurial antiseptic.

Nitrosourea Anteneoplastic agents including carmustine, lomustine, semustine and streptozocin.

Nitroxazepine Antidepressant.

Nitrous oxide Inhalation anesthetic used in conjuction with oxygen *SYN*—laughing gas.

Nocardiosis Infection with gram positive aerobic bacteria (often acid fast to be confused with tubercle bacillus), causing pulmonary infection or foot infection (maduramycosis).

Nociceptive reflex Reflex initiated by painful stimuli.

Nocturia Urination at night.

Nocturnal emission Involuntary semen discharge during sleep.

Nocturnal penile tumescence Penile erection during sleep, a normal phenomenon, when present excludes organic causes of impotency.

Nodal points A pair of points situated on the axis of optical system.

Nodal rhythm Cardiac rhythm originating at AV node.

Nodding Falling forward of the head.

Node A small swelling or constriction. *n. AV* The mass of purkinje fibers at lower end of interatrial septum giving origin to bundle of His. *n. Bouchard's* Bony enlargement of proxymal interphalangeal joint in osteoarthritis. *n. Heberden's* Nodes in terminal interphalangeal joints of hand in osteoarthritis. *n's of Ranvier* Constriction of myelin sheath along the course of medulated nerve fiber. *n's Osler* Tender nodes in pulp of finger and toes in subacute bacterial endocarditis. *n's of Parrot* Osteophytes around anterior fontanel in congenital syphilis. *n. Schmorl's* Prolapse of nucleus pulposus into vertebral body. *n. singer's* Small white nodes on vocal cords due to vocal abuse. *n. sinoatrial* Node in the wall of right atrium near entry of

SVC acting as the pacemaker of heart (*see* Figure).

Nodule A small node; collection of cells. *n. Aschoff's* Myocardial nodule with central fibrinoid necrosis with surrounding epithelioid cells, a feature of rheumatic carditis.

Nomogram Representation by graphs, diagrams.

Nonoxynol A spermicide.

Noonan's syndrome Congenital pulmonary stenosis with skeletal abnormalities.

Norepinephrine Vasopressor hormone secreted by adrenal medulla.

Norethandrolone An anabolic steroid.

Norethindrone Progestational agent.

Norfloxacin A quinolone with broad spectrum antibacterial activity.

Norgestrel A progestational agent.

Normetanephrine A metabolite of epinephrine.

Normoblast Type of nucleated red blood cell during erythropoiesis.

Normochromasia Normal staining capacity of tissue.

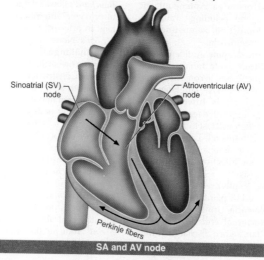

SA and AV node

Normocyte Averaged size RBC.

Normosthenuria Urine of normal amount and specific gravity.

Normotensive Normal blood pressure.

Norplant Implantable contraceptive system containing levogestrel.

Norrie's disease Sex-linked blindness with retinal malformation, vitreous opacity, often with hearing loss and mental retardation.

Norton Scale A widely used scale to determine a patient's risk to develop pressure sores or ulcers.

Nortryptyline Tricyclic antidepressant.

Norwalk agent A virus implicated in gastroenteritis .

Noscapine Antitussive opium alkaloid.

Nose The organ of olfaction, also warms, moistens and filters the air. Orifices of frontal, anterior ethmoid and maxillary sinuses open into middle meatus while posterior ethmoid and sphenoid sinuses open into superior meatus.

Nosocomial Hospital acquired infection.

Nosology The science of classification of diseases.

Nosophilia An abnormal desire to be ill.

Nostalgia Homesickness.

Notch Depression, narrow gap. *n. acetabular* Notch on the inferior border of acetabulum. *n. aortic* Notch of aortic valve closure in pulse tracing. *n. sciatic* Two in number, greater and lesser sciatic notches on hip bone.

Notifiable diseases All communicable and contagious diseases to be notified to local health authorities under the statutes of law.

Notochord The axial skeleton of embryo, its remnant in adult is nucleus pulposus of intervertebral disk.

Novocain Procaine hydrochloride.

Noxious Harmful.

NREM sleep Nonrapid eye movement sleep.

Nuck's canal A peritoneal pouch extending into labium in female, homologous to processus vaginalis of male.

Nuclear antigen Antigenicity of nuclear materials in some connective tissue disorders.

Nuclear magnetic resonance When certain atomic nuclei with odd number of protons or neutrons or both are subjected to strong magnetic field they absorb and reemit electromagnetic energy. Application of a radiofrequency pulse causes deflection in the net magnetization vector and image production. The technique is useful for imaging of brain, soft tissue and heart.

Nuclear medicine Medicine dealing with diagnostic, therapeutic and investigative aspects of radionuclides.

Nucleic acid A complex product consisting of pentose, phosphoric acid, purines and pyrimidines.

Nucleolus A spherical body within the nucleus.

Nucleoprotein Combination of nucleic acid with protein found in cell nuclei.

Nucleosidase Enzyme causing hydrolysis of nucleoside.

Nucleoside Glycoside formed by union of pentose sugar with purine or pyrimidine.

Nucleotide Compound containing phosphoric acid, pentose sugar and purine/pyrimidine.

Nucleus The central vital portion in a cell which controls metabolism, reproduction and transmission of cell characteristic. *n. ambiguous* Nucleus of 9th and 10th cranial nerves in the medulla. *n. caudate* The comma shaped constituent of basal ganglia. *n. cuneate* Nucleus in lower medulla in which end the fibers of fasciculus cuneatus. *n. Deiters* Lateral vestibular nucleus. *n. Dentate* The large nucleus in lateral part of cerebellar lobe giving rise to fibers of superior cerebellar peduncle. *n. Edinger Westphal* Nucleus in midbrain giving rise to parasympathetic fibers to innervate cilliary muscles and sphincter iris. *n. emboliform* Nucleus in cerebellum lying inbetween dentate and globose nuclei. *n. fastigial* Nucleus in medullary portion of cerebellum. *n. gracilis* Nucleus in lower portion of medulla where fibers of fasciculus gracilis terminate. *n. habenular* Nucleus in diencephalon functioning as olfactory correlation center. *n. pulposus* The central gelatinous remnant of notocord in intervertebral disks (*see* Figure on page 509).

Null hypothesis The hypothesis that the observed difference between two groups of patients studied is accidental.

Nullipara A woman who has not produced a viable child.

Numb Dead, insensible.

Numular Shaped like a coin.

Nurse Person providing health care.

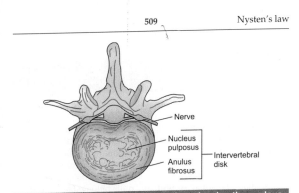

Intervertebral disk in transverse section, showing the nucleus pulposus and the anulus fibrosus: Normal disk

Nursery Newborn care center.

Nutrient Food constituents supplying body with essential elements of metabolism.

Nutrition The process involved in assimilation and utilization of food.

Nutritious Providing nutrition.

Nux vomica Poisonous seed containing strychnine.

Nyctalopia Night blindness as seen in avitaminosis A and retinitis pigmentosa.

Nyctamblyopia Poor night vision without any other eye changes.

Nyctaphonia Hysterical loss of voice only at night.

Nyctophilia Abnormal preference for darkness.

Nyctophobia Abnormal fear of darkness.

Nylidrin Peripheral vasodilator.

Nymph Wingless immature stage in developmental cycle of insects.

Nympha Labia minora.

Nymphomania Abnormal and excessive sexual desire in a female.

Nystagmograph Apparatus for recording nystagmus.

Nystagmus Involuntary to and fro movement of eyeball.

Nystatin Antifungal agent.

Nysten's law The law that states that rigor mortis begins with muscles of mastication and then progresses down.

O

Oat A cereal used as food.

Oatmeal Porridge of oat.

Obduction Autopsy.

Obese Fatty.

Obesity Weight in excess of 20% than the ideal weight for height, age and sex. *o. endogenous* Obesity caused by metabolic abnormality within the body. *o. exogenous* Obesity due to excess food calorie intake. *o. hypothalamic* Obesity resulting from hypothalamic dysfunction i.e., regulation of eating behavior.

O bfuscation Mental confusion.

Object Anything visible or appealing to senses.

Objective sign In reaching a diagnosis, a sign that can be seen, heard or felt by the examining doctor.

Objective symptoms Symptom apparent to physical means of diagnosis.

Obligate Necessary.

Oblique Slanting or diagonal.

Obliquity The state of slanting. *o. Litzmann's* Inclining of fetal head with posterior parietal bone presenting. *o. Naegele's* Inclining fetal head with oblique biparietal diameter in relation to pelvic brim.

Oblongata Oblong e.g., medulla oblongata.

Obscure Hidden, indistinct.

Obsession A mental state where one is occupied with uncontrollable desire, idea or emotion even though he knows fully about it.

Obsessive compulsive disorder A psychiatric disorder in which a person repeats same action or behavior for many hours which effects daily living.

Obstetrician A physician who treats a woman during pregnancy and child birth.

Obstetrics Branch of medicine dealing with childbirth, puerperium and management of pregnancy.

Obstipation Complete constipation without passage of flatus and feces.

Obstructive lung disease A group of diseases which cause increased resistance to passage of air in and out of the lungs, e.g. asthma, chronic bronchitis, etc.

Obstruent Blocking up.

Obtundent A soothing remedy.

Obturator Anything that closes a cavity or opening.

Obturator foramen An opening in the membrane.

Obturator muscle Muscle in the pelvis that rotates the thigh outwards.

Obturator sign Inward rotation of hip so as to stretch obturator internus, causes pain in acute appendicitis.

Occipital bone Bone in hind part of skull between parietal and temporal bones.

Occipital lobe Posterior lobe of cerebral hemisphere shaped like a three sided pyramid (*see* Figure).

Occiput The back part of skull.

Occlusion State of being closed.

Occult Hidden, concealed.

Occult blood test Examination of stool for microscopic hemorrhage.

Occupational neurosis Neurosis that develops in certain persons in particular occupations.

Occupational therapy Therapy aimed at making a patient independent and able for self care, and prevent disability.

Ochlesis Any disease caused by over crowding.

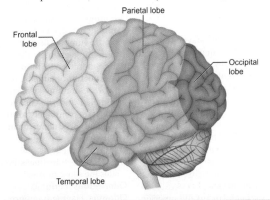

Parietal lobe
Frontal lobe
Occipital lobe
Temporal lobe

Occipital lobe

Ochlophobia Abnormal fear of populated places or crowds.

Ochronosis An inborn error of metabolism marked by dark pigmentation of cartilage, ligaments and skin with black coloration of urine due to excretion of homogentisic acid.

Octamethylpyrophosphoramide Anticholinesterage insecticide.

Octapeptide Peptide with eight amino acids.

Octogenarian A person in his/her eighties.

Octopanrine An adrenergic transmitter.

Octreotide Growth hormone antagonist.

Oculocardiac reflex Slowing of pulse following pressure on eyeball.

Oculocerebrorenal syndrome A sex-linked syndrome characterized by cataract, mental retardation, amino aciduria, vitamin D resistant rickets, etc.

Oculogyric crisis Involuntary upward gaze fixation lasting for minutes to hours in postencephalitic parkinsonism.

Oculomotor nerve The third cranial nerve arising from midbrain and supplying extrinsic muscles of eye excluding lateral rectus and superior oblique.

Odontitis Inflammation of tooth.

Odontoblast The dentin forming cells in dental papilla or pulp chamber.

Odontocele An alveodental cyst.

Odontoclast A class of cells that bring about resorption of roots of deciduous teeth.

Odontogenesis The formation/development of teeth.

Odontograph Equipment to determine the degree of uneveness of enamel.

Odontoid Tooth like.

Odontoid process Tooth like projection from 2nd cervical vertebra.

Odontology The art and science of dentistry.

Odontoma Tumor originating from dental tissue. *o. ameloblastic* Tumor of dental tissue containing enamel, dentine and odontogenic tissue but does not form enamel. *o. composite* Odontoma in which epithelial and mesenchymal cells are completely differentiated producing enamel and dentin.

Odor Any smell.

Odorant Anything that stimulates the sense of smell.

Odoriferous Perfumed.

Odorous Having fragrance.

Odynophagia Dysphagia.

Oedius complex Abnormally intense love of child for opposite sex parent.

Ogilvie syndrome Acute intestinal pseudoobstruction.

Ohm Unit of electrical resistance equal to current of 1 ampere produced by potential difference of one volt across the terminals.

Ohm's law The strength of an electric current expressed in amperes is equal to the electromotive force expressed in volts divided by resistance.

Ointment A medicated fatty soft substance for external application.

Olanzapine Anti-psychotic agent.

Olecranon The proximal bony projection of ulna at the elbow (*see* Figure).

Oleic acid Fatty acid.

Oleogranuloma Granuloma formation at the site of injection of oily substances.

Olfaction The act of smelling.

Olfactometer The apparatus for testing power of sense of smell.

Olfactory area Area in hippocampal convolution and uncus of brain.

Olfactory bulb Enlarged upper end of olfactory tract.

Olfactory membrane Membrane in the upper part of nasal cavity containing olfactory receptors.

Olfactory nerves Fine unmyelinated fibres arising from olfactory mucosa and ending in olfactory bulb after piercing cribiform plate.

Olfactory tract The tract that extends from olfactory bulb

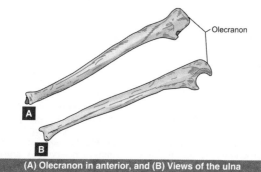

Olecranon

A

B

(A) Olecranon in anterior, and (B) Views of the ulna

to the anterior perforated substance where it divides into olfactory striae.

Olfactory trigone Small triangular area between lateral and medial olfactory striae.

Oligemia Low blood volume.

Oligodendroglia The neuroglial cell with long slender processes which maintains the myelin sheath.

Oligodendroglioma A malignant tumor of CNS, frequently calcified arising from oligodendrocytes.

Oligohydramnios Less than normal amniotic fluid, a feature of postmaturity.

Oligomenorrhea Scanty or infrequent menstruation.

Oligosaccharide Compound made-up of small number of monosaccharides.

Oligospermia Diminished sperm count.

Oligotrophy Inadequate nutrition.

Oliguria Decreased formation of urine.

Olivary body A rounded mass of nerve tissue in anterolateral portion of medulla oblongata. (*see* Figure).

Ollier's disease Chondrodysplasia.

Ollier's layer The deepest layer of periosteum containing bone forming osteoblasts.

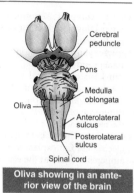

Cerebral peduncle
Pons
Medulla oblongata
Oliva
Anterolateral sulcus
Posterolateral sulcus
Spinal cord

Oliva showing in an anterior view of the brain

Olmesartan ACE receptor inhibitor.

Omental bursa The cavity in greater omentum.

Omentopexy Fixation of omentum to anterior abdominal wall.

Omentum A double fold of peritoneum attached to stomach, the portion attached to greater curvature of stomach extending to envelop the intestines is called greater omentum and the portion extending from lesser curvature of stomach to transverse fissure of liver is called lesser omentum.

Omeprazole Proton pump inhibitor, used in peptic ulcer, Zollinger-Ellison syndrome.

Ommaya reservoir A mushroom shaped reservoir with

a self sealing plastic dome and attached to a catheter. The reservoir is implanted under the skin flap in skull and catheter is put into lateral ventricle useful for measuring CSF pressure and administration of drugs.

Omnivorous Eating both meat and vegetables.

Omohyoid Concerning scapula and the hyoid bone, the muscle attached to these two structures.

Omphalitis Inflammation of umbilicus.

Omphalocele Congenital umbilical hernia.

Omphalotomy Cutting of umbilical cord afterbirth.

Onanist Person practising coitus interruptus.

Onanoff's reflex Contraction of bulbocavernosus muscle on pressing the glans penis.

Onchocerca volvulus Onchocerca invading the eye and causing blindness in Africa.

Oncogene Genes that can cause tumor formation.

Oncogenesis Tumor initiation and growth.

Oncology The branch of medicine dealing with tumors.

Oncotic pressure The osmotic pressure exerted by proteins in plasma.

Oncovin Vincristine sulphate.

Ondansetron Antiemetic.

Ondine's curse Primary alveolar hypoventilation due to reduced responsiveness of respiratory center to CO_2.

Oneirology The scientific study of dreams.

Oneiroscopy Dream analysis for study of one's emotional state.

Oniomania An irrepressible urge to spend money.

Onlay A graft applied to the surface of tissue e.g., bone graft applied to bone.

Ontogeny The history of development of an individual.

Onychia Inflammation of nailbed with loss of nail.

Onychodystrophy Maldevelopment of a nail.

Onychograph Device that records capillary blood pressure under the finger nail.

Onycholysis Losing and detachment of nail.

Onychomycosis Fungal infection of nails.

Oocyst Encysted form of zygote in certain sporozoa.

Oocyte Primitive ovum.

Oogenesis Growth and maturation of ovum.

Oogonium The primordial cell from which an oocyte originates.

Ookinesis Mitotic phenomena taking place within an ovum

during maturation and fertilization.

Ookinete Motile zygote of plasmodia.

Oophorectomy Surgical removal of one or both ovaries.

Oophorrhaphy Suture of displaced ovary to pelvic wall.

Opaque Not transparent; not allowing light rays to pass through.

Open heart surgery Surgery on heart or its blood vessels requiring cardiopulmonary bypass.

Open reduction Exposure of fractured ends of a bone for bringing reunion by suitable reduction.

Operant conditioning Conditioning or influencing behavior by rewarding for certain desired acts.

Operation The act of operating i.e., incision, excision, suture.

Opercular Concerning a covering structure.

Operculitis Inflammation of gingiva over a partly erupted tooth.

Operculum Any covering.

Operon A term used in genetics to mean a group of linked genes and regulatory elements functioning as an unit for transcription.

Ophiases A form of baldness of scalp.

Ophidism Poisoning from snake bite.

Ophritis Inflammation of eyebrow.

Ophthalmia Inflammation of the eye. *o. gonococcal* Severe purulent conjunctivitis. *o. neonatorum* Severe purulent conjunctivitis of newborn, usually gonococcal. *o. sympathetic* Uveitis of healthy eye following trauma to other eye.

Ophthalmic nerve A branch of trigeminal, having only sensory function.

Ophthalmitis Inflammation of eye.

Ophthalmodynamometer Instrument for measuring pressure in ophthalmic arteries.

Ophthalmologist A doctor who practises in the treatment of diseases of eye.

Ophthalmometer Instrument for measuring errors of refraction, size of eye and anterior curvature.

Ophthalmoplegia Paralysis of ocular muscles. *o. externa* Paralysis of extra ocular muscles. *o. interna* Paralysis of iris and ciliary body. *o. nuclear* Paralysis of 3rd, 4th and 6th cranial nerves due to a lesion involving their nuclei. *o. Parinaud's* Paralysis of conjugate deviation of eyes in upward direction.

Ophthalmoscope Instrument for examination of fundus and retina.

Ophthalmoscopy Examination of the interior of the eye using an ophthalmoscope.

Opiate receptor Specific receptors on cell surfaces to which combine the opiates, endorphins and encephalins for mediating their effects.

Opioid Synthetic narcotics or endogenous substances with opium like activity e.g. encephalins and endorphins.

Opisthotonus A form of tetanic spasm where the body bends backwards (*see* Figure).

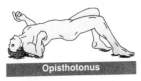

Opisthotonus

Opium Substance derived from juice of unripe capsules of poppy.

Oppenheim's disease *SYN—* myotonia congenita characterized by poor muscular development in the limbs.

Opponens digiti minimi Intrinsic muscle of hand that helps opposing little finger to thumb.

Opponens pollicis Muscle that places thumb opposite the little finger.

Opsin One of the colorless proteins in rods and cones.

Opsonin A substance present in blood that prepares bacteria for phagocytosis.

Opsonize To render microorganisms susceptible to phagocytosis.

Optic atrophy Atrophy of optic nerve head with sharply demarcated chalky white optic disc.

Optic axis The imaginary line passing through center of cornea and posterior pole of retina.

Optic canal The groove at the apex of orbit through which pass optic nerve and ophthalmic artery.

Optic chiasma The commissure anterior to hypophysis where there is partial decussation of fibers of optic nerve.

Optic disk The posterior pole in retina where the fibers from ganglion cell converge to form optic nerve.

Optic neuritis Involvement of optic nerve due to inflammation, degeneration, demyelination resulting in visual loss.

Optic radiation The geniculocalcarine tract connecting lateral geniculate body with area 17 and 19 of calcarine cortex.

Optic tract The visual path from optic chiasm to lateral geniculate body (*see* Figure).

Optic vesicle The embryonic evagination of diencephalon giving rise to pigmentary and sensory layers of retina.

Optical center The point where the secondary axes of a refractory system meet and cross the principal axis.

Optical index A constant applied to objectives for purpose of comparison taking into account the focal length.

Optical isomerism Substances having similar structural formula but differing rotation of polarized light.

Optics Branch of science relating to properties of light, its refraction, reflexion and relation to vision.

Optimal Most desirable.

Optokinetic Relating to eye movements in relation to movement of objects in visual field.

Optokinetic nystagmus Nystagmus occurring when moving objects traverse the field of vision or vice versa.

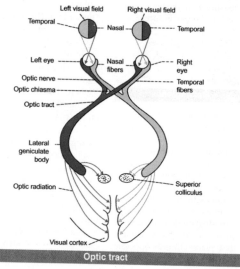

Optic tract

Optometer Instrument for measuring refractive error of eye.

Optometry Measurement of visual power.

Ora serrata Portion of retina behind ciliary body.

Oral contraceptive Contraceptives taken by mouth.

Orbicularis oculi The ring muscle of eye, causing its closure.

Orbicularis oris The ring muscle of mouth, causing pursing of lips.

Orbit The bony socket containing the eye formed by frontal, sphenoid, ethmoid, maxillary and palatal bone.

Orbital cellulitis Inflammation of soft tissue of orbit usually following sinusitis causing proptosis and diplopia.

Orbital index Orbital height to orbital breadth × 100.

Orbital lobe Part of frontal lobe that rests on orbital plate of frontal bone.

Orchic Testis.

Orchiopexy Surgical fixation of testis.

Orchitis Inflammation of testis.

Ordinate The vertical line of the two coordinates.

Orfenadrine Anticholinerigic agent.

Organelle Special structures of a cell e.g., mitochondria.

Organic 1. Pertains to living organisms. 2. In chemistry pertaining to compounds of carbon. 3. Physical not mental or psychogenic.

Organic acid Any acid containing carboxyl group.

Organic brain syndrome Diffuse impairment of brain function.

Organic disease Disease with recognizable structural changes in organs and tissues.

Organic murmur Murmur due to structural changes in heart valves.

Organism Any living entity capable of carrying on life process.

Organize To undergo organization i.e. repair process with growth of fibroblasts and capillaries.

Organizing pneumonia Pneumonia where the exudate undergoes organization and cicatrization rather than resorption.

Orgasm The intense pleasure of sexual intercourse at climax with pelvic throbbing, contraction of levator ani and anal sphincters to culminate in seminal ejaculation.

Orifice An opening or entrance to a cavity.

Origin The starting point.

Ormeloxifine Selective estrogen receptor modulator.

Ornidazole Antiamoebic agent.

Ornithine An amino acid in the urea cycle.

Ornithosis Psittacosis contracted from birds other than parrots.

Oropharynx Portion of pharynx below the level of soft palate.

Orosomucoid An acidic mucoprotein from nephrotic urine.

Orotic acid A pyrimidine precursor.

Oroya fever Bartonellosis.

Orphenadrine Antispasmodic antitremor drug.

Ortalani's sign Slipping of femoral head back to acetabulum with a snapping sound when congenitally displaced hip in full abduction is tapped.

Orthochromatic Having normal staining characteristics.

Orthodontics The branch of dentistry dealing with malocclusion and its treatment.

Orthograde Walking or standing in upright position.

Orthopedics That branch of surgery dealing with corrective treatment of deformities, diseases of locomotor apparatus.

Orthophoria Normal balance of eye muscles i.e., parallel.

Orthopnea Difficulty in breathing in lying down but not in sitting or upright position.

Orthoptics The training meant for making visual responses normal like esophoria.

Orthoscopy Examination of eye using orthoscope.

Orthostat Device for straightening curvatures of long bones.

Orthostatic Standing upright. *o. albuminuria* Albuminuria when assuming erect position. *o. hypotension* Fall in blood pressure while assuming erect position.

Orthotics Science of orthopedic appliance and their use.

Orthotonus Tetanic spasm that causes a rigid straightness of the body.

Orthotopic In the natural or normal position. *o. transplantation* Transplantation of an organ from a donor into its normal anatomical position in recipient.

Os Bone, mouth.

Oscillation A swinging or vibration.

Oscillopsia A form of visual aberration where stationary objects appear to move to and fro leading to blurred vision.

Oscilloscope A cathode ray vacuum tube to reflect oscillations of electromotive forces.

Osgood-Schlatter disease Osteochondritis of tibial tubercle.

Osler-Rendu-Weber disease Hereditary hemorrhagic telangiectasia.

Osler's disease Polycythemia vera.

Osler's node Painful indurated red areas on finger pulp in acute bacterial endocarditis.

Osmole The quantity of a solute existing in solution as molecules, commonly stated in grams, that is osmotically equivalent to one mole of an ideally behaving electrolyte.

Osmometer Instrument for measuring osmotic pressure.

Osmophobia Abnormal fear of odors.

Osmoreceptors Hypothalamic receptors that respond to changes in osmotic pressure of blood and hence influence ADH secretion.

Osmosis The passage of solvent through a membrane from a dilute solution into a more concentrated one.

Osmotic fragility The susceptibility of RBCs to lyse in hypotonic solutions.

Osmotic pressure The pressure developed when two solutions of different concentrations of some solute are separated by a semipermeable membrane.

Osseous Bony.

Ossicle A small bone, particularly that in middle ear.

Ossification The formation of bone.

Ossifying fibroma A benign tumor from connective tissue of bone.

Osteitis Inflammation of bone. *o. fibrosa cystica* Generalized bone demineralization with large osteoporotic areas resembling cyst as in hyperparathyroidism. *o. fragilitans* Osteogenesis imperfecta.

Osteoarthritis A progressive joint disease in which there is progressive cartilage deterioration in synovial joints and vertebrae (*see* Figure on page 522).

Osteoarthrosis Degenerative joint disease.

Osteoblast Cells of mesenchymal origin concerned in the formation of bony tissue.

Osteoblastoma Malignant tumor of osteoblasts SYN – Osteosarcoma.

Osteocarcinoma A condition of cancer of bone.

Osteochondral Composed of both bone and cartilage.

Osteochondritis dissecans A joint disease characterized by partial or complete detachment of a fragment of articular cartilage and underlying bone.

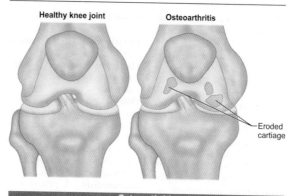

Healthy knee joint | **Osteoarthritis**

Eroded cartilage

Osteoarthritis

Osteochondrodysplasia Abnormal development of bony and cartilaginous structures.

Osteochondrodystrophy Morquio syndrome.

Osteochondroma Benign hamartomatous tumor of bone or cartilage.

Osteochondromyxoma An osteochondroma with myxoid component.

Osteochondrosarcoma An osteosarcoma with significant myxosarcomatous element.

Osteochondrosis A process involving ossification centers with avascular necrosis followed by slow regeneration.

Osteoclasis The fracture of a long bone without resorting to open surgery for correcting deformity.

Osteoclast Multinucleated cells responsible for bone remodelling.

Osteoclastoma Giant cell tumor.

Osteodystrophy Defective bone formation.

Osteofibroma A benign bone tumor with fibrous tissue component.

Osteogenesis imperfecta Autosomal dominant disease characterized by hypoplasia of bone and cartilage leading to fracture with minimal trauma, hypermobility, blue sclera.

Osteogenic sarcoma A malignant tumor composed of mesenchymal anaplastic cells with varying elements of osteogenesis, osteolysis, telangiectasis and bone cyst formation.

Osteoid The young hyaline matrix of true bone in which calcium is deposited.

Osteoid osteoma A benign hamartomatous tumor of bone composed of a nidus of well vascularized tissue with pain.

Osteolysis Bone resorption/degeneration.

Osteoma Benign bony tumor arising from membranous bones.

Osteomalacia Failure of ossification due to fall in serum calcium.

Osteomatosis Presence of multiple osteomas.

Osteometry The study of proportions and measurement of skeleton.

Osteomyelitis Inflammation of marrow and hard tissue of bone.

Osteopathy A school of healing art which teaches that the body is a vital mechanical organism whose structural and functional integrity are coordinated and interdependent.

Osteopenia Less bone tissue than normal.

Osteopetrosis A familial disease characterized by excessive radiographic density with a tendency towards fracture and obliteration of marrow cavity.

Osteophyte A bony outgrowth.

Osteopoikilosis Disease of unknown etiology with ellipsoidal dense foci in all bones of body.

Osteoporosis Absolute decrease in quantity of bone tissue with enlarging marrow cavity and haversian spaces.

Osteosclerosis Abnormal increase in density of bone.

Osteosis Metaplastic bone formation.

Osteotome An instrument for cutting bone.

Osteotomy Cutting of a bone (*see* Figure on page 524).

Osteotropy Nutrition of bony tissue.

Ostium A mouth or aperture.

Otic Pertaining to ear.

Otic capsule The cartilage capsule that surrounds developing auditory vesicle and later fuses with the sphenoid and occipital cartilage.

Otic ganglion The nerve ganglion immediately below foramen ovale of sphenoid bone giving rise to postganglionic parasympathetic fibers to parotid gland.

Otitic hydrocephalus Hydrocephalus associated with chronic ear infection, esp., mastoiditis.

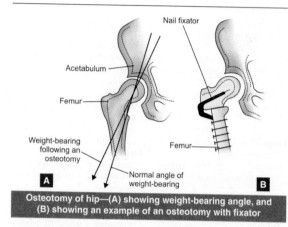

Osteotomy of hip—(A) showing weight-bearing angle, and (B) showing an example of an osteotomy with fixator

Otitis Inflammation of the ear.

Otitis externa Inflammation of external ear.

Otitis interna Inflammation of internal ear.

Otitis media Inflammation of middle ear.

Otogenic Originating or arising within the ear.

Otolaryngologist A physician who specializes in otolaryngology.

Otolaryngology Speciality dealing with diseases of ear, nose and larynx.

Otolith Calcareous concretions within membranous labyrinth.

Otology The science of ear and its diseases.

Otological Relating to study of diseases of the ear.

Otomycosis Fungal infection of ear canal.

Otorhinolaryngology The branch of medical science dealing with functions and diseases of ear, nose and larynx.

Otorrhea Discharge from external auditory meatus.

Otosclerosis A disease characterized by new bone formation around oval window with immobilization of foot plate of stapes and hence conductive hearing loss.

Otoscope Instrument for visualization of external ear and the tympanic membrane (*see* Figure on page 525).

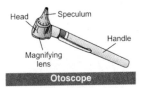

Otoscope

Ototoxic Agents toxic to the neural process of hearing.

Ouabain A digitalis glycoside, rapid acting.

Ounce An unit of measure equivalent to 28 grams.

Outer nuclear layer The layer of retina which contains rods and cones.

Outflow In neurology transmission of efferent impulses.

Outgrowth Growth or development from a preexisting structure or state.

Outline The shape.

Outpouching Evagination.

Ovale malaria Malaria caused by *Plasmodium ovale* with the red blood cells and trophozoites both being often oval in shape.

Ovalocyte Elliptocyte.

Ovarian agenesis Failure of development of ovaries. *SYN*—Turner's syndrome.

Ovarian follicle An ovum and the granulosa cell surrounding it occupying the cortex of ovary.

Ovarian graft A portion of ovary implanted commonly to abdominal wall to preserve hormone secretion.

Ovarian hormones 1. Follicular hormones-estradiol, estrone, and estriol 2. Luteal hormone-progesterone.

Ovarian ligament The terminal portion of genital ridge uniting the caudal end of embryonic ovary with the uterus.

Ovarian plexus A network of veins in the broad ligament or nerve plexus around the ovary.

Ovary The glandular female reproductive organ giving rise to ova (*see* Figure on page 526).

Overbite The extent to which the upper anterior teeth overlap the lower during occlusion.

Overriding The extent of overlapping of broken ends in a fracture.

Overweight Excessive weight of an individual by more than 10% than permissible for sex and age.

Oviparous Producing eggs.

Ovoid Egg shaped.

Ovotestis Ovarian and testicular tissue combined in the same gonad.

Ovulation The maturation and discharge of ovum (*see* Figure on page 526).

Ovum The female germ cell.

Oxalate Any ester or salt of oxalic acid.

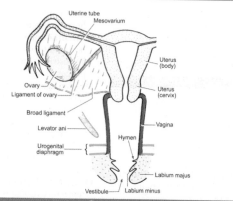

Ovary

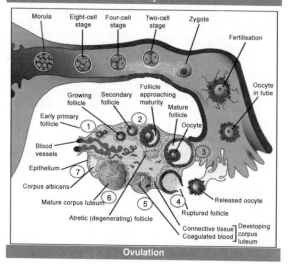

Ovulation

Oxalic acid An acid found in plants and vegetables, used as reagent.

Oxaloacetic acid A participant in citric acid metabolic cycle.

Oxalosis An inborn error of metabolism due to impaired glyoxylic acid metabolism with overproduction of oxalic acid and deposition of calcium oxalate in body tissues.

Oxaluria Presence of oxalic acid or oxalates in urine.

Oxandrolone Anabolic steroid.

Oxazepam A benzodiazepine, tranquilizer.

Oxcarbazepine Antiepileptic drug.

Oxethazaine Gastric mucosal anesthetic.

Oxidase Enzyme that promotes an oxidation reaction.

Oxidation An increase in positive valence of an element or decrease in negative valence occurring due to loss of electrons; the process of combining with oxygen.

Oxime Any compound resulting from action of hydroxylamine upon an aldehyde or ketone.

Oximeter Photoelectric instrument for measuring degree of oxygen saturation of blood.

Oxymetholone Anabolic steroid.

Oxprenolol A betablocker used in coronary artery disease.

Oxybutynin Urinary antispasmodic.

Oxycephaly A condition where head is conical in shape.

Oxycodone A narcotic analgesic, dihydro hydroxy codeinone.

Oxygen The colorless and odorless gas that supports combustion and essential to animal life. It constitutes one-fifth of atmosphere, eight-ninth of water and one half of earth's crust.

Oxygen hyperbaric Oxygen given at 1½-3 times of atmospheric pressure in gangrene, cyanide poisoning, burns, smoke inhalation, crush injury, etc.

Oxygen radicals Hydrogen peroxide, superoxide produced by incomplete reduction of oxygen that cause membrane damage.

Oxygen saturation Oxygen content divided by oxygen capacity expressed in volume per cent.

Oxygen tent A transparent air tight chamber, enclosing patient's head and shoulder, in which oxygen content can be maintained at a higher level.

Oxyhemoglobin Hemoglobin combined with oxygen.

Oxymetazoline A vasoconstrictor used topically to reduce nasal congestion.

Oxymetholone An anabolic steroid.

Oxymorphone A semisynthetic narcotic analgesic.

Oxyntic Secreting acid, e.g. parietal cells of stomach.

Oxyopia Unusual acuity of vision.

Oxyphenbutazone A metabolite of phenyl butazone used for its analgesic—antiinflammatory property.

Oxyphenisatin A cathartic.

Oxyphenonium bromide An anticholinergic agent used in peptic ulcer and gastrointestinal hypermotility or spasm.

Oxypurinol A xanthine oxidase inhibitor, used in gout.

Oxytetracycline An antibiotic of tetracycline group from *Streptomyces rimosus* where the hydrogen atom of tetracycline is replaced by a hydroxyl group.

Oxytocin An octapeptide secreted by posterior pituitary, causes uterine contraction and promotes lactation.

Ozone O_3. An allotropic form of oxygen, a powerful oxidizing agent, used as disinfectant.

Ozonide A compound of ozone with certain unsaturated organic substances that exert bactericidal effect from liberation of nascent oxygen.

P

Pachhionian bodies Pedunculated fibrous tissue growths along longitudinal fissure of cerebrum.

Pacemaker 1. Electronic device that controls rate and rhythm of heart. 2. The specialized cells in right atrium that generate impulse. *p. wandering* A form of arrhythmia where the origin of cardiac impulse shifts from place to place (*see* Figure).

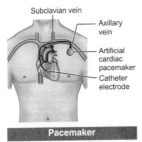

Subclavian vein

Axillary vein

Artificial cardiac pacemaker

Catheter electrode

Pacemaker

Pachyderma Unusual thickening of skin.

Pachymeningitis Inflammation of dura mater.

Pachyonychia Abnormal thickening of nails.

Pacing code A three letter code for describing pacemaker type and function. The first letter indicates the heart chamber paced (V = ventricle, A = atrium, D = dual), the second letter indicates the chamber from which electrical activity is sensed and the third letter indicates the response to sensed electrical activity.

Pacinian corpuscle Encapsulated sensory nerve endings of skin and internal organs sensitive to deep pressure.

Pack A dry or moist; hot or cold blanket or sheet used for therapeutic purpose.

Packed cell Blood containing cellular elements only, devoid of plasma.

PaCO$_2$ Partial pressure of CO_2 in arterial blood.

Pad Cushion of soft material used to apply pressure, or support on an organ.

Paget's disease Skeletal disease of elderly with thickening, softening and bending of bones. *P's disease of breast* Carcinoma of mammary ducts.

Pagophagia A form of pica where patient loves eating ice.

Pain Sensory and emotional experience associated with irritation/inflammation of tissue.

Paint Castellani's A germicide containing phenol, resorcinol, boric acid, etc.

Palatal reflex Soft palate contraction during attempt of swallowing.

Palate Roof of the mouth separating it from nasal cavity (*see* Figure).

Palatine arches Two arch like folds of mucous membrane (glossopalatine and pharyn-

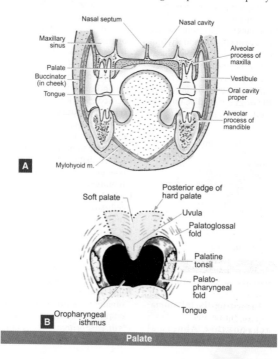

Palate

gopalatine) that form the lateral margin of faucial and pharyngeal isthmuses.

Palatine artery Branch of maxillary artery, supplying palate and pharynx.

Palatoglossus Muscle that arises from sides and undersurface of tongue and inserted to palatine aponeurosis. It acts as a constrictor of faucial isthmus by raising the root of tongue.

Palatography Recording of movement of palate during speech.

Palatopharyngeus Muscle that arises from thyroid cartilage and pharyngeal wall and inserted into aponeurosis of soft palate. It constricts pharyngeal isthmus and raises larynx.

Palatorrhaphy Operation for cleft palate.

Paclitaxel Antineoplastic agent.

Paleocerebellum The oldest portion of cerebellum that includes flocculi, and part of vermis concerned with equilibrium, and locomotion.

Paleothalamus Medial older parts of thalamus.

Palilalia Rapid repetition of same words and phrases.

Pallidectomy Surgical or cryogenic/laser destruction of globus pallidus.

Pallor Paleness.

Palm Anterior surface of hand from wrist to fingers.

Palmar reflex Grasping reflex in infants that disappears after 4-5 months of age.

Palm-chin reflex Contraction of superficial muscles of eye and chin on scratching of the-nar eminence of the same side. *SYN*—Palmomental reflex.

Palmitic acid A long chain fatty acid found in palm oil.

Palpable Perceptible to touch.

Palpation Examination by application of hand or fingers.

Palpebra An eyelid.

Palpebral commissure The union of the eyelids at each end of palpebral fissure.

Palpebral fissure Opening between the eyelids.

Palpebral ligament The medial and lateral ligaments that fix the two ends of tarsi to the orbital wall.

Palpitation Rapid throbbing pulsation of heart.

Palsy Paralysis/loss of ability to act. *p. Bell's* Lower motor facial palsy. *p. bulbar* Paralysis of lower cranial nerves. *p. cerebral* Nonprogressive palsy of childhood from developmental defect of brain, or birth asphyxia or trauma. *p. Erb's* Palsy of C_5C_6 due to lesion of brachial plexus. *p. shaking* Paralysis agitans.

Pamidronate A biphosphonate for osteoporosis.

Panitumumab Monoclonal antibody for colon cancer.

Pampiniform Convoluted like a tendril.

Pampinocele *SYN* – varicocele; swollen dilated veins of pampiniform plexus of spermatic cord.

Panangiitis Inflammation of all the three layers of a blood vessel.

Panarteritis Inflammation of all the three coats of an artery.

Pancarditis Inflammation of all the three layers of heart i.e., pericardium, myocardium and endocardium.

Pancoast's syndrome Tumor of lung apex that erodes into brachial plexus to produce Horner's syndrome.

Pancolectomy Surgical excision of entire colon.

Pancreas A compound acinotubular gland in front of L_1L_2 vertebra behind the stomach, secretes hormones like insulin, glucagon and digestive enzymes. *p. annular* A portion of pancreas encircles duodenum (*see* Figure).

Pancreatectomy Excision of a part or whole of pancreas.

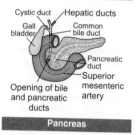

Opening of bile and pancreatic ducts

Pancreas

Pancreatic juice 500-800 ml of alkaline pancreatic secretion per day containing enzymes like trypsinogen, amylopsin, lipase, etc. Secretin and cholecystokinin secreted by duodenum stimulate pancreatic secretion.

Pancreaticoduodenostomy Surgical creation of an artificial tract between pancreas and duodenum.

Pancreatin A mixture of pancreatic enzymes like amylase, lipase and proteases.

Pancreatitis Inflammation of pancreas. *p. calcareous* Pancreatitis accompanied by pancreatic calcification. *p. chronic* Scarred pancreas due to chronic inflammation.

Pancreatolith Calculus within pancreas.

Pancreozymin Polypeptide that stimulates pancreas to secrete insulin; also found in brain.

Pancuronium bromide Neuromuscular blocking agent.

Pancytopenia Reduction in all cellular elements i.e., RBC, WBC, platelets in blood.

Pandemic Disease widely prevalent in population.

Pandiculation Yawning and stretching of limbs as on awakening from sleep.

Panencephalitis A diffuse inflammation of brain. *P. subacute sclerosing* a cerebral degenerative disease which in fatal in childhood and is due to chronic measles.

Paneth cells Secretory cells in the intestinal crypts.

Panic Sudden anxiety, terror or fright.

Panic attack Acute intense anxiety with sweating, palpitation, nausea, chest pain and feeling of approaching death.

Panniculitis Inflammation of fatty connective tissue.

Pannus Vascularization around cornea.

Pansinusitis Inflammation of all paranasal sinuses i.e. maxillary frontal, ethmoidal.

Panting Shallow rapid breathing.

Pantograph A device that reproduces figures or drawings.

Pantopaque Iophendylate, a radiographic contrast for myelography.

Pantoprazole Proton pump inhibitor.

Pantothenic acid A member of vitamin B complex group found in yeast, liver, eggs etc.

PaO2 Partial pressure of oxygen in arterial blood.

Papain Proteolytic enzyme from papaya.

Papanicolaou test A study for detection of cancer from examination of cells shed from abnormal mucosal growths.

Papaverine Smooth muscle relaxant.

Papilla Small elevation, nipple like. *p. circum vallate* Large papilla near base of tongue. *p. filiform* Small papilla at tip of tongue. *p. interdental* Triangular shaped gingiva between the teeth. *p. lacrimal* Small elevation at inner end of eyelid through which lacrimal duct opens. *p. of hair* A conical portion of dermis through which capillaries enter into hair root. *p. of Vater* Elevation in medial wall of second part of duodenum through which pancreatic and common bile duct open. *p. renal* Apex of renal pyramids.

Papillary muscle The two muscle groups in each ventricle of heart connecting to free margin of A-V valves.

Papilledema Edema of optic nerve head.

Papilliform Resembling papilla.

Papillitis Inflammation of optic nerve head.

Papilloma Benign epithelial tumors including wart, condyloma and polyp.

Papillomatosis Widespread formation of papillomas.

Papovavirus The group includes polyoma virus, papilloma virus which are incriminated in cancer.

Pappus The fine downy beard hair appearing at puberty.

Papule Solid circumscribed elevation of skin.

Papulosquamous Presence of papules and scales.

Para-aminobenzoic Used as sunscreen.

Para-aminohippuric acid Derivative of amino benzoic acid used for testing renal excretory function.

Para-aminosalicylic acid Bacteriostatic antituberculous agent.

Paracentesis Cavity puncture for draining fluid.

Paracentral Near to center. *p. lobule* Cerebral convolution on medial surface serving as motor area of leg.

Parachromatism Defective color perception.

Paracoccidioidomycosis Chronic granulomatous fungal disease of skin.

Paracrine Hormone secretion from non-endocrine cells.

Paradoxical respiration 1. Seen in open pneumothorax where lungs fill during expiration. 2. Moving up of diaphragm during inspiration in diaphragmatic palsy.

Paraffin Hydrocarbon derivative of petroleum. *p. liquid* Mineral oil. *p. soft petrolatum* Used for making creams and ointments.

Paraganglia Sympathetic ganglia akin to adrenal medulla.

Paraganglioma Tumor of adrenal medulla and paraganglia.

Paragonimiasis Infestation with fluke *P. westermanni,* transmitted through crabs and causing lung infection.

Paragranuloma Benign form of Hodgkin's disease only limited to lymphatic system.

Parainfluenza virus A group of viruses causing acute upper respiratory infection.

Parakeratosis A partial keratinization process where keratinocytes still contain nuclei

Paraldehyde Colorless liquid polymer of acetaldehyde used as a hypnotic, analgesic and anticonvulsant.

Paralexia Difficulty in comprehension of vocal/printed matter with substitution of meaningless words.

Parallax Displacement of objects by change in observer's position.

Paralysis Loss of muscular function usually due to nerve dysfunction; may be spastic or flaccid. *p. agitans* Parkinson's disease characterized by rigidity, akinesia, tremor and gait disorder. *p. Bell's* Lower motor facial palsy. *p. crossed* Paralysis of one side of body and opposite side of face, a feature of lesion in brainstem. *p. familial periodic* Flaccid palsy usually on awakening due to disturbances in serum potassium. *p. hysteric* Apparent paralysis due to psychiatric conflict. *p. Erb's* Paralysis of muscles of upper arm due to C_5C_6 root lesion. *p. Klumpke's* Birth injury causing paralysis of arm and hand muscles (Policeman's hand in bribe). *p. Pott's* Tuberculosis of spine causing paraplegia. *p. pseudobulbar* Upper motor palsy of cranial nerves due to central lesion. *p. Saturday night* Compression of radial nerve in spiral groove (usually due to alcoholic binge on saturday night). *p. Todd's* Transient muscular palsy (up to 24 hours) following epilepsy, due to neuronal exertion.

Paralytic ileus Intestinal palsy with distention of abdomen, vomiting and obstipation.

Paramagnetic Anything attracted by a magnet.

Paramedian Close to midline.

Paramedic A trained person to assist doctor.

Paramedical Supplementary to medical profession like occupational, speech and physiotherapy.

Paramethidione Anticonvulsant.

Parametritis Inflammation of parametrium.

Parametrium Loose connective tissue around uterus.

Paramnesia Use of words without meaning or recall of events that never occurred.

Paramyotonia Increased muscle tone and poor relaxation after contraction.

Paramyxoviruses Includes measles, mumps, parainfluenza and respiratory syncytial virus.

Paranasal sinuses Frontal, maxillary, ethmoidal and sphenoidal sinuses.

Paraneoplastic syndrome Symptoms of multiple organ dysfunction in a patient of cancer (lung, kidney) without actual metastasis.

Paranoia Paranoid schizophrenia.

Paranoid Ideas of persecution, suspicious thinking.

Paraphasia Misuse of spoken words or word combinations.

Paraphilia A psychosexual disorder that includes fetishism, transvestism, pedophilia, voyeurism which mean bizarre acts for sexual excitation.

Paraphimosis Inflamed or narrowed prepuce unable to be retracted over glans and strangulating it.

Paraphrasia Unintelligible speech due to incorrect and jumbling up of words used.

Paraplegia Paralysis of both legs. *p. dolorosa* Extremely painful paraplegia due to pressure of a neoplasm on nerve roots and spinal cord. *p. Pott's* Tuberculosis of spine with paraplegia.

Paraprotein Abnormal plasma protein like macroglobulin, myeloma protein.

Paraquat A weed killer that when ingested causes liver, renal and pulmonary damage.

Parasite Organism living at expense of another organism. *p. external* Parasite living on outer surface of host e.g., lice, fleas, ticks, etc. *p. facultative* Parasite capable of living independent of the host at times.

Parasitemia Presence of parasite in the blood.

Parasitize To infest with a parasite.

Parasitology The study of parasites and parasitism.

Parasternal Adjacent to sternum.

Parasympathetic nervous system The preganglionic fibers arise from midbrain, medulla and sacral portion of spinal cord through 3rd, 7th, 9th and 10th cranial nerves and S2-S4 somatic nerves to synapse with postganglionic neurones located in autonomic ganglia. Parasympathetic stimulation causes smooth muscle contraction, increased glandular secretion (except that of sweat) and slowing of heart.

Parasympatholytic Agents that have actions opposite to parasympathetic stimulation.

Parasympathomimetic Agent that produces actions similar to parasympathetic stimulation.

Parasystole Ectopic rhythm from ventricle.

Parathion Insecticide, toxic to humans.

Parathormone Parathyroid hormone controlling calcium and phosphorus metabolism.

Parathyroids Four small glands lying in neck adjacent

**to thyroid whose extirpation leads to hypocalcemia, carpopedal spasm, and tetany.

Paratrichosis Abnormality of hair or its growth pattern.

Paratyphoid fever A less severe form of typhoid caused by *Salmonella paratyphi*.

Parazoon An animal that lives as parasite on another animal.

Parecoxib Anti-iaflammatory, analgesic.

Paregoric 1. Soothing. 2. Tincture opium used for diarrhea.

Parenchyma The functional portion of an organ.

Parent A father or mother.

Parenteral Any route other than alimentary canal.

Paresis Partial or incomplete paralysis.

Paresthesia Sensation of numbness, pricking, needling, tingling due to irritation of a nerve or its central connections.

Parietal Forming wall of a cavity or outer shell. *p. cells* Large cells or oxyntic cells secreting HCl in stomach.

Parieto-occipetal Relating to parietal and occipital bones or lobes.

Perinaud's syndrome Paralysis of vertical gaze due to subthalamic bleed.

Pari passu Side by side, occurring at the same time/rate.

Parity Carrying pregnancy up to viability (28 weeks gestation).

Parkinson's disease See paralysis agitans.

Paromomycin Aminoglycoside antibiotic used to treat amebiasis.

Paronychia Infection of nail margin soft tissue.

Paronychosis Growth of nail in an abnormal position.

Paroophoron Vestigial structure consisting of minute tubules, the remains of caudal group of mesonephric tubules, homologous to paradidymis of male.

Parosmia Perversion of sense of smell where agreeable odors are considered offensive and vice versa.

Parosteal Connected to or arising from outer layer of periosteum.

Parotid duct The duct of parotid gland 2" long opening into mouth opposite second upper molar.

Parotid gland One of the salivary glands near angle of mouth secreting saliva.

Parotitis Inflammation of parotid gland.

Parovarium Vestigial remains of mesonephric tubules located in mesosalpinx between the ovary and fallopian tubes.

Paroxetine SSRI antidepressant.

Paroxysm Periodic recurrence of symptoms.

Paroxysmal cold hemoglobinuria Autoimmune hemolysis due to hemolysins occurring in syphilis and some viral infections, manifesting with chill, abdominal pain and fever with hemoglobinuria.

Parrot's node Bony outgrowths on the skull of infants with congenital syphilis.

Pars flaccida A portion of ear drum that is not taut SYN – Sharpnell's membrane.

Pars tensa Tightly stretched larger portion of tympanic membrane.

Parthenogenesis (Parthenos = virgin). Reproduction arising from unfertilized female egg.

Particle A tiny fragment or very minute piece. *p. alpha* A charged radioactive particle of low penetrability. *p. beta* A high speed electron emitted during decay of an atom. *p. Dane* HBsAg, serum hepatitis capsular antigen.

Parturient Concerning childbirth.

Parturition Delivery or childbirth.

Parvovirus A group of viruses pathogenic to humans and animals *P.V. B19-* causes benign rash (fifth disease) but in immunocompromised can cause aplastic anemia. Intrauterine infection can cause fetal hydrops.

Passion Great emotion or zeal usually concerning sexual excitement.

Passive exercise Exercise to muscle given by an assistant or machine.

Passive smoking Inhaling smoke by persons around the smoke.

Passivity Dependence upon others, not willing to take responsibility.

Pasteurization The process of sterilizing a fluid without changing its chemical composition.

Past pointing Inability to place fingers at a selected point in space, a feature of cerebellar disorder.

Patella A sesamoid bone in front of knee in the tendon of quadriceps femoris muscle. *P. alta-* Patella in placed high. *P. bipartite* – patella develops from two centeres, often mistaken for fracture.

Patellar ligament The extension of quadriceps femoris tendon beyond inferior pole of patella to be attached to tuberosity of tibia.

Patellar reflex Contraction of quadriceps on tap on patellar ligament.

Patency The state of being open.

Patent Open.

Patent ductus arteriosus Persistent communication between aorta and pulmonary artery after birth.

Paternity test Group of tests (blood group, HLA, and gene analysis) done to determine if a particular individual has fathered the specific child in question.

Pathetism Winning over and exploring some one's mind by suggestion.

Pathogen Any microorganism capable of causing disease.

Pathognomonic Discrete or characteristic symptom of a disease.

Pathology Branch of medical science dealing with nature and cause of disease and the functional/structural changes caused by the disease.

Pathophysiology Study of changes in physiology by the diseased process.

Patient One who is ill or sick, physically or mentally.

Patient-controlled analgesia A system of controlling pain by drugs whose delivery is controlled by the patient himself; usually helpful in obstetric pain of labor by epidural catheter drug delivery.

Patulous Open, spread apart.

Paul-Bunnell test Test for heterophil antibody in patients of infectious mononucleosis.

Peau d' orange Dimpled skin resembling orange as in carcinoma breast.

Pectin A carbohydrate obtained from peel of citrous fruits and apple pulp used as astringent.

Pectineal line The ridge of pubis bone.

Pectineus The quadrangular muscle at upper and inner thigh acting as a flexor and adductor of thigh.

Pectoralis Pertains to breast; the muscles on anterior chest wall. *p. major* Triangular muscle attached to upper humerus that draws the arm forward and downward.

Pectoriloquy The distinct transmission of vocal sounds to ear through the chest wall as in consolidation.

Pectus The chest or thorax. *p. carinatum* Abnormal prominence of sternum as in rickets *SYN* – Pigeon chest. *p. excavatum* Abnormal depression of sternum (*see* Figure on page 540).

Pedesis Brownian movement of particles in a system, may be liquid or gas.

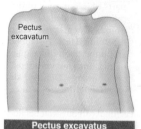

Pectus excavatum

Pectus excavatus

Pediatrics Medical science dealing with children below 14 years of age.

Pedicle The stem that attaches the tumor to the organ (*see* Figure).

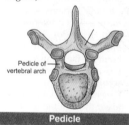

Pedicle of vertebral arch

Pedicle

Pedicle flap The skin flap used in plastic surgery which carries its blood supply.

Pediculosis Infestation with lice.

Pedigree The tree or chart involving one's ancestors as used for genetic analysis.

Pedodontist Dentist practising pediatric dentistry.

Pedograph Imprint of foot on paper.

Peduncle A connecting band of nervous tissue. *p. cerebellar inferior* Connects spinal cord and medulla with cerebellum. *p. cerebellar middle* Channel for pontocerebellar fibers. *p. cerebellar superior* Connects cerebellum with midbrain. *p. cerebral* A pair of white bundle connecting cerebrum to midbrain; the pathway for descending corticospinal and corticonuclear projection.

Pegrete The downward extension of thickened epidermis between the dermal papillae.

Pel-Ebstein fever Cyclic fever occurring in Hodgkin's disease.

Pelger-Huet anomaly A congenital inherited anomaly of neutrophils which have coarse chromatin in the nuclei but function in normal manner.

Peliosis Purple patches on skin and mucous membrane. *SYN*—purpura.

Pellagra Avitaminosis due to want of nicotinic acid manifesting with diarrhea, dermatitis and dementia.

Pellet A small ball of medicine or food.

Pelotherapy Therapeutic use of mud or hay to treat disease by application on body.

Pelvic inflammatory disease Infection of fallopian tubes, broad ligament and supporting tissues of uterus (*see* Figure).

Pelvic inlet Upper pelvic entry i.e., space between sacral promontory and upper aspect of symphysis pubis.

Pelvic outlet Lower pelvic outlet outlined by tip of coccyx, ischial tuberosities and lower margin of symphysis pubis.

Pelvimetry Measurement of pelvic dimension manually or by X-ray.

Pelvis The structure formed by iliac bones, sacrum and coccyx.

Inlet A-P diameter = 11 cm.

Diagonal conjugate = 13 cm. True conjugate = 11 cm. Transverse diameter = 11 cm. Outlet AP diameter = 11 cm. *p. android* Male type pelvis with shallow sacral hollow. *p. anthropoid* Long narrow pelvis. *p. contracted* Pelvis in which one or more diameters are less so as to impede birth of fetus. *p. funnel shaped* Pelvis with normal inlet but markedly contracted outlet. *p. Naegeles* Obliquely contracted pelvis. *p. Otto* Pelvis in which head of femur extends into pelvic cavity due to depressed acetabulum (*see* Figure on page 542).

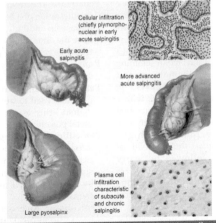

Early acute salpingitis

Cellular infiltration (chiefly plymorpho-nuclear in early acute salpingitis

More advanced acute salpingitis

Plasma cell infiltration characteristic of subacute and chronic salpingitis

Large pyosalpinx

Pyosalpinx associated with pelvic inflammatory disease

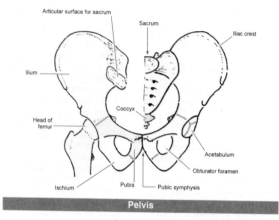

Articular surface for sacrum

Sacrum

Iliac crest

Ilium

Coccyx

Head of femur

Acetabulum

Obturator foramen

Ischium

Pubis

Pubic symphysis

Pelvis

Pemphigus A bullous disease that appears suddenly on normal skin and disappears leaving pigmented spots. *p. erythematous* Erythematous macules and blebs resembling lupus erythematosus and perphigus vulgaris. *p. foliaceus* Pemphigus with a chronic course and purulent bullous fluid from beginning. *p. vegetans* Pemphigus with pustules instead of bullae followed by warty vegetations. *p. vulgaris* Common form of bullous pemphigus with bilateral distribution.

Pemphigoid Skin lesion similar to pemphigus.

Penetrance The frequency of manifestation of a hereditary disease in individuals who have the dominant or double recessive gene.

Penfluridol Antipsychotic agent.

Penicillamine A derivative of penicillin used to treat rheumatoid arthritis and heavy metal poisoning.

Penicillin Antibiotic synthesized by various molds, bactericidal to gram positive cocci, spirochaetes and rickettsiae by inhibition of cell wall synthesis.

Penicillinase An enzyme that breaks up molecule of some penicillins.

Penicillium A genus of molds that occasionally produce infection of external ear, skin and respiratory passage.

Penicilloyl-polylysine A substance used to test sensitiveness of a person to penicillins by intradermal skin test or instillation to conjunctival sac.

Penile prosthesis Implantable device in the penis to achieve erection; the device is in form of inflatable plastic cylinders implanted to corpora cavernosa attached to a pump embedded in scrotal pouch. The fluid reservoir to fill the cylinders is implanted behind the rectus.

Penile reflex Contraction of bulbocavernosus muscle on percussion of dorsum of penis or compression of glans penis.

Penile ring A malleable ring that by preventing venus return from penis helps to maintain erection and delaying orgasm.

Penis The male organ of copulation consisting of root, body and glans penis. The body contains paired corpora cavernosa and the corpus spongiosum through which passes the urethra (*see* Figure on page 544).

Pentaerythritol tetranitrate Organic nitrate for angina pectoris.

Pentagastrin Synthetic gastrin to stimulate HCl secretion.

Pentamidine An antimonial used to treat leishmaniasis.

Pentavalent Having valency of five.

Pentazocine An analgesic with strong addictive potential.

Pentobarbital A hypnotic-sedative agent.

Pentolinium Ganglion blocking agent.

Pentosuria Excretion of pentose sugars in urine.

Pentothal sodium Thiopental sodium, used for induction of anesthesia.

Pentoxifylline Vasodilator improve haemorrheology.

Penumbra in radiology an area of blurring around the edge of a structure. *p. ischaemic* an area of moderately ischaemic zone around a more severely ischaemic zone.

Pepsin Proteolytic enzyme of gastric juice which converts proteins into proteoses and peptones.

Pepsinogen The inactive precursor of pepsin found as granules in chief cells of stomach.

Peptic ulcer An ulcer occurring at sites of peptic mucosa, i.e.

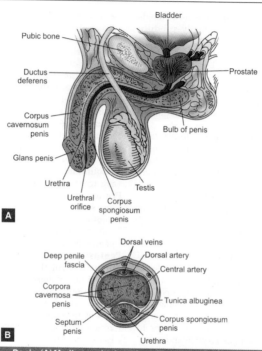

Penis. (A) Median sagittal section; (B) transverse section

lower end of esophagus, stomach, first part of duodenum.

Peptide Compound formed by combination of 2 or more amino acids.

Peptidoglycan The material making the cellwall of most microorganisms.

Peptidyl dipeptidase an enzyme of hydrolase class that converts angiotensin I to angiotensin II, hence called antiogensin converting enzyme (ACE).

Peptococcus Anaerobic grampositive cocci present in oral cavity, intestine and urinary tract.

Peptone Nitrogenous compounds formed by action of proteolytic enzymes on certain proteins.

Peptostreptococcus Gram-positive anaerobic cocci.

Per anum Through anus.

Percentile One of 100 equal divisions of a series of items or data.

Perception Process of being aware or being conscious.

Percolate To filter, to strain.

Percolator Apparatus used for extraction of a drug with a liquid solvent.

Percussion The use of finger tips to tap the body directly or indirectly to determine position, size and consistency of underlying structure (*see* Figure).

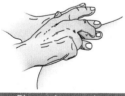

Bimanual percussion

Percutaneous Through skin.

Percutaneous transluminal coronary angioplasty (PTCA) A non-operative balloon dilata-tion of partially occluded coronary vessels.

Percutaneous ultrasonic litho-triptor Device using ultra-sound applied externally to break up kidney stone.

Perforation A hole.

Perfusion Supply of an organ/ tissue with blood.

Periactin Cypro heptadine hydrochloride, antiserotonin.

Periadenitis Inflammation of tissue surrounding a lym-phnode.

Perianal Around the anus.

Periarteritis Inflammation of outer coat of an artery.

Periarthritis Inflammation of joint capsule.

Peribronchial Surrounding the bronchus.

Pericardial rub Friction be-tween the inflamed layers of pericardium.

Pericardiectomy Excision of pericardium.

Pericardiocentesis Drainage of pericardial sac.

Pericardiopexy Increasing blood supply to heart by join-ing pericardium to adjacent tissue.

Pericarditis Inflammation of pericardium often with sero-fibrinous effusion and rarely constriction. *p. constrictive* Pericarditis leading to re-striction in ventricular filling with equalisation in diastolic pressure in both ventricles and atria.

Pericardium A bilayer fibroserous sac enclosing heart.

Pericholangitis Inflammation of tissue surrounding bile duct.

Perichondritis Inflamed perichondrium.

Perichondrium Fibrous membrane around the cartilage.

Pericranium Periosteum of skull.

Perimenopause The phase before menopause in which pattern of regular menstrual cycle changes to irregular cycles with increased period of amenorrhea.

Perinatal The period beginning after the 28th week of pregnancy and ending 28 days after birth.

Perindopril ACE inhibitor.

Perineoraphy Repair of perineal tear caused during parturition.

Perineotomy Incision into perineum to facilitate delivery as in rigid perineum of primi.

Perinephric Around the kidney.

Perineum The structures occupying the pelvic outlet and constituting pelvic floor. *p. tears of* First degree tear involves vaginal mucosa, second degree involves the musculature in addition and in third degree tear the anal sphincter is also torn (*see* Figure on page 547).

Perineural Around the nerve.

Perineurium Connective tissue sheath around bundle of nerve fibers.

Period The menstruation; the time interval between two events. *p. absolute refractory* The period during which any strong stimulus cannot bring about muscle contraction. *p. gestation* Period of pregnancy, i.e. 10 lunar months or 280 days measured from onset of last menstrual period. *p. incubation* Time from contacting infection till appearance of first symptom. *p. isoelectric* In ECG electrical neutrality or balancing positive and negative charges. *p. latent* Time between application of stimulus and onset of contraction. *p. missed* Nonoccurrence of menstruation at expected time. *p. puerperal* The six weeks period immediately following child birth. *p. safe* The period during the menstrual cycle during which intercourse cannot lead to conception. It usually includes the first 5 days after stoppage of period and the last 10 days prior to next period.

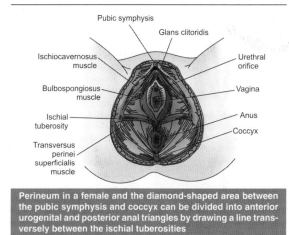

Pubic symphysis
Glans clitoridis
Ischiocavernosus muscle
Urethral orifice
Bulbospongiosus muscle
Vagina
Ischial tuberosity
Anus
Transversus perinei superficialis muscle
Coccyx

Perineum in a female and the diamond-shaped area between the pubic symphysis and coccyx can be divided into anterior urogenital and posterior anal triangles by drawing a line transversely between the ischial tuberosities

Periodic table The chart depicting chemical elements arranged by their atomic numbers.

Periodicity Recurring at more or less regular intervals.

Periodontal abscess Abscess formation in gingiva, periodontal pockets.

Periodontal disease Disease of supporting structure of teeth with bleeding gum, loosening of teeth, etc.

Periodontal ligament The fibrous bundles attaching tooth to alveolar bone.

Periodontics The branch of dentistry dealing with study and treatment of periodontal disease.

Periodontitis Inflammatory or degenerative disease of dental periosteum, alveolar bone, cementum and gingiva.

Periodontium The structures that support the teeth and firmly anchor it to alveolar bone (*see* Figure on page 548).

Periodoscope Pregnancy table for knowing expected date of delivery.

Perionychia Inflammation around a nail.

Perioperative Period immediately before or after an operation.

Perioral Around the mouth.

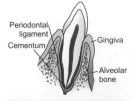

Periodontal ligament

Gingiva

Cementum

Alveolar bone

Peridontium—showing the peridontal ligament attaching the cemtnum of the tooth root to the alveolar bone of the socket and the collagen fibers of the ligament are grouped into bundles

Periosteitis Inflamed periosteum.

Periosteum A fibrous membrane covering the bone, supporting the blood vessels supplying bone and giving attachment to ligaments and muscles. Its inner cellular layer forms new bone.

Peripheral nervous system Included in this are 12 cranial nerves, 31 spinal nerves, sympathetic and parasympathetic nerves.

Periphlebitis Inflammation of outer coat of vein or tissue around the vein.

Peristalsis Wave like contraction occurring in hollow viscus.

Peristasis A temporary decrease in blood flow in early inflammation.

Peritomy Incision around cornea to treat pannus.

Peritoneal dialysis Removal of toxic metabolic byproducts and some poisons from body by irrigation of peritoneal cavity by dialysate and then draining out the dialysate.

Peritoneopexy Fixation of uterus by way of vagina.

Peritoneoscope An endoscope to visualize abdominal cavity through an incision in the abdominal wall.

Peritoneum A serous membrane reflected over abdominal viscera and lining the abdominal cavity.

Peritonitis Inflamed peritoneum manifesting with board like rigidity of abdomen and aperistalsis, commonly follows rupture of hollow organ, pelvic inflammation, or is primary; can be localized or generalized; acute or chronic, adhesive and aseptic.

Peritrichous Organism with cilia/flagella covering its entire body.

Periurethral Around the urethra.

Permeability The quality of being permeable that which can be traversed.

Pernicious anemia Vitamin B_{12} deficient anemia due to antibodies to gastric parietal cells leading to deficient intrinsic factor secretion.

Pernio Swelling of skin due to cold.

Peroneal Concerning fibula.

Peroneal sign In tetany tapping over peroneal nerve causes dorsiflexion and eversion of foot.

Peroral Through the mouth.

Peroxidase An enzyme essential for oxygen transfer, hence important in cellular respiration.

Peroxisome Granules in cell cytoplasm that contain a variety of enzymes.

Perphenazin e Antipsychotic agent.

Perseveration Repetition of meaningless words, phrases or answers.

Personality The composition of one's characteristics, behavior, grooming, etc. *p. compulsive* A type of personality where individual's perfectionism, indecisiveness hampers with social adjustment and interpersonal relationship. *p. extroverted* Individual's activities and libido are directed to other individuals or environment. *p. histrionic* Personality with self exaggeration, dramatisation, irrational and angry outbursts. *p. introverted* Per-

son's activities and libido are directed towards himself. *p. paranoid* Undue suspiciousness, mistrust and hypersensitiveness. *p. schizoid* Shyness, seclusiveness, eccentricity.

Perspiration Water loss from skin via evaporation of sweat; 1 liter of sweat evaporation removes 580 calories of heat from the body.

Perthe's disease Osteochondritis of femoral head due to compromised circulation.

Perturbation Agitated, uneasiness of mind.

Pertussis Acute infectious respiratory disease caused by *B. pertussis. SYN*—whooping cough.

Pertussis immune globulin Globulin derived from patients immunized with pertussis vaccine, used for passive immunization.

Pertussis vaccine Killed pertussis bacilli used for active immunization.

Perversion Deviation from normal accepted path. *p. sexual* Abnormal sexual behavior.

Pervert One who has deviated from normal path.

Pervious Capable of being permeated.

Pes Foot *p. cavus* Increased concavity of foot. *p. equinovalgus* Elevation and lateral rotation of heel. *p. equino varus* Elevation and internal rotation of heel. *p. equinus* Walking on forefoot, the heel not touching the ground.

Pessary Device inserted into vagina to support pelvic structures like uterus, urethra (*see* Figure).

Pessimism A state of mind where one feels dejected, hopeless and gloomy.

Pest Destructive insect.

Pesticide Chemicals used to kill pests.

Petechiae Hemorrhagic spots on the skin.

Pethidine Meperidine hydrochloride.

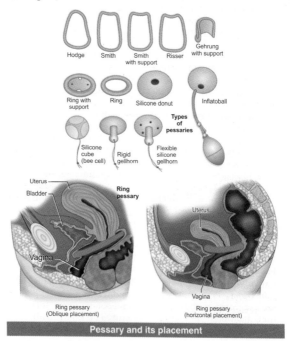

Hodge   Smith   Smith with support   Risser   Gehrung with support

Ring with support   Ring   Silicone donut   Inflatoball

Types of pessaries

Silicone cube (bee cell)   Rigid gellhorn   Flexible silicone gellhorn

Uterus
Bladder
Ring pessary
Vagina

Ring pessary
(Oblique placement)

Uterus
Vagina

Ring pessary
(horizontal placement)

Pessary and its placement

Petit's ligament Uterosacral ligament.

Petit's triangle An area on lateral abdominal wall bounded by iliac crest, posterior margin of external oblique and lateral margin of latissims dorsi.

Petitmal Little illness. A form of epilepsy.

Petri dish A shallow dish with a cover to hold solid media for culture.

Petrifaction Process of hardening.

Petrositis Inflammation of petrous part of temporal bone.

Peutz-Jegher's syndrome Small intestinal polyposis with hypermelanosis of skin and mucous membrane.

Peyer's patch Lymphoid tissue in small intestine as circular/oval patches in the mucosa-submucosa in the antimesenteric border.

Peyronie's disease Hardening of corpora cavernosa which leads to painful erection and a curved penis.

pH The degree of acidity or alkalinity based on hydrogen ion concentration. Maximum acidity is pH0 and maximum alkalinity in pH 14. Blood pH is 7.35-7.45.

Phacoemulsification A method of cataract removal by disintegrating it, followed by aspiration.

Phacomatosis A group of hereditary diseases manifesting with cutaneous and neurological symptoms. Included in this group are von-Recklinghausen's disease, Hippel-Lindau disease, Sturge-Weber syndrome, tuberous sclerosis and incontinentia pigmenti.

Phage Viruses that can lyse bacteria.

Phage typing A method of identifying particular strains of bacteria that are lysed by only strain specific bacteriophages.

Phagocyte A cell capable of ingesting and digesting cell debris, protozoa, bacteria, etc.

Phagocytic index Average number of bacteria ingested by each leukocyte.

Phagocytosis The process of ingestion and digestion of bacteria by phagocytes.

Phagolysosome The body formed when membrane bound phagosome inside a macrophage fuses with lysosome.

Phagomania Abnormal craving for food.

Phagosome A membrane bound vacuole inside a phagocyte containing matters to be digested.

Phakoma Microscopic gray white tumor of retina in tuberous sclerosis.

Phalanx Bones on finger and toes; proximal, middle and distal.

Phalloidin Poisonous peptide from mushroom *Amanita phalloides.*

Phallus Penis.

Phaneromania Abnormal tendency to bite nails, pull or play with hair, beard or moustache.

Phantasy A daydream or disregard for reality.

Phantom An appearance or illusion of body part. *p. limb* Following amputation, patient feels as if the limb exists. *p. tumor* Muscular contraction or abdominal fat mistaken as tumor.

Pharmaceutics Science of dispensing medicines.

Pharmacodynamics Study of drugs and their action on living organisms.

Pharmacognosy The science of natural drugs and their properties.

Pharmacokinetics Branch of pharmacology dealing with the fate of drug substances.

Pharmacology The science of drugs, their property and effect.

Pharmacy The practice of compounding and dispensing medicines; a drug store.

Pharyngeal bursa A small blind sac occasionally present in lower portion of pharyngeal tonsils.

Pharyngeal reflex Contraction of pharyngeal musculature following its stimulation by contact.

Pharyngismus Spasm of pharyngeal muscles.

Pharyngitis Inflammation of pharyngeal mucosa.

Pharyngocele Hernia through pharyngeal wall.

Pharyngoconjunctival fever An adenovirus infection.

Pharynx The common gateway in throat for food and air extending from base of skull to 6th cervical vertebra. Nasopharynx is the portion above palate; oropharynx lies between palate and hyoid bone and laryngo-pharynx below the hyoid bone (*see* Figure on page 553).

Phase A stage of development.

Phenacemide Anticonvulsant agent, rarely used because of serious side effects.

Phenacetin An analgesic and antipyretic agent.

Phenanthrene A coal tar derivative with high carcinogenic potential.

Phenazopyridine Urinary analgesic causing red urine.

Phencyclidine A hallucinogen, also used as anesthetic in veterinary medicine (angel dust).

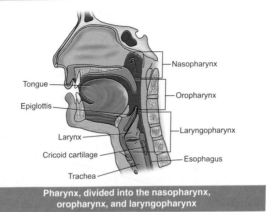

Pharynx, divided into the nasopharynx, oropharynx, and laryngopharynx

Phenelzine An antidepressant.

Phenergan Promethazine hydrochloride.

Phenformin An oral hypoglycemic agent, having propensity to cause lactic acidosis.

Phenindione An anticoagulant.

Pheniramine maleate An antihistaminic agent.

Phenmetrazine A sympathomimetic often used to treat obesity.

Phenobarbital Phenylethyl barbituric acid used as a hypnotic and anticonvulsant.

Phenol A coal tar derivative effective as a bacteriostatic agent (*SYN*—Carbolic acid).

Phenolphthalein A laxative.

Phenolsulphonphthalein A dye used for renal function test.

Phenomenon A change perceivable by senses. *p. Bell's* Rolling of eyeball upward and outward on attempting to close the affected eye in lower motor neurone facial palsy.

Phenothiazine The basic compound used for manufacture of tranquilizers, anthelmintics, dyes and some insecticides.

Phenotype The physical appearance or the sum total of visible traits which characterize the members of a group.

Phenoxyacetic acid A fungicide.

Phenoxybenzamine An alfa-adrenergic blocking agent that causes peripheral vaso-dilatation.

Phenozygous A developmental anomaly where the skull is much narrower than the face.

Phensuximide Anticonvulsant useful for petit mal.

Phentermine Sympathomimetic drug used as anorexic agent.

Phentolamine An alpha adrenergic blocking agent used in diagnosis of pheochromocytoma.

Phenylalanine An essential amino acid.

Phenylbutazone An analgesic anti-inflammatory agent sparingly used for adverse effects on marrow.

Phenylephrine Adrenergic agent used as nasal decongestant.

Phenylethyl alcohol An antibacterial agent used as a preservative.

Phenylhydrazine Used as a test reagent for detecting sugar in urine.

Phenylketonuria An autosomal recessive disease where due to defective enzyme system phenylalanine is not converted to tyrosine and there is likelihood of brain damage.

Phenylmercuric acetate A bacteriostatic agent, also fungicide and herbicide.

Phenylmercuric nitrate A bacteriostatic agent employed for wound dressing and preservation of IV solutions.

Phenylproparolamine Nasal decongestat.

Phenylpyruvic acid A metabolic derivative of phenylalanine.

Phenytoin Anticonvulsant drug, also antiarrhythmic.

Pheochromocyte The chromaffin cells of adrenal medulla giving yellowish reaction with chrome salts.

Pheochromocytoma A benign chromaffin cell tumor of adrenal medulla producing adrenaline and noradrenaline.

Pheromone A chemical substance which acts as a means of communication between species of insects through its smell.

Philadelphia chromosome Dislocation of long arm of chromosome 21 to chromosome-9, seen in 90% patients of chronic myelocytic leukemia (*see* Figure on page 555).

Philtrum The median groove on upper lip.

Phimosis Narrowing of prepucial orifice so that it cannot be retracted over glans penis.

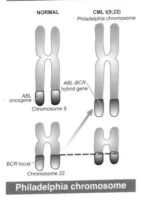

NORMAL   **CML t(9;22)**
             Philadelphia chromosome

ABL oncogene
Chromosome 9

ABL-BCR hybrid gene

BCR locus
Chromosome 22

Philadelphia chromosome

Phlebectomy Surgical resection of vein.

Phlebitis Inflammation of a vein.

Phlebogram A venous pulse tracing.

Phlebography X-ray imaging of the veins by contrast injection.

Phlebolith A concretion in a vein.

Phlebotom Lancent used in incising vein.

Phlebotomus A genus of sandflies, the blood sucking insects transmitting leishmaniasis, oroya fever.

Phlegm Thick mucus secreted by the respiratory tract.

Phlegmasia Inflammation. *p. alba dolens* Edema of leg due to thrombophlebitis.

Phlegmon Acute inflammation with suppuration of subcutaneous tissue.

Phlyctenula A tiny vesicle or pustule.

Phobia Irrational fear resulting in desire to avoid the feared object/situation.

Phocomelia Congenital malformation where proximal part of a limb is ill developed.

Pholcodine Morphine analog, high addictive potential.

Phonation Production of vocal sounds.

Phonetics Science of pronunciation and speech.

Phonocardiogram Graphic recording of heart sounds.

Phonophobia Morbid fear of sound or noise.

Phonophoresis Use of ultrasound to introduce drugs into tissue.

Phosgene A poisonous gas used in production of pharmaceutical and chemical products.

Phosphatase Enzymes that catalyze hydrolysis of phosphoric acid esters. *p. acid* Present in semen, prostatic secretion, osteoclasts and odontoclasts. *p. alkaline* Present in developing bone, plasma, and teeth; excreted by liver, increase in obstructive jaundice, bone metastasis and osteomalacia.

Phosphate Salt of phosphoric acid (PO_4). Monosodium and disodium phosphates help to maintain acid-base balance of blood. *p. acid* Phosphate in which one or two atoms of hydrogen in phosphoric acid are replaced by a metal. *p. triple* Calcium ammonium and magnesium phosphate.

Phosphaturia Increased excretion of phosphate in urine.

Phosphocreatine An important compound in muscle metabolism.

Phosphofructokinase A glycolytic enzyme.

Phosphorescence The emission of light without heat.

Phosphoric acid Principally used to etch enamel of teeth during restoration work.

Phosphorylase Enzyme catalyzing formation of glucose-1 phosphate from glycogen.

Phosphorylation The reaction of phosphate with an organic compound.

Photic epilepsy Convulsion following light stimulation.

Photocoagulation Light energy used to coagulate tissue proteins as in retinal detachment or diabetic proliferating retinopathy.

Photodermatitis Skin allergy due to ultraviolet light.

Photometer Device for measuring the intensity of light.

Photomicrograph Photograph of an object under microscope.

Photon Unit of energy of light ray.

Photophobia Intolerance to light, a feature of keratitis, uveitis, etc.

Photophone Instrument for production of sound by action of light.

Photopsia Subjective feeling of seeing flashes of light as in disease of hind brain (occipital cortex).

Photoptometer Instrument determining the smallest amount of light required to make an object visible.

Photoptometry Measurement of light perception.

Photoreceptor Sensory nerve endings or cells capable of being stimulated by light, e.g. rods and cones.

Photoretinitis Macular burn on exposure to intense light.

Photosensitizer Substance that compounds abnormal reaction of skin to light.

Photosynthesis The process by which plants combine water and trapped carbondioxide to produce carbohydrates.

Phototherapy Therapeutic use of sunlight or artificial blue light to reduce serum bilirubin in newborn.

Phototropism Tendency of plants and some microorganisms to grow towards light.

Phrenic Concerning diaphragm.

Phrenicotomy Severing the phrenic nerve to produce paralysis of diaphragm in order to provide rest to that lung.

Phthisic Concerning pulmonary tuberculosis.

Phycomycosis A fungal disease caused by inhalation of spores.

Phylogeny Growth and development of a race.

Phylum One of the primary divisions of animal or plant kingdom.

Physical Concerning body or material things.

Physical therapy Rehabilitation for restoration of function and prevention of disability by using exercise, heat, massage, ultraviolet, etc.

Physician A doctor practising medicine.

Physicist A specialist in physics.

Physics The science of laws of matter, their properties and various forms of energy.

Physiological Concerning normal body function.

Physiology The branch of science dealing with functions of living organisms.

Physiotherapy Treatment with physical means.

Physometra Distention of uterine cavity with gas.

Physostigmine Cholinergic agent, acts by destruction of cholinesterase in nerve ending; used in myasthenia gravis.

Phytin Calcium or magnesium salt of inositol and hexaphosphoric acid; present in cereals.

Phytobezoar An accumulated mass of vegetable matter found in the stomach.

Phytogenesis The origin and development of plants.

Phytohemagglutinin A plant lectin agglutinating red blood cells.

Phytonadione Synthetic vitamin K.

Phytophotodermatitis Dermatitis produced from exposure to certain plants and then to sunlight.

Phytosis Disease caused by vegetable parasite.

Phytotoxin Plant toxin.

Pica Perverted appetite with eating of uneatables like plastic, clay, plaster, etc.

Pickwickian syndrome Obesity with hypoventilation.

Pico = 10^{-12}

Picornavirus RNA virus group that includes coxsackie, Echo and rhinoviruses.

Picrotoxin A CNS stimulant, a shrub derivative not in use now.

Pierre Robin syndrome Small jaw, cleft palate and absent gag reflex.

Piezoelectricity Production of electricity by application of pressure to certain crystals like mica, quartz, etc.

Pigeon breast Sternum projecting forward due to rickets or childhood respiratory obstruction.

Pigeonbreeder's lung A form of hypersensitive pneumonitis due to exposure to excreta of pigeons and parakeets.

Pigeon toed *SYN*—Pes varus; walking with feet turned inward.

Pigment Any organic coloring material in the body. *p. bile* Bilirubin and biliverdin, the hemoglobin degradation products in blood secreted in bile, urobilin and bilifuscin excreted in stool and urine. *p. blood* Hematin, hemin, methemoglobin and hemosiderin, all derivatives of hemoglobin.

Pigmentophore A cell that carries pigment.

Pile Hemorrhoid. *p. sentinel* Thickened anal mucous membrane at the lower end of an anal fissure.

Pili Hairs.

Piliation Formation and development of hair.

Piliform Hair like.

Pill A medicine presented as a solid mass for swallowing; oral contraceptive.

Pillar An upright support/ column.

Pilobezoar Trichobezoar; hairball concretion in GI tract.

Pilocarpine A cholinergic causing pupillary contraction, used in glaucoma.

Piloerection Standing out of body hairs due to contraction of arrector pili muscles.

Pilojection Introduction of hair into aneurysm (usually intracranial) to promote blood coagulation.

Pilomotor reflex Goose flesh formation when cold is applied to skin or during emotion.

Pilonidal cyst Sacrococcygeal cyst from the entrapped epithelial tissue beneath the skin, a developmental defect.

Pimozide Antipsychotic agent.

Pimple A papule or pustule of the skin from blockage of sebaceous glands.

Pindolol A betablocker antihypertensive agent.

Pineal body A gland like structure near splenium of corpus callosum secreting melatonin.

Pinealoma Encapsulated tumor of pineal body usually causing precocious puberty.

Pinguecula Yellowish triangular thickening of bulbar conjunctiva adjacent to cornea.

Pinhole pupil Extremely contracted pupil as in opium poisoning and pontine hemorrhage.

Pink disease A disease of infancy characterized by pink and swollen extremities often with arthrosis, a hypersensitive reaction to mercury.

Pinna The auricle or external ear.

Pinocytosis A process by which cells absorb and ingest nutrients.

Pinosome The fluid filled vacuole formed during pinocytosis.

Pin's sign The disappearance of symptoms of pleurisy and pain in a patient of pericarditis when he leans forward in knee-chest position.

Pinta A nonvenereal skin disease caused by (*Treponema carateum*) and spreading by body contact.

Pinworm *Enterobius vermicularis.*

Pioglitazone Antidiebetic agent.

Piperazine Drug used for enterobiosis and ascariasis.

Piracetam Cerebral activator.

Pirenzepine Belladona alkaloid derivative, used in peptic ulcer.

Piriformis syndrome Pain in buttock, thigh and lower back due to sciatic nerve entrapment in piriformis muscle, common to women.

Piroxicam Nonsteroidal antiinflammatory agent.

Pisiform The smaller pea shaped carpal bone in proximal row of wrist.

Pitch The quality of sound dependent upon frequency.

Pithiatry Treatment of disease by suggestion or persuasion.

Pitressin Vasopressin secreted from posterior pituitary (contains ADH + pressor agent).

Pitting Removal of senesent RBC by spleen.

Pituitary Endocrine gland of size 1.3 cm. × 1 cm × 0.5 cm at base of brain secreting various hormones like TSH, GH, ACTH, LH, oxytocin and vasopressin (*see* Figure on page 560).

Pituitrin Posterior pituitary extract.

Pityriasis Skin disease with brany scales. *p. alba* Patches of macular scaly lesions, commonly in children. *p. rosea* Acute inflammatory skin disease with macular eruption,

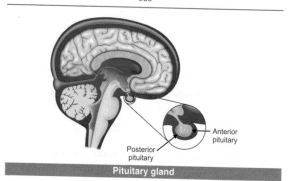

Anterior pituitary

Posterior pituitary

Pituitary gland

rose red in color, symmetrical distribution and a clearing center. *p. rubia pilaris* Persistent general exfoliative dermatitis. *p. versicolor* Superficial fungal infection caused by *Malassezia furfur.*

Placebo An inactive substance, used in controlled studies of drugs.

Placenta The oval structure in pregnant uterus through which fetus derives its nutrition. *p. accreta* Placenta whose cotyledons have invaded the uterine musculature so that placental separation after delivery is difficult. *p. circumvallate* Cup shaped placenta with raised edges. *p. percreta* Placental cotyledons invade uterus right up to serosal lining threatening rupture of uterus. *p. previa*

Placenta implanted to lower uterine segment, often causing painless profuse third trimester bleeding. *p. retained* Placenta not expelled even 2 hours after fetal delivery. *p. succenturiate* An accessory placenta having vascular connection with main placenta. *p. velamentous* Placenta where the umbilical cord is attached to membranes, so that the umbilical vessels enter placenta at its margins.

Placental souffle Auscultatory sound of placental blood flow.

Placido's disk A disk with black and white lines used to measure corneal astigmatism.

Plagiocephaly Irregular closure of cranial sutures resulting in deformed skull.

Plague Disease caused by *Pasteurella pestis. p. bubonic*

Common form of plague with suppurative lymphadenitis. *p. hemorrhagic* Rare form of plague with prominent hemorrhagic manifestations particularly into skin. *p. pneumonic* Virulent form of plague with extensive involvement of lungs.

Plane A smooth surface; imaginary cut through a body part. *p. coronal* Vertical plane at right angles to sagittal plane so that body is divided into anterior and posterior halves. *p. median* Antero-posterior plane dividing body or organ into two equal parts. *p. sagittal* Plane dividing body into equal right and left halves (*see* Figure).

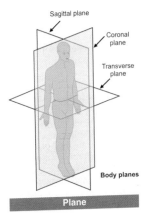

Plane

Planned parenthood The concept of choosing the time to have children.

Planoconcave An optical lens concave on one side but plane on the other side.

Planoconvex An optical lens convex on one side but plane on the other side.

Planorbis The genus of fresh water snails that serve as intermediate hosts for schistosoma.

Plantar arch The arch of the foot.

Plantaris A slim muscle in the calf.

Plantigrade The type of foot where the entire sole of foot touches the ground while walking.

Plaque A patch on skin or mucous membrane. *p. dental* A gummy mesh harboring microorganism growing on the crowns of teeth, a forerunner of dental caries.

Plasma The liquid portion of blood, the medium for transporting nutrients and suspending the corpuscles.

Plasmacyte A plasma cell as found in connective tissue with eccentric nucleus.

Plasmacytoma Myeloma arising from marrow.

Plasma exchange Removal of patient's, plasma with replacement by colloid solution.

This removes the immune complexes, excess antibodies or drugs and poisons.

Plasmapheresis Similar to plasma exchange.

Plasmid Extranuclear cell inclusion having genetic function; commonly seen in bacteria and used in DNA cloning and recombinant DNA technology.

Plasmin Fibrinolytic enzyme derived from plasminogen.

Plasmodium A genus of protozoa that includes causative agents of various types of malaria.

Plaster 1. Plaster of Paris used to immobilize a part or make an impression. 2. Medicinal agents formed into a tenacious mass, e.g. belladona plaster.

Plastic bronchitis Bronchitis with fibrin casts of bronchi.

Plastic surgery Surgery for reconstruction, repair or restoration of body parts.

Plate 1. A flattened part or portion. 2. Disk holding culture medium. *p. bite* In dentistry used for getting dental impression of bites. *p. epiphyseal* The cartilage between diaphysis and epiphysis on which depends the longitudinal growth of bone.

Plateau Elevated and flat area or steady and consistent phase of disease or fever.

Platelet Round or oval disk like cells in blood which help in blood coagulation and hemostasis.

Platelet concentrate Platelets prepared from few units of blood and suspended in plasma.

Platinum A hard heavy silver white metal.

Platybasia A developmental defect where the floor of posterior fossa of skull protrudes upwards often causing hydrocephalus and high cervical cord compression.

Platycephaly Flattening of the skull.

Platysma A thin aponeurotic muscle of neck which on contraction causes wrinkling of skin of neck and depression of jaw.

Platysmal reflex Dilatation of pupil on pinching platysma muscle of neck.

Plegia Suffix meaning paralysis.

Pleocytosis Increased number of lymphocytes in CSF.

Pleomorphism Having many shapes or forms.

Pleoptics A method of eye exercises to train and stimulate amblyopic eye.

Plethora Congestion with fluid.

Plethysmography The method of measuring volume of blood

flow through a part from change in volume.

Pleura A bilayered membrane that encloses the lungs (*see* Figure on page 564).

Pleural cavity Space between the fibrous parietal pleura and serous visceral pleura.

Pleural effusion Fluid collection in pleural cavity, may be serous, serofibrinous or hemorrhagic.

Pleural fibrosis Thickening of pleura from inflammation, irritation.

Pleurisy Inflammation of pleura; may be primary or secondary, acute or chronic, serous or sero sanguinous. *p. diaphragmatic* Inflammation of diaphragmatic pleura causing intense pain under margin of the ribs, hiccough, and often dyspnea. *p. dry* Pleurisy where a fibrinous exudate covers the pleural surface causing pain during respiration. *p. encysted* Pleurisy with effusion encysted by adhesion.

Pleurodesis Production of adhesion between visceral and parital pleura.

Pleurodynia Sharp pain in intercostal muscles due to fascitis of chest wall.

Pleurolysis Loosening of pleural adhesions.

Plexiform Resembling a network.

Pleximeter The one that receives the percussion.

Plexus A network of nerves, lymphatics or blood vessels. *p. enteric* One of the two plexuses of nerve fibers and ganglion cells lying in the wall of alimentary canal namely Auerbach's plexus and submucosal Meissner's plexus. *p. pampiniform* A network of veins draining the testis in male or ovary in the female.

Plica A fold.

Plicate Folded.

Plication The stitching of folds or tucks to reduce the size of an organ.

Ploidy The number of chromosome sets in a cell.

Plototoxin A toxic substance present in cat fish.

Plug A mass closing or intending to close a hole. *p. Dittrich's* A putrid mass of bacteria and fatty acids crystals in bronchiectasis.

Plumbism Lead poisoning.

Plummer-Vinson syndrome Iron deficiency anemia with dysphagia, achlorohydria, koilonychia and esophageal web, occurring commonly in women.

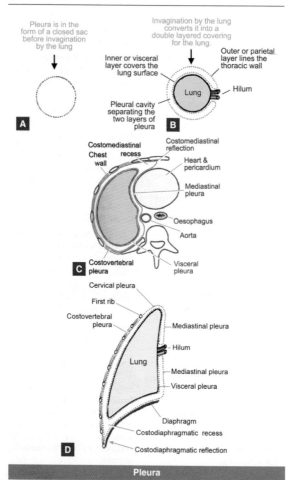

A Pleura is in the form of a closed sac before invagination by the lung

B Invagination by the lung converts it into a double layered covering for the lung.

Inner or visceral layer covers the lung surface

Outer or parietal layer lines the thoracic wall

Lung

Hilum

Pleural cavity separating the two layers of pleura

C

Costomediastinal recess

Chest wall

Costomediastinal reflection

Heart & pericardium

Mediastinal pleura

Oesophagus

Aorta

Costovertebral pleura

Visceral pleura

D

Cervical pleura

First rib

Costovertebral pleura

Mediastinal pleura

Hilum

Lung

Mediastinal pleura

Visceral pleura

Diaphragm

Costodiaphragmatic recess

Costodiaphragmatic reflection

Pleura

Pluripotent An embryonic cell having power to differentiate into different kinds of cells.

Plutomania Delusion of richness.

Plutonium A fissile material derived from uranium.

Pneodynamics The dynamics of breathing.

Pneumarthrogram X-ray of joint after air injection.

Pneumatics Branch of physics dealing with properties of gases.

Pneumatization Formation of airfilled cavities especially of mastoid.

Pneumatocele A swelling containing gas or air.

Pneumatosis Presence of air or gas in abnormal location of body.

Pneumaturia Presence of gas in urine due to vesicovaginal fistula.

Pneumococcal vaccine polyvalent A vaccine containing 23 of the known 83 pneumococcal capsular polysaccharides; providing immunity for 3-5 years. The vaccine is particularly useful in patients with sickle cell disease, immunodeficiency and post- splenectomy.

Pneumococcus Encapsulated nonspore forming gram-positive organism causing pneumonia, meningitis, otitis, mastoiditis, keratitis, etc.

Pneumoconiosis Occupational diffuse lung disease due to inhalation of mineral dusts.

Pneumocystis carinii A protozoan parasite causing pneumonia in AIDS patients.

Pneumocystography Cystogram after injection of air into bladder.

Pneumoencephalogram X-ray for subarachnoid cisterns and ventricles of brain after injectin of air into subarachnoid space via lumbar puncture.

Pneumohemopericardium Presence of air and blood in the peritoneal cavity.

Pneumohydrothorax Presence of air and fluid in the thoracic cavity.

Pneumomediastinum Presence of gas in the mediastinum.

Pneumomelanosis Pigmentation of lung as seen in pneumoconiosis.

Pneumonectomy Excision of lung.

Pneumonia Inflammation of lung tissue. *p. alba* Pneumonia of newborn due to congenital syphilis. *p. aspiration* Pneumonia following aspiration of purulent matter from throat/mouth or gastric content.

p. caseous Pneumonia associated with tuberculosis. *p. interstitial* Pneumonia with infiltration of pulmonary interstitium. *p. eosinophilic* Pneumonia with eosinophilia as during migration of round worm larva, microfilaria or due to drugs like nitrofurantoin, penicillin. *p. Friedlander's* Lobar pneumonia caused by *Klebsiella pneumoniae*. *p. giant cell* An interstitial pneumonia of childhood with infiltration of lung by multinucleated giant cells, e.g., postmeasles. *p. hypostatic* Pneumonia of aged and debilitated patients due to congestion of one part of lung at all times. *p. atypical* Mild pneumonia but with radiological evidence of extensive lung infiltration as caused by *Mycoplasma pneumoniae*. *p. woolsorter's* Pulmonary anthrax.

Pneumonitis hypersensitive Diffuse granulomatous disease due to inhalation of organic dusts.

Pneumonosis Any noninfective lung disease.

Pneumoperitoneum Presence of air in the peritoneal cavity.

Pneumoradiography Injection of air into a part for X-ray examination.

Pneumorrhachis Presence of gas in the spinal canal.

Pneumothorax Presence of air in pleural cavity. *p. artificial* Intentionally induced pneumothorax to cause pulmonary collapse as a treatment option in pulmonary tuberculosis. *p. tension* A type of pneumothorax where air enters pleural space with each act of respiration but without an exit leading to high pleural pressure and collapse of lung (*see* Figure).

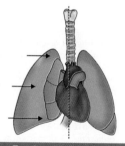

Tension pneumothorax

Podagra Gout involving great toe or foot.

Podalic version Rotating the fetus to bring feet to the lower pole.

Podiatrist A specialist in diagnosis, treatment and care of diseases of foot.

Podocyte A special type of epithelial cell lining the glomeruli.

Podology The study of anatomy and physiology of foot.

Podophyllum Preparation from roots of *Podophyllum peltatum* to treat warts.

Poikilocyte Red blood cells of abnormal shape.

Poikiloderma A skin disorder characterized by pigmentation, telangiectasia, purpura, pruritus and atrophy.

Poikilothermy The condition of having same temperature as that of the environment.

Point A minute spot, sharp end of any object. *p. Boa's* A tender spot on left of 12th thoracic vertebra in patients of gastric ulcer. *p. far* Point (20 feet or more) at which normal eye does not use accommodation. The far point is less than 20' in myopia and there is no far point for hypermetropic eye. *p. McBurney's* Point 4-5 cm above the right anterior superior iliac spine on the line joining it to umbilicus, the point of tenderness in appendicitis (*see* Figure).

Poison Any substance which when inhaled, ingested or injected disturbs normal body function.

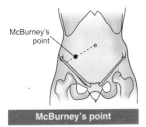

McBurney's point

McBurney's point

Poison Ivy A climbing vine which on contact produces severe dermatitis.

Poison Oak A climbing vine producing dermatitis similar to ivy.

Policosanol Mixture of plant alcohols for hyperlopridemia.

Poliomyelitis Acute viral disease that causes destruction of anterior horn cells in spinal cord and often cranial nerve nuclei with ensuing palsy. *p. ascending* The paralysis begins in lower extremity and then ascends up trunk often to involve respiratory muscles. *p. bulbar* Paralysis of cranial nerves and the respiratory center. *p. nonparalytic* Pain and stiffness in muscles but no paralysis.

Poliosis Whiteness of hair.

Poliovaccine Available as oral live attenuated vaccine or injectable killed vaccine prepared from types I, II, III polioviruses, given in 3 doses starting at $1^{1}/_{2}$ months of age and then repeated for 2 more doses at 4-6 weeks interval.

Politzer bag Rubber bag used for inflating middle ear.

Pollen The microspores of a seed plant constituting the male gametocyte. Many airborn pollens are allergens.

Polyandry Having more than one husband.

Polyarteritis nodosa Inflammation of medium and small vessels segmentally with necrosis, an autoimmune disorder.

Polyarthritis Inflammation of more than one joint.

Polychromasia Having many colours.

Polychromatophilia The quality of a cell being stainable with more than one stain.

Polyclinic A clinic catering for many variety of ailments.

Polycystic Having many cysts.

Polycystic ovary An endocrine disorder with anovulation and multiple cysts in the ovaries (*see* Figure).

Polycythemia An excess of red blood cells. *p. rubra vera* A malignant disorder of marrow with increase in RBC mass, WBC and platelets.

Polydactylism Having supernumerary fingers or toes (*see* Figure on page 569).

Polydipsia Excess thirst.

Polydystrophy Condition of having multiple congenital anomaly of connective tissue.

Polyendocrine deficiency syndrome Hypofunction of many endocrine glands; may be type I or type II; Type I-hypoparathyroidism, adrenal

Normal and polycystic ovary

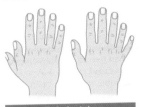

Polydactyly

insufficiency, mucocutaneous candidiasis, Type II: IDDM, thyroid deficiency and adrenal insufficiency.

Polyethylene A polymer used in production of IV tubing.

Polyethylene glycol Used as ointment base.

Polygamy Practice of having several wives or husbands.

Polygraph Machine that records arterial and venous pulse.

Polyhydramnios Excess of amniotic fluid.

Polymenorrhea Menses occurring at rapid frequency.

Polymer A synthetic substance made of two or more molecules.

Polymerase An enzyme catalyzing polymerization of nucleosides to form DNA.

Polymerization The process of changing a simple chemical substance into another of higher molecular weight.

Polymorph A polymorphonuclear leukocyte.

Polymorphism Appearing in many forms.

Polymyalgia rheumatica A connective tissue disorder of autoimmune nature affecting women with high ESR, weakness of proximal muscles and prompt response to low-dose corticosteroids.

Polymyoclonus Muscular contraction proceeding in wave form to involve many muscle groups.

Polymyositis A connective tissue disorder characterized by inflammation and degeneration of muscles and dermatitis.

Polymyxin Aminoglycoside antibiotic designated polymyxin A, B, C, D, E, highly nephrotoxic.

Polyneuropathy Involvement of many peripheral nerves.

Polyneuroradiculitis Inflammation of nerve roots, peripheral nerves and spinal ganglia.

Polynucleotide Nucleic acid composed of one or more nucleotides.

Polyomavirus A papovavirus family causing malignancy in lower animals.

Polyopsia Multiple images seen of the same object.

Polyorchidism Condition of having more than two testicles.

Polyostotic Concerning many bones.

Polyp A tumor with a pedicle.

Polypeptide Union of two or more amino acids.

Polyphagia Frequent and excess eating.

Polypharmacy Concurrent use of number of drugs.

Polyphenon E Tea extract for warts.

Polyphrasia Talkativeness.

Polyploidy Condition characterized by twice or more number of normal haploid chromosome numbers of gametes.

Polyposis Presence of many polyps. *p. familial* Multiple polyps in colon with rectal bleeding and chances of malignant changes.

Polysaccharide Complex sugars which on hydrolysis yield more than 2 molecules of simple sugar.

Polyserositis Inflammation of many serous cavities, e.g. pleural effusion, ascites, pericardial effusion.

Polystyrene A synthetic resin.

Polythiazide A mercurial thiazide diuretic.

Polyunsaturated Pertains to fatty acids having many carbon atoms joined by double or triple bonds.

Polyuria Excessive passage of urine of low specific gravity.

Polyvalent Substance with combining power of more than two atoms of hydrogen.

Polyvinyl alcohol A water soluble synthetic resin used for preparation of ophthalmic solutions.

Polyvinyl pyrrolidine Povidone.

Pompe's disease Glycogen storage disease type II.

Pompholyx Deep seated vesicles of palm and sole associated with contact allergy or fungal infection.

Ponderal index Height in inches/cube root of weight in pounds.

Pontic An artificial tooth set in a bridge.

Pontcaine hydrochloride Topical or spinal anesthetic.

Popliteal Concerning back of knee (*see* Figure on page 571).

Popliteus Muscle that flex the knee.

Poppy Any plant of genus Papaver; opium is obtained from juice of unripe pods.

Porcine Piglike, obtained from porks.

Pore A small opening.

Porencephaly A congenital brain anomaly where ventricles extend up to subarachnoid space.

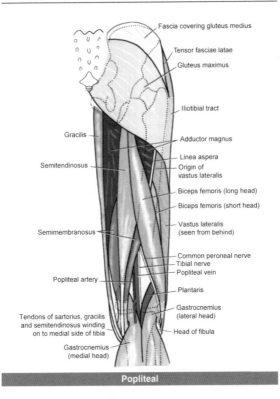

Fascia covering gluteus medius

Tensor fasciae latae

Gluteus maximus

Iliotibial tract

Gracilis

Adductor magnus

Linea aspera

Semitendinosus

Origin of vastus lateralis

Biceps femoris (long head)

Biceps femoris (short head)

Semimembranosus

Vastus lateralis (seen from behind)

Common peroneal nerve

Tibial nerve

Popliteal vein

Popliteal artery

Plantaris

Gastrocnemius (lateral head)

Tendons of sartorius, gracilis and semitendinosus winding on to medial side of tibia

Head of fibula

Gastrocnemius (medial head)

Popliteal

Pornography Sex stimulating photographs or literature.

Porphobilinogen An intermediate product in heme biosynthesis, often present in urine in patients of porphyria, when exposed to air for long- time changes to porphobilin imparting red colour to urine.

Porphyria A group of disorders of porphyrin metabolism. *p. acute intermittent* Autosomal dominant trait characterized by abdominal pain, photosensitivity and neurological disturbances. *p. congenital erythropoietic* Autosomal recessive trait with hemolysis, splenomegaly and skin reaction. *p. variegate* Hepatic porphyria with fragile skin, recurrent episodes of abdominal pain and neuropathy.

Porphyrin Nitrogen containing organic compounds obtained from hemoglobin and chlorophyll.

Porphyrinuria Excess excretion of porphyrin in urine.

Porta Point of entry for nerves and vessels.

Portal circulation The circulation of blood in liver via portal vein and hepatic vein.

Porta hepatis The transverse fissure on visceral surface for entry of hepatic artery and portal vein and exit of hepatic ducts.

Portal hypertension Increased pressure in portal vein due to obstruction to portal blood flow in liver.

Portal system The portal vein and its branches which drain the abdominal viscera and carry the blood to liver to be

drained to inferior vena cava via hepatic vein.

Portal vein The vein formed from union of superior and inferior mesenteric, splenic, gastric and cystic veins.

Portography X-ray of portal vein after injection of contrast.

Portwine mark Superficial purple red birthmark.

Position Manner in which the body of patient is put. *p. Fowler's* The position where head end of bed is elevated by $1^1/_2$ feet and knees are elevated. *p. left lateral recumbent* Patient lies on left side; right knee and thigh drawn up. *p. lithotomy* Patient lies on back with thighs drawn on abdomen and abducted. *p. Trendelenburg* Dorsal position with patient supine on a bed tilted to about 45° with head low (*see* Figure on page 573).

Positive end expiratory pressure A method to prevent collapse of alveoli at end expiration.

Positron Positively charged particle.

Positron emission tomography A method of demonstrating brain image by use of positron emitting radionuclides.

Possum Device that permits a disabled individual to per-

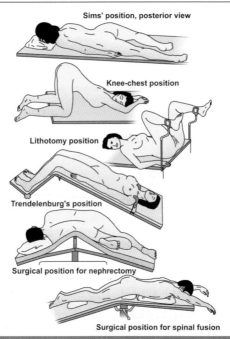

Sims' position, posterior view

Knee-chest position

Lithotomy position

Trendelenburg's position

Surgical position for nephrectomy

Surgical position for spinal fusion

Various positions used in examination or treatment

form some job by force fully breathing into master control apparatus.

Postcibal After meals.

Postclimacteric After menopause.

Postcoital After sexual intercourse.

Postconnubial After marriage.

Posterior Situated at back or behind; dorsal.

Posterior drawer sign A test for posterior cruciate ligament tear of knee.

Posteroanterior Movement from back to front.

Posteromedial On the back towards midline.

Postfebrile After fever.

Postganglionic fiber The autonomic nerve fiber passing from ganglia to visceral effector.

Posthaemorrhagic Occurring after a bleeding episode.

Posthetomy Circumcision, removal of fore skin of penis.

Posthitis Inflammation of prepuce.

Postictal Following an attack of epileptic fit.

Postmature Infant born after 42 weeks of gestation.

Postmortem After death.

Postmortem examination Dissection of dead body to determine the cause of death and pathological changes.

Postnasal Located behind the nose.

Postnatal Occurring after birth.

Postpalatine Behind the palate.

Postpaludal After an attack of malaria.

Postpartum After childbirth.

Postpartum depression Depression occurring in puerperium.

Postpartum hemorrhage Bleeding after childbirth in excess of 500 ml. usually due to uterine atony, or cervical laceration.

Postpartum psychosis Psychosis occurring within the six months following childbirth. The symptoms and signs are hallucination, delusion, preoccupation with death, etc.

Postprandial After a meal.

Postpubescent Following puberty.

Poststenotic Distal to a stenosed site.

Post-term pregnancy Pregnancy which has continued beyond 42 weeks from the onset of the last menstrual period or 40 completed weeks from conception.

Posttransfusion syndrome Fever, splenomegaly, atypical lymphocytosis that follow blood transfusion.

Postulate Supposition.

Postural Related to posture or body position.

Postural drainage Drainage of secretion from bronchi or pus from a cavity by positioning the patient so that gravity allows free drainage; usually done in bronchiectasis; lung abscess and following any prolonged surgery.

Postural hypotension Severe drop in blood pressure on assuming erect posture.

Posture Attitude or position of body.

Postviral fatigue syndrome Muscle fatigue unrelieved by rest after attack of viral fever.

Post-void residual Amount of urine that remains in the bladder after urination.

Potable Water free from impurities and hence fit for drinking.

Potash Potassium carbonate. *p.caustic* Potassium hydroxide.

Potassium Mineral element found in combination with other elements in the body. *p.bicarbonate* Used to neutralize acid in stomach. *p. chloride* Used in IV solutions and as oral preparation to supplement during digoxin and diuretic therapy. *p. citrate* Used as alkalizer. *p. iodide* Used in expectorant preparations. *p. permanganate* Topical astringent and antiseptic, antidote for phosphorus poisoning. *p. tartarate* A cathartic.

Potency Strength, power, ability to perform sexual intercourse in case of male.

Potent Powerful, highly effective.

Potentiate To augment or increase the potency.

Potion Liquid medicine.

Pott's disease Tuberculosis of vertebra.

Pott's fracture Fracture of medial malleolus of tibia with lower end of fibula and outward and backward dislocation of foot (*see* Figure).

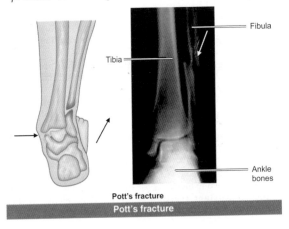

Pott's fracture

Pott's fracture

Pouch Any pocket or sac. *p.Rathke's* An embryonic out-pocketing that forms anterior lobe of pituitary.

Poultice Counter irritant preparation in the form of plaster.

Poupart's ligament The rolled up lower end of external oblique aponeurosis stretching between anterior superior iliac spine and pubic tubercle. *SYN* – Inguinal ligament.

Povidone A synthetic polymer.

Povidone iodine A complex of povidone and iodine used for skin preparation prior to surgery, as vaginal tablets, as lotions and ointments for antiseptic purposes.

Pox Pustular lesion.

Praecox Early.

Praevia Going before in time or place.

Pragmatagnosia Inability to recognize even familiar object.

Pragmatic Pertains to practical aspect of anything.

Pralidoxime A cholinesterase reactivator used in organophosphorus poisoning.

Pramipexole Dopamine receptor agonist for parkinsonism.

Provastatin Lipid lowering agent.

Pramoxine A topical anesthetic.

Prandial Related to meal.

Prausnitz-Kustner reaction Intracutaneous transfer of antibody to a healthy person followed by application of suspected allergen to produce wheal and flare. Not recommended nowadays because of fear of AIDS and viral hepatitis.

Praxiology Study of behavior.

Praxis Planning and execution of coordinated movements.

Prazepam Antianxiety medicine.

Praziquantel Broad-spectrum antihelminth and antischistosomal drug.

Prazosin Alpha-adrenergic receptor blocker; antihypertensive agent.

Precancerous Any growth or lesion that will probably become cancerous.

Precentral convolution The frontal convolution or motor area.

Precipitate The process of deposition of substances from solutions.

Precipitin An antibody in animal, due to soluble protein antigen.

Precipitin test The formation of precipitate in a solution containing soluble antigen on addition of antibody.

Precocious Development, physical or mental earlier than expected.

Precordium The area of chest overlying the heart.

Precornu Anterior horn of lateral ventricle of brain.

Precursor A substance that precedes another substance, e.g. angiotensinogen is a precursor substance of angiotensin.

Prediabetes The stage or condition prior to development of clinical diabetes.

Predisposing A susceptibility to disease.

Predisposition The potential to develop a certain disease.

Prednisolone A glucocorticoid.

Preeclampsia Toxemia of pregnancy with albuminuria, hypertension and edema.

Preeruptive Before eruption in exanthema.

Preexcitation Premature excitation of the ventricle by an impulse by-passing A-V node.

Preganglionic fibers Fibers transmiting autonomic impulse from CNS to peripheral autonomic ganglia.

Pregnancy The condition of development of embryo in the uterus. *p. abdominal* Development of embryo in the abdominal cavity drawing its blood supply from omentum. *p. ampullar* Implantation of ovum in the ampulla of fallopian tube. *p. cornual* Pregnancy in one of the horns in a bicornuate uterus. *p. ectopic* Condition where ovum develops outside the uterus. *p. molar* Pregnancy where ovum degenerates into moles (*see* Figure on page 578).

Pregnancy test Tests employed to confirm pregnancy by using patient's urine or blood which assess the chorionic gonadotrophins. The test is positive beginning 40th day from the last menstrual period. Radioimmunoassay is better and more accurate.

Pregnanediol Progesterone metabolite (end product) in urine.

Pregnanetriol An intermediate metabolite of progesterone.

Pregnenolone A synthetic corticosteroid.

Prehension The primary functions of hand that includes pinching, grasping, etc.

Preleukemia Some blood changes that may be fore warners of leukemic process, i.e. unexplained anemia, purpura, mucositis.

Preload In cardiac physiology it is ventricular wall stretch at end diastole.

Premarin Conjugated estrogen.

Premature Before full development.

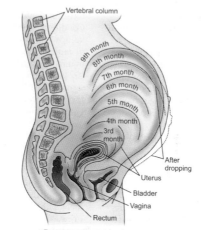

Pregnancy–Uterine levels

Pregnancy—Uterine levels

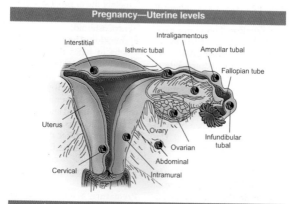

Locations of ectopic, i.e. extrauterine pregnancy

Premature ejaculation Ejaculation shortly after the onset of sexual excitement.

Premature infant Infant with birth weight below 5 lb or born prior to 37 weeks of gestation.

Premature rupture of membrane Rupture of amniotic membranes during pregnancy before 37 weeks of gestation.

Premenstrual tension syndrome The syndrome of irritability, anxiety, depression, rage, edema and breast tenderness prior to the onset of menstruation.

Premolar One of the permanent teeth occurring between canine and molar.

Premonition A feeling of an impending event.

Premorbid Prior to onset of disease.

Prenatal care Regular monitoring and management of pregnant woman and her child.

Prenatal diagnosis Diagnosis of developmental defects and diseases while the baby is *in utero* by use of chemical tests, ultrasound, amnioscopy and amniocentesis.

Preoperative care Care preceding an operation like preparation of operation site, sedation, bowel wash, breathing exercise, etc.

Preoptic area The anterior portion of hypothalamus.

Prepatellar bursitis Inflammation of bursa in front of patella. *SYN* – Housemaid's knee.

Preprandial Before a meal.

Prepubescent Just prior to puberty.

Prepuce The foreskin or skinfold over glans penis.

Prepucial glands Sebaceous glands at corona of penis secreting smegma. *SYN—* Tyson's glands.

Prepyloric Preceding the pylorus of stomach.

Prerenal 1. In front of kidney. 2. Uremia or any condition occurring prior to defects or changes affecting the kidney.

Presbycusis Sensory neural deafness of old age.

Presbyopia Recession of near point of eye with advancing age due to loss of elasticity of crystalline lens.

Prescribe To advise or indicate medicines/treatment to be taken.

Prescription A written order or direction for using a drug. A prescription consists of four main parts, i.e. superscription, inscription, subcription and signature.

Presenile Premature old age.

Presenium Prior to onset of senility.

Presentation In obstetrics the fetal part presenting at the pelvic inlet; can be breech, vertex, face, brow (*see* Figure).

Preservative A chemical additive to drug preparations and food stuffs that prevents growth of molds and fungi.

Pressure Compression, force exerted on any body tissue, e.g. blood vessel. *p. blood* Pressure exerted by moving column of blood against arterial wall. *p. central venous* Pressure in the right atrium. *p. end diastolic* Pressure in the ventricles at the end of diastole. **p. intracranial** Pressure to which CSF is subjected in subarachnoid space. *p. intraocular* Pressure within the eye ball, maintained by vitreous and aqueous humor, usually 10-20 mmHg. *p. negative* Pressure less than atmospheric pressure. *p. oncotic* Osmotic pressure exerted by colloids in a solution. *p. osmotic* The force at which solvent like water passes through a semipermeable membrane separating solutions of

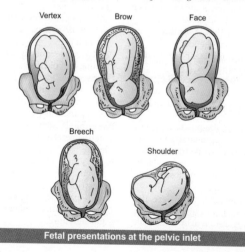

Vertex   Brow   Face

Breech

Shoulder

Fetal presentations at the pelvic inlet

different concentrations.

p. wedge Pressure obtained by wedging a fluid filled catheter in a distal branch of pulmonary artery which is equivalent to left atrial pressure.

Pressure palsy Temporary palsy due to pressure on a nerve, e.g. saturday night palsy.

Pressure point Areas where pressure is applied to control bleeding. These points are where the bleeding artery passes over a bone little above the site of bleed, e.g. common carotid artery-2" above clavicle, temporal artery—in front of ear, subclavian artery—behind clavicle, brachial artery—midarm or just above elbow; radial artery at wrist against radius and ulnar artery at wrist against ulna; femoral artery—compression of artery against femoral head in abduction and external rotation of limb; popliteal artery in popliteal space; anterior tibial artery at ankle in front; and posterior tibial artery behind.

Pressure sore A sore caused by pressure of splint or other appliance or pressure of body on bed at contact points particularly when the skin is insensitive or person is in coma or lies immobile for longtime.

Preterm In obstetrics labor occurring before 37th week of gestation.

Prevalence The number of cases of a disease present in a specified population at a given time.

Preventive medicine The branch of medicine concerned with prevention of mental and physical illness and disease.

Prevertebral In front of vertebra.

Prevesical In front of bladder.

Priapism Painful sustained penile erection without any sexual desire.

Prickle cell A cell with rod shaped processes.

Prickly heat The blockage of sweat pores with escape of sweat to epidermis and formation of itchy tiny vesicles.

Primaquine Antimalarial, for radical treatment of *P. vivax*.

Primates An order of vertebrates highly developed in respect to nervous system and brain, e.g. monkey, apes and man.

Prime Period of greatest health and strength.

Primidone An anticonvulsant.

Primigravida Woman conceiving for first time.

Primipara Woman who has delivered a viable baby.

Primitive Early in point of time.

Prinzmetal's angina Angina of coronary spasm with ST elevation.

Prion The proteinaceous infections agent, without any detectable nucleic acid, and immune response causing degenerative neurological diseases.

Prism A transparent solid, three sides of which are parallelograms. Light rays passing through a prism are split into primary colors. *p. maddox* Two base together prisms used in testing cyclophoria or torsion of eyeball.

Privacy Right of the patient to revelation of data concerning illness.

Private practice Medical practice not under external policy control other than professional ethics.

Privileged communication Confidential information given by patient to treating doctor which is not to be divulged by the latter.

Proactivator A substance that contains a portion which can be split off and then it is able to activate another substance.

Proantithrombin The substance of plasma which is converted to thrombin by action of heparin.

Probability The ratio that expresses the likelihood of occurrence of specific event important in health statistics.

Proband The initial person with disease who serves as nucleus to study the same disease in his family and subsequent generations.

Probang A device to apply medicines in larynx.

Probanthine Propantheline bromide, an anticholinergic agent.

Probe An instrument for knowing depth and direction of sinus and wound (*see* Figure).

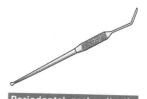

Periodontal probe, its tip marked in millimeter gradations

Probenecid A benzoic acid derivative, uricosuric and delays excretion of penicillin and its derivatives.

Probiotic Bacteria having health promoting effect on living organisms.

Probucol An antihyperlipidemic drug.

Procainamide Drug used for ventricular arrhythmia.

Procaine A local anesthetic used in infiltration anesthesia, nerve block, and spinal anesthesia.

Procarbazine A cytotoxic agent used in treatment of lymphomas.

Procedure A way of accomplishing a task to obtain desired result.

Proceious Concave anteriorly.

Procerus muscle A muscle that arises in the skin over the nose and is connected to forehead.

Process A projection or outgrowth of tissue; the steps or method of action. *p. alar* Process of cribiform plate of ethmoid articulating with frontal bone. *p. alveolar* Inferior border of maxilla or superior border of mandible containing tooth sockets. *p. ciliary* About 70 meridional ridges projecting from the corona ciliaris to which suspensory ligament of lens is attached. *p. clinoid* The anterior, middle and posterior clinoid processes of sphenoid bone. *p. condyloid* The process from mandible articulating with temporal bone. *p. coracoid* A beak shaped process extending from neck of scapula. *p. coronoid* Sharp

projection from semilunar notch of ulna. *p. odontoid* Tooth like extension from axis (*see* Figures).

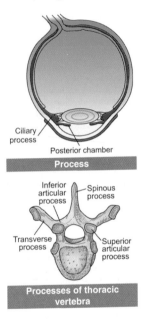

Ciliary process
Posterior chamber

Process

Inferior articular process — Spinous process
Transverse process — Superior articular process

Processes of thoracic vertebra

Prochlorperazine A phenothiazine derivative for treating nausea and vomiting.

Procidentia Complete prolapse of uterus where it completely protrudes outside the introitus.

Procollagen Precursor of collagen.

Proconvertin Coagulation factor VIII.

Procreate To give birth.

Proctalgia Pain in and around anus and rectum.

Proctitis Inflammation of anus and rectum.

Proctoclysis Infusion into rectum and anus.

Proctocolitis Inflammation of rectum and colon.

Proctology Branch of medicine dealing with diseases of rectum, colon and anus.

Proctoscopy Instrument for examination of rectum.

Proctosigmoidoscopy Visual examination of rectum and sigmoid colon by sigmoidoscope.

Procyclidine Antiparkinsonian drug.

Prodromal Initial stage of disease before appearance of distinguished features.

Prodrome A symptom heralding an approaching ailment.

Prodrug Chemicals which exhibit their pharmacologic property after biotransformation in the body.

Proenzyme Inactive form of an enzyme.

Proerythroblast The earliest bone marrow precursor of erythrocyte.

Proestrus The period before menstruation.

Profunda Deep seated especially blood vessel.

Progenitor An ancestor.

Progeny Offspring.

Progeria Premature senility occurring in childhood.

Progestational Concerned with luteal phase of menstrual cycle; action of hormone progesterone.

Progesterone Hormone secreted by placenta, corpus luteum and adrenal cortex; essential for secretory phase of endometrium, mammary growth and development and growth of placenta.

Progestin Group of synthetic drugs having progesterone like effect on uterus.

Proglotid A segment of tapeworm containing both male and female reproductive organs.

Prognathism Prominent jaws projecting beyond line of face.

Prognosis Prediction of course and outcome of a disease.

Prognosticate To state about outcome of a disease.

Progranulocyte Promyelocyte.

Progress notes Notes endorsed by doctors and nurses during course of treatment.

Progressive Advancing as bad to worse.

Progressive muscular atrophy
Gradually advancing muscle
atrophy due to disease of
spinal cord.

Proguanil Antimalarial
agent.

Prohormone Precursor of hormone.

Proinsulin Insulin precursor
produced in pancreas.

Projectile vomiting Vomiting
where the stomach content is
ejected with great force.

Projection A part extending
beyond the level of its
surrounding; referral of
peripheral sensory stimuli
to higher centers in CNS for
interpretation.

Prokaryote Organism with a
single circular chromosome
without mitochondria and
lysosomes, e.g. bacteria and
algae.

Prolabium Central portion of
upper lip.

Prolactin Hormone of anterior
pituitary that helps in milk
production.

Prolapse Falling down of a
body part or organ (see Figure).

Proliferate To increase by
reproduction of similar forms
as to the parent source.

Proliferous cyst Cyst with
epithelial lining which
proliferates and protrudes
from its inner surface.

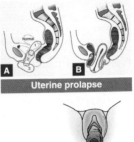

Uterine prolapse

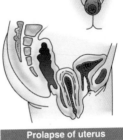

Prolapse of uterus

Proline An amino acid.

Promazine An antipsychotic
agent, often used in obstetrics
for sedation and tranquility
during labor.

Promegakaryocytes Precursor
cell of platelets.

Prometaphase A stage in mitosis when the nuclear membrane disintegrates and the
chromosomes move towards
the equatorial plate.

Promethazine An antihistaminic agent.

Promine A tissue extract that promotes growth of certain tumors in mice.

Prominence A projection or eminence.

Promonocyte Precursor of monocyte.

Promontory A projecting surface or part. *p. of sacrum* The anterior projecting surface of sacrum (*see* Figure).

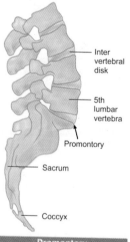

Inter vertebral disk

5th lumbar vertebra

Promontory

Sacrum

Coccyx

Promontory

Pronation The position of face downwards or palm facing downwards.

Pronator syndrome Syndrome of median nerve entrapment at elbow with paresthesia, thumb weakness, and tenderness in thenar muscles.

Pronephric duct Duct that connects posteriorly to cloaca and to which pronephric tubules are connected.

Pronephric tubules Tubules that open into cranial portion of pronephric duct and communicate with coelom.

Pronephros The earliest and simplest type of excretory organ in vertebrates.

Pronestyl Procainamide hydrochloride.

Pronormoblast An early precursor of red blood cells.

Pronucleus Nucleus of ovum or spermatozoa after fertilization.

Propantheline Anticholinergic agent.

Propafenone Anti-arrhythmic agent.

Proparacaine Topical anesthetic.

Properdin A serum protein with some bactericidal property.

Prophase First stage of mitotic cell division.

Prophylaxis Prevention of disease.

Propiolactone A disinfectant used in preparing certain viral and bacterial vaccines.

Propiomazine A sedative agent.

Propionic acid A constituent of sweat.

Propositus Index case or proband in investigation of hereditary disease.

Propoxycaine hydrochloride Local anesthetic agent.

Propoxyphene hydrochloride Analgesic agent.

Propranolol Beta-adrenergic blocking agent used for hypertension, arrhythmias, angina pectoris, portal hypertension, etc.

Proprietary medicine Any preparation used in treatment of diseases and has patent and copyright.

Proprioception Knowledge of body position, movement.

Proprioceptor Receptors responsible for body position and equilibrium, e.g. muscle spindles, pacinian corpuscles and labyrinthine receptors.

Proptometer Instrument for measuring degree of exophthalmos.

Proptosis Protrusion of eyeball as in exophthalmic goiter, retroorbital mass or cavernous sinus thrombosis.

Propylene glycol A demulcent agent used as solvent.

Propylhexedrine A sympathomimetic used as inhalation for nasal congestion.

Propyliodone Radiopaque dye used in bronchography.

Propylparaben An antifungal agent used as preservative.

Propylthiouracil Antithyroid drug for hyperthyroidism.

Prosection Dissection for demonstrating anatomic structures.

Prosector One who dissects body for demonstration.

Prosencephalon Embryonic forebrain giving rise to telencephalon and diencephalon.

Prosody The normal rhythm, melody and articulation of speech.

Prosopagnosia Inability to recognise a person from face.

Prosopectasia Abnormal enlargement of face.

Prosoplasia Progressive development of cells to produce cells with higher degree of function.

Prospective study A clinical or epidemiological investigation over a period of time.

Prostacyclin The precursor intermediate of prostaglandins; vasodilator.

Prostaglandin A group of 20 carbon unsaturated fatty acids, metabolites of arachidonic acid, e.g. PGD_2, PGE_2, PGF_2, PGI_2.

Prostate The musculoglandular organ of the size of 2 × 4 ×

3 cm that surrounds neck of urinary bladder and urethra in male (*see* Figure).

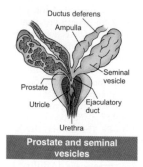

Prostate and seminal vesicles

Prostate cancer Malignant tumor of prostate gland.

Prostatic plexus Plexus of nerves and veins that lie in the capsule of prostate.

Prostatic urethra That portion of urethra surrounded by prostate.

Prostatism Symptoms of nocturia, increased frequency and dribbling of any cause.

Prostatitis Inflammation of prostate, whether acute or chronic with aching pain in perineum, urethral discharge often with fever, dysuria, chills and constipation.

Prostatosis Any non-inflammatory and non-malignant condition of prostate.

Prosthesis An artificial part or organ.

Prosthetics Branch of surgery dealing with prosthesis.

Prostitute Woman who sells herself for sexual exploitation, the major cause of spread of AIDS and other venereal diseases.

Prostration Extreme exhaustion.

Protal Existing before birth, i.e. congenital.

Protamine A simple strongly basic protein used to neutralize excess heparin or to slow down absorption of insulin.

Protanopia Red color blindness.

Protean Variable.

Protease Protein splitting enzyme.

Protein Complex nitrogenous compounds which are essential for growth and development. *p. Bence Jones* A light chain protein found in urine in patients of myeloma, lymphoma, etc.

Protein C A blood protein which on conversion to protein *Ca* inhibits blood coagulation. Its deficiency leads to thrombotic tendency.

Protein-calorie malnutrition Symptoms complex due to deficiency of protein and calorie in small children. *SYN*—kwashiorkor.

Protein hydrolysate A solution of amino acids and short chain peptides.

Protein losing enteropathy Excessive protein loss into G.I. tract as in extensive G.I. ulceration or constrictive pericarditis.

Proteinosis Accumulation of excess proteins in tissues.

Proteinuria Loss of protein usually albumin in urine. *p. orthostatic* Proteinuria occurring on assuming erect posture but not during recumbency. Hence morning urine is protein free but urine of daytime contains albumin.

Proteolysis Hydrolysis of proteins.

Proteose An intermediate product of proteolysis.

Proteus A genus of enteric bacillus, *P. vulgaris* causes urinary infection while *P. morgagni* in addition causes enteritis, *P. mirabilis* is usually saprophytic.

Prothrombin A blood coagulation factor synthesized in liver which is converted to thrombin.

Prothrombin time The time taken for decalcified plasma to clot on addition of thromboplastin and calcium. Usually employed to evaluate effects of anticoagulants.

Prothrombinase An enzyme that catalyzes conversion of prothrombin into thrombin in presence of calcium and platelets.

Protocol Description of steps to be taken in an experiment.

Protodiastole The first phase of diastole occurring immediately after closure of aortic and pulmonary valves.

Protoduodenum The upper half of duodenum.

Proton A positively charged particle in the atom.

Protoplasm A thick viscous colloid, the physical basis of all living organisms.

Protoporphyrin A tetrapyrole, derivative of hemoglobin.

Protoporphyrinuria Protoporphyrin in urine.

Protozoa Unicellular organism multiplying by binary fission.

Protractor Instrument for removing foreign bodies from wounds.

Protriptyline An antidepressant.

Protrude To project.

Protuberance A prominent part.

Provitamin Any substance which is converted to vitamin within body, e.g. carotene as precursor of vitamin A.

Prurigo A chronic skin disease with recurrent discrete deep-seated itchy papules usually on extensor surfaces, of unknown etiology.

Pruritus Itching. *p. senilis* Pruritus in aged due to degeneration of skin. *p. vulvae* Itching around vulva, a feature of diabetes.

Prussak's space Tiny space in middle ear between Sharpnell's membrane laterally and neck of malleus medially.

Prussic acid Hydrocyanic acid, a potent poison.

Psammoma A small tumor of choroid plexus and other areas of brain containing sandlike calcareous particles.

Psammoma bodies Laminated concretions in pineal body.

Psammoma sarcoma Sarcoma with psammoma bodies.

Psammotherapy Use of sand-baths as therapy.

Psammous Sandy-gritty.

Pseudacusis Hearing of false sounds.

Pseudoarthrosis Development of false joint consequent to nonunion of a fracture.

Pseudoacanthosis nigricans Velvety pigmented thickening of flexure surfaces as occurring in obese persons.

Pseudoaneurysm Dilatation of vessel giving impression of aneurysm.

Pseudocyesis Symptoms of pregnancy like amenorrhea, abdominal enlargement, morning sickness, etc. in absence of uterine enlargement as occurring in women who are too keen to have pregnancy.

Pseudocyst A dilatation resembling cyst.

Pseudodementia Social withdrawal but without mental deterioration.

Pseudoephedrine Vasoconstrictor, nasal decongestamt.

Pseudofracture A line of decalcification as seen in osteomalacia.

Pseudogeusia A subjective sensation of taste in absence of any stimulus to taste buds.

Pseudoganglion Local thickening of nerve resembling ganglion.

Pseudogout Joint pain resembling gout but caused by calcium pyrophosphate dihydrate crystals.

Pseudohermaphrodite Individual with sex chromatin and sex organs of one sex but with some of the physical appearance of opposite sex. *p. male* Genetically male with a small rudimentary penis and a scrotum without testes resembling labia; usually occurs due to disease of adrenals or feminizing tumors of undescended testis. *p. female* A genetically female with large clitoris resembling penis and hypertrophied labia mimicking scrotum.

Pseudohypertrophy Increase in size of tissue but with diminished function.

Pseudohypoparathyroidism Features of hypoparathyroidism due to tissue resistance to parathormone. Features are short stature, cataract, tetany, etc.

Pseudojaundice Yellow coloration of skin due to carotinemia.

Pseudomania Pathological lying or a form of psychosis where patient falsely accuses himself for crimes which he has not committed.

Pseudomembrane A false membrane as in diphtheria.

Pseudomenstruation Bleeding from uterus without menstrual changes of endometrium.

Pseudomonas A genus of motile gram-negative bacilli some of which produce yellow and blue pigments. *p. aeruginosa* Causes urinary tract infection and wound infection. *p. pseudomallei* Causes melioidosis.

Pseudomyxoma A peritoneal tumor containing a thick viscid fluid resembling myxoma.

Pseudoneuroma A tumor forming at the end of amputation stump.

Pseudopapilledema Optic neuritis causing swelling of optic nerve head.

Pseudoparesis Hysterical palsy.

Pseudopodium Any temporary outpouching of cell membrane in protozoa for locomotion.

Pseudopolyp Hypertrophied area of mucous membrane resembling polyp.

Pseudotuberculosis A group of diseases resembling clinically tuberculosis but caused by gram-negative organism, *Yersinia pseudotuberculosis*.

Pseudotumor cerebri Benign intracranial hypertension of unknown cause, most patients recover spontaneously.

Pseudoxanthoma elastium Chronic degenerative skin disease with angioid streaks in retina, degeneration of vessel walls.

Psilocybin A hallucinogen obtained from mushrooms.

Psi phenomena Events without explanation, e.g. telepathy.

Psittacosis Fever with pulmonary symptoms caused by *Chlamydia psittaci.*

Psoas A muscle in the loin, inserted to lesser throchanter of femur. It flexes the thigh, adducts and rotates it medially.

Psoas abscess A cold abscess in the sheath of psoas major muscle often noticed above inguinal ligament or near attachment of psoas muscle to femur.

Psoralen Plant derivatives causing phototoxic dermatitis; used in psoriasis and vitiligo.

Psoriasis A chronic itchy disorder of skin marked by lesions on extensor surfaces with silvery yellow white scales. A psoriatic skin produces nearly 2700 cells/cm^2 in comparison to 1250/cm^2 per day in normal person and cell cycle is reduced to 36 hours in comparison to the normal of 311 hours.

Psyche Mind.

Psychedelic Drugs producing visual hallucinations like LSD.

Psychiatry The branch of medicine dealing with diagnosis, treatment and prevention of mental illness.

Psychoanalysis A method of obtaining detailed account of past and present experiences and repressions.

Psychodynamics The scientific study of mental force.

Psychogenesis The origin and development of mind.

Psychogenic Of mental origin.

Psychograph A chart that lists personality traits.

Psychokinesis Impulsive maniacal behavior caused by defective inhibition.

Psycholepsy Sudden alteration of mood.

Psychologist Person trained in methods of psychological analysis, therapy and research.

Psychology Branch of science dealing with mental processes and their influence on behavior.

Psychometry The measurement of psychological variables like intelligence, aptitude, behavior and emotion.

Psychomotor epilepsy Temporal lobe epilepsy.

Psychomotor retardation Generalized slowing of physical and mental reactions.

Psychoneurosis Emotional mal-adaptation due to unresolved emotional conflicts.

Psychopathy Any mental disease.

Psychopharmacology The science of drugs effecting behavior and emotions.

Psychoplegic Drug reducing excitability.

Psychosexual Pertains to mental and emotional aspects of sexuality.

Psychosexual disorders Disorder of sexual function not due to organic causes, e.g. paraphilias, transvestism, pedophilia, etc.

Psychosis An impairment of mental function to the extent of interfering with individual's adaptation to family, society, self care and ordinary demands of life. There is personality disintegration and loss of contact with reality; hallucinations and delusions.

Psychosomatic Pertains to body and mind , i.e. a disease producing physical symptoms due to some disturbance in emotional state.

Psychotherapy A method of treating disease by mental means like suggestion, hypnotism rather than physical means.

Psyllium seeds Used as mild laxative.

Pterygium Triangular thickening of bulbar conjunctiva with apex towards pupil (*see* Figure).

Pterygoid Wing shaped.

Pterygoid process Downward projection from sphenoid bone at junction of body and greater wings.

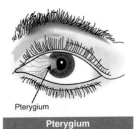

Pterygium

Pterygium

Ptomaine A nitrogenous putrefactive product from bacterial action on proteins.

Ptosis Drooping of an organ or eyelid (*see* Figure below).

Ptyalagogue Agent that stimulates secretion of saliva.

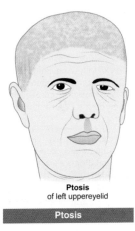

Ptosis
of left uppereyelid

Ptosis

Ptyalin A salivary enzyme that hydrolyzes starch and glycogen to maltose and glucose.

Ptyalism Excessive secretion of saliva.

Ptyalography X-ray of salivary glands and ducts.

Puberty The period of sexual maturity between 13-15 years in boys and 9-16 years in girl, probably related to decrease in secretion of pineal gland. *p. precocious* Onset of puberty earlier than normal.

Pubescence Puberty.

Pubic hair Hair in pubic region, appearing on sexual maturity.

Pudenda External genitalia especially of female.

Puerile Concerning puerperium.

Puerperal sepsis Infection of genital tract in the puerperium.

Puerperium Period of six weeks following childbirth.

Pulmometer Spirometer; device to measure lung capacity.

Pulmometry Determination of lung capacity.

Pulmonary alveolar proteinosis Eosinophilic material deposition in alveoli causing dyspnea.

Pulmonary arterial webs Web like deformities in pulmonary angiogram at the site of previous thromboembolism.

Pulmonary artery wedge pressure Pressure at the capillary end of pulmonary arterial system usually below 16 mmHg, is equal to mean left atrial pressure and left ventricular end diastolic pressure.

Pulmonary function tests Tests done to measure functional ability of lungs, e.g. total lung capacity, vital capacity, peak flow rate, gas exchange.

Pulmonary insufficiency Failure of pulmonary valve to close completely during diastole.

Pulmonary mucociliary clearance Removal of inhaled particles and sputum from bronchial tree by ciliary action of bronchial mucosa.

Pulmonary stenosis Narrowing of pulmonary valves.

Pulmonary valve The valve between right ventricle and pulmonary artery, has three cusps 2 posterior and one anterior.

Pulmonary veins Four set of veins draining the lungs into left atrium.

Pulp Soft vascular portion of the center of tooth; the soft part of fruit.

Pulp capping Covering and protecting the exposed or infected pulp by metal cap thus allowing it to heal and be protected by formation of secondary dentin.

Pulpectomy Extirpation of dental pulp.

Pulpitis Inflammation of pulp.

Pulsate To throb, or beat.

Pulsation The rhythmic beat.

Pulse The wave form of blood passing through an artery as a consequence to cardiac contraction. *p. alternating* Pulse with weak and strong beats. *p. anacrotic* Pulse with a secondary wave on ascending limb. *p. bigeminal* Pulse where every third beat is irregular. *p. collapsing* Pulse striking the finger with force but then abruptly subsiding. *p. corrigans* Bounding and forceful pulse of aortic regurgitation. *p. deficit* Pulse rate counted from wrist and cardiac rate auscultated over chest differ as in atrial fibrillation. *p. paradoxical* Pulse disappearing at the end of inspiration as in pericardial tamponade. *p. thready* Barely perceptible pulse. *p. waterhammer* Sudden jerky pulse with immediate collapse.

Pulse generator The component of cardiac pacemakers that provides electrical discharge.

Pulseless disease Aortoarteritis causing absence of brachial and radial pulse.

Pulse pressure Difference between systolic and diastolic pressure. Pulse pressure above 50 and below 30 are considered abnormal.

Pulverization To crush any hard substance into powder form.

Punchdrunk Boxers with repeated head trauma leading to multiple scars and intellectual deterioration and Parkinsonian features.

Punched out Small clearly defined hole like appearance.

Punctate Pinpoint punctures or depressions.

Punctate rash Minute rash.

Puncture To make a hole, or wound by a sharp pointed instrument. *p. cisternal* Puncture of cerebromedullary cisterns through suboccipital space to obtain CSF. *p. lumbar* Puncture of subarachnoid space between L_3-L_4 vertebrae to obtain CSF for analysis, or to do myelogram. *p. sternal* Aspiration of bonemarrow from sternum.

Pupil The opening at the center of iris. *p. Argyl Robertson* Pupil that reacts to accommodation but with loss of light reflex. *p. Hutchinson's*

One side dilatation of pupil with contraction on other side due to intracranial space occupying lesion. *p. pinpoint* Excessively constricted pupil in opium poisoning, myopias and in pontine hemorrhage.

Pupillary reflex Constriction of pupil upon stimulation of retina by light.

Pupilometer Instrument for measuring diameter of pupil.

Purgative Drug stimulating bowel movement.

Purge To evacuate the bowel.

Purine End products of nucleo-protein digestion consisting of adenine, guanine and uric acid.

Purine free diet Diet devoid of meat, liver, kidney, poultry, fish, condiments, alcohol, sweets, pastries, fried foods.

Purine low diet Diet that excludes foods like meat, fish, fowl, spinach, lentils, mushrooms, peas, aspargus.

Purkinje Anatomist and physiologist. *p. cells* Large neurons that have dendrites extending from cortex to deep white matter. *p. fibers* A type of muscle fibers which conduct electrical impulse to ventricular muscle. *p. network* Fibrous network of large muscle cells beneath the endocardium.

p. phenomenon The maximum pupillary movement while dark adaptation occurs in green rather than yellow light.

Purpura Hemorrhages into skin, mucous membrane first appearing as red, then purple and finally brownish yellow before disappearing; can be allergic to food, drugs, microorganisms, and idiopathic as well as due to other causes like thrombocytopenia and vasculitis.

Purpurin An acid dye used to stain nuclei, a red pigment often present in urine.

Purulent Containing pus, suppurative.

Pus Liquid product of inflammation containing albuminous substances, leukocytes and organisms. Blue or green pus is due to infection by pseudomonas group and fetid pus is due to growth of anaerobes.

Puscells Dead and degenerated leukocytes.

Pustule Small elevated skin lesion containing pus, may be flat, round or umbilicated.

Putrefaction Decomposition of protein with production of malodorous and toxic products like ptomaines, mercaptans, hydrogen sulphide, caused by bacteria and fungi. Decomposition occurring spontaneously in sterile tissue is called autolysis.

Putrefy To undergo putrefaction.

Putrescence Decay, rottenness.

Putrescine A poisonous polyamine formed by bacterial action on arginine.

Pyarthrosis Pus in a joint.

Pyelocystitis Inflammation of renal pelvis and bladder.

Pyelogram X-ray of ureter and renal pelvis.

Pyelolithotomy Operation to remove stone from renal pelvis.

Pyelonephritis Inflammation of kidney substance and pelvis, in 85% caused by *E. coli.*

Pyemia Presence of pus forming organisms in blood, a form of septicemia, causing metastatic abscess.

Pygmy A very small person or dwarf.

Pygodidymus Conjoined twins with fusion of chest and head but free abdomen and limbs.

Pyknocyte A form of spiculated red cell.

Pyknodysostosis A form of osteopetrosis, but without hematologic and neurologic abnormalities.

Pyknosis Shrinking of cell through degeneration and becoming thick.

Pyopoiesis formation of pus Also known as pyesis, suppuration and pyosis.

Pyosalpingitis This refers to the suppurative inflammation of the fallopian tube.

Pyosalpinx Distension of uterine tube due to collection of pus.

Pyosis *See* pyopoiesis.

Pylephlebitis Inflamed portal veins.

Pylethrombosis Occlusion of portal vein.

Pylon A temporary artificial leg.

Pyloric antrum First part of pylorus leading into pyloric canal.

Pyloric canal The short narrow lowermost portion of stomach entering into duodenum.

Pyloric stenosis Narrowing of pyloric orifice due to peptic ulcer or postpyloric duodenal ulcer or congenital hyperplasia of pyloric circular muscles (*see* Figure on page 598).

Pyloroplasty Surgical enlargement of the opening of pylorus.

Pylorospasm Contraction of pyloric orifice secondary to ulcer in pyloric antrum or duodenum.

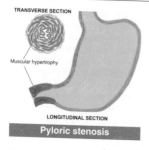

Pyloric stenosis

Pylorotomy Incision into pyloric submucosa to relieve hypertrophic stenosis.

Pylorus The lower orifice of stomach which opens intermittently to allow partly digested food to enter into duodenum (*see* Figure).

Pyocele Any cavity distended with pus.

Pyoderma Purulent lesions in skin. *p. gangrenosum* Pyoderma of skin associated with ulcerative colitis or any chronic wasting disease.

Pyogenic Pus producing.

Pyometra Pus in the uterus.

Pyovarium Pus in the ovary.

Pyopneumothorax Pus and gas present in pleural cavity.

Pyorrhea A discharge of purulent matter. *p. alveolaris* A periodontal inflammatory disease with resorption of alveolar bone, and loosening of teeth.

Pyramid An object whose three triangular sides meet at an apex. *p. of medulla* A pair of elongated prominences on the anterior surface of medulla oblongata representing descend-

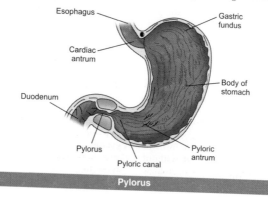

Pylorus

ing corticospinal tract. *p. renal* Cone shaped structures making the medulla of the kidney, the apex that projects as renal papilla into the renal sinus.

Pyramidal tract One of the three descending tracts (lateral, ventricular, and ventrolateral) of the spinal cord whose fibers are axons of giant Betz cells of motor cortex.

Pyrantel pamoate Drug used in helminthiasis especially ascariasis and enterobiasis.

Pyrazinamide Bactericidal antitubercular drug, very effective in killing intracellular slowly growing bacilli.

Pyrethrum Compounds having antipeduculosis property and insecticidal.

Pyrexia Fever.

Pyrexin A substance isolated from inflammatory exudate that produces fever.

Pyridium Urinary antiseptic and soothing agent.

Pyridostigmine An anticholin esterase drug used in myasthenia.

Pyridoxal-5 phosphate A derivative of pyridoxine acting as a coenzyme.

Pyridoxamine One of the vitamin B₆ group.

Pyridoxine Vitamin B₆ that includes pyridoxal and pyridoxamine.

Pyriform Shaped like a pear.

Pyrilamine maleate Antihistaminic agent.

Pyrimethamine Antimalarial agent (Daraprim).

Pyrimidine Nitrogenous compound containing uracil, cytosine and thymine.

Pyritinol Cerebral activator.

Pyrogen Agent that produces fever.

Pyrophosphatase An enzyme that catalyzes splitting of phosphoric groups.

Pyrophosphate Any salt of phosphoric acid.

Pyrosis Burning in epigastrium and lower chest. *SYN* —heart burn.

Pyrrobutamine phosphate An antihistaminic agent.

Pyrrole A heterocyclic substance acting as a building block for hemoglobin and others.

Pyrrolidine Substance obtained from pyrole or tobacco.

Pyruvate Ester of pyruvic acid.

Pyruvic acid An intermediate product in metabolism of carbohydrates and fats. Its blood level increases in thiamine deficiency.

Pyrvinium pamoate A drug for pinworms.

Pyuria Pus in the urine.

Q

Q fever Acute infectious disease caused by *Coxiella burnetti*, a rickettsial organism, characterized by fever, sweating, myalgia.

QNST *Quick neurological screening test* An assessment tool for neurological functions that evaluates attention, balance, motor planning, coordination, and spatial organization in people of age 5 years and older.

QRS complex A group of waves depicted on an electrocardiogram; called also the QRS wave. It actually consists of three distinct waves created by the passage of the cardiac electrical impulse through the ventricles and occurs at the beginning of each contraction of the ventricles. In a normal Electrocardiogram the R wave is the most prominent of the three; the Q and S waves may be extremely weak and are sometimes absent (*see* Figure).

QT segment In ECG the period from beginning of Q wave to the end of T wave.

Quack Person who pretends to have knowledge and skill of medicine.

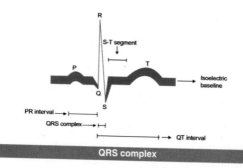

QRS complex

Quadrangular lobe A region on superior surface of each cerebellar hemisphere.

Quadrangular membrane Upper portion of elastic membrane of larynx extending from aryepiglottic folds above to the level of ventricular folds below.

Quadrantanopia Diminished vision or blindness in one quadrant of visual field.

Quadrate lobe A small lobe of liver on the visceral surface lying in contact with pylorus and duodenum.

Quadriceps Four headed muscle of thigh consisting of rectus femoris, vastus lateralis, vastus medialis, and vastus intermedius.

Quadriceps reflex Extension of leg following contraction of quadriceps muscle.

Quadriplegia Paralysis of all four extremities and the trunk usually due to injury to spinal cord above C_5 segment. Lesion above C_3 causes death due to diaphragmatic palsy.

Quadruped Four footed animal.

Quadruplet Giving birth to 4 children at a time.

Quantum mottle Mottle caused by the statistical fluctuation of the number of photons absorbed by the intensifying screens to form the light image on the film.

Quarantine The period of isolation when one is exposed to infectious disease which is the longest incubation period of disease.

Quartan Occurring every fourth day.

Quartz Silicon dioxide.

Queckenstedt's test Rise in cerebrospinal fluid pressure on compression of jugular veins of neck. A failure in rise of pressure means spinal subarachnoid block.

Quervain's disease Chronic tenosynovitis of abductor pollicis longus and extensor pollicis brevis.

Quetiapine Antipsychotic agent.

Quickening Feeling of first movements of fetus *in utero* usually between 18-20 weeks of pregnancy.

Quick lime Calcium oxide.

Quick's test A liver function test for measuring hippuric acid after a dose of sodium benzoate.

Quiescent Inactive, dormant.

Quinacrine hydrochloride An agent sparsely used for treatment of malaria and often *Giardia lamblia.*

Quincke's disease Giant urticaria.

Quincke's pulse Capillary pulsation in finger nails, a sign of aortic incompetence.

Quinethazone A diuretic.

Quingestanol A progestational agent.

Quinghasu A plant product for resistant malaria.

Quinidine sulfate Antiarrhythmic agent from cinchona bark.

Quinine An antimalarial alkaloid from cinchona bark used orally as sulfate, bisulfate and hydrochloride and parenterally as dihydrochloride. Quinine tannate is tasteless, best for giving to young children, used for falciparum malaria.

Quinoline An amine from coaltar whose salts are used as analgesic, antipyretic and in amebiasis.

Qinolone A class of compounds whose well -known derivatives are norfloxacin, ciprofloxacin, pfloxacin and ofloaxacin.

Quinquad's disease Purulent folliculitis of scalp with cicatrization of the skin.

Quinsy Peritonsillar abscess.

Quintan Occurring every fifth day.

Quintuplet Birth of 5 children at same time to a mother.

Quotidian Occurring daily.

Quotient Number of times a number is contained in another. *q. intelligence* Division of one's mental age by actual age. *q. respiratory* Division of amount of CO_2 in expired air by the oxygen. Normal value is 0.9.

Q wave The downward defection before R wave in ECG. Prominent Q waves indicate myocardial necrosis.

R

Rabeprazole A proton pump inhibitor for hyperacidity.

Rabid One having rabies.

Rabies An acute infectious CNS disease with fatal outcome; transmitted to humans by bite of rabid animals like dogs, foxes and cats. Bats, foxes and raccoons serve as reservoir of infection.

Rabies immune globulin Antibodies against rabies isolated from plasma of those immunized with rabies vaccine. It is used for imparting passive immunity.

Race A distinct ethnic group who originated from a common ancestor, or a taxonomic classification of individuals within the same species who exhibit distinct genetic characteristics.

Racemase An enzyme that helps in production of an optically active compound.

Rachi graph Device for outlining the spinal curvature.

Rachial Concerning spine.

Rachilysis Mechanical treatment of scoliosis by traction and pressure.

Rachiometer Device for measuring curvature of spine.

Rachischisis Spina bifida.

Rachitis Rickets.

Rachitome Instrument for opening spinal canal.

Radial reflex Flexon of forearm on percussion on lower end of radius.

Radiant Transmitted by radiation; coming out from a common center.

Radiation The process by which energy is propagated through space or matter. Ionizing radiation is used for therapeutic and diagnostic purposes. *r. auditory* Fibers fanning out from medial geniculate body of thalamus to auditory cortex. *r. electromagnetic* Rays travelling at speed of light (186000 miles/sec) exhibiting both electrical and magnetic properties. *r. optic* The fibers extending from lateral geniculate body of thalamus to visual cortex. *r. ultraviolet* Radiant energy from 2900-3900 AU. *r. visible* Visible spectrum of light: Violet (3900-4550 AU); blue

(4550-4920 AU); green (4920-5770 AU); yellow (5770-5970 AU); orange (5970-6220 AU) and red (6220-7700 AU).

Radiation absorbed dose The quantity of ionizing radiation absorbed by any material per unit mass measured as ergs per gram.

Radiation carcinoma Squamous cell carcinoma of skin attributed to radiation injury.

Radiation injury Injury to cells by ionizing radiation which can lead to cell death or malignancy.

Radiation protection Preventive measures against radiation like shielding of source, keeping appropriate distance, use of protective clothing, dosimeter, lead appron and limiting the dose and duration of exposure.

Radiation sickness Acute nausea and vomiting following therapeutic radiation. Prolonged exposure may lead to sterility, carcinogenesis, leukemia and bone marrow aplasia.

Radical A group of atoms acting as single unit. *r. free* A molecule containing an odd number of electrons and an open bond, hence highly reactive to cause myocardial injury.

Radical treatment Treatment, medical or surgical aimed at providing absolute cure.

Radicle Rootlet.

Radiculitis Inflammation of spinal nerve roots.

Radiculomyelopathy Any disease involving spinal cord and nerve roots.

Radiculopathy Disease of nerve roots.

Radioactive Capable of emitting radiant energy.

Radioactive decay The decrease in number of radioactive atoms in a substance with passage of time.

Radioactive patient A patient who was treated with radioactive substance or was accidentally contaminated with radioactive material and hence remains radioactive to be a source of radiation injury to family and friends.

Radioactivity The ability of a substance to emit rays or particles (alpha, beta or gamma) from its nucleus.

Radioallergosorbent test A test to measure the quantities of IgE.

Radioautograph Photograph of tissue section to show distribution of radioactive substances.

Radiobiology Branch of biology dealing with effects of

Radium

ionizing radiation on living organisms.

Radiode The metal container for radium.

Radiodermatitis Inflammation of skin on exposure to X-ray or radioactive elements.

Radioimmunoassay A method for determining concentration of substances particularly protein bound hormones to the range of picograms.

Radioimmunodiffusion Study of antigen-antibody interaction by use of radioisotope labelled antigens or antibodies diffused through a gel.

Radioimmunoelectrophoresis Electrophoresis involving use of radioisotope labelled antigens or antibody.

Radioiodine Radioactive isotope of iodine[131] used in diagnosis of thyroid disorders.

Radioisotope A radioactive form of an element.

Radiologist A doctor practising the art of diagnosis and treatment by use of radiant energy.

Radiolucency The property of being partly or fully permeable to radiant energy.

Radiolucent Permitting the X-rays to pass through.

Radiometer Equipment for measuring the intensity of radiation.

Radiomimetic Imitating the biological effects of radiation, e.g. alkylating agents.

Radionecrosis Tissue destruction on exposure to radiant energy.

Radionuclide Atom that disintegrates by emission of electromagnetic radiation.

Radiopaque Impermeable to X-ray or other form of radiation.

Radiopelvimetry Measurement of pelvis by use of X-rays.

Radiopharmaceuticals Radioactive chemicals or their combination with carriers. Used for determining size and function of body organs.

Radioresistant Tumors that cannot be destroyed by radiation, and hence are radio resistant.

Radiotelemetry Transmission of data via radio from a patient to a remote monitor for analysis.

Radiotherapist Doctor trained in therapeutic use of radiant energy.

Radiotherapy The treatment of disease by application of X-rays, radium, ultraviolet or other forms of radiations.

Radium A radioactive and fluorescent metallic element with half life of 1622 years.

Radium needles Metallic needle shaped containers which contain radium and are inserted to tissue to destroy malignant growths.

Radon A radioactive gaseous element resulting from disintegration of radium. It occurs in nature and is estimated to cause 5-10% of lung cancers occurring in general population.

Raffinose A trisaccharide which on hydrolysis yields fructose and melibiose.

Raimiste's phenomenon In hemiplegia resistance to hip abduction or adduction in the noninvolved extremity evokes same response in involved limb.

Rale Abnormal sound heard during auscultation of chest produced by passage of air through diseased bronchi, (means both rhonchi and crepitation); can be dry or moist, coarse, crackling, bubbling, clicking, amphoric, sibilant and sonorous.

Raloxifene Selective estrogen receptor modulator.

Ramipril ACE inhibitor.

Ramus A branch or division of a forked structure.

Rancid Disagreeable smell or taste from decomposition of fatty substances.

Random controlled trial An experimental study for testing the effectiveness of a drug or treatment regime in which subjects are divided at random into two groups: experimental and control.

Randomization SYN – double blind technique; a method used to assign subjects into treatment or non treatment group by procedures like tossing a coin or use of numbers.

Random sample The selection of samples from population where each individual in the group has same opportunity of being selected.

Ranitidine H_2 receptor blocker, used in peptic ulcer.

Ranula A blue cystic swelling in mouth under the tongue due to obstruction of sublingual or submandibular ducts.

Ranvier's nodes Constriction in myelin sheath of nerve fibers at regular intervals.

Rape Intercourse, homosexual or heterosexual, against consent or with consent which is obtained by force. The age of victim for consent varies from countries to countries. In India it is 16 years.

Raphe A ridge, crease or point of joining of two halves of a part.

Rapport A relationship of mutual trust.

Rarefaction Decreased density, e.g. of bone due to mineral loss.

Rash Any eruption of skin usually associated with communicable disease. *r. butterfly* Skin rash on cheeks and over the bridge of nose as seen in systemic lupus erythematosus. *r. diaper* Skin inflammation in diaper areas in infants. *r. drug* Rash due to drugs like ampicillin, sulphas, iodides and bromides. *r. macular* Flat rash not protruding above the skin surface. *r. mulberry* Dusky rash in typhus fever. *r. nettle* Smooth, elevated itchy rash SYN—urticaria.

Rat A rodent of genus *Rattus* that serve as reservoirs of many infections and infestations, e.g. ratbite fever.

Ratbite fever Fever, bodyache and joint pain caused by *Streptobacillus moniliformis* and *Spirilium minus* transmitted by bite of rat.

Rate The frequency of occurrence of an event expressed with respect to time or some other standard. *r. birth* The number of live births per 1000 in a given population per year. *r. case fatality* The ratio of the number of deaths caused by a disease to the total number of people who contracted the disease. *r. death* The number of deaths in a year per a specified population. *r. glomerular filtration* Rate of filtrate formation in glomeruli of the kidneys; normal 120 ml/min. *r. heart* The number of heart beats per minute.

Rathke's pouch A depression in the embryo giving origin to anterior lobe of pituitary.

Ratio Relationship between two substances. *r. albumin globulin* Ratio of albumin to globulin in blood; usually 1.3:1 or 1.4:1. *r. arm* In chromosome the ratio of long arm to short arm. *r. lecithin-sphingomyelin* The ratio of lecithin to sphingomyelin in amniotic fluid, an indicator of fetal maturity, usually at term. *r. Odd's* In epidemiological and case control studies a relative measure of disease occurrence. *r. therapeutic* A ratio of effective therapeutic dose to minimum lethal dose.

Ration Fixed food and drink per day/month.

Rational Logical.

Rationale The reasoning for course of action.

Rationalization In psychology, a justification for an unreasonable or illogical act or idea to make it appear reasonable.

Rattle A gurgling sound. *r. death* The crepitant rale heard due to fluid accumulation in trachea in a dying person.

Rattle snake A poisonous snake that produces a characteristic rattle.

Raucous Hoarse or harsh.

Rauwolfia The dried roots of *Rauwolfia serpentina* from which are extracted the potent hypotensive agents like reserpine.

Rave Irrational talk, as in delirium.

Ray Any narrow beam of light, the line of propagation of any radiant energy. *r. alpha* The less penetrative rays composed of positively charged particles of helium having powerful fluorescent, photographic and ionizing properties. *r. beta* Negatively charged electrons of disintegrating radioactive elements. *r. gamma* High velocity and penetrating rays coming from nucleus of radioactive elements with wavelength of 1.4 to 0.00 1AU.

Raynaud's disease Intermittent pallor and cyanosis of digits on exposure to cold in females due to abnormal vascular response.

Raynaud's phenomenon Intermittent attacks of pallor followed by cyanosis, occurring in emotional stress or secondary to myxedema, pulmonary hypertension, systemic sclerosis, thoracic outlet syndrome.

React To respond to stimulus; to participate in chemical reaction.

Reaction Response of an organism to a stimulus.

r. antigen-antibody reversible binding of homologous antigen to antibody. *r. Arias-Stella* endometrial changes of cytoplasmic vacuolization with loss of cell polarity in response to chorionic gonadotropin. *r. Arthus* development of induration edema, erythema and haemorrhagic necrosis on intradermal antigen injection in a previously sensitized animal (Class III hypersensitivity reaction). *r. Jarisch-Herxheimer* Commonly seen with antibiotic treatment of early syphilis causing fever, arthralgia and exacerbation of skin lesion, attributed to production of endotoxin by dying organism. *r Mazzotti* reaction following intake of DEC in oncocerciasis with fever, arthralgia eosinophilia, etc. *r. Prausnitz Kustner* a form of type I hypersensitivity reaction produced by intradermal injection of serum from an atopy patient to a healthy one followed by challenge with an antigen. *r. quellung* pneumococci and other capsulated organism swell up when mixed with antisera. *r. Russo* addition of 4 drops of methylene blue to 15 ml of urine of a patient of typhoid fever–urine becomes light green in early disease, emerald colour at peak disease and bluish during recovery. *r. Shwartzman* localized cutaneous reaction with leucocyte infiltration, hemorrhagic necrosis at the skin site of endotoxin injection when the same endotoxin is given 24 hours after.

Reaction time The time interval between application of stimulus and response to it.

Reactive depression Depression following situations like bereavement, financial loss, slander, etc.

Reading lip Interpretation of ones speech from movement of his lips.

Read only memory The part of computer's memory that contains permanent instructions in contrast to random access memory which holds only a temporary memory (program).

Reagent A substance that reacts in a chemical reaction to detect presence of another substance.

Reagin IgE antibody.

Reamer Instrument of dentists for enlargement of root canal.

Reanimate To revive, resuscitate.

Rebound phenomenon When a limb or part is moved against resistance and the resistance is suddenly withdrawn, the limb moves abruptly in the direction of effort, a feature of cerebellar disease.

Recall Recapitulation.

Receptaculum chyli Inferior pear shaped expanded portion of lower end of thoracic duct in abdomen.

Receptor In pharmacology, a cell component that combines with a drug or hormone to alter the function of the cell.

Recess A small depression or indentation.

Recession In dentistry, the atrophy of gingival tissue leading to exposure of the roots.

Recessive gene Gene that does not express itself in presence of its dominant allele.

Recidivism Habitual criminality; repetition of criminal act.

Recidivity Tendency to relapse or to return to a former position/condition.

Recipe A medicine formula.

Recipient One who receives, e.g. blood kidney, heart-lungs, etc.

Reciprocal Mutual, complementary.

Recklinghausen German pathologist. *R's disease* Multiple neurofibromata of nerve sheath, arising from cranial and spinal nerve roots and peripheral nerves.

Recline To lie down; to be in recumbent position.

Reclus' disease Multiple benign cystic growth in the breast.

Recombinant DNA Insertion of DNA segment from one organism into DNA of another organism.

Recombination In genetics, the joining together of gene combinations in the offspring that were not present in the parents.

Recon In genetics, the smallest unit that can enter into recombination.

Recover To regain lost health after the illness.

Recovery The process of becoming well after illhealth.

Recovery room The room where patients are kept to recover from effects of anesthesia after the surgery.

Recrudescence Relapse or return of symptoms after a remission.

Recruitment 1. In audiology, an increase in the perceived intensity of sound out of proportion to the actual increase in the sound level, failure of recruitment indicates lesion. 2. Increase in the intensity of a reflex by activation of greater number of motor neurones by a reflex action even though strength of stimulus remains unchanged, e.g. patellar reflex augmented by clasping/pulling the hands apart.

Rectal crisis Rectal pain and tenesmus in CNS disorders.

Rectal reflex Desire to defecate when rectum is filled with stool.

Rectified Made pure or set right.

Rectifier In electricity, a device for transforming alternating current into direct current.

Rectocele Prolapse of posterior vaginal wall along with anterior wall of rectum.

Rectoclysis Slow introduction of fluid into rectum.

Rectopexy Surgical fixation of rectum.

Rectosigmoid Upper portion of rectum and adjoining sigmoid colon.

Rectourethral Concerning rectum and urethra.

Rectouterine Concerning rectum and uterus.

Rectovaginal Concerning rectum and vagina.

Rectovesical Concerning rectum and bladder.

Rectum The lower 5″ of large intestine, responsible for initiation of defecation reflex through $S_1S_2S_3$ sacral segments of spinal cord.

Rectus muscle 1. The short muscles of eye. 2. Two long midline muscles of abdominal wall stretching from pubic bone to ensiform cartilage and 5th, 6th and seventh ribs (*see* Figure).

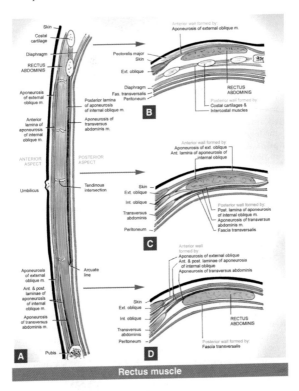

Rectus muscle

Recumbent Lying down.

Recuperation To recover, restoration to normal health.

Recurrence Return of symptoms after a period of quiescence or relapse.

Recurrent Returning at intervals.

Red cross Internationally recognized sign of medical installation or a medical personnel bearing impunity against attack in war.

Redia A stage in lifecycle of trematode following sporocyst which develop into infecting cercaria.

Red nucleus Gray matter in the tegmentum of midbrain.

Redox Combined form to indicate oxidation reduction reaction.

Reduce 1. To restore to normal apposition as in fracture. 2. In chemistry a type of reaction in which a substance gains electrons.

Reducing agent A substance that loses electrons easily, e.g. hydrogen sulfide, sulphur dioxide.

Reductase An enzyme accelerating the process of reduction in a chemical reaction.

Reduction division Cell division occurring in gametogenesis so that the chromosome number is reduced to half.

Redundant Superfluous, more than necessary.

Reed-Sternberg cells Giant connective tissue cells with large nuclei (owleye), characteristic of Hodgkin's disease.

Reentry In electrophysiology of heart, a mechanism to explain tachyarrhythmias where a stimulus passing down the conduction system is blocked in one pathway but travels down in an alternative pathway and again ascends up in previously blocked pathway to give rise to a circus movement.

Reference man A concept employed in nutritional investigation and surveys where a man weighing 70 kg, of 22 years of age engaged in light physical activity consumes 2800 kcal/day.

Reference woman Woman of around 22 years of age weighing 58 kg and consuming 2000 kcal/day.

Referred pain Pain felt at a point remote from point of origin due to similar segmental inervation.

Reflection 1. The condition of being turned back on itself, e.g. peritoneum. 2. In psychology mental consideration of something already considered.

Reflex Involuntary instantaneous response to a stimulus; usually purposeful and adaptive. In a simple reflex the reflex circuit consists of a sensory receptor, afferent neuron, reflex center in brain or spinal cord, efferent neurone supplying the organ (muscle or gland). *r. Babinski* Flexion of great toe and fanning out of other toes on stroking the lateral aspect of sole of foot in healthy persons. *r. Bainbridge* Acceleration of heart rate with ventricular distention. *r. grasp* Grasping reaction of finger on stimulation of hollow of palm, its presence in adults is evidence of diffuse cerebral disease, e.g. G.P.I, dementia, etc. *r. hung up* Abnormal slowness of relaxation phase of deep tendon reflex, e.g. hung up ankle jerk in hypothyroidism. *r. light* Contraction of pupil on focussing a bright light on it. *r. mass* A condition following complete transsection of cord where a weak stimulus brings about widespread responses (muscle contraction, defecation, urination, etc.), due to release from inhibition of higher cortical centers. *r. Moro's* flexion of thighs and knees, fanning out and then clenching of fingers, the arms first thrown outward and then moved inwards in an infant up to 3 months of age produced by sudden strucking next to child. *r. neck righting* Turning of the body in the direction of head rotation in supine infants elicited between 4 months to 2 years of age. *r. parachute* Extension of arms, hands and fingers when the infant is suspended in prone position and dropped a short distance to a soft surface. Asymmetrical response indicates motor abnormality in children above 9 months of age. *r. rooting* Stroking the cheek of the infant causes turning of mouth towards the stimulus. It is present up to 7th month of age. *r. stepping* Leg movements simulating walking when the infant is held erect, inclined forward with sole of feet touching a flat surface. The reflex is present at birth and is gone by 6 weeks of age. *r. tonic neck* In the infant forcibly turning the head causes extension of extremities on the side to which head is turned with flexion of extremities on the other side.

Reflex arc The neural pathway or circuit between the point of stimulation and the responding organ (*see* Figure on page 614).

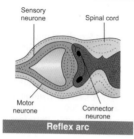

Reflex arc

Reflex center An area in the brain or spinal cord where afferent input initiates impulses in the efferent pathway.

Reflux Regurgitation or backward flow.

Refraction The change in the direction of light rays while passing from one medium to another medium of a different density. *r. errors of* Pathological condition where parallel rays of light are not brought to focus on retina because of defect in refractive media, i.e. cornea and lens.

Refractive power The degree to which a transparent object deflects a ray of light from its straight path.

Refractometer Instrument for measuring refractive power.

Refractometry Measurement of refractive power of lenses.

Refractory period Period of relaxation of a muscle during which excitation is not possible.

Refrigerant Agent producing cooling.

Refrigeration Cooling.

Refsum disease A hereditary disorder of phytanic acid metabolism manifesting with ataxia, neuropathy, visual disturbances (night blindness) and heart disease.

Regeneration Regrowth, repair.

Regimen A systematic plan of therapy.

Region A body part or area.

Regression Return to a former state.

Regulation The state of being controlled.

Regurgitation Backward flow. *r. aortic* Backflow of blood from aorta to left ventricle during diastole due to incompetent aortic valve. *r. duodenal* Reflux of duodenal secretions and bile into stomach. *r. mitral* Backflow of blood from left ventricle into left atrium during ventricular systole due to incompetent mitral valve. *r. pulmonary* Backflow of blood from pulmonary artery into right ventricle. *r. tricuspid* Regurgitation of blood from right ventricle into right atrium.

Rehabilitation The processes of treatment and education for a disabled patient to achieve maximum function and independent living. *r. cardiac* A combination of psychological support, progressive exercise and patient education to achieve maximum functional ability after one has had myocardial infarction.

Rehydration Restoration of body hydration or water balance.

Reichert's cartilage The second branchial arch in embryo giving rise to stapes, styloid process, stylohyoid ligament, etc.

Reimplantation Replacement of a part from where it was taken out, e.g. tooth, finger, ear.

Reinfection A second infection by the same organism.

Reinforcement Augmentation or strengthening.

Reissner's membrane The thin membrane separating the cochlear canal from the scale vestibule.

Reiter's syndrome A symptom complex consisting of urethritis, arthritis and conjunctivitis commonly occurring in young men with a preceding history of gastrointestinal upset.

Rejection Destruction of transplanted tissue/organ due to host immune response. Rejection can be hyperacute, acute or chronic.

Relapse Reappearance of symptoms after apparent cure.

Relapsing fever Infectious disease caused by *B. recurrentis.*

Relative risk In epidemiological studies it is the ratio of incidence rate of a disease in the exposed group to that in the unexposed group.

Relax To diminish anxiety, tension, nervousness.

Relaxant An agent decreasing tension, tone of a muscle.

Relaxin A polypeptide hormone secreted by corpus luteum of ovary during pregnancy that inhibits uterine contraction.

Relieve To provide relief.

Remedy Cure.

Remission Abatement in severity of symptoms.

Remittent fever Fever alternately increasing and decreasing but not touching the normalcy.

Remodelling The reshaping or reconstructing of a part or area.

Renal failure Failure of kidneys to perform excretory and metabolic functions resulting in anuria/metabolic changes.

Renal transplant Surgical implantation of donor kidney to replace a diseased host kidney.

Renal tubular acidosis A group of four diseases, in

which acidosis is due to excess bicarbonate excretion and excess chloride reabsorption.

Reniform Shaped like a kidney.

Renin An enzyme secreted by juxtaglomerular apparatus of kidneys that converts angiotensinogen to angiotensin.

Renin substrate Alpha-2 globulin.

Rennin An enzyme present in gastric juice of animals that coagulates milk.

Renography X-ray of kidneys.

Renshaw cells Small cells with short axons connecting motor nerve axons with each other and thereby inhibit motor neurons.

Reovirus A class of viruses found in the intestinal and respiratory tract of healthy humans.

Repellent An agent that repels insects, ticks and mites, e.g. dimethypthalate.

Repletion Complete fullness or satisfied.

Replication The process of doubling of tissue, cell, genetic material.

Repolarization Restoration of basal electrical status in muscle or nerve fiber after excitation.

Reposition Restoration of an organ or tissue to its original position.

Repositor Instrument for reposition.

Reproduction The process by which plants and animals give rise to offsprings. *r. asexual* Reproduction by fission or budding without involvement of sex cells.

Repulsion Act of driving back or use of force to cause separation.

Research Scientific and diligent study, investigation and experimentation to establish facts and intelligently analyze them to derive conclusion.

Resect To cut out, e.g. a part of intestine in gangrene of bowel.

Resection Partial excision. *r. wedge* Resection of a piece of tissue in form of a wedge as in polycystic ovary.

Resectoscop e Instrument for resection of prostate through urethra.

Reserpine Derivative from plant *Rauwolfia serpentina* acting as a hypotensive agent.

Reserve That which is held back for future use. *r. alkali* Alkali content of body available for neutralization of acid. *r. cardiac* The ability of heart to increase cardiac output during strenuous physical work.

Reserve air Additional amount of air that can be expelled from lungs over the normal quantity.

Reservoir Any human being, animal or insect in which an infecting agent lives, multiplies and reproduces for transmission to susceptible host.

Resident A doctor under training after internship.

Residual Relates to that left as a residue.

Residual urine Urine left in bladder after urination; commonly it is less than 50 ml.

Residue-free diet Diet free of cellulose or roughage.

Resilience The property of coming back to original shape after stretch is released.

Resin 1. Some natural substances obtained as exudation from plants. 2. A class of solids or soft organic compounds that includes most polymers like polyethylene, polystyrene and polyvinyl. *r. ionexchange* Ionizable synthetic substances either anionic or cationic, used to remove acid or basic ions from solutions.

Resistance 1. Power of resisting. 2. In psychology, the force which prevents repressed thoughts from entering conscious mind from the unconscious. 3. The power of body to withstand infection.

Resolution 1. The subsidence of inflammation and return to normalcy, 2. The ability of a ultrasonic transducer system to show fine details of organ scanned.

Resolve To return to normal after pathological process subsides.

Resonance The musical quality elicited on percussing an air containing cavity. *r. vocal* The vibrations of voice transmitted to ears during auscultation. It is increased in consolidation, and over cavities in communication with bronchus.

Resorb To absorb again or to undergo resorption.

Resorbent An agent that promotes absorption of blood and exudates.

Resorcinol A mild antiseptic, keratolytic and fungicidal agent.

Resorption Act of removal by absorption, e.g. callus following bone fracture, root of deciduous tooth, blood from hematoma.

Respiration The act of breathing for interchange of gases, i.e. O_2 and CO_2. *r. abdominal* Use of diaphragm and abdominal muscles for respiration as in rib fracture, pleurisy. *r. paradoxical* A condition seen in paralysis of diaphragm whereby the affected side diaphragm moves up during inspiration and moves down during expiration. *r. Cheyne-Stokes* Abnormal bizarre breathing with periods of apnea followed by gradually increasing depth of respiration followed by a slow decline to end in apnea; seen in diencephalic dysfunction. *r. Kussmaul's* Deep gasping respiration of diabetic ketoacidosis. *r. thoracic* Respiration performed entirely by expansion of chest as in peritonitis, diaphragmatic inflammation.

Respirator An apparatus which rhythmically inflates and deflates the lungs; either pressure cycled or volume cycled.

Respiratory center The centers in medulla oblongata controlling the act of respiration. Consists of an inspiratory center in rostral half of reticular formation overlying olivary nuclei, an expiratory center dorsal to it and a pneumotaxic center in the pons.

Respiratory distress syndrome Dyspnea in newborn due to deficient pulmonary surfactant, causing atelectasis, commonly seen in prematures *SYN*—hyaline membrane disease.

Respiratory failure Inability of lungs to perform ventilatory function with PaO_2 of ≤ 60 mmHg and PCO_2 ≥ 50 mmHg.

Respiratory quotient The relationship between CO_2 produced and oxygen consumed.

Respiratory syncytial virus A virus that induces formation of syncytial masses in infected cell cultures; causes acute respiratory disease in children.

Response The reaction like that of muscle or gland following a stimulus. *r. triple* Three phases of vasomotor response following skin injury, i.e. red reaction, flare or spreading of flush and wheal.

Restiform Rope like.

Restiform body Inferior cerebellar peduncle on lateral border of 4th ventricle.

Resting potential The potential difference existing between inside and outside of a cell membrane while the cell is at rest.

Restitution Return to a former status.

Restless leg Irrepressible ache in the legs of unknown etiology compelling the patient to move the legs to bring some relief.

Restoration Return of anything to its previous state; in dentistry material or device that restores or replaces a tooth.

Restraint Preventing or restricting from any action.

Resuscitation Restoration of life or consciousness one who is apparently dead by artificial respiration and cardiac massage.

Retardation Slowing down, delayed mental or physical response.

Retch To make an involuntary attempt to vomit.

Rete A network of vessels and nerves. *r. testes* A network of tubules in mediastinum testis that receives sperms from seminiferous tubules. From rete testis efferent ducts convey sperm to epididymis.

Retention 1. Keeping within body of substances like urine, stool. 2. Holding back.

Retention cyst Cyst caused by retention of secretion in a gland due to closure of the duct.

Retention enema Enema retained in colon to provide medication or nutrition.

Reticular In the form of a network

Reticular activating system The system essential in maintaining wakefulness. It consists of reticular formation, hypothalamus and medial thalamus.

Reticular cells Phagocytic cells present in bone marrow and lymphnodes, constitute the reticular tissue.

Reticular formation The group of cells and fibers forming a diffuse network in brainstem and connecting to the ascending and descending tracts around. Responsible for wakefulness and sleep.

Reticular layer Connective tissue layer in deeper portion of dermis beneath the papillary layer.

Reticulation Formation of a network.

Reticulin A proteinacious substance in the connective tissue.

Reticulocyte Immediate precursor of mature RBC, contains a network of granules or filaments, constitute 1% of circulating RBC.

Reticulocytosis Raised number of reticulocytes in peripheral blood indicating active erythropoiesis; occurs after hematinics in treatment of anemia, following bleeding episode.

Reticuloendothelial cell A phagocytic cell of reticuloendothelial system.

Reticuloendothelial system The phagocytic cell system of body capable of ingesting particulate matter like bacteria, colloid particles. It includes macrophages (both fixed and wandering), reticular cells, Kuffer cells of liver and spleen, microglia of CNS, adventitial cells of blood vessels and dust cells of lungs.

Reticulosarcoma A malignant tumor composed of large monocytic cells originating from reticuloendothelial system.

Reticulosis Reticulocytosis, a fatal lymphoma, often familial, with hepatosplenomegaly, lymphadenopathy, anemia and granulocytopenia.

Retina The innermost light sensitive layer of eye extending from optic disk to margin of pupil. The various layers of retina from without inward are: pigment epithelium, rods and cones, external limiting membrane, external nuclear layer, external plexiform layer, internal nuclear layer, internal plexiform layer, layer of ganglion cells, layer of nerve fibers, internal limiting membrane.

Retinaculum A band or membrane holding any organ or part in its place.

Retinal detachment Separation of inner sensory layer of retina from outer pigment layer with visual loss.

Retinene Orange-yellow carotenoid pigment formed by action of light on rhodopsin.

Retinitis Inflammation of retina. *r. pigmentosa* A degenerative condition, usually hereditary, beginning in childhood with pigmentary changes. Manifests with defective night vision due to degeneration of rods followed by constricted field of vision.

Retinoblastoma Malignant glioma of retina giving yellow reflex (cat's eye reflex).

Retinodialysis Peripheral retinal detachment.

Retinoic acid Vitamin A breakdown product.

Retinoid Resembling a resin.

Retinol A form of vitamin A.

Retinopathy Any disorder of retina; may be arteriosclerotic, diabetic, hypertensive, syphilitic, etc.

Retinoscopy A method of determining refractive power of the eyes.

Retinosis Noninflammatory degeneration of retina.

Retort Long necked glass vessel used in distillation.

Retractile Capable of being drawn back.

Retraction Shortening, state of being drawn back.

Retraction ring A ridge of uterus separating upper contractile segment from lower dilating segment.

Retractor Instrument for holding back a tissue.

Retreat Act of withdrawal.

Retrieval The process of recalling past memory.

Retro Situated behind or backward in position, e.g. retroocular, retrobulbar, retrocecal, etc.

Retroflexed Bent backwards, a retroflexed uterus is the state where uterine body is bent backwards on cervix (*see* Figure).

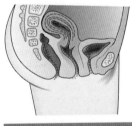

Retrograde Moving backward.

Retrograde amnesia Memory loss for events just preceding the time of patient's illness.

Retrograde ejaculation Semen discharge into bladder rather than through urethral meatus as in diabetic neuropathy.

Retrograde pyelography Pyelography by injection of dye through ureters.

Retrolental fibroplasia Bilateral retinal vessel occlusion followed by fibrous proliferation often involving the vitreous in premature newborns exposed to high concentration of oxygen.

Retroperitoneal fibrosis Fibrotic tissue growth in retroperitoneal space often compressing ureters, vena cava and aorta, a sequel to mathysergide treatment of migraine. *SYN*—Ormond's syndrome.

Retroposition Backward displacement of an organ.

Retropulsion Moving backward involuntarily as in Parkinson's disease.

Retrospective study A study where patient's records are analyzed after they have experienced the disease.

Retroversion of uterus Backward tilting of entire uterus including cervix so that the latter points towards symphysis pubis (*see* Figure on page 622).

Retroviruses A group of viruses containing reverse transcriptase, e.g. RNA containing tumor viruses causing leukemia, lymphoma, in lower animals and AIDS infection in human.

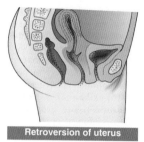

Retroversion of uterus

Rett's syndrome Genetic disorder commonly affecting females between the age of 6 and 18 months characterized by loss of language and motor skills and abnormally small development of head.

Retzius Swedish anatomist.

Revascularization Restoration of blood flow to a part.

Reverberation 1. Repeated echoing of a sound. 2. In neurology the process by which a single applied impulse causes continuous discharge of impulses from collaterals of the neurones.

Revirapine Factor Xa inhibitor, anti-coagulant.

Reye's syndrome A syndrome characterized by encephalopathy, and hepatic failure in children in consequence to viral infection, aspirin use.

Rhabdomyolysis A disease with destruction of muscle cells, common sequence to snake venom.

Rhabdomyoma Benign tumor of striated muscle.

Rhabdovirus Rod shaped RNA virus, e.g. Rabies virus.

Rhachischisis Congenital cleft in spinal canal.

Rhaphe A ridge.

Rh. blood group A blood group antigen on human RBCs, in common with rhesus monkeys. A Rh –ve mother if bears a Rh +ve fetus, Rh antibodies produced in mother may cross the placenta to destroy the fetal RBCs.

Rheology Study of deformation and flow of materials.

Rheostosis A form of osteitis occurring in streaks in long bones.

Rheumatic fever A systemic illness that follows streptococcal sore throat manifesting with carditis, fleeting polyarthritis, chorea, erythema marginatum, subcutaneous nodules, etc. believed to be an autoimmune phenomenon.

Rheumatism A generic term to denote inflammation of muscle, joint pain. *r. palindromic* A disease of unknown etiology manifesting with joint pain, joint swelling lasting from few hours to days with periods of complete normalcy. *r. soft tissue* Pain around a joint not related to any joint pathology, e.g. bursitis, tendinitis, perichondritis, Tietz syndrome, etc.

Rheumatoid Resembling rheumatism.

Rheumatoid arthritis Bilaterally symmetrical polyarthritis involving the fingers and toes with bony erosion, joint deformity and involvement of great vessels, vertebra, etc.

Rheumatoid factor An IgM autoantibody present in up to 75% of patients suffering from rheumatoid arthritis.

Rheumatology Branch of medicine dealing with rheumatic diseases.

Rh immune globulin Anti-Rh gammaglobulin, usually given to Rh –ve mothers within 72 hours of giving birth to a Rh +ve baby or following abortion.

Rhinecephalon The part of brain concerned with reception and integration of olfactory impulses.

Rhinitis Inflammation of nasal mucosa, can be allergic, atrophic (rusting and bad odor), hyperplastic, etc.

Rhinologist A specialist dealing with diseases of nose.

Rhinomiosis Reduction in size of nose by surgery.

Rhinophyma Hypertrophy of tissue over the nose with congestion and retention of sebum.

Rhinoplasty Plastic surgery of nose.

Rhinorrhea Thin watery nasal discharge.

Rhinosalpingitis Inflammation of nasal mucosa and eustachian tube.

Rhinoscleroma An infective disease of nose caused by *Klebsiella rhinoscleromatis* manifesting with hard nodular growth often spreading to lower respiratory tract.

Rhinoscopy Examination of nasal passage.

Rhinosporidiosis A fungal disease caused by *Rhinosporidium seberi* characterized by growth of pedunculated polyps in nose, larynx and genital tracts.

Rhinovirus A subgroup of picorna virus causing common cold.

Rhitidectomy Removal of wrinkles by plastic surgery.

Rhitodosis Wrinkling of cornea, a feature of approaching death.

Rhizo Root.

Rhizoid Root like.

Rhizometic Concerning hip and shoulder joints.

Rhizotomy Section of nerve roots.

Rhodopsin The purple pigment of rods responsible for vision in dimlight.

Rhombencephalon A primary division of embryonic brain giving rise to brainstem and cerebellum.

Rhomboid An oblique parallelogram.

Rhonchis Rattling sound resembling snoring; pleural = rhonchi.

Rhubarb Extract from root and stem of plant used as cathartic and astringent.

Rhythm Regularity of occurrence of an action or movement or impulse. *r. alpha* In EEG a rhythm of 8-12 per second. *r.beta* Rhythm frequency of 15-30 per second in EEG, predominantly in frontomotor leads. *r.cicardian* The recurrence of biological activities every 24 hours not being influenced by environment. *r.delta* A slow EEG rhythm of 4 or less per second with relatively high voltage, usually recorded over tumor or hematoma. *r. ectopic* Impulse originating outside SA node. *r.escape* An impulse originating from a site other than SA node when the latter fails to initiate the impulse.

r. gallop Three heart sounds heard ($S_1S_2S_3$) in sequence in each cardiac contraction resembling gallop of horse. *r. gamma* In EEG 50/second rhythm. *r. idioventricular* Impulse originating from bundle of His or myocardium in consequence to complete A-V block. *r. theta* An EEG rhythm of 4-7 cycles/sec. *r. tic-tac* A rhythm where S_1, and S_2 are of same quality usually in cardiac distress or in fetus.

Rib One of the 12 pairs of narrow curved bones of chest wall connecting sternum to vertebra. *r. cervical* A super numerary rib arising from 7th cervical vertebra and often causing thoracic inlet syndrome by compression of lower cord of brachial plexus.

Ribavirin Antiviral agent.

Riboflavin Yellow-orange crystalline powder of B complex group functioning as coenzyme in cellular oxidation; Richly found in milk and milk products, green leafy vegetables, fish and meat; deficiency causes glossitis, seborrhea, cheilosis and corneal vascularization.

Ribonuclease An enzyme that breaks down RNA.

Ribonucleic acid (RNA) RNA differs from DNA in that

its sugar is ribose and the pyrimidine compound it contains is uracil rather than thymine. RNA is principal constituent of cytoplasm and of certain viruses. Messenger RNA carries the transcription code for specific amino acid sequences from DNA to cytoplasmic reticulum for protein synthesis. Transfer RNA carries the amino acid groups to the ribosomes for incorporation into proteins.

Ribose A pentose sugar present in RNA and riboflavin.

Ribosome A constituent of cell cytoplasm that receives genetic information and translates them into synthesis of proteins.

Ricin A white highly toxic protein of castor beans.

Ricinoleic acid An unsaturated fatty acid with a strong laxative action, principally found in castor oil.

Rickets A vitamin D deficiency disease in children where mineralization of newly formed osteoid tissue is defective. The child is restless with aches and pains, hepatosplenomegaly, delayed dentition, soft skull bones with proneness to skeletal deformities like kyphoscoliosis, bow leg, pigeon chest. *r. renal* Rick-

ets in chronic renal failure primarily due to inadequate formation of active vitamin D₃ and accompanying acidosis causing bone dissolution. *r. vitamin D resistant* Defects of renal tubular function causing excessive renal calcium and phosphorus loss so that the accompanying ricket responds poorly to vitamin D (*see* Figure).

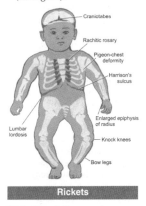

Craniotabes
Rachitic rosary
Pigeon-chest deformity
Harrison's sulcus
Enlarged epiphysis of radius
Lumbar lordosis
Knock knees
Bow legs

Rickets

Rickettsia Microscopic organism in between viruses and bacteria causing typhus fever, Q fever, rocky-mountain spotted fever; transmitted by arthropods.

Rickettsial pox A self-limited acute, febrile disease caused by *Rickettsia akari*.

Rider's bone Bone formation in adductor longus muscle of thigh in horse riders.

Ridge Long projecting surface or crest.

Riedel's lobe A tongue-shaped process of liver.

Rifampin An antibiotic from streptomyces, used in treatment of mycobacterial diseases (leprosy, tuberculosis) and meningitis prophylaxis. Other congeners are rifabutin and rifapentia.

Right handedness Proneness of a person to dominantly use the right hand.

Rigidity Stiffness; one who resists all changes. *r. cerebellar* Stiffness of body parts from disease of middle lobe of cerebellum. *r. clasp knife* Rigidity seen in pyramidal disease where flexion of a limb causes increased resistance of extensors but if flexion is continued, there is a sudden giving way. *r. cogwheel* Jerky resistance felt while stretching a hypertonic muscle. *r. decerebrate* Sustained contraction of extensor muscles from lesion of brainstem.

Rigor Paroxysmal chill.

Rigor Mortis Temporary rigidity of the muscles occurring after 3–4 hours in humans after death due to the chemical changes in the muscles.

Rima A fissure or crack.

Rimiterol A beta$_2$ agonist for use in bronchial asthma.

Rimantadine An analog of amantadine, the antiviral agent.

Ring Band around circular opening, circular form. *r. abdominal* Apertures in abdominal wall, often producing herniations, e.g. inguinal, femoral etc. *r. Bandl's* Retraction ring of uterus. *r. lymphoid* Lymphoid tissue in a ring fashion in pharynx consisting of palatine, pharyngeal and lingual tonsils. *SYN*— Waldeyer's ring.

Ringer's solution A sterile aqueous solution containing 8.6 g sodium chloride, 0.3 g potassium chloride and 0.33 g calcium chloride used especially to replenish fluids and electrolytes by intravenous infusion or to irrigate tissues by topical application.

Ringworm Dermatomycosis caused by trichophyton and microsporum group of fungi.

Rinne test Tuning fork test for testing bone and air conduction. The base of vibrating tuning fork is held in contact with the mastoid process till vibrations are no longer heard by the patient, then it is held close to external ear. If patient still hears the vibration it is called positive Rinne test. When the patient does not hear the vibrations once shifted from mastoid process to external ear, air conduction is tested first by placing the vibrating fork in front of external ear until the sound is no longer heard, then the stem of the fork is placed on mastoid. If vibration is still heard it is called negative Rinne test. All normal persons are Rinne positive and those with defective air conduction are Rinne negative.

Ripening 1. Softening and dilatation of cervix during labor. 2. Maturation of cataract.

Risedronate Bisphosphonate.

Risk-benefit analysis In medicare the analysis of risk and benefit from a procedure discussed between patient, doctor and relations.

Risk factor Factors that predispose a person to development of a disease, e.g. hypertension, diabetes, hyperlipidemia, cigarette smoking, etc. are high risk factors for developing coronary artery disease.

Risperidone Antipsycnotic agent.

Ristocetin An antibiotic obtained from cultures of *Nocardia lurida*.

Risus Laughter. *r. sardonicus* A peculiar grin as in tetanus due to spasm of facial muscles.

Ritgen's maneuver An obstetric procedure aimed to assist the delivery of the head of the fetus and protect the structure of perineum of the mother by applying an upward pressure from the coccygeal region to extend the head of the fetus (*see* Figure on page 628).

Ritodrine- Beta$_2$ agonist for use in bronchial asthma.

Ritonavir Anti-HIV agent.

Ritualistic surgery Surgery without scientific justification performed in primitive societies.

Rivastigmine Cholinergic for brain.

Rizatriptan Antimigraine agent.

Rocking A technique to increase muscle tone in hypotonic muscles through vestibular stimulation.

Rocky-Mountain spotted fever A tick born typhus with fever, rash and myalgia caused by *Rickettsia ricketsii*.

Rodent Mammals like mice, rats and squirrel.

Rodenticide Chemicals that kill rodents.

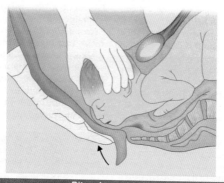

Ritgen's maneuver

Rodent ulcer Basal cell carcinoma commonly occurring on upper face with destruction of underlying tissue and bone.

Roentgen German physicist who discovered roentgen rays, (X-rays) and won noble prize in 1901.

Rokitansky's disease Acute yellow atrophy of liver.

Rolando's fissure Fissure between parietal and frontal lobes.

Romberg's sign Inability to stand still with the eyes closed and feet drawn together in patients of sensory ataxia.

Ropinirole Antiparkinsonian agent.

Root canal The pulp cavity in root of a tooth.

Rosacea A disease of unknown etiology manifesting with papules, pustules and hyperplasia of sebaceous glands principally affecting face.

Rosary Resembling a string of beads. *r. rachitic* Swollen costochondral junctions in rickets.

Rose bengal Iodine-131 along with ^{131}I rose bengal used for liver scanning.

Rosenmuller's body A rudimentary structure in mesosalpinx homologous to head of epididymis in male.

Roseola Rose colored rash. *r. infantum* Noninfectious rose colored rash appearing in infants with splenomegaly, high fever.

Rose's position A supine position with head and

neck extended to perform a surgery within the mouth and fauces to prevent aspiration or swallowing of blood (*see* Figure).

Rosette Something resembling a rose.

Rosiglitazone Antidiabetic agent.

Ross bodies Copper color round bodies with dark granules seen in blood and tissue fluids of syphilis.

Rossolimo's reflex Plantar flexion of second to fifth toes in response to percussion on plantar surface of toes.

Rostellum A fleshy protrusion on anterior end of scolex of tapeworm bearing spines or hooks.

Rostral Towards cephalic end of body.

Rostrum Any hooked or beaked structure.

Rosuvastatin Lipid lowering agent.

Rotavirus Virus causing epidemic and sporadic enteritis.

Roth spots Small white spot on retina close to optic disk in acute infective endocarditis.

Rotoxamine tartarate An antihistaminic drug.

Roughage Fibers in cereals, fruits and vegetable, essential for patients of diabetes and those with constipation but inadvisable for patients of colitis.

Round ligament Round cord like structures passing from uterus in the broad ligament and then through the inguinal canal to end in soft tissues of labia majora.

Roxatidine H_2 receptor blocker used in peptic ulcer.

Rub The sound of friction of one roughened surface moving on another, e.g. pleural rub, pericardial rub.

Rubefacient Agents causing redness of skin by vasodilatation, e.g. liniments of turpentine.

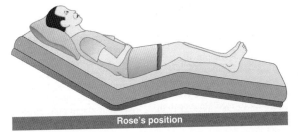

Rose's position

Rubella Acute infectious disease of viral origin causing rash, cervical and postauricular lymphadenopathy, in first trimester can cause fetal anomalies and in pubertal girls can cause oophoritis.

Rubeola *SYN*—measles.

Rubeosis iridis Vascularization of anterior surface of iris with retinal vein thrombophlebitis often responsible for hemorrhagic glaucoma in diabetics.

Rubidium A soft silvery metal that bursts into flames spontaneously in air.

Rubin's test Carbondioxide/air uterine insulflation to test tubal patency.

Rubor Redness caused by inflammation. The other three classical signs of inflammation are calor (heat), dolor (pain) and tumor (swelling).

Rubrospinal The descending tract from rednucleus of midbrain to gray matter of spinal cord.

Rudiment 1. Remnant of a part which was functional in earlier stage of development or in ancestors. 2. Undeveloped.

Ruffini's corpuscles Encapsulated sensory nerve endings of skin to mediate sensation of warmth.

Ruga A fold of mucous membrane, e.g. of stomach or vagina.

Ruggeri's reflex Rise in pulse rate on convergence of eyes on a near object.

Rugose, rugous Having many wrinkles or creases.

Rugosity Condition of having wrinkles or being folded.

Rule of nine Formula for estimating percentage of body surface area, where head represents 9%, front and back of trunk 18% each, each lower extremity 18%, each upper extremity 9% and perineum 1%.

Rum fits Convulsion occurring within 48 hours following abstinence in habitual drinkers.

Rumination 1. Regurgitation of previously swallowed food. 2. Obsessional preoccupation with thoughts.

Rump Gluteal region or buttocks.

Rumpf's symptom In neurasthenia, rise in pulse rate on pressure over a painful spot.

Rupatadine Antihistamine.

Rupia A thick cutaneous syphilitic erruption often with extensive ulceration.

Rupture Breaking apart of any organ or tissue, e.g. of amniotic membrane, uterus, intestines fallopian tubes.

Rush The first spell of pleasure produced by a narcotic drug.

Russel bodies Small spherical hyaline bodies in cancerous and simple inflammatory growths.

Russian bath Steam bath followed by friction and plunge in cold water.

Rust's disease Tuberculosis of cervical vertebrae and their articulations.

Rutin A crystalline glucoside derived from buckwheat closely related to hesperidin, used in hemostatic preparations.

Rye A cereal used for food and beverages.

Saber sin Convex prominent anterior border of tibia in congenital syphilis.

Sabin vaccine Oral polio vaccine containing inactivated polio- virus.

Sabulous Sandy, gritty.

Sac A cavity or pouch often containing fluid. *s. yolk* The extraembryonic membrane that connects with midgut through long narrow yolk stalk and is first hematopoitic organ of the embryo (*see* Figure).

Saccades Fast involuntary movements of eyes while changing gaze from one point to another.

Saccate Enclosed in a sac.

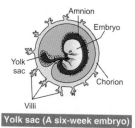

Yolk sac (A six-week embryo)

Saccharase An enzyme catalyzing breakdown of disaccharides to monosaccharides.

Saccharic acid A dibasic acid produced by action of nitric acid on dextrose.

Saccharide A group of carbohydrates including mono, di, tri, and polysaccharides.

Saccharin A coal tar product, 300-500 times sweeter than sugar, used as artificial sweetner.

Saccharolytic Capable of splitting up sugar.

Saccharomycosis A disease due to yeasts.

Saccharose Sucrose, or cane-sugar.

Saccular Resembling a sac.

Sacculation Group of sacs or formed into group of sacs .

Saccule A small sac.

Sacculus Singular of saccule.

SACH foot *Solid ankle cushioned heel.* A prosthetic foot designed to absorb shock and allow movement of the shank while walking (*see* Figure on page 633).

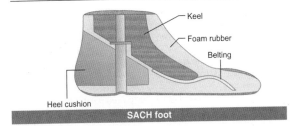

SACH foot

Sacralization Fusion of the sacrum and the 5th lumbar vertebra.

Sacral nerves The 5 pairs of mixed nerves emerging through sacral foramina.

Sacral plexus Plexus of sacral nerves giving rise to sciatic nerve.

Sacrococcygeus One of the two muscles, anterior and posterior extending from sacrum to coccyx.

Sacroiliitis Inflammation of sacroiliac joint.

Sacrospinalis A large muscle lying on either side of vertebral column, consists of iliocostalis and longissimus.

Sacrovertebral angle Angle formed between base of sacrum and fifth lumbar vertebra.

Sacrum The triangular bone of buttock lying in between the two iliac bones forming sacroiliac joints. Male sacrum is narrower and more curved.

Saddle A seat for horse riders.

Saddle area The areas of buttocks coming in contact with the saddle during horse riding.

Saddle joint A joint where the articulating surfaces are convex and concave.

Saddle nose A depressed nasal bridge, due to congenital absence of bony or cartilaginous support or destructive disease like leprosy and syphilis.

Sadism Sexual pleasure from inflicting physical or mental torture on others.

Sadist One who practises sadism.

Sadness Feeling of dejection or melancholy.

Safelight Darkroom lights whose wavelength does not hamper undeveloped X-ray film.

Sagittal Anteroposterior direction.

Sagittal plane The plane that divides body into left and right halves.

Sagittal sinus The superior longitudinal sinus.

Sagittal suture Suture between two parietal bones.

Sago A starch preparation; when taken as food, leaves little residue.

Saint Vitus' dance Sydenham's chorea.

Salam spasm Infantile epilepsy with nodding of head due to spasm of sternocleidomastoids.

Salbutamol Beta₂ agonist bronchodilator.

Salacious Lustful.

Salicylate Salt of salicylic acid. Methyl salicylate is a counter irritant whereas sodium salicylate is analgesic and antipyretic.

Salicylic acid A phenol derivative used for making aspirin and used as keratolytic and antifungal agent.

Saline Solution of salt or salty; can be hypertonic > 0.9% or hypotonic < 0.85% concentration.

Saline enema 1 teaspoon of salt dissolved in a pint of water to which is added magnesium sulfate (epsum salt) to induce catharsis.

Saliva Colourless, odorless, weakly alkaline secretion of salivary glands. Contains ptyalin, maltase and lyso-zymes. Daily secretion is up to 1500 ml.

Salivant Agents that stimulate flow of saliva.

Salivary glands The parotid, sublingual and submandibular paired glands and the unpaired palatal, buccal, lingual glands secreting saliva.

Salk vaccine Formalin inactivated poliomyelitis vaccine for intramuscular use.

Salmeterol Beta₂ adrenergic stimulant.

Salmonellosis Infection with salmonella group of organism producing typhoid fever, gastroenteritis and septicemia.

Salmonpatch Salmon colored areas of cornea in syphilitic keratitis.

Salpingectomy Surgical removal of fallopian tubes.

Salpingitis Inflammation of fallopian tubes usually due to gonococci, tuberculosis, strepto and staphylococci.

Salpingography Imaging of fallopian tubes by injection of radio-opaque dye in investigation of infertility.

Salpingolysis Surgical procedure to free the fallopian tubes of adhesions.

Salpingo-oophorectomy Excision of ovary and fallopian tube.

Salpingo-oophoritis Inflammation of fallopian tube and ovary.

Salpingopexy Surgical fixation of fallopian tube.

Salpingoplasty *SYN* – Tuboplasty; plastic surgery of fallopian tube to promote fertility.

Salpingorrhaphy Ligation of fallopian tube.

Salpingostomy Surgical opening up of a fallopian tube.

Salpingotomy Incision on a fallopian tube.

Salpinx The fallopian or eustachian tube.

Salsalal Salicyl-salicylic acid.

Salt 1. Sodium chloride. 2. A chemical compound formed from action of an acid with a base. *s. bile* Salt of glycocolic and taurocolic acids present in bile, help in absorption of fat. *s. iodized* Salt containing 1 part of sodium or potassium iodide per 10,000 parts of sodium chloride for iodine deficiency. *s. smelling* Aromatized ammonium carbonate.

Saltatory Dancing or leaping movement.

Saltatory conduction Nerve conduction where impulse skips from node to node.

Salt free diet Diet containing <500 mg salt/day.

Salubrious Good for health, wholesome.

Saluresis Excretion of salt in urine.

Salutary Promoting health.

Salvarsan Arsenic salt previously used for syphilis.

Sample A portion of population or any substance that is representative of entire population or that substance.

Sampling The process of selecting a portion or part to represent the whole.

Sanatorium A place or establishment for promotion of good health or treatment of chronic ailments, e.g. tuberculosis.

Sand Fine particles from disintegration of rock. *s. auditory* Calcareous concretions in inner ear. *s. pineal* Calcium deposit near base of pineal gland.

Sandflies Flies belonging to genus *Phlebotomus* transmitting sandfly fever, oroya fever and various forms of leishmaniasis.

Sandfly fever An arbovirus disease mimicking influenza but without respiratory symptoms, transmitted by sandflies.

Sandhoff's disease A gangliosidosis where enzymes hexosaminidase A and B are absent.

Sane Mentally sound.

Sanfilippo's disease A form of mucopoly saccharidosis with mental retardation, dwarfism, hepatosplenomegaly and skeletal defects.

Sanguine Pertains to blood, cheerful.

Sanguinous Bloody.

Sanies Wound discharge which is thin, fetid and green.

Sanitary Clean; conditions conducive to good health.

Sanitary napkin Perineal pad used during menstruation.

Sanitation Establishment of conditions favorable to health.

Sap Any fluid essential for life.

Saphenous nerve A deep branch of femoral nerve supplying innerside of foot and leg.

Saphenous veins The long saphenous vein extends from foot to saphenous opening in upper thigh where as short saphenous vein runs up behind lateral malleolus to join popliteal vein.

Saponification 1. Conversion into soap, i.e. hydrolysis of fat by an alkali yielding glycerol and salts of fatty acid. 2. In chemistry hydrolysis of an ester into corresponding alcohol and acid.

Saponin Some plant glycosides that produce gastroenteritis.

Saporific Imparting taste or flavor.

Saprogen Any microorganism causing or produced by putrefaction.

Saprophyte Organisms living on decaying or dead organic matter.

Saquinavir Anti-HIV agent.

Saralasin Converting enzyme inhibitor for hypertension.

Sarcoblast Embryonic cell that develops into a muscle cell.

Sarcocele A fleshy tumor of testicle. *Sarcocystis* a genus of *Coccidian protozoan*, forms sarcocysts in human muscle. *Sarcocystosis* Usually transmitted by eating undercooked pork or beef containing sporocysts or ingestion of sporocysts in the feces of animal.

Sarcoid 1. Resembling flesh 2. Small tubercle like lesion characteristic of sarcoidosis.

Sarcoidosis A granulomatous disease of unknown etiology affecting lungs, lymph nodes, skin, eyes, small bones of hand and feet.

Sarcolemma A thin membrane surrounding each striated muscle fiber.

Sarcoma Cancer of connective tissue like muscle and bone. *s. Ewing's* A fusiform swelling of long bones containing round endothelial cells. *s. Kaposi's* A skin sarcoma in AIDS victims. *s. osteogenic* Sarcoma in metaphysis of long bones containing variously shaped cells. *s. reticulum cells* A form of malignant lymphoma.

Sarcomere That portion of a striated muscle fibril lying between two adjacent dark lines (*see* Figure).

Sarcoplasm The cytoplasm inside muscle cells.

Sarcoptes A genus of *Acarina* that includes mites. e.g., *Sarcoptes scabiei* causing scabies.

Sartorius The thin longest muscle of body in the thigh acting as weak knee flexor.

Satellite A small structure attached to a larger one.

Satiety Feeling satisfied with food.

Satranidazole Antiprotozoal agent.

Saturated compound Any compound with all its carbon bonds saturated.

Saturation A state in which all of a substance, that can be dissolved in a solution. Adding more of the substance will not increase its concentration.

Saturday Night Palsy Paralysis of radial nerve in alcoholics from its compression against the chair.

Satyriasis Uncontrollable or excessive sexual urge in males.

Saucerization Surgical creation of a shallow area in tissue.

Sauna An enclosure where a person is exposed to high temperature and humidity for brief period and then he is given cold bath; a process to relieve aches and pains, loosen stiff joints and loose weight.

Savory Appetizing taste or odor.

Saxifragant Dissolving or breaking of bladder stones.

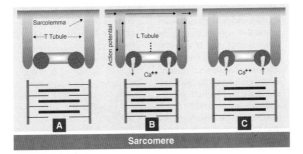

Sarcomere

Scab Crust formed on a wound, pustule or ulcer.

Scabicide Agents effective against scabies organism, i.e. *Sarcoptes scabiei*.

Scabies A mite borne contagious skin disease characterized by papule, vesicle, pustule, with intense itching.

Scala One of the three spiral passages of cochlea: the scala media, scala tympani and scala vestibuli.

Scald Burn caused by moist heat or hot vapors.

Scalded skin syndrome Staphylococcal necrotizing skin infection.

Scale Thin dry exfoliation from upper layers of skin, maximum in psoriasis, eczema, seborrhea sicca, etc.

Scalenotomy Division of scalenus muscle to contain apical tuberculosis of lungs.

Scalenus Scalenus anterior, medius and posterior muscles originating from transverse processes of C_3-C_6 vertebra and inserted to 1st and 2nd ribs.

Scalenus syndrome Thoracic inlet syndrome due to compression of brachial plexus and subclavian artery manifesting with pain, paresthesia in upper limb with atrophy of small muscles of hand.

Scaler An instrument used for removing dental calculus.

Scaling Removal of calculus from teeth.

Scalp The hairy portion of head, consisting from out to inwards: skin, dense subcutaneous tissue, occipitofrontalis muscle with the galea aponeurotica, and periosteum.

Scalpel A straight surgical knife with a convex edge (*see* Figure below).

Scalp tourniquet Tourniquet applied to scalp during IV administration of antineoplastic drugs to prevent alopecia.

Scanning electron microscope An electron microscope that provides three dimensional views of an object.

Scanning speech A symptom of cerebellar disease where words are pronounced by syllables, slowly and hesitantly.

Scaphoid Boat shaped.

Scapula The flat triangular bone at the back of shoulder articulating with clavicle and humerus. *s winged* Paralysis of serratus anterior or tra-

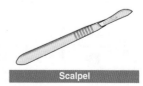

Scalpel

pezius causing prominence of medial border of scapula (*see* Figure).

Scar Healing of wound or injury leaving a mark on skin or internal organs.

Scarlatina Scarlet fever.

Scarlatiniform Resembling scarlet fever or its rash.

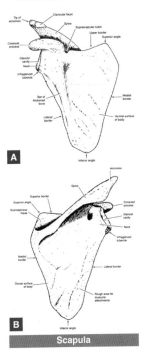

Scapula

Scarlet fever A streptococcal infection characterized by sore throat, strawberry tongue, rose colored rash and fever.

Scattergram Display of data on a paper where each value is indicated by a symbol and the individual symbols are not connected by a line.

Schatzki ring A mucosal web like ring at the squamocolumnar junction of lower esophagus often causing dysphagia.

Schick's test Skin test in diphtheria to determine immunity status. 1 ml. of diphtheria toxin is injected intradermally and result is read after 72 hours. Presence of immunity is indicated by absence of any erythema and inflammation at point of injection.

Schiller's test A test to demonstrate superficial cancer cervix. Iodine is applied on the cervix. As the cancer cells do not contain glycogen, they fail to stain with iodine.

Schilling test A test using radioactive B_{12} for assessment of vitamin B_{12} absorption and diagnosis of intrinsic factor deficiency as in pernicious anemia.

Schistocyte Fragmented red-blood cells of various shapes and irregular surfaces.

Schistosoma A genus of blood flukes living in blood vessels of internal organs and discharging eggs through urine and feces. *s. haematobium* The schistosoma inhabit in vesical plexus and discharge egg in urine; produce hematuria, cystitis and bladder wall calcification. *s. japonicum* Adults live in branches of superior mesenteric vein and produce dysentery. *s. mansoni* Adults live in branches of inferior mesenteric veins.

Schistosomiasis Infestation with the blood flukes, the schistosoma.

Schizencephaly Deformed fetus with a longitudinal cleft in the skull.

Schizogony Asexual reproduction by binary fission as in case of malarial parasite.

Schizoid Resembling schizophrenia.

Schizoid personality disorder A personality cult with difficult interpersonal relationship, and a limited range of emotional experience and expression; the cold, lonely, aloof personality.

Schizont A stage in lifecycle of sporozoa when it reproduces asexually to 12-24 merozoites inside RBC.

Schizophrenia A form of psychosis with disorder of thinking, affect and behavior. Patients have delusions and hallucinations with loss of self identity. *s. catatonic* Patients have catatonic stupor or mutism, catatonic rigidity, catatonic posturing, etc. *s. paranoid* Patient has delusions of persecution, jealousy.

Schlemm's canal Canaliculi or spaces at sclerocorneal junction of eye in anterior chamber for drainage of aqueous.

Schmorl's nodes Herniation of nucleus pulposus into vertebral body producing X-ray density.

Schonlein's disease Allergic or anaphylactoid purpura in response to serum sickness, sensitiveness to drugs or most often idiopathic.

Schuffner's dots Minute granules present within RBC infected by *Plasmodium vivax*.

Schwann cell Cells of ectodermal origin, form neurilemma.

Schwannoma Benign tumor of Schwann cells.

Sciatic Pertains to hip or ischium.

Sciatica Pain along the course of sciatic nerve from back of thigh along lateral border of leg to little toe usually due to disk prolapse at L_5-S_1.

Sciatic nerve The largest nerve in body ($L_{4-5}S_{1,2,3}$) passing from pelvis through greater sciatic foramen down the back of the thigh where it divides into tibial and peroneal nerves. Its lesion cause paralysis of hamstrings, peroneal and calf muscles and toe extensors (*see* Figure).

Science Branch of knowledge utilizing systematic study and intelligent analysis to understand, explain, quantitate and predict the phenomena of life and natural laws.

Scintiphotography Photography of scintillations emitted by radioactive substances injected into body.

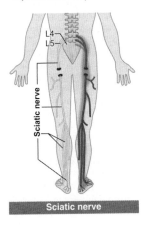

L4
L5

Sciatic nerve

Sciatic nerve

Scintiscan The scintiphotography record to indicate the differential accumulation of a substance in various parts of body.

Schiller's test A test performed in the diagnosis of cervical cancer in which the cervix is painted with iodine solution. The cancerous tissues are stained white or yellow because of their inability to take up the stain due to glycogen deficiency in the cells.

Schirrhus Hard cancerous overgrowth of fibrous tissue.

Scission To divide, split or cut.

Scissor gait Crossing of the legs while walking as in cerebral diplegia.

Scissor leg Contraction of thigh adductor causing the legs to have abnormal tendency to cross to the other side.

Scissors A cutting instrument with two opposing blades with handles held together by a pin.

Sclera The outer tough white fibrous tissue of eyeball extending from optic nerve to corneal margin. *s. blue* Abnormally thin sclera with visible choroid as in osteogenesis imperfecta.

Scleredema A benign self-limited skin disease characterized by edema and induration of skin.

Sclerema Hardening of the skin.

Scleritis Inflammation of sclera, can be anterior (adjacent to cornea), posterior or annular (in ring fashion around cornea).

Sclerodactyly Hardening of skin of fingers and toes.

Scleroderma A chronic disease of unknown etiology causing sclerosis of skin, esophageal dysmotility, pulmonary fibrosis, etc. The skin is tough, taut, hard and leather bound.

Scleroma Circumscribed indurated area of granulation tissue in skin or mucous membrane.

Scleromalacia Softening of sclera as in late rheumatoid arthritis.

Sclerophthalmia A congenital condition where opacity of sclera advances over the cornea.

Scleroproteins A group of insoluble proteins found in cartilage, hair, nails and skeletal tissue.

Sclerosent Any substance that produces sclerosis.

Sclerosis Hardening or induration of a tissue due to excessive growth of fibrous tissue, a feature of degeneration. *s. amyotrophic lateral* A form of motor neurone disease which results in atrophy of anterior horn cells and the pyramidal tracts. *s. multiple* A slowly progressive disease of central nervous system marked by widespread demyelination producing visual disturbances, sensory motor deficit, and cerebellar symptoms.

Sclerosing agents Urea, alcohol, polydachonol tetradecyl sulphate.

Sclerotherapy Use of sclerosing agents for hemorrhoids and bleeding varices.

Sclerothrix Brittleness of hair.

Sclerotome Knife used for incision of sclera.

Scolex The head of tapeworm possessing hooks, suckers or grooves for attachment.

Scoliosis Lateral curvature of spine; the abnormal curve and the compensatory curve in opposite direction; can be congenital, myopathic, ocular, paralytic, etc (*see* Figure on page 643).

Scombroid poisoning Poisoning by histamine like toxin present in the undercooked fish of suborder scombroidea.

Scoop Spoon shaped surgical instrument.

Scopalamine A plant alkaloid producing smooth muscle relaxation and twilight sleep.

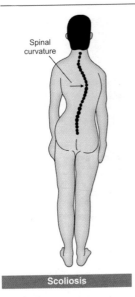

Spinal
curvature

Scoliosis

Scopophilia Sexual pleasure obtained from seeing nude and obscene picture.

Scorbutic Concerning scurvy.

Score A rating or grade as compared to standard. *s. Apgar* A scoring system for evaluation of neurological maturity of newborn from pulse, respiration, reflexes, skin color, grimace, etc.

Scorpion sting Symptoms from scorpion bite resembling spider bite or of strychnine poisoning. The venom contains neurotoxin, hemolysins and agglutinins. Stings are fatal to children below 3 years. As the venom is heat labile emersion of part bitten in hot water for 30-90 minutes neutralizes the toxin.

Scoto Pertains to darkness.

Scotochromogen Microorganisms that produce color when grown in darkness.

Scotoma Dark or blind areas in visual field, can be annular, arcuate, central (around point of fixation), centrocecal (covering point of fixation to blindspot), peripheral. *s. scintillating* An irregular outline around a luminous patch in the visual field as seen in migraine.

Scotopic vision Dark adaptation.

Scotopsin The protein portion of rods of retina that combines with retinol to form visual purple, i.e. rhodopsin.

Scratch test An allergy test where the allergen is placed over a skin scratch. In sensitive persons wheal develops within 15 minutes.

Screen 1. A flat surface for projecting slides or movies or visualizing X-ray films. 2. To make fluoroscopic examination. 3. To thoroughly examine and investigate a person for a disease. 4. Materials used to protect the body parts from ionizing radiation/X-rays. **s. Bjerrum** One meter square surface which is viewed from one meter to chart blind spot, scotoma and extent of visual field.

Scrofula Tubercular cervical lymphadenopathy.

Scrotal reflex Contraction of scrotal muscle (dartos) on stroking the perineum.

Scrotum The double cavity male pouch containing testicles and epididymis, composed of layers of skin, nonstriated dartos muscle, cremasteric, infundibular and spermatic fascia, cremasteric muscle and tunica vaginalis.

Scrubbing Thorough washing of hands and finger nails before performing any surgical procedure.

Scrub typhus Typhus fever caused by *Rickettsia tsutsugamushi* transmitted by mites.

Scum The floating impurities in surface of a culture.

Scurvy Vitamin C or ascorbic acid deficiency manifest with bleeding spongy gums, subperiosteal hemorrhage, muscle pain and induration, loosening of teeth and poor wound healing (*see* Figure).

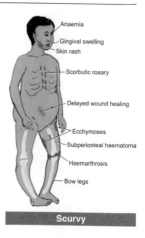

Anaemia
Gingival swelling
Skin rash
Scorbutic rosary
Delayed wound healing
Ecchymoses
Subperiosteal haematoma
Haemarthrosis
Bow legs

Scurvy

Scybala Hard rounded masses of fecal matter.

Sea-sickness Akin to motion sickness with giddiness, nausea, vomiting and headache while travelling in ship.

Sebaceous cyst Sebum filled cyst of sebaceous gland with a black head, may need complete extirpation rather than drainage.

Sebaceous gland Holocrine glands (secretion arising from complete disintegration of cells) in the skin that open into hair follicle and secrete oily substance, the sebum.

Seborrhea A functional disease of sebaceous glands marked by increased secretion of altered quality sebum. Commonly affects scalp (dandruff), face and trunk. *s. sicca* Seborrhea with gray brown or yellow scale and crust.

Sebum A fatty secretion from sebaceous gland, that from the ear is called cerumen and from pepuce is called smegma.

Secnidazole Antiprotozoal agent.

Secobarbitol Short acting barbiturate used for its hypnotic effect.

Secondary areola Pigmentation around nipple during pregnancy.

Secondary hemorrhage Hemorrhage occurring after 48 hours of injury or operation commonly due to sepsis.

Secondary intention Healing by formation of granulation tissue that fills the gap between torn or incised edges.

Secondary nursing care Nursing care aimed at early recognition and treatment of a disease.

Secretin A hormone secreted from duodenum that stimulates secretion of pepsinogen and inhibits secretion of acid by stomach.

Secretion Substances produced or the process of glandular secretion. *s. apocrine* A process by which the secreting cell breaks off to extrude the secretion, e.g. milk production. *s. holocrine* The process where the entire cell and its contents are extruded, e.g. sebum. *s. merocrine* The process where the cell remains intact and discharges its secretion through cell membrane.

Secretogogue Agent that stimulates secretion.

Secretomotor Nerve fibers that promote glandular secretion.

Sector The area within a circle between two radii and the arc.

Sectorial Having cutting edges like teeth.

Sedative Agent that soothes, quietens or brings tranquility.

Sedentary Work with minimal physical exertion.

Sediment The substance settling at the bottom of a liquid.

Sedimentation rate A test to determine the speed at which RBCs settle down when suspended in a test tube. The speed depends upon the size of RBC aggregate which is further dependent upon fibrinogen content of blood. Fibrinogen is an acute phase reactant and is increased in infection, inflammation of any etiology. ESR is reduced in polycythemia, congenital cyanotic heart disease and microcytic hypochromic anemia. Normal ESR is 10-15 mm/hr. in male and slightly higher in female.

Segment A portion.

Segmentation Division into similar parts; division of fertilized egg into many smaller cells.

Segregation Separation.

Seizure A sudden attack of pain, disease or certain symptoms like convulsion, epilepsy.

Seldinger technique A method of introducing a catheter into a vein or artery. The vessel is punctured with a needle that contains a wire. The needle is removed and the catheter is then advanced over the wire, the latter being finally withdrawn.

Selegiline Anti-Parkinsonian drug.

Selenium sulfide Drug used in treatment of tinea versicolor and dandruff.

Self-limited A disease which without treatment pursues a definite course within a limited time.

Sella turcica The concavity on superior surface of body of sphenoid that holds the pituitary gland.

Sellick's maneuver Technique used during endotracheal intubation by applying pressure on the cricoid cartilage to

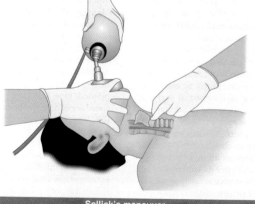

Sellick's maneuver

prevent regurgitation or better visualization of the glottis by the doctor.

Selzer water Naturally occurring water with high CO_2 and mineral content.

Semantics The field of language concerning meaning.

Semen Thick viscid fishy odor discharge per male urethra during sexual climax. It contains the sperms 60-150 million/ml. Eighty percent are motile and normal in morphology. Semen is alkaline without any leukocytes, volume per ejaculation is 2-5 ml.

Semi Prefix meaning half.

Semicircular Half of a circle. *s. canals* The superior, inferior and posterior structures of inner ear for maintenance of body posture.

Semicoma Mild degree of impaired consciousness.

Semilunar Shaped like a crescent. *s. cartilage* The medial lateral, fibrocartilages of knee between tibia and femur.

Semilunar valves The pulmonary and aortic valves.

Semimembranosus A large muscle at inner and back portion of thigh, a knee flexor.

Seminal vesicle Two sac like structures close to prostate in the male giving rise to ductus deference. Act to store semen and secrete a thick viscus fluid that forms part of semen.

Seminiferous tubule Tubules in testes forming and conducting semen.

Semitendinosus Fusiform muscle of posterior and inner part of thigh.

Senescence The process of growing old or period of old age.

Sengstaken-Blakemore tube A three lumened tube used to stop bleeding from esophageal varices (*see* Figure).

Senility Pertains to old age and its changes, physical and mental.

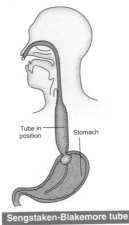

Tube in position • Stomach

Sengstaken-Blakemore tube

Senna Leaves of a plant, used as cathartic.

Sennosides Anthraquinone glucosides present in senna, used as cathartic.

Sensation Feeling or awareness.

Sense 1. The general faculty responsible for perceiving the outside world. 2. To perceive. 3. Normal power of understanding.

Sensible 1. Reasonable. 2. Can be perceived by senses.

Sensitive 1. Able to feel a sensation. 2. Abnormal response to substances like drugs and foreign proteins.

Sensitivity 1. The term is employed in relation to accuracy of diagnostic tests/observations. It is the proportion of people who truely have a specific disease as identified by the test. 2. Susceptibility of bacteria to antimicrobials.

Sensitization Making a person susceptible to a substance by its repeated injection.

Sensitizer A substance that makes the susceptible individual react to same or another irritant.

Sensorium The sensory apparatus of body or consciousness.

Sensory area The postcentral gyrus of cerebral cortex responsible for analysis of somatosensory input.

Sensory integration Skill and performance required in the development and coordination of sensory input and motor output.

Sensory nerve A nerve conveying afferent impulses to brain.

Sensualism State of emotions dominating one's actions.

Sensuous Affecting senses or susceptible to influence through the senses.

Sentiment Mental feeling or opinion, an emotional attitude towards an object.

Sentinel node Cancer metastasis into supraclavicular nodes.

Separator Any device or instrument used for separating two substances, e.g. cell separators.

Sepsis A pathological state due to bacterial multiplication and toxin production. *s. puerperal* Infection of genital passage resulting from childbirth. Common infecting agents are strepto, staphylo and *Escherichia coli*.

Septa Partition.

Septate Having a partition or wall.

Septic Infected

Septicemia Multiplication of pathogenic bacteria in

peripheral blood producing toximia, disseminated cellulitis, lymphangitis, etc.

Septic fever Fever due to presence of pathogenic organisms or their products in blood, producing shaking chills with abrupt rise in temperature and sweating.

Septoplasty Plastic surgery on nasal septum for deviated nasal septum.

Septostomy Surgical formation of an opening in septum.

Septulet Seven children in one pregnancy.

Septum A partition wall dividing two cavities, e.g. interatrial, interventricular, atrioventricular, nasal septum, rectovaginal. *s. pellucidum* A thin triangular sheet of nervous tissue forming the medial wall of the lateral ventricles. *s. primum* The embryonic septum dividing the two atria in a developing heart.

Sequela The final outcome of a disease with or without treatment.

Sequestration Formation of sequestrum. *s. pulmonary* A nonfunctioning area of the lung receiving blood from systemic circulation.

Sequestrum The necrotic bone separated from adjacent healthy bone in osteomyelitis.

Serine An amino acid found in urine of healthy humans.

Seroconversion Appearance of antibodies to an infecting agent or vaccine.

Serodiagnosis Diagnosis from tests involving patient's serum.

Seroepidemiology Epidemiological study of a disease by investigating for presence of diagnostic characteristic in the serum.

Serology The scientific study of serum.

Seroma A localized collection of serum resembling a tumor, commonly after stitching of operational wounds.

Serosa A serous membrane like pleura, pericardium and peritoneum.

Serosanguinous Discharge containing serum and blood.

Serositis Inflammation of serous membrane.

Serotherapy Treatment of disease by injection of serum containing antibodies thereby conferring passive immunity.

Serotonin 5 hydroxy tryptamine present in platelets, mastcells, argentaffin cells of carcinoid tumors. A potent vasoconstrictor incriminated in migraine.

Serotype A classification of microorganisms based on antigenic structure of cell.

Serous cavity Cavity lined by serous membrane like pleural, pericardial and peritoneal cavities.

Serpiginous Creeper like course.

Serpin Serine-protease inhibitor involved in coagulation, complement activation, fibrinolysis etc. They include alfa$_2$, antitrypsin, alfa$_1$, antiplasmin, PAI-I, C1 inhibitor, etc.

Serrate Tooth like, notched. *Sarcocystosis* usually transmitted on eating under cooked pork or beef containing sporocysts or ingestion of sporocysts in the feces of animal. *Serratia* Gram-negative facultative anaerobic enterobacteria producing white, pink or red pigment; cause nosocomial bacteremia, endocarditis and pneumonia in immune compromised.

Serratus A muscle arising or inserted by a series of tooth like processes.

Sertoli's cells Supporting cells in the seminiferous tubules that nourish the spermatids.

Sertraline Anti psychotic agent.

Serum The straw coloured fluid after blood coagulates.

Serum sickness A type III hypersensitivity immune response following vaccination or drugs with fever, arthralgia.

Serum glutamic-oxaloacetic transaminase (SGOT) *SYN* – aspartate transaminase (AST). An intracellular enzyme present in muscle, liver and brain. Its serum level is increased in necrosis of above tissues.

Serum glutamatepyruvate transaminase (SGPT) *SYN* – Alanine amino transferase (ALT) Like SGOT, this enzyme is also present in muscle, liver and brain tissue and its level increases in necrosis of above tissues.

Sesamoid bone A bone developing under a cartilage, e.g. patella.

Sewer gas Methane and hydrogen sulphide produced in sewage, may be used as fuel.

Sex The distinctive characteristics that separate living beings and plants into males and females.

Sex chromatin *SYN* – Barr body. It represents the inactivated 'X' chromosome in female somatic cells (Lyon hypothesis).

Sex chromosome The X and Y chromosomes which determine the sex of an individual.

Sex-linked A character controlled by genes on sex chromosome.

Sextuplet Six children in one pregnancy.

Sexual dysfunction Sexual dissatisfaction due to defective arousal, orgasm, pain or penetration.

Sexually transmitted diseases (STD) Diseases acquired during sexual intercourse with partner. They include syphilis, gonorrhea, lymphogranuloma venereum, granuloma inguinale, chancroid, acquired immunodeficiency syndrome, genital herpes and warts, viral hepatitis B, chlamydia urethritis, etc.

Sexual reflex Erection and ejaculation from sexual stimulation (whether direct or indirect) irrespective one is asleep or awake.

Sezary cells An atypical mononuclear cell containing mucopoly saccharide filled cytoplasmic vacuoles.

Sezary syndrome Exfoliative skin disease characterized by infiltration of skin by sezary cells; a variant of mycosis fungoides.

Shakes Shivering or tremulousness.

Shaking palsy Parkinson's disease.

Shaman A traditional healer who while in a trance, uses spirits to cure diseases.

Shagreen patch Thick granular grayish green skin of tuberous sclerosis.

Shear A force applied parallel to the planes of an object but opposite in direction to existing force.

Sheath A connective tissue covering. *s. carotid* Enclosure of carotid artery, vagus nerve and internal jugular vein by cervical fascia. *s. myelin* Layers of lipid and protein forming a semifluid covering of nerves, an extension of plasma membrane of Schwann cells. *s. synovial* Double walled tube like bursa enclosing the tendon of hands and feet.

Shedding Casting off surface layer of epidermis.

Sheehan's syndrome Hypopituitarism secondary to pituitary infarction following postpartum hemorrhage and shock.

Sheep cell agglutination test (SCAT) A test for rheumatoid factor when sheep erythrocytes sensitized with rabbit anti sheep RBC immunoglobulin are agglutinated by patient's serum containing rheumatoid factor.

Sheet Linen. *s. draw* Folded linen placed under a patient which can be withdrawn without lifting the patient.

Shield A protective device.

Shigella Nonmotile gram-negative bacilli causing bacillary dysentery and alimentary disturbances, e.g. S. boydii, S. dysenteriae, s. flexneri, S. sonnei.

Shigellosis Disease produced by Shigella.

Shin Anterior edge of tibia.

Shingles SYN – Herpes zoster producing painful vesicles along course of a nerve.

Shirodkar operation Placement of purse-string suture around cervix to prevent premature delivery in incompetent cervix.

Shiver Involuntary muscle contraction during cold, fear or at onset of some fevers.

Shock A state of poor tissue perfusion due to deficient circulating blood volume, pump failure or sudden fear, anaphylaxis, overwhelming infection, drugs, toxins. s. anaphylactic Shock following injection of foreign substances to a sensitized patient. s. cardiogenic Shock due to pump failure following myocardial infarction or electrical disturbances. s. endotoxic Shock from endotoxins of gram- negative bacteria. s. spinal Acute flaccid paralysis with loss of all sensations and reflexes following complete transection of spinal cord.

Shohl's solution Solution of citric acid and sodium citrate used for acidosis.

Short bowel syndrome Poor absorption of nutrients following resection of sizeable length of small intestine.

Shortsightedness SYN—myopia. A condition where parallel rays are brought to focus in front of retina.

Shot A subcutaneous injection.

Shoulder The junction of upper arm with collar bone and scapula. s. dislocation Slipping of humeral head from glenoid cavity of scapula.

Show Blood mixed thick mucoid discharge from vagina during first stage of labor.

Sharpnell's membrane The triangular portion of tympanic membrane lying above the malleolar fold. SYN – pars flaccida.

Shred Thin strand of mucus.

Shrink To reduce in size.

Shudder Convulsive tremor from fear, aversion.

Shunt Diversion of flow. s. arteriovenous Congenital abnormal arteriovenous communication or the one done for hemodialysis. s. Blalock-Taussig-side to side, anastomosis of left subclavian artery to left pulmonary artery, done in TOF to increase pulmonary blood flow. *s. left to right* Passage of blood from left side of heart to right side chambers as in VSD, ASD, PDA. *s. right to left* Reverse of the above occurring in Fallot's tetralogy, transposition of great vessels, single ventricle, DORV and Eisenmenger syndrome. *s.* *transjugular intrahepatic portosystemic* (TIPS) percutaneous creation of shunt between hepatic and portal vein to reduce portal pressure in cirrhosis. (*see* Figure).

Shy Drager syndrome Chronic orthostatic hypotension due to primary autonomic failure.

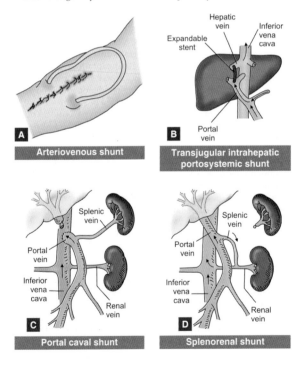

| **A** Arteriovenous shunt | **B** Transjugular intrahepatic portosystemic shunt |

Hepatic vein
Inferior vena cava
Expandable stent
Portal vein

| **C** Portal caval shunt | **D** Splenorenal shunt |

Splenic vein
Portal vein
Inferior vena cava
Renal vein

Sialism Excessive salivary secretion.

Sialoadenitis Inflammation of salivary gland.

Sialogogue An agent that promotes salivary secretion.

Sialography X-ray examination of salivary ducts and the gland by die injection through the duct opening.

Sialoporia Deficient secretion of saliva.

Siamese twins (Named after Chang and Eng joined Chinese twins born in Siam), cogenitally joined twins.

Sib A blood relative, brother or sister.

Sibilant Hissing or whistling sound.

Sibilismus A hissing sound.

Sibling Children of same parent.

Sibutramine Antiobesity agent.

Siccus Dry.

Sick Not well, ill.

Sickle cell Crescent shaped RBC.

Sickle cell anemia A form of congenital hemolytic anemia where there is abnormal hemoglobin (Hbs) resulting in sickling during splenic hypoxic conditioning.

Sickle cell crisis Capillary plugging by sickle cells causing joint pain, abdominal pain, renal pain, etc. due to infarction.

Sickling Tendency of RBC to assume sickle shape.

Sickness Illness. *s. motion* Nausea and vomiting experienced during motion by road, air or water. *s. morning* Nausea and vomiting of early pregnancy. *s. mountain* Nausea, anorexia, insomnia and dyspnea of high altitude due to oxygen lack. *s. sleeping* 1. Trypanosomiasis involving CNS (Chaga's disease), transmitted by testsefly. 2. Encephalitis lethargica. *s. serum* Joint pain, fever, lymphadenopathy following injection of serum.

Sick-sinus syndrome SA node dysfunction manifesting as excessive bradycardia, brief periods of sinus arrest or tachybrady syndrome.

Side effect Undesirable effects of a drug.

Sidenafyl A phosphodiesterage inhibitor used in impotency (viagra).

Sideroblast Ferritin containing normoblast in bone marrow that constitute 20-90% of bone marrow normoblasts. The ferritin gives prussian blue reaction indicating presence of ionized iron.

Siderocyte RBC containing iron in any form other than hemoglobin.

Siderophil A cell having affinity for iron.

Siderosis A form of pneumoconiosis due to inhalation of iron dusts/fumes.

Siderosome A reticulocyte with iron containing granules.

Sieve A mesh with uniform sized pores.

Sigh A deep inspiration followed by a slow but loud expiration.

Sight Vision.

Sigmoid Shaped like capital greek letter sigma.

Sigmoid flexure Lower part of sigmoid colon shaped like S.

Sigmoidoproctostomy Artificial communication of sigmoid flexure with colon.

Sigmoidoscope Tubular instrument for examination of rectum and sigmoid colon.

Sigmoidoscopy Examination of rectosigmoid by sigmoidoscope.

Sigmoidosigmoidostomy Artificial creation of communication between two segments of colon.

Sign Any objective evidence or manifestation of disease. *s. Aaron's* pain in epigastrium on pressure at Mc Burney's point in appendicitis. *s. Auenbrugger's* bulging of epigastrium due to pericardial effusion. *s. Babinski's* when a hemiplegia patient whistles, there is good contraction of platysma on healthy side. *s. Battle's* discolouration of skin over mastoid region with ecchymosis on tip of mastoid process in fracture base of skull. *s. Beevor's* a sign of functional paralysis, patient unable to inhibit the antagonistic muscle. *J. Braunwal's* occurrence of a weak pulse after a instead of strong one immediately after VPB; *s. Brudzinski's* in meningitis flexion of neck causes flexion of hip and knee. *s. Carvallo's* in tricuspid regurgitation augmentation of pansystolic murmur by inspiration. *s. Chadwilk's* congested dark bluish vaginal mucosa, an indication of pregnancy. *s. Chvostek's* taping of facial nerve causes spasm of facial muscles in tetany. *s. Cullen's* bluish discolouration around umbilicus in haemorrhagic pancreatitis/ectopic pregnancy rupture. *s. Dejerine's* aggravation of symptoms of radiculitis by coughing, sneezing, straining. *s. Ewart's* bronchial breathing and dullness on percussion at the lower angle of left scapula in pericardial effusion. *s. Ewing's* tenderness at upper inner angle of orbit, a feature of frontal sinus obstruction.

s. Federici's on auscultation of abdomen, the cardiac sounds are heard in intestinal perforation. *s. fissure of 3* seen in aortic coarctation in X-ray. *s. Gower's* a sign of pseudo-hypertrophic muscular dystrophy in which to stand from supine position patient rolls to prone position kneels and then rises. *S Graefe's* failure of upper eyelid to move downward promptly on looking down, a feature of Graves' disease. *s. Hamman's* precordial chronching sound synchronous with each heart beat as in pneumomediastinum. *s. Hell's* disproportionate systolic femoral hypertension as seen in aortic incompetence. *s. Hoffmann's* sudden nipping the main of index finger causes flexion of terminal phalanx of thumb in hemiplegia. *s. Hoover's* a lying patient when presses one leg on to bed, the other leg lifts up-a feature of normalcy is absent in hysteria. *s. Kehr's* severe pain in left shoulder in rupture of spleen. *s. Kernig's* a sign of meningitis-thigh flexed on abdomen cannot be extended. *s. Kussmaul's* distention of jugular veins on inspiration in constrictive pericarditis. *s. Lhecmitte's* sudden electric like shock on head flexion in multiple sclerosis. *s. Lloyd's* pain on loin on deep percussion but not pressure, in renal calculus. *s. Mercedes Benz* the MB logo on gall-bladder X-ray due to gas filled fissures in gallstones, the gallstones being invisible. *s. Mobius's* inability to keep the eyeballs converged in Graves' disease. *s. Müller's* pulsation of uvula in aortic insufficiency. *s. Murphy's* in terruption of deep inspiration when finger is pressed below hepatic margin in acute cholecystitis. *s. Musset's* rhythmical jerking movement of head in aortic aneurysm and incompetence. *s. Nikolsky's* ready separation of outer layer of epidermis with minor trauma/rubbing in pemphigus. *s. Ortolani's* click on hip reduction by abduction in congenital hip dislocation. *s. Osler's* painful small erythematous swellings on hands and feet in bacterial endocarditis. *s. Puddle* a method of detecting free fluid in abdominal cavity. *s. Queckenstedt's* compression of neck veins increases spinal CSF pressure normally but not with spinal block. *s. Romberg's* swaying of body when standing feet togethers with eyes closed in diseases involving posterior column. *s. Rovsing's* pressure on left flank produces pain in right flank in acute appendicitis. *s. Spalding's* overriding of fetal skull bones in X-ray abdomen indicating death *in utero*. *S. Square root* a cardiac cath sign in constrictive pericarditis. *s. Stelwag's* infrequent blinking in Grave's disease. *S. string of beads* in X-ray abdomen due to round-worms causing obstruction. *Ds. Tinel's* tingling in distal limb when a divided nerve is percussed indicating regeneration. *s Turner's* bruising of skin at costovertebral angle in acute haemorrhagic pancreatitis (*see* Figure A below and Figure B on page 658).

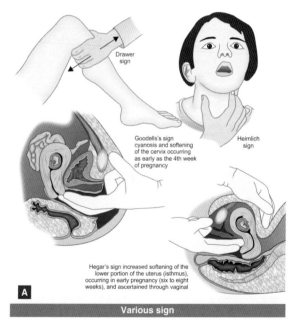

Drawer sign

Goodells's sign cyanosis and softening of the cervix occurring as early as the 4th week of pregnancy

Heimlich sign

Hegar's sign increased softening of the lower portion of the uterus (isthmus), occurring in early pregnancy (six to eight weeks), and ascertained through vaginal

A

Various sign

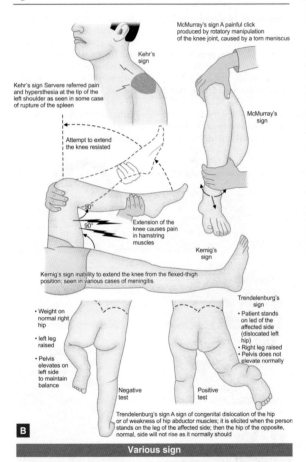

Kehr's sign

Kehr's sign Servere referred pain and hypersthesia at the tip of the left shoulder as seen in some case of rupture of the spleen

McMurray's sign A painful click produced by rotatory manipulation of the knee joint, caused by a torn meniscus

McMurray's sign

Attempt to extend the knee resisted

-90°

90°

Extension of the knee causes pain in hamstring muscles

Kernig's sign

Kernig's sign inability to extend the knee from the flexed-thigh position; seen in various cases of meningitis

Trendelenburg's sign

• Weight on normal right hip

• left leg raised

• Pelvis elevates on left side to maintain balance

Negative test

• Patient stands on led of the affected side (dislocated left hip)

• Right leg raised

• Pelvis does not elevate normally

Positive test

Trendelenburg's sign A sign of congenital dislocation of the hip or of weakness of hip abductor muscles; it is elicited when the person stands on the leg of the affected side; then the hip of the opposite, normal, side will not rise as it normally should

B

Various sign

Silastic Silicone material which are usually inert and hence compatible with body and used in reconstructive surgery.

Silent Mute.

Sildenafil a phosphodiesterage 5 inhibitor, vasodilator used for impotency and pulmonary hypertension.

Silent angina Angina pectoris without subjective symptoms like precordial pain.

Silent period Period in a tendon reflex immediately following muscle contraction when another neural impulse entering the reflex center cannot excite efferent motor neurone.

Silica Silicon dioxide.

Silicate A salt of silicic acid.

Silicon A nonmetallic element constituting 25% of earth's crust.

Silicone A group of polymeric organic compounds used in adhesives, lubricants and prosthesis.

Silicosis A form of pneumoconiosis resulting from inhalation of silica (quartz) dusts producing nodules, fibrosis and often emphysema.

Silo-filler's disease Hypersensitive pneumonitis in workers working in silos caused by nitric acid and nitrogen dioxide that are produced by fermenting organic matter.

Silver White malleable metal used for astringent and antiseptic effect. *s. amalgam* Alloy of silver with tin or copper used as a dental restorative material. *s. halide* The coating on radiographic films which when exposed to radiant energy forms the image. *s. sulfadiazine* Used for topical application on burn.

Silver-fork deformity Malunited Colle's fracture resembling back of the fork.

Silver nitrate A germicide and local astringent used for throat cauterization; causes grayish discoloration of mucous membranes.

Silvester's method A method of artificial respiration where patient lies on back with arms raised to the sides of head, then brought down and pressed against the chest.

Silymarin Hepatoprotective agent.

Simethicone Dimethyl polysiloxanes, an antifoaming agent used to treat intestinal gas.

Simian crease A single transverse crease on palm as in monkeys. Its presence may signify Down's syndrome, rubella syndrome, Turner's syndrome, Klinefelter's syndrome (*see* Figure).

Similimum A therapeutic concept in homeopathy where a medicine produces symptoms similar to that of the disease for which it is prescribed.

Simmond's disease Hypopituitarism due to pituitary atrophy.

Simon's position An exaggerated lithotomy position with elevation of buttock and abduction of thighs, employed for operation of vagina.

Sim's position A semiprone position with patient lying in left side with right knee and thigh drawn up, best for rectal examination and giving enema.

Simulation Imitation, pretention.

Simulator Any device that creates a situation similar to one that might be encountered, a technique useful in teaching in flying practice, engine testing.

Simulium A genus of insects that includes black flies, *S. damnosum,* serves as intermediate host of *Onchocerca volvulus.*

Simvastin Lipid lowering agent.

Sinciput Front and upper part of head.

Sinemet Combination of levodopa and carbidopa.

Singer's node A swelling between arytenoid cartilages in singers.

Sinister Evil, wickedness; in anatomy left or present on left side of body.

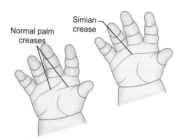

Normal palm creases

Simian crease

Simian crease

Sinistrous Awkward, clumsy, unskilled; opposite to dextrous.

Sinoatrial node Node at entry of superior venacava into right atrium, the pace maker of heart.

Sinogram X-ray of sinus after radiopaque dye injection.

Sinuous Winding, wavy, tortuous.

Sinus A cavity within bone, dilated venous channel, a cavity with small opening. *s. cavernous* The intracranial sinus extending from sphenoidal fissure to the apex of the petrous portion of temporal bone. *s. circular* A venous sinus around pituitary body communicating on each side with the cavernous sinus. *s. coronary* The vein in the atrioventricular groove of heart draining into right atrium. *s. inferior petrosal* A large venous sinus along lower margin of petrous part of temporal bone draining into cavernous sinus. *s. maxillary* Cavity in the maxilla communicating with middle meatus of nose. Both maxillary sinuses are usually symmetrical. *s. sigmoid* Continuation of transverse sinus along posterior border of petrous part of temporal bone to the jugular foramen to continue as jugular vein. *s. superior sagittal* A straight sinus along upper border of falx cerebri from the crista galli to the internal occipital protuberance where it joins transverse sinus, the left or right.

Sinus arrhythmia Rise and fall in heart rate in inspiration and expiration respectively; usually innocuous.

Sinusitis Inflammation of paranasal sinuses, the maxillary, frontal, ethmoidal and sphenoidal with headache, fever and chills. A consequence to chronic allergic rhinitis, deviated nasal septum, or nasal polyp.

Sinusoid A large blood channel with reticuloendothelial lining found in liver, spleen, adrenal and bone marrow.

Sinus rhythm The normal cardiac rhythm originating from SA node.

Siphon A tube bent at an angle with two unequal parts for transferring liquids from one container to another.

Sipple syndrome Multiple endocrine neoplasia type III.

Sirolimus Immunosuppressant.

Sitagliptin Antidiabetic.

Site Position or location.

Sitophobia Abnormal psychic aversion for particular food.

Sitosterols A mixture of saturated sterols that increase fecal elimination of cholesterol and therefore used as lipid lowering agent.

Sitting height In anthropometry a vertical height taken from the table on which patient is sitting to the vertex.

Situational crisis In psychiatry any brief transient period of psychological stress.

Situs A position. *s. inversus* An anomaly where visceral positions are reversed.

Sitz bath Emersion of patient's buttocks and perineal region in hot water.

Sixth cranial nerve Abducent nerve that supplies the external rectus.

Sjögren's syndrome A combination of rheumatoid arthritis with xerostomia, keratoconjunctivitis sicca and parotid enlargement.

Sjögren-Larsson syndrome Mental retardation, ichthyosis, spastic diplegia, inherited as an autosomal recessive trait.

Skatole A nitrogenous decomposed product of protein formed from tryptophan with bad odor.

Skeletal muscle A muscle attached to bone and involved in body movements.

Skeletal survey X-ray of entire skeleton to detect any metastasis or disease.

Skeletal traction Traction applied directly to bone through inserted pins and needles.

Skeleton The bony framework supporting and protecting the viscera. It consists of 206 bones, 80 axial and 126 appendicular (*see* Figure on page 663).

Skene's glands Paraurethral glands opening to the floor of terminal urethra. Constantly involved in gonococcal infection.

Skew Asymmetrical, to slant.

Skew deviation A condition where one eyeball is deviated upward and outward, the other being inward and downward.

Skin The integument covering the body. It is the largest organ system consisting of epidermis and dermis. The layers of epidermis are stratum corneum, statum luciderm, stratum granulosum, stratum basale (*see* Figure on page 663).

Skin clip An alternative to sutures to close the skin wound.

Skin fold thickness Measuring thickness of subcutaneous fat over triceps, in upper abdomen and in subscapular

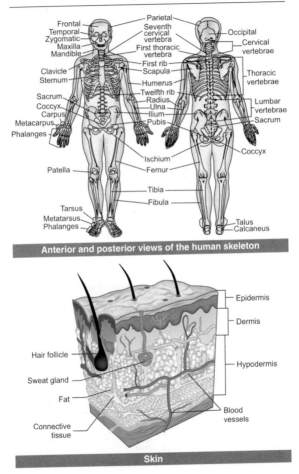

Anterior and posterior views of the human skeleton

Skin

region to assess the nutritional status.

Skull The bony structure of the head of many animals. Not only does the skull support the facial structures, it also protects the brain from injuries. In humans the adult skull is composed of 22 bones (*see* Figure).

Sleep The periodic state of rest in which there is diminution of consciousness and relative inactivity.

Sleep paralysis Transient paralysis with spontaneous recovery occurring while falling asleep or on awakening.

Sleeping sickness African trypanosomiasis, encephalitis lethargica.

Sleep spindle In electroencephalography, the bursts of about 14 per second waves occurring during sleep.

Slide A piece of glass on which specimens are examined under microscope.

Sliding hernia A variety of indirect irreducible inguinal hernia in which a section of viscus forms one wall of the sac.

Sling A bandage usually slung from neck to support the arm (*see* Figure).

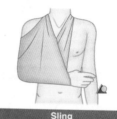

Sling

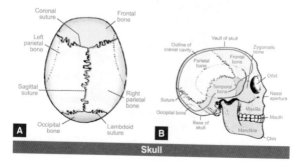

Skull

Slipped disk Herniated intervertebral disk.

Slipped epiphysis Displacement of upper femoral epiphysis, common to children.

Slit A narrow opening.

Slit lamp An instrument consisting of a light source providing a narrow beam of high intensity light and a microscope for better visualization of anterior segment of eye.

Slough A mass of necrotic tissue, to cast off a mass of necrotic tissue.

Slow reacting substance of anaphylaxis A chemical substance (leukotriene) produced by mast cell degranulation in allergic conditions. It causes smooth muscle contraction, e.g. bronchospasm.

Slow virus infection Virus infection manifesting after long latency period, e.g. kuru.

Sludge Any solid, semisolid or liquid waste arising from municipal, commercial or industrial waste water treatment; gallbladder sludge.

Slurry A thin watery mixture.

Smallpox Synonym variola, a viral exanthema with papulovesicular lesions on skin and constitutional symptoms.

Smegma The thick odorous secretion from Tyson's glands under prepuce and under labia minora.

Smellies forceps Obstetric forcep for delivery of aftercoming head in breech presentation.

Smellies scissors Special scissors with external cutting edges for fetal craniotomy.

Smelling salt A preparation containing ammonium carbonate and stronger ammonia water scented with aromatic substances.

Smelter's chills Zinc poisoning.

Smith-Hemli-Optiz syndrome Small stature, mental retardation, crypto-orchidism, and failure to thrive.

Smith-Hodge pessary A retroversion pessary.

Smith fracture Fracture of lower end of radius with forward displacement of lower segment.

Smith-Petersen nail A special nail that on cross-section has three flanges, used for stabilization of fracture neck of femur (*see* Figure on page 666).

Smog Dense fog combined with smoke.

Smokeless tobacco Tobacco used for chewing or as snuff. They irritate oral mucosa and increase the risk of oral cancer.

and opening of mouth due to displaced meniscus of temperomandibular joint.

Snapping knee An audible snapping sound on sudden extension of knee caused by slipping of biceps femoris tendon or displaced menisci.

Snare An instrument with a wire loop to remove polyps, tonsils and small growths with a pedicle.

Sneeze A sudden spasmodic expiration through nose.

Snellen chart A chart for testing visual acuity using letters that subtend an angle of 5° (*see* Figure on page 667).

Snore The noise produced while breathing through mouth during sleep.

Snout reflex A variant of sucking reflex in which sharp tapping of mid upper lip results in exaggerated contraction of the lips, positive in infants and in diffuse brain disease.

Snuff Powdered form of tobacco inhaled through nose.

Snuff box anatomical Triangular area at the base of thumb. Tenderness in this area indicates scaphoid fracture.

Soap A salt of one or more higher fatty acids with an alkali or metal. Soluble soaps are detergents and are

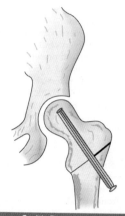

Smith-Petersen nail

Snake venom A secretion of posterior superior labial glands of poisonous snake containing neurotoxin, hemolysins, cytolysins and hemocoagulins.

Snap A sharp cracking sound. *s. opening* A high pitched sound heard during opening of diseased valves, e.g. mitral stenosis.

Snapping hip Presence of an abnormal tendinous band on gluteus maximus muscle which slips to produce a snap during certain hip movements.

Snapping jaw An audible and palpable snap on closing

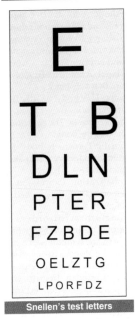

Snellen's test letters

prepared from alkali metals sodium and potassium.

Soap liniment A solution of soap and camphor in alcohol and water. Used as a stimulant and rubefacient.

Sociology Study of human social behaviour and the origin, institutions and functions of human groups and societies.

Sociopathy The condition of being antisocial.

Socket A hollow in a joint or bone. *s. alveolar* The bony space occupied by tooth and periodontal ligament.

Soda Salts of sodium. *s. baking* Sodium bicarbonate. *s. caustic* Sodium hydroxide. *s. lime* Mixture of calcium hydroxide and sodium hydroxide used to absorb carbon dioxide.

Soda ash Commercial sodium carbonate.

Soda water A solution of carbon dioxide under pressure.

Sodium Light, silvery white alkali metal which violently decomposes water forming sodium hydroxide and hydrogen. *s. acetate* Systemic and urinary alkalizer. *s. alginate* A food additive. *s. benzoate* A food preservative. *s. bicarbonate* Used IV to treat acidosis. *s. carbonate* Washing soda. *s. chloride* Table salt; 0.9% solution is osmotically compatible with blood. *s. lactate* In one sixth or one fourth molar solution used IV to correct acidosis. *s. monofluorophosphate* For topical application on teeth to prevent caries. *s. morrhuate* A sclerosing agent used to obliterate varices. *s. nitrite* Antidote for cyanide poisoning. *s. nitroprusside* A powerful vasodilator. *s. polystyrene sulphonate* Cation exchange resin used to lower body potassium. *s. propionate* Possesses antifungal action. *s. salicylate* Analgesic and antipyretic. *s. thiosulphate* Antidote for cyanide poisoning.

Sodium chromoglycate Mast cell stabilizer used in asthma as acrosol.

Soft palate The posterior portion of roof of mouth.

Soft sore Venereal ulcer caused by Ducrey's bacillus.

Soleus The flat broad muscle at back of calf of leg.

Solitary Single or lonely.

Solubility Capable of being dissolved.

Solute The substance that is dissolved in a solution.

Solution A homogeneous mixture of solid, liquid or gaseous substance in a liquid from which the dissolved substance can be recovered by crystallization or other physical process.

Solution aqueous Solution containing water as the solvent. *s. buffer* Solution of weak acid and its salt solvent for maintaining constant pH. *s. hypertonic* Solution with greater osmotic pressure than that of bodyfluids. *s. hypotonic* Solution with osmotic pressure less than that of body fluids. *s. isotonic* Solution with similar osmotic pressure as that of body fluids. *s. Ringer's* Solution containing chlorides of sodium, calcium and potassium.

Solvent A liquid that dissolves another substance.

Soma The body as distinct from mind.

Somatesthesia The consciousness of the body.

Somatic Pertains to body, the nonreproductive cells, skeletal muscles.

Somatization Expression of emotional conflicts as bodily ailment.

Somatoform disorders A group of disorders in which there are symptoms of a disease but no objective evidence to explain the symptoms.

Somatomedin Insulin like growth factors derived from liver (Somatomedin C and A) that stimulate growth under influence of growth hormone.

Somatostatin A hypothalamic hormone that inhibits release of somatotropin, insulin, and gastrin.

Somatotropin Growth hormone.

Somite Paired masses of mesoderm arranged segmentotally alongside neural tube of the embryo (*see* Figure on page 669).

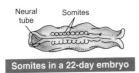

Somites in a 22-day embryo

Somnambulism Sleep walking, the performance of any fairly complex act while in a sleep like state or trance.

Somniferous Promoting sleep.

Somniloquism Talking during sleep.

Somnolence Sleepiness.

Somogyi phenomenon In diabetes mellitus, rebound hyperglycemia following an attack of hypoglycemia that triggers release of counter regulatory hormones. Reduction in dose of insulin helps to control the hyperglycemia by abolishing hypoglycemia.

Sonogram Ultrasonography record.

Sonolucent Condition of not reflecting the ultrasound wave back to the source.

Sonorous rale Low pitched rale caused by mucous secretion in bronchus.

Soporific A drug producing sleep, narcotic.

Sorbitol A crystalline alcohol used as sweetening agent.

Sordes Foul brown crusts about the lips in some fever.

Sore Painful lesion of skin or mucous membrane.

Sotalol Beta-adrenergic blocking agent used as antihypertensive agent, antiarrhythmic too.

Souffle A bruit, soft blowing sound. *s. uterine* Blood flow within uterine arteries producing the sound.

Sound Auditory sensation produced by vibrations, noise, measured in decibels. *s. heart* The first heart sound indicates mitral and tricuspid valve closure and the second heart sound indicates closure of aortic and pulmonary valves, third heart sound occurs during rapid ventricular filling and fourth heart sound occurs with atrial contraction. *s. Korotkoff's* Sounds heard over an artery during blood pressure measurement. *s. succussion* Splashing sound heard over a cavity filled with fluid. *s. tubular* Breath sound heard over trachea and large bronchi. *s. urethral* a long slim slightly conical instrument for exploring and dilating urethra. *s. uterine* like urethral sound for knowing uterine length.

Souque's phenomenon A phenomenon seen in incomplete hemiplegia, consisting of involuntary extension and separation of the fingers when the arm is raised.

Southey's tube Fine caliber tubes used to drain fluid from the subcutaneous tissue in the condition of edema or anasarca (*see* Figure).

Space dead In respiratory physiology, the area from nose to bronchioles which do not take part in exchange of oxygen and carbondioxide.

Space medicine Branch of medicine dealing with pathological and physiological problems encountered by humans in the space.

Sparfloxacin Quinolone, used for enteric fever.

Spargosis 1. Swelling of skin as in elephantiasis. 2. Distention of lactating breast with milk.

Spasm Sudden involuntary muscle contraction, can be clonic (alternate contraction and relaxation) or tonic (sustained contraction).

Spasmophilia A tendency towards spasm and convulsion as in rickets.

Spastic colon A motility disorder of colon with lower abdominal pain and alternating constipation and diarrhea.

Spasticity Increased muscle tone with muscular stiffness as in upper motor neurone lesions.

Spatial Pertaining to space.

Spatula Flat instrument for mixing or spreading semi-solids.

Specific gravity Weight of a substance compared with equal volume of water. Specific gravity of water is taken as 1000.

Spectinomycin Injectable antibiotic used for gonorrhea.

Spectrometer An instrument to measure wavelength based on the principle of prism or diffraction grating.

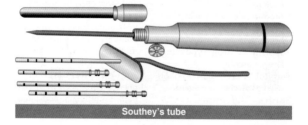

Southey's tube

Spectrophotometry Estimation of depth of colour by using spectrophotometer.

Spectroscope An instrument for separating radiant energy into its component frequencies or wavelengths.

Spectrum The series of components or images obtained when a beam of electromagnetic wave is dispersed and the constituent waves are arranged according to their frequencies or wavelengths. *s. invisible* Spectral portion below the red (infrared) or above violet (ultraviolet) which is invisible to the eyes lying below 3900 angstrom units and above 7700 angstrom units. *s. visible* Colors from red to violet with wavelengths of 3900-7700 AU.

Speculum Instrument for examination of canals, e.g. ear speculum, vaginal speculum (*see* Figure).

Speech Expression of thoughts by spoken words or sound symbols. *s. ataxic* Defective speech due to muscular incoordination as in cerebellar ataxia. *s. scanning* Speech with pauses in between syllables. *s. staccato* Slow and labored speech with each syllable being pronounced separately.

Spermatic cord The cord suspending the testis and is composed of vas deferens, spermatic arteries, veins and lymphatics.

Spermatic vein The vein draining the testis. The left vein drains into left renal vein while the right vein empties into inferior vena cava.

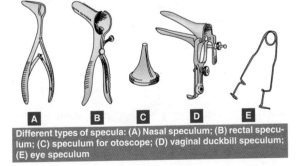

Different types of specula: (A) Nasal speculum; (B) rectal speculum; (C) speculum for otoscope; (D) vaginal duckbill speculum; (E) eye speculum

Spermatid A precursor cell of spermatozoon derived from secondary spermatocyte.

Spermatin A mucilaginous substance present in semen.

Spermatocele A cystic tumor of epididymis.

Spermatocyte The cell arising from spermatogonium that forms the spermatids.

Spermatogenesis The process of formation of mature spermatozoa, i.e. spearmatogonium-primary spermatocyte-secondary spermatocyte-spermatid-motile functional spermatozoa.

Spermatorrhea Involuntary loss of semen without orgasm.

Spermatozoon The mature male germ cell formed within the seminiferous tubules of testis, freely mobile resembling a tadpole (*see* **Figure**).

Spermaturia Semen passed with urine.

Spermicide Agent that kills spermatozoa.

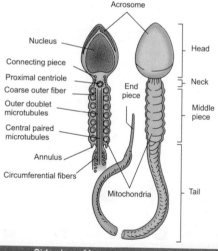

Side view of human spermatozoon:
(in cross-section) and flat view

Sphenoid Wedge-shaped.

Sphenoid bone Large bone placed at base of skull between the parietal and temporal bones laterally, occipital bone behind and ethmoid in front.

Sphenoiditis Inflammation of sphenoidal sinus cells.

Sphenoid spine Downward projection from the posterior extremity of greater wing of sphenoid, giving attachment to sphenomandibular ligament.

Sphenosis Condition in which fetus becomes wedged in the pelvis.

Sphere Globe like structure.

Spherocyte Erythrocyte assuming globular shape.

Spherocytosis A form of congenital hemolytic anemia characterized by hemolysis, anemia, splenomegaly and jaundice with increased red cell fragility.

Spherule A very small sphere; the structure present in tissues infected with *Coccidiodes imitis*, each spherule containing hundreds of endospores.

Sphincter Circular muscle fibers that close an orifice when contracted, e.g. anal sphincter, lower esophageal sphincter, pyloric sphincter and sphincter of Oddi.

Sphingolipid Lipid containing sphingosine bases.

Sphingolipidosis Hereditary disease with defective metabolism of sphingolipids. Included in this group are Tay-Sach's disease, Fabry's disease, Kufs' disease, Krabbe's disease and Niemann-Pick disease.

Sphingomyelins Phosphorus containing sphingolipids principally found in nervous tissue. They are derived from choline phosphate and a ceramide.

Sphygmo Pulse.

Sphygmograph Instrument for recording shape and force of pulse wave.

Sphygmomanometer Instrument for indirect measurement of arterial blood pressure, can be aneroid or mercurial.

Spica A reverse spiral bandage, the turn of which crosses like letter V.

Spicule Small needle shaped.

Spider black widow Black female spider with four pairs of legs and poison fangs. Its bite causes excruciating abdominal pain and ascending motor palsy.

Spider finger Abnormally long phallanges of hand.

Spider nevus Branched capillary growth in the skin

resembling a spider as in cirrhosis of liver.

Spigelian line The line in abdomen, that marks lateral border of rectus.

Spike The main peak, or a rapid sharp wave appearing suddenly in the background slow wave rhythm.

Spill Overflow.

Spillway The contour of teeth allowing food to escape from the cusps during mastication.

Spina The spine. *s. bifida* Congenital nonunion between the laminae of vertebra (*see* Figure).

Spinal anesthesia Anesthesia produced by injection of anesthetic agents into spinal canal.

Spinal canal The canal bounded by vertebral body and vertebral arches that contains the spinal cord.

Spinal column The vertebral column consisting of 33 vertebra: 7 cervical, 12 thoracic, 5 lumbar, 5 sacral and 4 in the coccyx.

Spinal cord The nervous tissue contained in spinal canal extending from medulla to lower border of first lumbar vertebra. The gray matter within spinal cord is in the form of H.

Spinal curvature Curvature of spine which is often

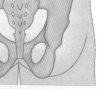
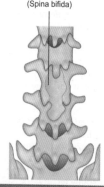

Vertebrae

Opening (Spina bifida)

Spina bifida

physiological like cervical and lumbar lordosis and thoracic kyphosis.

Spinal fluid Cerebrospinal fluid lying in the central canal and around the spinal cord within the subarachnoid space.

Spinal nerves 31 pairs of nerves arising from spinal cord; 8 cervical, 12 thoracic, 5 lumbar 5 sacral and coccygeal. Each nerve has a ventral efferent motor root and an afferent dorsal sensory root. Each nerve has white and gray rami communicant which pass to the ganglia of sympathetic trunk.

Spinal shock Complete arcflexic flaccid palsy following complete transection of spinal cord.

Spinal stenosis Narrowing of spinal canal due to trauma or degeneration of vertebral column.

Spindle A fusiform shaped body.

Spine A sharp process from a bone.

Spiral Coiling around a center like the thread of screw.

Spiramycin Antibiotic used in toxoplasmosis, respiratory infections.

Spirillum minus A flagellated aerobic bacteria in blood of rats causing rat bite fever.

Spirochaeta A genus of slender spiral motile microorganism causing diseases like syphilis, pinta, yaws.

Spirogram A record made by a spirograph depicting respiratory movements.

Spirograph Graphic record of respiratory movements.

Spirometer An apparatus for measuring the air capacity of the lungs.

Spironolactone Aldosterone antagonist that excretes sodium but conserves potassium, useful in cirrhotics.

Spissated Thickened.

Spit To expectorate.

Splanchnic Pertains to viscera.

Spleen A lymphoid vascular organ in left hypocondrium at the tail of pancreas, consisting of red and white pulp, functions as erythropoietic organ in embryo, and filtrates bacteria, senescent red blood cells, inclusion bodies from the blood (*see* **Figure** on page 676).

Splenectomy Surgical removal of spleen.

Splenic flexure Junction of transverse colon with descending colon.

Splenitis Inflammation of the spleen, acute or chronic, hypertrophic or suppurative.

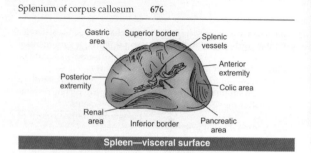

Labels: Gastric area, Superior border, Splenic vessels, Anterior extremity, Colic area, Posterior extremity, Renal area, Inferior border, Pancreatic area

Spleen—visceral surface

Splenium of corpus callosum
The thickened posterior end of corpus callosum.

Splenius A flat muscle in upper back on either side.

Splenoportogram Radiographic picture of spleen and portal vein after injection of radioopaque material into spleen.

Splenorenal shunt Anastomosis of splenic vein to renal vein as in portal hypertension.

Splenorrhagia Bleeding from ruptured spleen.

Splenorrhaphy Suturing of any splenic wound.

Splint An appliance used for protection, fixation or union of injured part, can be movable or immovable. *s. Thomas* A long wire splint with a proximal ring that fits into upper thigh, used for fracture femur (*see* Figure).

Splinter hemorrhage Small linear bleeding under the

nail as in subacute bacterial endocarditis.

Splinting Fixation of injured part with a splint.

Split Division or fissure.

Split tongue Bifid tongue.

SPO2 Saturation of arterial blood with oxygen.

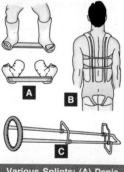

Various Splints: (A) Denis Browne splint; (B) Taylor splint; (C) Thomas knee splint

Spondylos Vertebra.

Spondylitis Inflammation of vertebra.

Spondylolisthesis Forward subluxation of lower lumbar vertebra on sacral vertebra.

Spondylosis Degenerative disease of vertebra and the intervertebral disk with new bone formation at vertebral margins and facet joint arthropathy.

Spondylotherapy Spinal manipulation in treatment of disease.

Sponge An absorbent pad made-up of cotton and gauze to absorb fluids and blood, used in wound dressing. *s. gelatin* Spongy substance of gelatin used to stop internal bleeding.

Spongiform Having appearance or quality of a sponge.

Spongioblast The precursor cell of astrocytes and ependymal cells that develop from neural tube.

Spongioblastoma A glioma arising from spongioblasts.

Spontaneous fracture Fracture of a osteoporotic bone.

Spoon nail Concave nail of iron deficiency anemia.

Sporadic Occurring occasionally.

Spore An asexual reproductive unit of plants, some protozoa and bacteria.

Sporocyst A reproductive cell containing spores.

Sporogony Reproduction by development of spores.

Sporothrix A genus of fungi.

Sporotrichosis A chronic granulomatous fungal infection involving skin and lymphnodes with abscess formation, nodularity and ulceration.

Sporozoa A subdivision of protozoa that includes plasmodia, toxoplasma and isospora.

Sporozoite Infective form of malarial parasite injected by mosquito bite.

Sports medicine Application of medical knowledge for treatment and prevention of sports injuries and improvement of training methods.

Sporulation Production of spores.

Spot A small area distinguishable from surrounding area. *s. blind* The optic disk containing opaque optic nerve fibers. *s. cherry-red* Red spot in retina in Tay-Sach's disease. *s. Koplik* Bluish white spots on oral mucous membrane before appearance of rash of measles. *s. Mongolian* Blue or mulbery coloured spots in sacral region present at birth that disappear later.

Spotted fever Name for eruptive fevers like typhus, and other rickettsial fevers.

Spotting Appearance of blood tinged discharge from vagina in between periods or at onset of labor.

Sprain Trauma to the ligamentous capsular support of a joint with tearing of fibers and haemorrhage.

Sprain fracture Separation of a tendon or ligament from its bony insertion site taking along with it a piece of bone.

Spray A jet of fine medicated vapor.

Spring ligament Calcaneoscaphoid ligament in the sole of foot.

Sprue Intestinal malabsorption disorder often due to dietary factors, folic acid deficiency producing bulky, frothy, offensive stool.

Spur A sharp bony outgrowth. *s. calcaneal* An exostosis from calcaneus.

Spurious False, adulterated.

Spurling's maneuver Manuever used to assess the nerve root pain by putting axial load on head with neck extension and lateral rotation towards each shoulder (*see* Figure).

Sputum Material expelled by coughing containing bronchial secretions, alveolar collections. *s. numular* Round coin shaped flat forms of sputum sinking in water as seen in bronchiectasis.

Squalene An unsaturated carbohydrate present in vegetable oils, precursor of cholesterol.

Squamous Scale like.

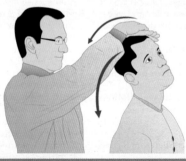

Spurling's maneuver

Squamous bone Upper anterior portion of temporal bone.

Squamous cell Flat scaly epithelial cell.

Square knot Double knot in which ends and standing parts are together and parallel to each other.

Squatting Sitting on ones haunches and heels.

Squint An abnormality where visual axes do not converge on a single point.

Stab Piercing with a sharp pointed instrument.

Staccato speech Jerky pronunciation with separation of each syllable and word by pauses.

Stachyose A nonabsorbable carbohydrate present in beans; hence causing flatulence.

Staging The process of classifying tumors with respect to their degree of differentiation, response to therapy and prognosis.

Stain A dye used to colour objects for microscopic examination. *s. acid-fast* Staining for mycobacteria which retain carbolfuschin even when washed with acid-alcohol. *s. dental* Staining of enamel or denture due to tea, coffee or tobacco or inhalation of metals like copper (green) manganese (black), iron (brown).

Stalk An elongated structure that attaches or supports an organ. *s. infundibular* Stalk connecting diencephalon with pituitary.

Stamina Strength, endurance.

Stammering Speech disorder with hesitation, mispronunciation, made worse by anxiety and fear.

Standard deviation In statistics, it is the square root of variance.

Standard error A measure of variability; the difference between means of two samples.

Standstill Cessation of activity.

Stannous fluoride A fluoride compound in toothpaste that prevents dental caries.

Stanolone Anabolic steroid.

Stanozolol Anabolic steroid, used for muscle building.

Stapedectomy Excision of stapes as in otosclerosis.

Stapedius A small muscle in the middle ear attached to stapes.

Stapes Ossicle in middle ear whose foot plate fits into oval window.

Staphyle Uvula, the fleshy mass hanging from soft palate.

Staphylococcus Gram-positive cocci appearing as bunch of grapes. Cause boils, carbuncles, internal abscess, food poisoning, toxic shock syndrome and scalded skin syndrome (*see* Figure).

Staphyloderma Cutaneous infection with staphylococci.

Staphyloma Protrusion of sclera or cornea.

Staphylopharyngeus Muscle of soft palate whose contraction narrows the fauces and occludes the nasopharynx.

Staphylotoxin Toxins produced by staphylococci, e.g. the enterotoxin, hemotoxin, dermonecrotic toxin, etc.

Staple food Any principal food item of a community supplying more than 25% of calorie and eaten regularly.

Stapling Fastening of incised wounds by metal staples.

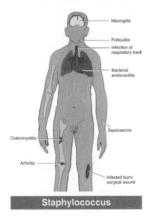

Meningitis
Folliculitis
Infection of respiratory tract
Bacterial endocarditis
Septicaemia
Osteomyelitis
Arthritis
Infected burn/surgical wound

Staphylococcus

Starch A plant polysaccharide of high molecular weight which on absorption is reduced to simple sugars to provide energy. Starch is converted to sugar when some fruits ripen while peas and corn change sugar into starch as their seeds develop.

Stare Fixed gaze at any object.

Starling's law Starling law of heart depicts that the force of contraction of heart muscle is directly related to length of muscle fiber at beginning of contraction.

Starvation Food deprivation.

Stasis Stagnation in the flow.

State A condition.

Static electricity Electricity produced by friction.

Stationary Fixed.

Statistics The systematic collection, organization and analysis of data and their interpretation.

Statoconia Minute beats of calcium adhering to the hair cells of macule and utricle responsible for maintenance of posture. *SYN*—statolith.

Stature Height of body in standing position.

Status A state or condition. *s. asthmaticus* Persistent and intractable asthma. *SYN* – acute severe asthma. *s. epilepticus* Recurrent convulsive episodes without regain of consciousness in between.

Steapsin *SYN* – Lipase, the pancreatic lipolytic enzyme.

Stearate Salt of stearic acid.

Stearic acid A fatty acid mainly found in animal fats.

Stearin Ester of stearic acid and glycerine.

Steatorrhea Fatty diarrhea of pancreatic enzyme deficiency; increased secretion of sebaceous glands.

Stein-Leventhal syndrome Polycystic ovary syndrome with amenorrhea and infertility.

Steinmann's extension Traction applied to a limb by applying weight to a pin placed through the bone at right angles to the direction of pull of the traction force.

Steinmann's pin A metal pin inserted into bone for application of traction.

Stellate Star shaped. *s. fracture* Fracture with radiating fracture lines from center of trauma. *s. ganglion* A sympathetic ganglion formed by fusion of inferior cervical and first thoracic ganglions.

Stellwag's sign Widening of palpebral fissure with infrequent blinking, a feature of Grave's disease.

Stem Stalk like structure.

Stem cell The cell which is initial precursor of specific differentiated red blood cells.

Stenosis Constriction or narrowing.

Stensen's duct Parotid duct.

Stent Any material used to hold tissue in place, provide support for graft, to keep a passage open, e.g. prostatic stent, esophageal stent and coronary stents (*see* Figure on page 682).

Stercobilin A brown pigment derived from bile that imparts the color to feces.

Stercolith A fecal concretion.

Stercus Feces.

Stereognosis Ability to recognize objects by touch.

Stereoisomerism Compounds having same number of atoms but in differing arrangement, e.g. dextrose and levulose.

Stereophotography Photography that gives depth, i.e. three dimensional picture.

Stereoscope Instrument that gives three dimensional view of objects seen by combining images of two pictures.

Stereotaxis A method of precisely locating areas of brain concerned with a particular function by moving a probe or electrode along coordinates

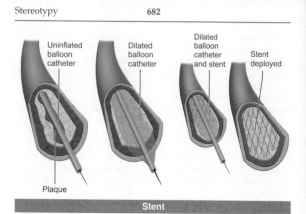

Uninflated balloon catheter | Dilated balloon catheter | Dilated balloon catheter and stent | Stent deployed

Plaque

Stent

for measured distances from certain external landmarks.

Stereotypy Persistent repetition of words, posture or activity.

Sterile Free from living microorganism; unable to procreate.

Sterility The state of being free from living microorganisms; state of being sterile.

Sterilization The process of destroying all microorganisms either by heat, chemical or ionizing radiation.

Sterilizer Appliance used for achieving sterilization.

Sternal puncture Removal of bone marrow for examination by pressing wide bore needle into sternum.

Sternoclavicular Relating to sternum and clavicle.

Sternocleidomastoid Muscle arising from sternum and clavicle, attached to the mastoid, helps in rotation of the head.

Sternohyoid Muscle attached to medial end of clavicle and sternum and the hyoid bone.

Sternum The narrow fat bone in the midline of thorax in front.

Steroid Any organic compound containing cyclopentano-perhydrinophenanthrine ring.

Steroidogenesis Production of steroid hormones.

Sterols Group of substances related to fats. They are alcohols with CPPP nucleus.

Stertorous Snoring sound.

Stertorous respiration Respiration characterized by a heavy snoring or gasping sound.

Stethoscope Instrument used to appreciate internal body sounds, i.e. respiratory, cardiovascular and intestinal (*see* Figure).

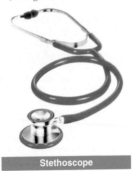

Stethoscope

Stevens-Johnson syndrome Erythema multiforme.

Stibium Antimony.

Stibophen Trivalent antimony compound used in treatment of schistosomiasis.

Stiff man syndrome A disease of unknown etiology manifesting with muscle stiffness that limits voluntary movements.

Stigma Any mark, spot on the skin, the spot on ovarian surface where graffian follicle ruptures.

Stillbirth Birth of dead fetus.

Still's disease Juvenile rheumatoid arthritis with prominent visceral involvement.

Stimulant Agent that increases functional activity.

Stimulus Any agent or factor that brings changes in living tissue, e.g. muscular contraction, secretion from gland, initiating an impulse.

Sting Punctured wound made by an insect.

S-T interval Time between completion of QRS complex and beginning of T-wave and represents the initial slow phase of ventricular repolarization.

Stippling Spotted appearance.

Stitch To unite skin or flesh; suture material; sharp spasmodic pain.

Stockinet Tubular woven elastic material to place uniform pressure around a body part.

Stock The original individual or tribe from which others have descended.

Stoke A unit of viscosity.

Stokes-Adam's syndrome Feeling of light headedness and becoming unconscious due to poor blood supply to brain as in complete heart block.

Stokes' law Paralysis of a muscle lying adjacent to inflamed serous or mucous membrane.

Stoma A mouth or opening.

Stomach The most dilated saclike portion of alimentary tract in between esophagus and duodenum, secretes hydrochloric acid and pepsinogen, destroys the microorganisms and subserves as a reservoir.

Stomachic Medicine that stimulates actions of stomach.

Stomatitis Inflammation of mouth. *s. aphthous* Development of minute tiny painful ulcers on mucosa of mouth and tongue.

Strabismus An abnormality of the eyes in which optic axes do not meet at the desired point due to incoordinate action of extraocular muscles.

Strabometer Instrument for measuring degree of strabismus.

Strachan syndrome Neuropathy and orogenital lesions in avitaminosis.

Strain Excessive use of a muscle or joint; to pass through a filter, to make great effort as in affecting bowel movement; a stock of bacteria.

Strait A narrow passage.

Strangle To choke or suffocate.

Strangury Painful and interrupted urination.

Strap A band to hold parts together.

Stratum A layer.

Strawberry tongue Red papillated tongue.

Streak A line or stripe.

Streptobacillus Bacilli found in chains.

Streptococcus Gram-positive cocci occurring in chains differentiated into alpha, beta and gamma types based on their reaction on agar plates. Those of alpha type (*St. viridans*) produce a greenish coloration about colonies and partially hemolyze the blood; those of beta type (*St. pyogenes*) form a clear zone about colonies and completely hemolyze the blood, gamma type (*St. faecalis*) are nonhemolytic and produce grayish discoloration about the colonies. *St. pneumoniae* Gram-positive spherical capsulated cocci causing lobar pneumonia, otitis media. *St. pyogenes* Hemolytic streptococci producing rheumatic fever, scarlet fever, puerperal sepsis. *St. viridans* Organism producing endocarditis (*see* Figure on page 685).

Streptodornase Enzyme secreted by hemolytic streptococci which along with streptokinase is used for enzymatic debridement of infected tissue.

Streptokinase Catalytic enzyme produced by hemolytic streptococci. It activates blood fibrinolytic

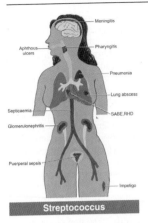

Streptococcus

system, used for dissolution of coronary thrombus.

Streptolysin Hemolysin (O and S) produced by *Streptococcus pyogens*.

Streptomyces A genus of aerobic nonacid-fast nonfragmenting organisms with branching filaments occupying a position between bacteria and fungi. They serve as source of antibiotics.

Streptomycin Aminoglycoside antibiotic from *Streptomyces griseus* used for pulmonary tuberculosis and gram-positive cocci.

Streptozocin Antineoplastic drug, used in pancreatic cancer.

Stress Any stimulus that tends to disrupt body homeostasis to cause disease/disability.

Stress fracture Hairline fracture often only visible 3-4 weeks after undue muscle stress as in runners.

Stress test Method of evaluating cardiovascular fitness by exercise on treadmill or bicycle ergometer or after drugs (dipyridamole, dobutamine).

Stress ulcer Peptic ulcer caused by excessive stress as in burn, head trauma.

Stretch To lengthen.

Stretcher A litter or carriage for patients.

Stretch receptor Proprioceptors in muscle or tendon that are stimulated by stretch or pull.

Stretch reflex Contraction of a muscle as a result of pull exerted on its tendon.

Stria A line or band differing in color and texture from surrounding tissue.

Striatal epilepsy A form of epilepsy characterized by tonic seizure of arm and leg due to disease of corpus striatum.

Striated muscles Skeletal muscles consisting of fibers marked by cross striations.

Striatum The caudate and lentiform nuclei of brain taken together.

Stricture Narrowing or constriction.

Stridor High pitched respiratory sound resembling blowing wind due to obstruction in air passage.

Strio nigral Tract arising from putamen and caudate nucleus and ending in substantia nigra.

Stroboscope A device by which moving object may appear to be at rest; a rapid motion may appear to be slowed.

Stroke 1. A sharp blow. 2. Sudden neurological deficit with or without unconsciousness due to cerebral thrombosis, hemorrhage or embolism.

Stroke volume Amount of blood ejected from ventricle during systole.

Stroma Supporting framework of an organ including its connective tissue, vessels and nerves.

Stromatosis Presence of mesenchyma like tissue throughout the endometrium of uterus.

Strongyloides stercoralis A round worm that inhabits human intestine and its motile larvae are passed in stool.

Strontium Radioactive isotope fall out from atomic explosions, principally stored in bone.

Struma Enlarged thyroid gland. *s. ovarii* Form of ovarian teratoma composed of thyroid follicles filled with colloid.

Strumpell's sign Dorsiflexion of foot when thigh is flexed on abdomen.

Struvite Crystals of magnesium ammonium phosphate.

Strychnine A poisonous alkaloid from plant nux vomica, a potent CNS stimulant.

Stryker frame A frame for holding the patient in position and rotating to various planes without the motion of individual parts.

Stuart-Prower factor Factor x of blood coagulation. *SYN*—thrombokinase.

Stupe Counter irritant for topical use.

Stupor A state of lessened responsiveness.

Sturge-Weber syndrome A form of neurocutaneous dysplasia with facial naevus, intracranial rail-road calcification, angiomas of leptomeninges and choroid, epileptic seizures, and mental retardation.

Stuttering Speech defect with stumbling and spasmodic repetition of same syllable.

Stye Inflammation of glands of Zeis and Moll at the edge of the lid. Internal stye involve meiobomian or tarsal glands.

Stylet A thin probe.

Styloglossus Muscle connecting tongue and styloid process that helps to retract and raise the tongue.

Styloid process Pointed process of temporal bone, distal end of radius.

Stylopharyngeus Muscle that elevates and opens up the pharynx.

Stylus A probe or slender wire for stiffening or clearing a canal or catheter.

Styptic Anything that stops bleeding by contracting blood vessels or by astringent action.

Sub Under, beneath, less in quantity.

Subacute myelo-optic neuropathy Neurological disease characterized by sensory motor disturbances, impaired vision, abdominal pain and ataxia occurring as a toxicity of chinoquinol (iodochlorhydroxyquin).

Subacute sclerosing panencephalitis A cerebral degenerative disease with decreasing mental function, and myoclonic jerks and rigidity. Probably related to chronic measle virus infection of CNS.

Subarachnoid hemorrhage Bleeding into the sub-arachnoid space (the area between the arachnoid membrane and pia mater surrounding the brain).

Subclavian artery Left subclavian is a direct branch of aortic arch while right subclavian is a branch of innominate artery; gives rise to vertebral arteries and terminates as brachial vessels supplying the arm.

Subclavian steal syndrome Shunting of blood away from cerebral circulation via vertebral artery to subclavian when subclavian is occluded at its origin. Exercise of involved arm then produces dizziness due to cerebral anoxia.

Subclavian triangle Triangle shaped part of neck formed by clavicle and the omohyoid and sternomastoid muscles.

Subclavius A tiny muscle from first rib to under surface of clavicle.

Subclinical Pertains to period before the appearance of typical symptoms.

Subcutaneous Beneath the skin.

Subdural space Space between dura and arachnoid.

Suberosis Hypersensitive pneumonitis in workers exposed to cork.

Subfamily In taxonomy between family and a tribe.

Subjective Concerned with the individual or perceived by individual himself but not by examiner.

Sublimate A solid or condensed substance obtained by heating a solid material which passes to vapor phase and then back to solid phase.

Sublingual gland Salivary gland situated at the floor of mouth.

Subluxation A partial or incomplete dislocation.

Submandibular gland Salivary gland about the size of wallnut that lies in digastric triangle beneath the mandible. Its main duct (Wharton's duct) opens by side of frenulum linguae.

Submerge To dip in water.

Submucosa Connective tissue layer below the mucosa containing vessels and nerves.

Submucous resection Resection of cartilaginous tissue below the mucosa for correction of deviated nasal septum.

Subphrenic Below the diaphragm.

Subscription That part of prescription containing directions for compounding ingradients.

Subsidence Gradual disappearance of symptoms of disease.

Subsistence Minimum or barely needed essentials for life.

Substance P A 11 amino acid peptide acting as neurotransmitter in pain fiber system.

Substitute Something used in place of another.

Subthalamic nucleus An elliptical mass of gray matter lying in ventral thalamus above the cerebral peduncle and rostral to substantia nigra.

Subtle Very fine or delicate; causing injury without attracting attention.

Subtraction A method of removing overlying shadows in radiography.

Succedaneum Something which can be used as a substitute.

Succenturiate Acting as a substitute.

Succinylcholine A neuromuscular blocking agent used as muscle relaxant during anesthesia.

Succus A juice or fluid secretion.

Succussion Shaking up a person to detect fluid in body cavity from presence of splashing sound.

Suck To draw fluid into mouth.

Suckle Breastfeed.

Sucralfate Drug used in peptic ulcer.

Sucrase Enzyme present in intestinal juice which splits cane sugar into glucose and fructose.

Sucrose A disaccharose which is broken down into glucose and fructose.

Suction The act of sucking, e.g. suction abortion, suction biopsy.

Sudan Biological stain for fat.

Sudanophilic Staining easily with sudan stain.

Sudeck's atrophy Acute atrophy of bone at the site of injury.

Sufentanil An opioid analgesic.

Suffocation Feeling choked.

Suffusion Spreading or extravassation of body fluid or blood; pouring of water on body as a treatment method.

Sugar Sweet tasting carbohydrate either monosaccharose or disaccharose.

Suggestion Imparting an idea indirectly or the psychological process of having an individual accept an idea without hesitation.

Suicide Voluntarily bringing an end to one's own life.

Suit An outer garment.

Sulbactam Beta lactamase inhibitor.

Sulbutiamine Rejuvenant agent.

Sulcus A furrow, groove, depression (*see* Figure).

Sulfacetamide A sulfonamide for ophthalmic use particularly in trachoma.

Sulfadiazine An absorbable sulfa which penetrates well

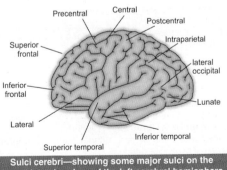

Sulci cerebri—showing some major sulci on the superolateral surface of the left cerebral hemisphere

into brain, hence was previously used in meningococcal meningitis, now chiefly used in rheumatic fever prophylaxis.

Sulfadoxine Sulfa used in malaria.

Sulfamerazine A derivative of sulfadiazine.

Sulfamethizole Sulfa for urinary tract infection.

Sulfamethoxazole Sulfa usually combined with trimethoprim for broad spectrum action and complimentary bactericidal effect.

Sulfanilamide A formerly used coaltar product for infections.

Sulfapyridine Sulfonamide used in the treatment of dermatitis herpetiformis.

Sulfasalazine Poorly absorbable sulfa used in treatment of ulcerative colitis.

Sulfatase An enzyme that hydrolyzes sulfuric acid esters.

Sulfathiazole A rapidly absorbable sulfa.

Sulfatide Any cerebroside with a sulfate radical esterified to galactose.

Sulfhemoglobin A form of greenish hemoglobin formed by action of hydrogen sulfide on blood, causes cyanosis if in excess.

Sulfinpyrazone Antigout agent.

Sulfisoxazole Sulfa used in urinary tract infection.

Sulfonamide Amides of sulfanilic acid, derived from their parent compound sulfanilamide. They are bacteriostatic.

Sulphonyl urea Group of drugs for NIDDM (*see* table).

Sulfoxone sodium A drug for treatment of leprosy and dermatitis herpetiformis.

Sulfur Yellow inflammable element. *s. dioxide* A bactericide and disinfectant. *s. precipitated* A keratolytic agent. *s. sublimed* A scabicide and keratolytic agent.

Sulfuric acid 10% solution used as an astringent and for gastric hypoacidity.

Sulindac Nonsteroidal antiinflammatory drug.

Sulphonyl ureas for NIDDM	
	Daily dose
Tolbutamide	0.5-2 g
Tolazamide	0.1-1 g
Acetohexamide	0.25-1.5 g
Chlorpropamide	0.1-0.5 g
Glyburide	1.25-20 mg
Glipizide	2.5-40 mg
Glimeperide	1-4 mg
Glicazide	80-320 mg

Sulpiride Agent used in peptic ulcer.

Summation Cummulative action or stimuli.

Sunburn Solar keratitis due to ultraviolet (290-320 nm).

Sunscreen Agents like PABA used for protection against solar dermatitis.

Sunscreen protective factor index The ratio of the amount of exposure needed to produce minimal erythema response with the sunscreen in place divided by amount of exposure required to produce the same reaction without the sunscreen.

Sunstroke Hyperpyrexia with cessation of sweating, headache and stupor due to failure of heat regulating mechanism.

Super ego The portion of personality associated with ethics, self-criticism, and moral standards of community, usually developed in childhood.

Superfecundation The fertilization of two or more ova ovulated more or less simultaneously by two or more coital acts, not necessarily involving the same male.

Superfetation Fertilization of two ova in the same uterus at different menstrual periods within a short interval.

Superinfection A new infection caused by a different organism from that which caused initial infection.

Superior Situated above or higher.

Supernatant The clear liquid remaining at top as the heavy particles settle down below.

Supernumerary In excess of regular number, e.g. supernumerary teeth and supernumerary breast.

Superoxide A highly reactive form of oxygen (oxygen with single electron) produced during phagocytosis and bacterial digestion by neutrophils, lipid metabolism.

Superoxide dismutage Enzyme that destroys superoxide, being tried in myocardial infarction.

Superscription The beginning of prescription marked by letter Rx meaning "you take".

Superstructure Any visible part external to the main structure.

Supination Turning the palm or foot upward, lying on the back.

Supinator Muscle causing supination of forearm.

Suppository A substance in the form of semisolid introduced into the vagina or rectum serving as vehicle for medicine (*see* Figure on page 692).

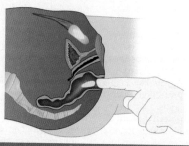

Suppository

Suppurate To form or generate pus.

Suppuration The process of pus formation.

Supra Meaning above, beyond.

Supraclavicular fossa Depression on either side of neck above the clavicle.

Suprahyoid muscles The digastric, geniohyoid, myohyoid and stylohyoid muscles.

Suprapubic cystostomy Surgical opening of urinary bladder from an approach above the symphysis pubis.

Suprarenal Gland lying superior and medial to kidney secreting adrenaline and nor adrenaline.

Sura Calf or calf muscles.

Suramin A urea derivative used in treatment of trypanosomiasis.

Surfactant An agent that lowers surface tension.

Surgery Branch of medical science dealing with operative procedures for diagnosis or treatment of diseases, and deformities.

Surgical dressing Sterile gauze or other material for wound dressing.

Surgical neck Constricted part of shaft of humerus below the tuberosities, the common site for fracture.

Surrogate Someone or something replacing another.

Surrogate mother Mother who bears a child for another couple. She is impregnated with the fertilized ovum from that couple.

Surveillance The monitoring of some programme.

Susceptible More prone to disease, suggestion; easily influenced or impressed.

Suscitate To stimulate or reactivate.

Suspensory bandage A sling/bag for support of testicles.

Sustentaculum Supporting structure.

Suture 1. The line of bony union as in skull bones. 2. To unite by stitching. 3. The thread, wire or other material used to stitch body parts together. *s. absorbable* Sterile strand from mammalian collagen. *s. catgut* Suture made from sheep's small intestine. *s. coronal* Suture between the frontal and parietal bones. *s. lamboid* Suture between parietal bones and superior border of occipital bones. *s. nonabsorbable* Suture materials like silk, silkworm gut, horse hair, synthetic material and wire. *s. purse string* Suture around the periphery of a circular opening which when drawn taught closes the opening. *s. sagittal* Suture between the parietal bones. *s. mattress* An interrupted suture where the needle pierces both flaps of wound and then reenters to emerge at the same side of insertion and then tied. Particularly useful in holding together thick fragile tissues (*see* Figure).

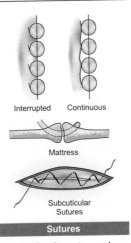

Interrupted   Continuous

Mattress

Subcuticular
Sutures

Sutures

Suxamethonium A muscle relaxant used during anesthesia. *SYN* – Succinylcholine.

Swab Cotton or gauze on end of a slender stick used for cleaning wounds, applying medicines or obtaining secretion for bacteriological culture.

Swallowing The act that enables passage of food or drink from mouth along esophagus into the stomach.

Swan-Ganz catheter A soft flexible catheter with a balloon at its tip. The balloon helps to guide the catheter into pulmonary artery. The balloon is inflated in distal pulmonary artery and the pressure is recorded which is pulmonary wedge pressure equivalent to left atrial pressure.

Swan-neck deformity Deformity of hand in rheumatoid arthritis with hyperextension of proximal interphalangeal joints due to tight interossei. Swan-neck deformity of renal tubules is a feature of adult Fanconi syndrome.

Sweat A salty aqueous slightly turbid fluid secreted by sweat glands.

Sweat gland Simple coiled tubular glands present all over body surface except in glans penis and inner surface of prepuce. The glands lie in dermis and the duct passes through epidermis to open outside. Most sweat glands are merocrine but those of axilla, labia majora and perianal region are apocrine.

Sweet's syndrome Painful skin plaques due to neutrophilic infiltration.

Swelling Enlargement mostly localized.

Swimmer's itch Itchy eruptions on skin due to swim in water containing cercariae of schistosomes.

Sycophant Flatterer, praiser of persons in command of wealth or influence.

Sycosis Chronic inflammation of hair follicle. *s. barbae* Sycosis of beard with papulo-pustular eruptions.

Sydenham's chorea Involuntary purposeless repetitive movements of distal parts as a remote manifestation of rheumatic fever.

Sylvian fissure The fissure separating temporal lobe from frontal and parietal lobes.

Symbiosis Living in perfect harmony in case of two organisms, a state beneficial to both.

Symblepharon Adhesion of lids to eyeball.

Syme's amputation Amputation just above ankle joint with removal of malleoli.

Sympathectomy Surgical excision of part of sympathetic system; either nerve, ganglia or plexus.

Sympathomimetic Producing effect similar to stimulation of sympathetic nerves.

Symphysiotomy Section of symphysis pubis to increase capacity of contracted pelvis to facilitate childbirth.

Symphysis Fibrocartilaginous union of bones.

Symptom Subjective description or manifestation of disease.

Synapse The point of junction between two adjacent neurones (*see* Figure on page 695).

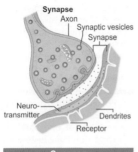

Synapse

Axon

Synaptic vesicles

Synapse

Neuro-transmitter

Dendrites

Receptor

Synapse

Synarthrosis A type of joint where skeletal elements are joined by a continuous intervening cartilage, fibrous tissue or bone. Hence movement is limited or absent and joint cavity is lacking, e.g. chondrosis, suture joints.

Synchondrosis A joint in which the surfaces are connected by plate of cartilage.

Synchysis Degenerative condition of vitreous.

Syncope Transient loss of consciousness due to inadequate blood supply to brain. *s. cardiac* Syncope of cardiac origin as in Stokes-Adam's attack, tachycardia, tight aortic stenosis, HOCM. *s. carotid sinus* Hypersensitive carotid sinus being stimulated by neck movement or tight collar producing bradycardia and syncope. *s. vasovagal* Syncope occurring due to abrupt fall in blood pressure due to fall in peripheral resistance and hence reduced venous return.

Syncytiotrophoblast Outer layer of chorionic villi.

Syncytium A mass of cytoplasm with numerous nuclei but no division into separate cells.

Syndactyly persistence of web between fingers/toes an autosomal dominant trait.

Syndesmology Study of ligaments, joints, their movements and disorders.

Syndesmosis A form of articulation where bones are united by cartilages.

Syndrome A group of signs and symptoms that provide a framework of reference to investigate as they characterize a definite lesion or pathology. *s. adrenogenital* Syndrome characterized by early puberty, over masculization, hirsutism, etc. due to excess production of adrenocortical hormones. *s. dumping* Palpitation, diarrhea, sweating and syncope occurring after food intake in patients of partial gastrectomy due to rapid emptying of food into jejunum. *s. Frohlich's* Obesity, genital atrophy, due to hypothalamic pituitary lesions. *s. Gradenigo's* Infection of petrous temporal bone causing 6th nerve paralysis as in otitis media. *s. Horner's* Ptosis, myosis, enophthalmos, and lack of sweating on affected side of face due to paralysis of cervical sympathetic. *s. Korsakoff's* A form of psychosis in chronic alcoholism with disorientation, loss of recent memory, confabulation, insomnia and hallucinations. *s. Marfan's* A connective tissue disorder with long arm span, spider finger, lax ligaments, dislocation of lens, high arched palate, aorticroot dilation and mitral valve prolapse. *s. Weber's* A form of crossed paralysis caused by a lesion in the upper border of pons involving cerebral peduncle and oculomotor nucleus. Hence there is third nerve palsy on one side with spastic hemiplegia on the opposite side.

Synechia Adhesion of iris to lens and cornea.

Synergetic Working together in cooperation, e.g. muscle groups.

Synergism Harmonious action of two agents to produce an effect greater than that produced by either agents singly.

Synergist A muscle acting in cooperation with another.

Synergy Coordinated action of two or more agents.

Syngamy Union of gametes in fertilization.

Syngeneic Individuals or cells without tissue incompatibility.

Synkaryon A nucleus resulting from fusion of two pronuclei.

Synkinesis An involuntary movement of one part occurring simultaneously with reflex or voluntary movement of another part.

Synonym Having the same or similar meaning.

Synopsis A summary; general review.

Synorchidism Partial or complete fusion of two testicles within scrotum or abdomen.

Synovectomy Excision of synovial membrane.

Synovia A colourless viscid lubricating fluid in the joint cavity, bursae and tendon sheaths.

Synovial cyst Accumulation of synovia in a bursa.

Synovial folds Smooth folds of synovial membrane inside joint cavity.

Synovial villi Slender avascular processes on the surface of synovial membrane.

Synovioma A tumor of synovial membrane.

Synthesis Union of elements to produce new compounds.

Synthetase An enzyme that acts as a catalyst to unite two molecules.

Syphilis Chronic venereal disease involving all tissues in body caused by *Treponema pallidum*, the spirochaete.

Syphilitic macules Small red non-itchy eruptions all over the body in secondary syphilis.

Syringe Instrument for injecting fluids or wash out purpose.

Syringomyelia A chronic progressive disorder with formation of cavities with surrounding gliosis in the spinal cord.

Syrinx Eustachian tube; pathological cavity within spinal cord, a fistula.

Syrup Concentrated sugar in water.

System A group of cells/organs that perform a particular function. *s. autonomic nervous* the sympathetic and parasympathetic nervous system controlling cardiac muscle, vascular smooth muscles, glandular secretions and urinary bladder; *s. cardiovascular* heart and blood vessels maintaining circulation; *s. central nervous* brain and spinal cord; *s. endocrine* glands autocrine or paracrine whose secretion act on distant sites, e.g. thyroid, parathyroid adrenal, pituitary, etc. *s. extrapyramidal* part of CNS like thalamus, caudate nucleus, substantia nigra and caudate nucleus that control muscle tone and posture. *s. hexaaxial reference* used in ECG interpretation of heart axis; *s. hypothalamohypophysial portal* The venules connecting the capillaries in the median eminence of the hypothalamus with the sinusoidal capillaries of adenohypophysis; *s. immune* cellular and molecular components that distinguish self from not self and provide defense against foreign organisms and substances; *s. limbic* The hippocampus, amygdala and cingulate gyrus that control emotion and behavior; *s. respiratory* organs like nose, larynx, trachea, bronchi and alveoli that take part in ventilation and gas exchange; *s. reticular activating* the reticular formation of medulla oblongata that maintain arousal, attentiveness and sleep; *s. reticuloendothelial* the macrophages lining sinusoids of liver, spleen and bone marrow that sequester inert particles.

Systemic circulation Blood flow from left ventricle to aorta and to arteries and return to heart via the superior and inferior vena cava (*see* Figure).

Systole The period of myocardial contraction, usually of 0.3 seconds in a heart beat.

Systolic pressure Maximum blood pressure during cardiac contraction.

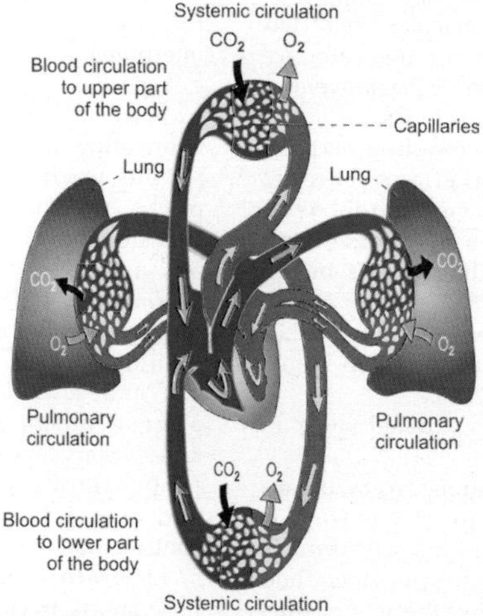

Systemic circulation

CO_2 O_2

Blood circulation to upper part of the body

Capillaries

Lung

Lung

CO_2

O_2

CO_2

O_2

Pulmonary circulation

Pulmonary circulation

CO_2 O_2

Blood circulation to lower part of the body

Systemic circulation

Systemic circulation

T

Tabes Chronic progressive wasting disease. *t. dorsalis* Degeneration of posterior column of spinal cord in syphilis.

Tabetic crises Paroxysms of pain occurring during course of tabes dorsalis.

Tablespoon A rough measure equivalent to 15 ml.

Taboo Setting apart of thing as sacred, thus forbidden for general use.

Taboparaesis Tabes dorsalis associated with general paralysis.

Tabular bone A flat bone composed of an outer and an inner table of compact bone with cancellous or diploe between them.

Tachogram A graphic tracing of rate of blood flow.

Tachyarrhythmia Abnormally rapid heart rate with or without irregularity.

Tachycardia Rapid heart rate; can be atrial, nodal, ectopic, ventricular or sinus depending upon the site of origin of the impulse.

Tachyphrasia Rapidity of speech.

Tachypnea Abnormally rapid respiration.

Tachysterol One of the isomers of ergosterol.

Tacrine Parasympathomimetic agent for Alzheimer's disease.

Tacrolimus Immunosuppressant.

Tactile Perceptible to touch.

Tactile discrimination The ability to localize two points of touch on skin surface as two discrete sensations.

Tactile localization Ability to accurately identify the site of tactile stimulation (touch, pain or pressure).

Tactometer Instrument for determining acuity of tactile sensitiveness.

Tadalafil Anti-impotency agent.

Taenia A genus of parasitic, elongated ribbon like worms, the body being segmented. *t. saginata* Tapeworm whose larvae live in flesh of cattle and adult worms (15 to 20 feet long) in human intestine.

Men acquire the infestation by eating undercooked beef. *t. solium* Tapeworm whose larval stage is in pigs and adult worms in human intestine. The disease is acquired by eating undercooked pork containing *Cysticercus cellulosae*.

Taenia coli Three bands in large intestine into which muscular fibers are collected.

Tag A small polyp or growth; a label.

Tag skin Small outgrowth of skin.

Tagging Incorporating radioactive isotope into chemical compounds to trace the metabolism.

Takayasu arteritis Aortic branch occlusion of unknown origin, often involving ophthalmic artery.

Talc Hydrous magnesium silicate, used as dusting powder.

Talipes Congenital nontraumatic abnormal deviation of foot. *t. calcaneus* The heel alone touches the ground. *t. equinus* The person walks on the toes; can be varus or valgus depending on whether the heel is turned inward or outward (*see* Figure on page 701).

Talus The ankle bone articulating with tibia fibula above and calcaneus and navicular bone below.

Tamm-Horsfall mucoprotein A Mucoprotein secreted from renal tubules.

Tamoxifen Antiestrogen drug used in adjuvant therapy of breast cancer.

Tampon A roll or pack made of various absorbent substances used to absorb body secretions or arrest hemorrhage, e.g. menstrual tampon.

Tamponade Pathologic compression of an organ or part. *t. balloon* Used to arrest variceal bleed. *t. cardiac* Increased pericardial pressure due to pericardial bleed or excess fluid causing compression of heart to the extent of compromising its function.

Tamsulosin Alfablocker for prostatic hypertrophy.

Tangier disease A syndrome of HDL deficiency first discovered in Tangier island. Symptoms and signs include polyneuropathy, lymphadenopathy, orange tonsils, hepatosplenomegaly.

Tannin An acid substance found in tea and an astringent, topical hemostatic and antidote for various poisons.

Tantrum Bad temper or anger.

Tapeworm Parasitic worms belonging to class cestoda having a scolex with hooks and suckers and a

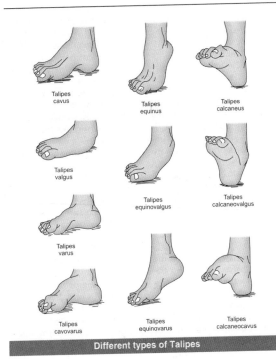

Talipes cavus

Talipes equinus

Talipes calcaneus

Talipes valgus

Talipes equinovalgus

Talipes calcaneovalgus

Talipes varus

Talipes cavovarus

Talipes equinovarus

Talipes calcaneocavus

Different types of Talipes

series of proglottids. *t. beef* Taenia saginata. *t. broad* Diphylobothrium latum. *t. dog* Dipylidium caninum. *t. dwarf* Hymenolepis nana. *t. pork* Taenia solium.

Tapia syndrome Paralysis of pharynx, larynx and atrophy of tongue due to paralysis of tenth and twelfth cranial nerves.

Tapping Removal of fluid from cavity, percussion in massage.

Tar Thick brown to black liquid obtained from distillation of carbonaceous matter.

Tardieu's spot Subpleural spots of ecchymosis following death by strangulation.

Tardive Tending to be late.

Target cell An abnormal erythrocyte which when stained shows a central and peripheral rim of hemoglobin with intermediate unstained area resembling a target.

Tarnier's sign A sign of impending abortion; the disappearance of angle between upper and lower uterine segments of uterus.

Tarnish Discoloration.

Tarsal glands Branched sebaceous alveolar glands in the eyelids. *SYN*—meiobomian glands.

Tarsal tunnel In the ankle, the bony fibrous passage for the posterior tibial vessels, nerves and flexor tendons.

Tarsal tunnel syndrome Weakness of plantar flexion of toes and numbness of sole of foot due to compression of tibial nerve in the tarsal tunnel.

Tarsectomy Excision of one or more bones of tarsus.

Tarsitis Inflammation of margin of eyelid; inflammation of tarsal bones (the seven bones of ankle).

Tarsorrhaphy The procedure of suturing the edges of upper and lower eyelids for purpose of reducing width of palpebral fissure.

Tarsus The ankle with its seven constituent bones, i.e. talus, calcans, cuboid, navicular and the three cuneiform bones.

Tartar A form of hardened dental plaque.

Tartrazin A pyrazole aniline dye used to colour foods, cloth and drugs.

Taste A sensation produced by stimulation of taste buds by sweet, sour, bitter and salty substances.

Taste buds Sensory end organs located on surface of tongue, on soft palate that mediate the sensation of taste.

Tattooing Production of permanent colors on the skin by introducing vegetable and mineral pigments.

Taurocholic acid Bile acid that yields taurine and cholic acid on hydrolysis.

Taxis The response of an organism to its environment.

Taxonomy Laws and principles of classification of animals and plants.

Tay-Sachs disease Autosomal recessive form of gangliosidosis (lipid storage disease) manifesting with mental retardation, blindness, cherry red spot in macula, etc. due to deficiency of hexosaminidase. A leading to accumulation of sphingolipid in CNS.

T cells Thymus derived lymphocytes consisting of helper inducer cells (T_4), killer T-cells and suppressor T-cells.

Tea black Tea made from the leaves that have been fermented before they are dried.

Tea green Tea made by heating the leaves in open trays.

Tear A watery saline solution secreted by lacrimal glands that lubricates the eyeball and eyelids.

Teaspoon Measure equivalent to 5 ml.

Teat The nipple of mammary gland.

Technetium Compounds used as radiopharmaceuticals. *Tc-99m albumin* Cardiac blood pool imaging. *Tc-99m albumin aggregated* Lung imaging. *Tc-99m bicisate* Brain imaging. *Tc-99m albumin colloid*-Liver imaging. *Tc-99m disofenin* Hepatobiliary imaging. *Tc-99m etidronate/medronate/oxidronate* Skeletal imaging. *Tc-99m ferpentetate/mertiatide* Renal imaging. *Tc-99m furifosmin* Myocardial perfusion imaging. *Tc-99m mebrofenin* Hepatobiliary imaging. *Tc-99m pertechnetate* Brain, parathyroid, thyroid,

Meckel's diverticulum imaging. *Tc-99m pyrophosphate* Cardiac/skeletal imaging. *Tc-99m sestamibi/teboroxime/tetrofosmin* Myocardial perfusion imaging.

Technetium -99m An isomer of technetium that emits gamma rays with a half-life of 6 hours, used for vascular imaging.

Technology The scientific knowledge and its practical application.

Tectocephaly Boat shaped head.

Tectospinal tract A descending tract from tectum of midbrain to spinal cord.

Tectum Structure resembling a roof; dorsal midbrain consisting of superior and inferior colliculi.

Teenage Age bracket of 13-19 years.

Teeth Hard bony projections from jaw helping in mastication. *t. deciduous* Milk teeth which are shed and replaced by permanent teeth. *t. Hutchinson's* Notched upper central incisors and peg-shaped lateral incisors. *t. wisdom* The third molar of permanent dentition, last to errupt.

Tegaserol Serotonin agonist for IBS.

Tegmen A structure that covers a part.

Tegmentum The dorsal portion of midbrain containing red nucleus and oculomotor nuclei.

Tegument The skin covering of body.

Teichopsia Zigzag lines bounding a luminous object in visual field as in migraine.

Teicoplanin Higher antibiotic.

Tela Any web like structure.

Telangiectasia Dilatation of group of capillaries to form elevated dark red wart like spots.

Telediagnosis Diagnosis based on data transmitted electronically to the doctor.

Telemedicine Exchange of medical information from one site to another through the use of telecommunication and information technologies.

Telemetry Transmission of data to a distant place by electronic means.

Telencephalon The embryonic forebrain that develops into olfactory lobes, cerebral cortex and corpora striate.

Teleology The belief that everything in nature is directed towards some final purpose.

Teleopsia A visual perceptive disorder where objects appear

to have excess depth or close objects appear to be away.

Telepaque Iopanoic acid.

Telepathy Communication of one's thought and mental process to another at a distance.

Teleradiography Radiography with radiation source at about 2 meters away from body.

Teletherapy Treatment of cancer in which source of radiation is placed at some distance from body.

Telmisartan ACE receptor antagonist for hypertension.

Telbivudine Anti-HIV drug.

Telogen Resting stage of hair growth.

Telophase The final stage of mitosis.

Temper State of one's mood, disposition and mind.

Temperament The combination of intellectual, emotional and physical characteristic of an individual.

Temperate Moderate.

Temperature The degree of intensity of heat. *t. ambient* Temperature of surrounding. *t. inverse* A state where morning body temperature is higher than evening body temperature. *t. normal* Oral temperature of 98.6°F (37°C). *t. rectal* More accurate than oral or axillary temperature.

It is about 1°F higher than oral temperature, whereas axillary temperature is 1°F lower than oral temperature.

Temper tantrums Spells of uncontrollable anger especially in children.

Template A pattern, form or mold used as a guide in duplicating, e.g. in preparation of denture.

Temple Forehead, the portion lying in front of ear and above the zygomatic arch.

Temporal Related to or limited in time.

Temporal fossa The fossa above ear that contains temporalis muscle.

Temporalis The muscle in temporal fossa inserted into coronoid process of mandible, a muscle of mastication.

Temporal lobe Lobe of cerebrum concerned with olfaction.

Temporoparietal Relating to temporal and parietal bones.

Tenacious Adhesive, sticky.

Tenacity Condition of being tough, stubborn.

Tenaculum Sharp hook like instrument (*see* Figure).

Tenderizer Preparations containing proteolytic enzymes like papain to make the meat more tender.

Tenderness Sensitive to pain on pressure. *t. rebound*

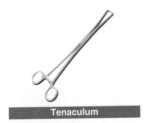

Tenaculum

Intensification of pain during release of pressure, a feature of peritonitis.

Tendinitis Inflammation of a tendon.

Tendinous synovitis Inflammation of tendon's synovial sheath.

Tendon Fibrous connective tissue attaching a muscle to bone. *t. Achilles* The thickest and strongest tendon of gastrocnemius muscle attached to calcaneus.

Tendovaginitis Inflammation of tendon and its sheath.

Tenesmus Ineffectual painful effort in bladder and bowel evacuation.

Teniposide Antineoplastic agents of podophylotoxin group.

Tennis elbow Pain over lateral epicondyle of humerus at the site of attachment of extensor tendons.

Tenon's capsule Connective tissue covering of eyeball.

Tenon's space Space between the posterior surface of eyeball and Tenon's capsule.

Tenosynovectomy Excision of tendon sheath.

Tenosynovitis Inflammation of tendon sheath.

Tenotome Instrument for cutting tendon.

Tenotomy Surgical section of a tendon.

Tenoxicam Analgesic anti-inflammatory.

Tension Expansive force that stretches; a state of mental strain. *t. premenstrual* Nervous instability, irritability, headache and depression occurring few days before menstruation.

Tension headache Headache caused by sustained contraction of muscles of head and neck.

Tension suture Suture used to reduce pull of the edges of wound.

Tensor Any muscle that makes a part tense.

Tensor vali palatini A muscle of soft palate arising from cartilaginous medial end of auditory tube and inserted into palatal aponeurosis.

Tentacle A slender projection of invertebrates used for tactile purposes or feeding.

Tentative Provisional.

Tenth cranial nerve Vagus nerve supplying heart, lungs, abdominal viscera, esophagus, etc.

Tentorial notch An arched cavity formed by anterior and inner border of tentorium cerebelli.

Tentorial pressure cone The herniation of uncus of temporal lobe and midbrain through tentorial notch due to raised intracranial pressure.

Tentorium cerebelli The process of dura mater between cerebrum and cerebellum supporting the occipital lobes.

Tepid Lukewarm.

Teratoblastoma A tumor containing embryonic tissue.

Teratocarcinoma Carcinoma developing from epithelial element of a teratoma.

Teratogen Any substance capable of disrupting fetal growth and producing fetal malformation.

Teratogenesis The development of abnormal structures in an embryo.

Teratology Scientific study of teratogens and their mode of action.

Teratoma Congenital tumor containing one or more of three embryonic germ layers.

Teratosis Deformed fetus.

Terazosin Alfa-blocker, used in hypertension and BPH.

Terbinafine Antifungal agent.

Terbutaline Synthetic sympathomimetic amine used as bronchondilator.

Terconazole A ketoconazole derivative, antifungal agent.

Teres Round and smooth.

Terfenadine H_1 receptor blocker, antiallergic agent.

Terlipressin Synthetic antidiuretic hormone.

Terminal Pertains to end or placed at the end.

Terminal arteriole Arteriole without any branches which ends in capillaries.

Terminal cancer An advanced stage of cancer from which patient cannot recover.

Terminal illness Illness from which recovery is impossible, hence death is imminent.

Terminal infection An acute infection that appears at late stage of another disease and often prove fatal.

Terminology Nomenclature, a system of technical terms used in arts, science and trade.

Terpene A hydrocarbon used as an expectorant.

Terracing Suturing in several rows through thick tissues in wound closure.

Terramycin Oxytetracycline, synthesized by *Streptomyces rimosus,* effective against bacteria, rickettsia and chlamydia.

Terror Great fear.

Tertian Occurring every third day as in malaria.

Tertiary Third in order.

Tertiary care A level of medicare.

Tertiary syphilis Third and most advanced stage of syphilis with general dissemination.

Testis The male reproductive gland located in scrotum about 4 cm long and 2 cm wide (*see* Figure on page 708).

Testmeal A meal of definite quality and quantity given for analysis of stomach function.

Testosterone An androgenic hormone secreted by Leydig cells of testes.

Test (1) An examination or trial (2) a chemical reaction. *t. acid elution* done for fetal hemoglobin which resists elution at pH 3.3 (citric acid—sodium phosphate). *t. acidified serum* (Ham test) done for paroxysmal haematuria. *t. acoustic reflex* done to differentiate conductive and sensory neural deafness and to diagnose acoustic neuroma from contraction of stapedias muscle in response to sound. *t. alkali denaturation* a spectrophotometric method

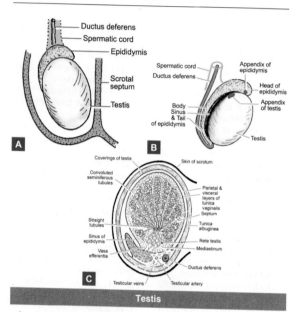

Testis

for determination of HbF. *t. Anes* a test for mutagenicity of chemical compounds using special strains of *Salmonella typhimurium*. *t. antiglobulin* a test for the presence of nonagglutinating antibodies against red cells. *t. Apt* a test for differentiating fetal from adult haemoglobin. *t. bentonite flocculation* any agglutination test using antigen adsorbed on bentonite to detect antibodies from flocculation. *t. benzidine* done for detection of occult blood in urine and stool. *t. caloric* done for occular and vestibular functioning. Irrigation of normal ear with warm water produces rotation nystagmus towards irrigated ear but opposite occurs with cold water. *t. Casoni's* done for hydatid disease. *t. chemiluminiscence* a test for neutrophil microbicidal function. *t. Chi square* a test for statistical use. *t. cocaine* in Horner syndrome cocaine fails to dilate the pupil of the affected eye. *t. contraction* the monitoring of fetal heart rate response to uterine contractions by cardiotocography. *t. Donath Landsteiner* test for paroxysmal nocturnal haemoglobinuria. *t. drawer's* a test for intactness of cruciate ligaments of knee. *t. euglobulin lysis* a test that evaluates for haemorrhagic tendencies by measuring time of fibrinolysis. *t. Fouchets'* done for presence of bilirubin in urine, the urine turning green on addition of Fouchet's reagent. *t. Gerhardt's* done for detection of acetoacetic acid in urine. *t. glucose tolerance* done for diabetes mellitus, patient given 1.59/kg mm 75 gm glucose to drink followed by serial blood sugar every 30 minute till 2½ hours. *t. glycosylated Hb* used to know % of HbA having keto-amine linkage between betachain and glucose in patients of diabetes mellitus. *t. Gmelin's* formation of coloured rings on addition of boiling nitric acid to urine containing bile pigment. *t. Guthrie's* for phenyl ketonuria. *t. haemagglutination inhibition* a sensitive procedure for measurement of soluble antigens in biologic specimens. *t. histamine flare* done for leprosy and post-herpetic neuralgia. *t. Hoppe Seyler* for carbon monoxide in blood. *t. hydrogen breath* done for deificiency of lactase, or other hydrolases or colonic overgrowth of bacteria. *t. kveim* skin test for sarcoidosis. *t. lepromen* intradermal test to differentiate various forms of leprosy from immune status. *t. limulus* to test presence of endotoxin from gelation of blood of horse shoe crab. *t. Lindenann's* for detection of acetoacetic acid in urine. *t. Lundh* a test of pancreatic function. *t. Mantoux* a skin test to know if one is exposed to tuberculosis. *t. Mazzotti* done for oncocerciasis. *t. methyl red* done for differentiation of enterobacteriacae. *T. Nagel's* a test for colour vision. *t. neostigmine* done for myasthenia gravis. *t. nitroblue tetrazolium* a test of neutrophil microbicidal function. *t. nonstress* monitoring of fetal heart rate in response to fetal movement.

t. osmotic fragility done for spherocytosis where osmotic fragility is increased. *t. Papanicolaou* an exfoliative cytological staining procedure for diagnosis of cervical cancer, and endometrial cancer. *t. patch* skin test for allergy. *t. Paul Bunnell* for detection of heterophil antibodies as in infectious mononucleosis from agglutination of sheep RBCs. *t. Perthe's* a test for collateral circulation in patients with varicose veins. *t. pulmonary function* the tests to measure capacities, flow rates and volumes of lungs, gas exchange, pulmonary blood flow and pH. *t. radioimmunosorbent* radioimmunoassay for IgE in serum. *t. rollover* test to assess risk of preeclampsia in pregnant women, increase in blood pressure in supine than lateral position indicates preeclampsia. *t. Romerg's* the test differentiates between cerebellar ataxia and ataxia of posterior column disease/peripheral nerves. *t. Rose Waaler* an agglutination test for rheumatoid factor. *t. Rubin's* tubal insuflation with CO_2 to know tubal patency. *t. Schiller's* test for cancer cervix, where painting of cervical mucosa with iodine gives yellow or white as the cancer cells do not have glycogen. *t. Shick* a test to know immunity status to diphtheria. *t. Schilling* a test for gastrointestinal absorption of B_{12}. *t. Trendelenberg's* a test of varicosity. *t. urea breath* a test for detection of urea splitting organisms like *H. pylori. t. VDRL*, the standard nontreponemal antigen test for syphilis. *t. Wada's* a test for cerebral dominance of language function. *t. Weil Felix* for diagnosis of typhus and other rickettsiosis. *t. Widal* a test for presence of aglutinins against O and H antigens of *S typhi*.

Test tube baby A baby born to a mother whose ovum was removed, fertilized outside her body and implanted in her uterus.

Tetanolysin A hemolytic component of the toxin produced by *Clostridium tetani*.

Tetanospasmin The toxin of *Clostridium tetani* responsible for spasm.

Tetanus An acute infectious disease caused by anaerobe *Clostridium tetani* manifesting with painful tonicclonic spasm of voluntary muscles.

Tetanus antitoxin Serum containing antibody against tetanus obtained from immunized horses or humans.

Tetanus toxoid Modified tetanus toxin capable of promoting active immunity.

Tetany A state of increased neuromuscular excitability caused by decreased serum ionized calcium or phosphorus and in alkalosis.

Tetracaine Local anesthetic used topically.

Tetrachlorethylene A clear colorless bitter liquid used as anthelmintic, potentially hepatotoxic.

Tetracycline A broad spectrum antibiotic.

Tetrad A group of four things.

Tetradactyly Having four digits on a hand or foot.

Tetrahydrocanabinol Principal active component of *Canabis indica*.

Tetrahydrozoline A vasoconstrictor used in ophthalmic and nasal drops.

Tetraiodothyronine One of the principal hormones secreted by thyroid. *SYN* – thyroxine (T_4).

Tetralogy A combination of four symptoms or elements. *t. of Fallot* Congenital heart disease with infundibular pulmonary stenosis, right ventricular hypertrophy, overriding aorta, and high ventricular septal defect (*see* Figure).

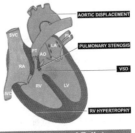

Tetralogy of Fallot

Tetramisole Anthelmintic.

Tetraparesis Paresis of all four limbs.

Tetraplegia *SYN*—quadriplegia.

Thalamic nuclei The anterior, lateral, medial and posterior thalamic nuclei.

Thalamic syndrome Severe sharp boring and burning pain caused by vascular lesions of thalamus.

Thalamotomy Destruction of thalamus by several means to treat psychosis or intractable pain.

Thalamus Large ovoid masses of gray matter on either side of third ventricle, serving as gateway for all sensory projections to brain.

Thalassemia A group of congenital hemolytic anemia due to impaired synthesis of hemoglobin polypeptide chains, alpha or beta. *t. major* The homozygous form of deficient beta chain synthesis manifesting with severe microcytic anemia, splenomegaly, jaundice, gallstones, leg ulcers and thickened cranial bones. *t. minor* Heterozygous state for alpha or beta chain production with mild microcytic hypo–chromic anemia and raised Hb A$_2$ (*see* Figure).

Thalidomide Alfa glutarimide previously used as sedative but now only used in lepra reaction; causes severe birth defects if given to pregnant mothers.

Thallium A metallic element used as rodenticide.

Thanatology The science of death.

Thanatophobia Morbid fear of death.

Theaism Chronic poisoning from excessive intake of tea.

Thebaine An alkaloid present in opium.

Thebesian valve An endocardial fold at entrance of coronary sinus into right atrium.

Thebesian vein Small veins draining blood from myocardium directly into heart chambers.

Theca A sheath.

Thecoma A benign tumor of ovary.

Thecomatosis Increased connective tissue in the ovary.

Thelalgia Pain in the nipples of breast.

Thelarche The beginning of breast development during puberty.

Thelothism Nipple erection by contraction of its smooth muscles.

Thenar Palm of hand or sole of foot; fleshy eminence at base of thumb.

Thenar muscles Abductor and flexor muscles of thumb.

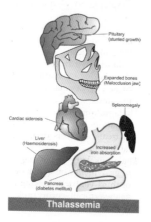

Pituitary (stunted growth)

Expanded bones (Malocclusion jaw)

Splenomegaly

Cardiac siderosis

Liver (Haemosiderosis)

Increased iron absorption

Pancreas (diabetes mellitus)

Thalassemia

Theobromine A smooth muscle dilator, used as a mild stimulant and diuretic.

Theomania Religious insanity.

Theophylline A plant product and bronchodilator. *t. ethylenediamine* Aminophylline.

Theorem A proposition proved by logic or argument.

Theory An assumption based on certain evidence or certain observations but lacking scientific proof.

Therapeutic A curative. *t. abortion* Termination of pregnancy that disrupts mother's physical or mental health (as a sequence of rape) or is likely to produce a physically or mentally handicapped child. *t. index* The ratio of toxic dose of a substance to its therapeutic dose; an index of safety of the drug.

Therapeutics The branch of medical science dealing with treatment of disease.

Therapist Practitioner of some kind of therapy.

Therapy The means employed to effect a cure or manage a disease. *t. collapse* Production of pneumothorax to effect pulmonary collapse as a method of treatment of non- healing cavitary pulmonary tuberculosis. *t. electroconvulsive* Passing of electric current in the convulsive dose to treat psychosis or suicidal depression. *t. photodynamic* Method of treating cancer by using light absorbing chemicals that are selectively retained by malignant cells. *t. physical* Use of physical agents such as massage, heat, hydration, electricity, exercise in the treatment of disease. *t. replacement* Therapeutic use of medicine as substitute for natural body substances, e.g. thyroid hormone, insulin.

Thermalgesia Pain caused by exposure to heat.

Thermesthesia Capability to perceive heat and cold.

Thermic Pertains to heat.

Thermistor An apparatus for determining small changes in temperature.

Thermoanaesthesia Insensitiveness to heat.

Thermocautery Cautery by using heat.

Thermocoagulation Coagulation or destruction of tissue by passage of high frequency current.

Thermocouple Device for measuring slight temperature changes.

Thermodilution A technique for determination of cardiac output from injection of cold saline into bloodstream and measuring the temperature change downstream.

Thermogenesis Production of body heat.

Thermography A technique to study blood flow into limbs and to detect breast cancer.

Thermoluminescent dosimeter A monitoring device that stores energy of ionizing radiation. When heated it emits light proportional to the amount of radiation to which it has been exposed, used by radiographers and those working near radiation source.

Thermometer Instrument for recording temperature.

Thermometry Measurement of temperature.

Thermophilic Thriving best in environment of raised temperature.

Thermoregulation Heat regulation.

Thermoregulatory center Hypothalamic center that regulates heat production and heat loss.

Thermostasis Maintenance of body temperature.

Thermostat A device that automatically regulates temperature.

Thiabendazole Anthelmintic used for strongyloidiasis and cutaneous larva migrans.

Thiazolidinediones A group of antidiabetic agents.

Thiamine Vitamin B_1 present in wheat germ, rice water, animal and plant foods. Acts as a coenzyme in carboxylation of pyruvic acid. Deficiency produces beriberi.

Thiersch's graft Partial thickness skin graft.

Thio Prefix meaning sulfur.

Thioguanine An antimetabolite and immunosuppressant.

Thiopental sodium An ultrashort acting barbiturate used for inducing surgical anesthesia.

Thioridazine Antipsychotic agent.

Thiotepa An alkylating agent, antineoplastic drug.

Thiothixene An antipsychotic drug.

Thiouracil Antithyroid agent.

Thiourea Antithyroid drug.

Third degree burn Burn involving entire thickness of skin and deeper structures.

Third degree heart block Complete heart block.

Third heart sound Heart sound occurring at the end of rapid ventricular filling.

Thirst Desire for water or the sensation arising out of lack of body fluids.

Thomas splint A splint with a proximal ring with two long steel rods used to place traction on the leg in long axis.

Thomsen's disease Myotonia congenita.

Thoracectomy A process of making incision in chest wall and resecting a portion of rib.

Thoracentesis Puncture of chest wall to drain out pleural fluids.

Thoracic cage The bony structure surrounding the chest.

Thoracic duct The main lymphatic duct of body arising at cisterna chyli, ascending up to join left subclavian vein near its junction with left internal jugular vein.

Thoracic outlet syndrome Compression of the neurovascular structures at the superior thoracic outlet located just above the first rib and behind the clavicle leading to various symptoms like pain in the neck and shoulder, numbness and tingling of the fingers and a weak grip.

Thoracocentesis Drainage of thoracic cavity through needle puncture.

Thoracolumbar Relating to the thoracic and lumbar parts of the spinal cord.

Thoracoplasty Partial resection of ribs to induce collapse of underlying lung as in lung abscess, or empyema.

Thoracoscopy Endoscopic examination of pleural cavity.

Thoracostomy Surgical resection of chest wall for drainage.

Thoracostomy tube A tube inserted into the chest wall to drain air or fluid from pleural space.

Thorax The part of the body between diaphragm below and base of the neck above. *t. barrel shaped* Rounded chest as in emphysema.

Thorium Radioactive metallic substance.

Thoron A radioactive isotope of radon.

Threadworm *Enterobius vermicularis.*

Threonine Alpha-amino-beta- hydroxybutyricacid, an essential amino acid.

Threshold 1. Point at which physiological response is produced. 2. A measure of sensitivity of an organ or function.

Threshold dose Minimum dose that will be effective.

Thrill A palpable murmur.

Thrix Hair.

Throat The pharynx and the fauces.

Throbbing Pulsatile.

Thrombasthenia A platelet disorder with prolonged bleeding time, and abnormal clot retraction.

Thrombectomy Excision of a thrombus.

Thrombin An enzyme derived from prothrombin by action of thromboplastin.

Thromboangitis Inflammation of blood vessel with thrombus formation. *t. obliterans* Chronic occlusive vascular disease common to cigarette smokers commonly affecting the feet with propensity for gangrene formation. *SYN* – Buerger's disease.

Thrombocythemia Absolute increase in platelet count.

Thrombocytopenia Decrease below normal in number of platelets ($\geq$ 50,000 cmm).

Thrombocytosis Increase in number of platelets ($\geq$ 400,000 cmm).

Thromboembolism A detached thrombus causing occlusion of a vessel.

Thrombogenesis The process of formation of blood clot.

Thrombokinase Factor 'x' or Stuart factor.

Thrombolysis Dissolution of blood clot.

Thrombophlebitis Inflammation of vein with thrombus formation.

Thromboplastin The coagulation factor III present in most tissues which accelerates clot formation by converting prothrombin to thrombin.

Thrombosis The formation or existence of thrombus or clot within the vessel.

Thrombus A blood clot (*see* Figure).

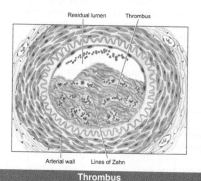

Residual lumen Thrombus

Arterial wall Lines of Zahn

Thrombus

Thrush Infection caused by *Candida albicans* in mouth and throat with formation of white patches and ulcers.

Thrust The sudden move forward.

Thumb The short thick first finger on radial side of hand having two phallanges in place of 3.

Thumb sucking Habit of sucking thumb.

Thymectomy Surgical removal of thymus.

Thymine A base present in DNA.

Thymocyte A lymphocyte that migrates from bone marrow to thymus where it matures and is released to blood as T-lymphocyte.

Thymoma Tumor from epithelial tissue of thymus.

Thymopoietin A substance produced by thymus gland that helps in differentiation of thymocytes.

Thymus The capsulated bilobed organ in anterior mediastinum which is essential for immune function of body.

Thyroepiglottic muscle Muscle arising from inner surface of thyroid cartilage and inserted into epiglottis. Acts to depress the epiglottis.

Thyroglobulin Iodine containing protein secreted by thyroid gland and stored within the colloid.

Thyroglossal duct A duct which in the embryo connects the thyroid diverticulum with the tongue.

Thyroid cartilage The V shaped principal cartilage of larynx, known as Adam's apple.

Thyroidectomy Excision of thyroid gland, usually done in hyperthyroidism.

Thyroid function tests A group of tests done to assess the level of functioning of thyroid gland. They include thyroid radioiodine uptake studies, estimation of T_3, T_4 and TSH.

Thyroid gland The bilobed gland joined by isthmus located at the base of the neck, secreting T_3 and T_4.

Thyroiditis Inflammation of thyroid gland. *t. giant cell* Thyroiditis characterized by presence of giant cells, round cell infiltration, fibrosis and destruction of the follicles. *t. Hashimoto's* A form of autoimmune thyroiditis common to women. There is thyromegaly and hypothyroidism.

Thyroid stimulating hormone (TSH) Hormone secreted by anterior pituitary which stimulates thyroid to secrete T_3 and T_4.

Thyroid storm A complication of thyrotoxicosis precipitated by infection, surgery; manifests with high fever, restlessness and congestive failure.

Thyromegaly Enlarged thyroid gland.

Thyroptosis Downward displacement of thyroid.

Thyrotoxic Pertains to hyperactivity of thyroid gland.

Thyrotoxicosis Hyperfunctioning of thyroid gland with tachycardia, fine tremor, anxiety, nervousness, diarrhea, etc.

Thyrotropic Agent that stimulates thyroid gland.

Thyrotropin Thyroid stimulating hormone.

Thyroxine Tetraiodothyronine, the principal hormone of thyroid gland.

Tianeptine Antidepressant agent.

Tibia The inner larger bone in the leg. *t. saber* Gummatous periosteitis of tibia with increased outward curvature.

Tic A sudden involuntary muscle contraction. *t. douloureux* Lightening pain along the branches of trigeminal nerve due to degeneration or pressure on the nerve.

Ticarcillin A semisynthetic penicillin effective against pseudomonas.

Tick A group of blood sucking acarids; can be hard tick or soft tick; transmit typhus group of fevers, Q fever, Lyme's disease, babesiosis, bereliosis, tularemia, etc.

Tickling Gentle stimulation of sensitive surface and the reflex thereof.

Ticlopidine Antiplatelet agent.

Tidal Periodically rising and falling.

Tietze syndrome Sternal costochondritis of unknown etiology, often requiring injection procaine and steroids locally.

Timolol Beta-blocker.

Tincture An alcoholic extraction of animal or vegetable substance.

Tincture of iodine A skin disinfectant containing a mixture of sodium iodide in an alcohol-water solution. This term is not used nowadays.

Tinea Fungus infection. *t. capitis* Fungal infection of head. *t. corporis* Fungal infections of body with scaly eruptions and clearing center. *t. cruris* Fungal infection of genital area. *t. nigra* Superficial fungal infection of palm with pigmented nonitchy nonscaly macules. *t. pedis* Fungal infection of foot (*SYN*-athlete's foot). *t. versicolor* Yellow or fawn colored skin patches due to *Malassezia furfur*.

Tinel's sign Tingling sensation on pressing or tapping a damaged or degenerating nerve.

Tingle Pricking or stinging sensation.

Tinidazole An imidazole used in amebiasis.

Tinnitus Ringing sensation in the ear.

Tinocordin Immunostimulant.

Tiotropium Antiasthmatic inhaler.

Tissue A group or collection of similar cells performing a particular function.

Tissue macrophage A large wandering branched cell with single nucleus capable of ingesting particulate matter.

Tissue plasminogen activator (TPA) A thrombolytic agent that is clot specific, acting on plasminogen causing breakdown of fibrin.

Titanium dioxide Used in solutions for protection against sunburn.

Titillation Sensation produced by tickling.

Titration 1. Determination of quantity of antibody in the serum. 2. Estimation of the concentration of chemical solution by adding known amount of standard reagent.

Titubation Unsteadiness of posture, swaying of trunk and head while sitting, staggering gait.

Tizanidine Muscle relaxant.

TNM classification Method of calssifying malignant tumors based on local characteristics of the tumor, involvement of lymph nodes and distant metastasis.

Toad skin Excessive dryness, wrinkling and scaling of skin as in vitamin A deficiency (phrynoderma).

Tobacco Dried leaves of the plant *Nicotiana tobacum* containing nicotine, picoline, pyridine, collidin, etc. Tobacco chewing is related to oropharyngeal cancer and tobacco smoking to lung cancer, hypertension, heart attack, vasoocclusive disease, etc.

Tobramycin Aminoglycoside antibiotic.

Tocainide A lidocaine analog, antiarrhythmic drug used for VT.

Tocodynamometer Device for estimating force of uterine contraction. *SYN*—tocometer.

Tocograph Device for recording force of uterine contraction.

Tocology Science of parturition.

Tocolysis Suppression of uterine contraction.

Tocopherol Compounds with vitamin E activity.

Tocophobia A fear of child birth or pregnancy.

Todd's paralysis Focal weakness in a part of the body after a seizure.

Toilet Wound cleaning.

Toe Any of the five digits of foot. *t. claw* dorsal subluxation of toes 2-5 in rheumatoid arthritis. *t. hammer* proximal phalanx is extended and 2nd and third are flexed.

Toilet training Teachings for a child to achieve control over urination and defecation.

Tolazamide An oral hypoglycemic agent.

Tolazoline An alfa-adrenergic blocking agent used for causing peripheral vasodilatation as in chilblain.

Tolbutamide An oral hypoglycemic agent.

Tolerance Progressive decrease in the effectiveness of a drug.

Tolfenamic acid A fenamate anti-inflammatory drug.

Tolnaftate Synthetic antifungal agent used topically.

Tolterodine Antimuscarinic agent.

Tomography A method of X-ray that shows details of image of structures at a particular plane of tissue by blurring images of structures in all other planes.

Tone 1. A state of partial contraction of muscle. 2. Normal tension in arterial wall.

Tongue A fleshy leafy organ lying in floor of mouth. Helps in mastication, deglutition, speech production and taste. *t. smooth* A tongue with atrophy of papillae as in anemia and malnutrition. *t. strawberry* A bright red tongue with prominent papillae as in scarlet fever.

Tongue tie Congenital shortness of frenum linguae with poor protrusion, difficulty in articulation and sucking.

Tonicity Property of possessing tone.

Tonography The recording of changes in intraocular pressure.

Tonometer Instrument for measuring intraocular pressure.

Tonometry Measurement of intraocular tension.

Tonsil 1. A mass of lymphatic tissue located in the fauces. 2. Two rounded masses projecting from inferior surface of cerebellum. 3. Lymphatic tissue near the opening of eustachian tube into pharynx.

Tonsillar fossa Depression between the glossopalatine and pharyngopalatine arches accommodating the tonsils.

Tonsillar ring Ring of lymphoid tissue encircling the pharynx, e.g. palatine and lingual tonsils and the adenoids.

Tonsillar sinus Space between the plica triangularis and anterior surface of tonsils.

Tonsillectomy Surgical removal of the tonsils.

Tonsillitis Inflammation of tonsils. *t. follicular* Tonsillitis principally affecting the crypts.

Tooth The hard structure in the jaw for mastication (*see* Figure).

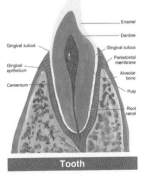

Tooth

Toothache Pain within or around a tooth.

Toothbrushing The act of using a soft brush for cleaning the teeth and gums.

Topagnosis Loss of ability to localize site of tactile sensation.

Tophaceous Related to tophus.

Topiramate Anticonvulsant.

Tophus Deposits of sodium biurate in tissue adjacent to a joint.

Topical Local.

Topotecan Anti-cancer agent.

TORCH An acronym standing for Toxoplasmosis, Other transplacental infections, Rubella, Cytomegalovirus and Herpes simplex. TORCH infections can attack an embryo or fetus.

Torpent Medicine that modifies irritation.

Torpidity Sluggishness, inactivity.

Torque A force producing rotary motion.

Torr The pressure of 1/760 of standard atmospheric pressure or simply 1mm of Hg.

Torsade-de-pointes Polymorphic rapid ventricular tachycardia with changing QRS configuration.

Torsemide Diuretic.

Torsion Rotation of the vertical meridians of eye; rotation of tooth along its long axis.

Torticollis Spasmodic contraction of neck muscles causing head to tilt to one side and chin pointing to other side.

Tortuous Having many bends or twists and turns.

Torture Infliction of mental or physical pain.

Torula Yeastlike organism, now called *Cryptococcus*.

Total hip replacement Replacement of acetabulum and head of femur by metallic or silicone prosthesis in the treatment of advanced disabling hip disease.

Total parenteral nutrition (TPN) Provision of total electrolyte, protein, calorie, vitamin and mineral need via intravenous route.

Totipotent A cell capable of dividing into a large variety of cells.

Touch Tactile sense or perceive from palpation.

Tourniquet Any item used to exert pressure over an artery to stop bleeding. *t. rotating* A technique of applying tourniquets to three extremities in rotation to reduce venous return to heart as in pulmonary edema (*see* Figure).

Tourniquet test Test for determining capillary fragility from their ability to withstand pressure.

Touton cells Giant multinucleated cells found in lesions of xanthomatosis.

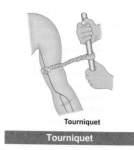

Tourniquet

Tourniquet

Toxemia Circulation of toxins throughout the body producing symptoms like fever, diarrhea, vomiting, hypotension, flushing tachycardia, etc. *t. of pregnancy* A series of changes occurring in pregnancy leading to hypertension, proteinuria, convulsion and intrauterine growth retardation.

Toxic allergic syndrome A disease caused by ingestion of adulterated rapeseed oil with aniline producing respiratory distress, eosinophilia, hepatosplenomegaly, etc.

Toxicity Quality of being poisonous.

Toxicology Branch of science dealing with toxic substances, their detection, pharmacological action, selection of suitable antidotes, treatment and prevention of their symptoms.

Toxicosis A diseased condition resulting from poisoning.

Toxic shock syndrome Fever, diffuse macular erythematous rash, syncope due to toxins produced by *Staphylococcus aureus*.

Toxiferous Containing a poison.

Toxigenic Producing toxins or poisons.

Toxigenicity The virulence of a toxin producing pathogenic organism.

Toxin A poisonous substance of animal or plant origin.

Toxoid A toxin without toxicity but with intact antigenicity so that when injected can produce antibodies.

Toxocariasis Infection with toxocara organism.

Toxolysin Substance capable of destroying toxin.

Toxoplasma A form of protozoa, e.g. *T. gondii* causing toxoplasmosis.

Toxoplasmosis A disease due to infection with *Toxoplasma gondii* manifest with pneumonitis, hepatitis, encephalitis (in the severe form) or mild fever and malaise in mild form. In congenital form the newborn may have encephalopathy, jaundice, anemia, hepatosplenomegaly and generalized lymphadenopathy.

Trabecula Fibrous cord of connective tissue extending into an organ from its capsule or wall.

Trace 1. Very small quantity. 2. A visible mark or sign.

Trace elements Organic elements normally present in minute quantity but very essential for plant or animal life.

Tracer An isotope which due to its unique physical properties, can be detected in extremely minute quantity, and hence is used to trace the chemical behavior of natural element; used in absorption and excretion studies for identifying intermediary products of metabolism and determination of distribution of various substances in the body. Commonly used tracers are ^{14}C and ^{131}I.

Trachea The round cartilaginous air tube extending from larynx to bronchi (6th cervical to 5th dorsal vertebra).

Trachealis Smooth muscle fibers extending between the ends of tracheal rings whose contraction narrows the lumen.

Tracheal ring C-shaped fibrous rings of trachea.

Tracheal tug The downward tugging movement of larynx in thoracic aortic aneurysm.

Tracheitis Inflammation of trachea.

Trachelectomy Amputation of uterine cervix.

Trachelitis Inflammation of cervix.

Trachelology Scientific study of neck, its diseases and injuries.

Tracheobronchomegaly Congenital enlargement of trachea and bronchi.

Tracheocele Protrusion of tracheal mucous membrane through its wall.

Tracheomalacia Softening of cartilaginous framework of trachea.

Tracheostomy Surgical opening up of trachea to put an airway to facilitate respiration in laryngeal obstruction or a condition requiring prolonged respiratory assistance (*see* Figure).

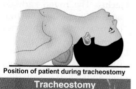

Position of patient during tracheostomy

Tracheostomy

Tracheotomy tube A tube inserted in trachea to get control of breathing obstruction.

Trachitis Inflammation of trachea.

Trachoma A form of chronic follicular conjunctivitis caused by *Chlamydia trachomatis*.

Tracing A graphic record of some events like respiration, electrical activity of heart and brain.

Tract 1. A pathway. 2. Bundle of nerve fibers within spinal cord or brain acting as an anatomical and functional unit.

Traction The act of drawing or pulling. *t. axis* Traction in line with the long axis of the part. *t. aneurysm* An aneurysm due to traction on artery, e.g. traction on aorta by an incompletely atrophied ductus. *t. diverticulum* A circumscribed sacculation usually of the esophagus due to pull of adhesions. *t. headache* Pain arising from traction on intracranial structures by tumors, hematoma, abscess, etc.

Tract of Schuz Periventricular tract.

Tractotomy Surgical section of a tract in CNS, e.g. for pain relief.

Tragus Cartilaginous projection in front of external auditory meatus.

Training 1. An organized system of instruction. 2. Systematic exercise for physical development or some specialized aim.

Trait A characteristic or property of an individual.

Tramadol Anti-inflammatory pain killer.

Trance The state of hypnosis resembling sleep or a state of being mentally out of touch with the environment.

Trandolapril ACE inhibitor.

Tranquilizer A drug reducing mental tension and anxiety without interfering with normal mental activity.

Transabdominal Across the abdominal wall or through the abdominal cavity.

Transaminase An enzyme that catalyzes transamination, i.e. transfer of amino group of an amino acid to a ketoacid. *t. glutamic-oxaloacetic* (SGOT) Highest concentration in heart muscle and liver; hence raised in myocardial infarction and hepatitis. *t. glutamic-pyruvic* Highest concentration in liver. Injury to hepatic cells liberates the enzyme to bloodstream.

Transamination Resuscitation by mouth to mouth respiration.

Transatrial Procedure done through or across the atrium.

Transcortin A corticosteroid binding globulin.

Transcriptase A polymerase that transcripts by converting a DNA base sequence into its complementary RNA base sequence.

Transcription The DNA directed synthesis of messenger RNA.

Transcutaneous nerve stimulation (TNS) Application of mild electrical stimulation to skin electrodes placed over a painful area to block transmission of pain sensation into CNS.

Transducer Device that converts one form of energy into another, e.g. ultrasonic transducers that convert sound energy to electrical energy.

Transection Cutting across the long axis.

Transexamic acid Antifibrinolytic agent used to stop bleeding.

Transfer factor A factor present in antigen sensitized lymphocytes.

Transferrin Iron transporting globulin in plasma.

Transfixion The act of piercing through and through.

Transfixion sutures A method of closing a wound by the use of suture which is placed through both wound edges in a figure of eight fashion.

Transformation Change of shape or form, in oncology the change of one tissue into another; a type of mutation occurring in bacteria.

Transfusion Injection of blood, blood products or IV solutions into vein. *t. exchange* Transfusion of blood and withdrawal of blood at same time until blood volume is entirely replaced as in hemolytic disease of newborn.

Transfusion reaction A variety of reactions including fever, chill, hemolysis, jaundice, shock and anaphylaxis occurring during transfusion.

Transgrow A special medium for culture of *N. gonorrhea*.

Transient ischaemic attack (TIA) Symptoms of neurological deficit lasting for few hours without residual damage due to transient interference with blood supply to brain.

Transillumination Inspection of a cavity or organ by passing a light through its wall, e.g. examination of paranasal sinus by means of a light placed across mouth; examination of hydrocele contents in scrotum and examination of brain in hydrocephalus in infants.

Transition Passing from one state or position to another.

Translation Protein synthesis under direction of RNA.

Translocation The displacement of part or whole of chromosome to another.

Translucent Permitting a partial transmission of light; somewhat transparent.

Transmethylation Transfer of a methyl group from a donor to a receptor compound. Methionine and choline serve as donors of methyl group.

Transmigration A wandering across or through as that of ovum or leukocytes across the capillary wall.

Transmissible Capable of being transmitted from one person to another; communicable, infectious.

Transmission Transfer of anything; like disease or hereditary characteristics. *t. mechanical* Passive transfer of causative agent of disease, especially by arthropods, e.g. fly-borne diseases. *t. placental* Transmission of disease from mother to fetus via the placenta. *t. synaptic* The mechanism by which an impulse in one neurone gives rise to impulse in another neurone. *t. transovarian* Transmission of a diseased agent to offspring from mother from infection of ovary of latter as in ticks and mites.

Transmural Across a wall, e.g. myocardial infarction involving full thickness of wall in a given area.

Transparent Permitting passage of light rays without obstruction.

Transpeptidase An enzyme that catalyzes the transfer of a peptide from one compound to another.

Transplant To transfer tissue or organ from one part to another.

Transplantation The operation of transplanting an organ or tissue from one person to another, e.g. heart, lung, kidney, liver and bone marrow. *t. heteroplastic* Transplantation of a part from one individual to another of the same or closely related species. *t. heterotopic* Transplantation in which transplant is placed in a different location in host than it had in donor.

Transport Movement or transfer of substances in biological system; transport may be active, passive or carrier mediated.

Transposition A change in position of an organ or viscera usually to opposite side.

Transposition of great vessels A congenital cardiac anomaly where aorta arises from right ventricle and pulmonary artery from left ventricle.

Trans-sexual An individual who has overwhelming desire or feels psychically to be of opposite sex or has got his external sex changed by surgery.

Transudate A fluid that passes through the capillary wall.

Transudation Oozing of fluid through the membrane.

Transurethral An operation performed through urethra, e.g. transurethral prostatectomy.

Transverse arrest In obstetrics, arrest of transverse axis of descending fetal head in maternal pelvis.

Transverse mesocolon The transverse portion of mesentery connecting transverse colon with posterior abdominal wall.

Transverse myelitis Inflammation of spinal cord involving entire cord substance at a particular level, usually of unknown etiology.

Transverse sinus A sinus of dura mater running from internal occipital protuberance along attached margin of tentorium cerebelli to reach jugular foramen.

Transvestism Dressing or masquerading in the clothing

of opposite sex to be accepted as a member of opposite sex.

Tranylcypromine An antidepressant of MAO inhibitor group.

Trapezium The first bone of the second row of carpal bones.

Trapezius The muscle arising from occipital bone, nuchal ligament and the spines of thoracic vertebra and inserted into clavicle, acromion and spine of scapula.

Trauma A physical injury or wound caused by external force or violence. *t. psychic* A painful emotional experience.

Trauma score A numerical grading system that assesses neurological and cardiopulmonary functions to assess severity of trauma and prediction of survival.

Traumatology The branch of surgery dealing with wounds and their care.

Tray A flat surface with raised edges. *t. impression* In dentistry U shaped receptacle to carry impression material and support it in contact with teeth.

Trazodone Antidepressant.

Treacher Collins syndrome Mandibulofacial dysostosis.

Treatment Any specific procedure employed for amelioration of a disease or pathological condition. *t.*

empiric Treatment based on observation and experience rather than having a scientific basis. *t. expectant* Relief of symptoms that arise during an illness but treatment not directed at specific cause of illness. *t. palliative* Symptomatic treatment rather than a cure.

Trematoda A class of flat worms commonly known as flukes.

Tremble Involuntary shaking or quivering.

Tremor Involuntary movement resulting from alternate contraction of opposing muscle groups. *t. action* Tremor when voluntary motion is attempted. *t. alcoholic* Visible tremor in alcoholics. *t. cerebellar* Intention tremor of 3-5 Hz frequency seen in cerebellar disease. *t. essential* Benign tremor usually of head, chin, outstretched hands, 8-10 cycles per second, made worse by anxiety and action, usually familial. *t. flapping* Coarse tremor with momentary loss of tone in muscle groups followed by return of tone. *SYN*—asterixis, seen in hepatic encephalopathy. *t. parkinsonian* A rest tremor which is suppressed briefly during voluntary activity, usually pill rolling type. *t. physiologic* Tremor occurring in normal persons during anger, anxiety, fatigue and hypoglycemia.

Tremulous Trembling or shaking.

Trench fever The disease caused by *Rickettsia quintana,* transmitted by body louse.

Trench foot A condition akin to frost bite due to keeping of feet in wet socks and shoes for prolonged period.

Trench mouth Painful pseudomembranous ulceration of mucous membrane of mouth.

Trend The tendency to proceed in a certain direction.

Trendelenburg's position Position in which patient's head is low and the legs are on an elevated and inclined position.

Trendelenburg's sign A pelvic drop on the side of elevated leg indicating weakness of gluteus medius when one stands on one leg.

Trephination The process of cutting a piece of bone from skull by a trephine.

Trephine A cylindrical saw for cutting circular piece of bone out of skull.

Trepidation Fear, anxiety, trembling motion.

Treponema A genus of spirochetes causing infections in man, e.g. syphilis (*T. pallidium*), pinta (*T. carateum*), frambesia (*T. pertenue*).

Tretinoin Transretinoic acid used topically for acne.

Triacetin Antifungal agent used topically.

Triad Any three things having or denoting something in common.

Triage The screening and classification of sick, wounded or injured during war or disaster to assign priority for medical and nursing attention.

Triamcinolone Synthetic glucocorticoid used for skin conditions.

Triamterene A potassium sparing diuretic.

Triangle An area formed by three angles and three sides.

Triangular bandage A bandage folded diagonally.

Triangular ligament The ligaments left and right connecting right and left lobes of liver with corresponding portions of diaphragm.

Triatoma A genus of blood sucking bugs, one variety of it transmits *Trypanosoma cruzi,* causative agent of Chaga's disease.

Triazolam Benzodiazepine anxiolytic.

Tribadism A condition where women attempt to imitate

heterosexual intercourse with each other.

Tribasic Composed of three replaceable hydrogen atoms.

Tribe A taxonomic division between genus and family.

Tribromoethanol An anesthetic agent.

Tricarboxylic acid cycle The metabolic cycle of pyruvic acid breakdown for production of energy; the terminal pathway where by fats, carbohydrates and proteins are utilized.

Triceps A muscle arising by three heads.

Triceps reflex Extension of forearm on tapping the triceps tendon while the elbow is flexed.

Trichiasis Inwardly directed eye lashes that rub against cornea.

Trichinella A genus of nematode. *Trichinella spiralis* of this genus causes trichinosis from ingestion of undercooked pork containing the cyst.

Trichinellosis Disease caused by *Trichinella spiralis* SYN − trichinosis. Symptoms are swelling of face, firm, tender swollen muscles, fever and eosinophilia.

Trichloracetic acid The caustic agent used for cauterization of warts, condylomata and hyperplastic tissue.

Trichlorethylene Inhalational anesthetic that supplements nitrous oxide.

Trichobezoar A hair ball in the stomach.

Trichogen An agent stimulating hair growth.

Trichology Study of hair, its growth and care.

Tricholine Hepatic stimulant.

Trichomatosis Entangled matted hair due to fungal disease.

Trichomonas Genus of flagellated protozoa. *T. hominis* Intestinal flagellate causing diarrhea and bacillary dysentery like disease. *T. vaginalis* Flagellate inhabiting vagina causing profuse white watery often blood stained discharge and intense itching (*see* Figure).

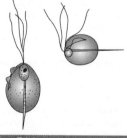

Trichomonas vaginalis

Trichomycosis Any fungal disease of hair.

Trichophytobezoar A hair ball found in the stomach along with vegetable fiber and other debris.

Trichophyton Parasitic fungus living on skin or its appendages.

Trichorrhexis Splitting of hair.

Trichosis Any disease of the hair and its abnormal growth at some abnormal place.

Trichosporon A genus of fungi growing on hair.

Trichotilomania Unnatural impulse to pull out one's own hair.

Trichromatic Able to differentiate three primary colors, which means normal color vision.

Trichuriasis Infestation with *Trichuris trichura.*

Trichuris trichura A nematode that inhabits large intestine and causes diarrhea and abdominal pain.

Tricitrates oral solution Solution of sodium citrate, potassium citrate and citric acid.

Triclophos sodium A sedative-hypnotic preparation.

Triclosan Gum antiseptic.

Tricuspid Having three cusps, e.g. tricuspid valve, tricuspid tooth.

Tricuspid atresia Congenital atresia of tricuspid valve with cyanosis and clubbing.

Tricuspid valve Right atrioventricular valve.

Trident Having three prongs.

Tridihexethyl chloride An anticholinergic agent.

Triethylenemelamine One member of nitrogen mustard group of antineoplastic agent.

Triethylenethiophosphoramide An alkylating agent used in cancer chemotherapy. *SYN* – thiotepa.

Trifluoperazine An antipsychotic agent (Espazine).

Trifluperidol Antipsychotic.

Triflupromazine Antipsychotic agent used mainly for nausea and vomiting (Siquil).

Trifluridine Antiviral agent.

Trifurcation Division into three branches.

Trigeminal nerve The fifth cranial nerve, the sensory-motor nerve dividing into 1. ophthalmic (supplies upper part of face, nasal mucosa, cornea and conjunctiva). 2. maxillary (supplies gums and teeth of upper jaw, upper lip and orbit) and 3. mandibular supplying muscles of mastication, gum and teeth of lower jaw.

Trigeminal neuralgia Neuralgic pain (burning and tingling) in distribution of trigeminal nerve due to any lesion of Gasserian ganglion or compression of its large sensory root by an aberrant artery and often idiopathic.

Trigger To initiate with suddenness. An event or impulse that initiates other events or actions.

Trigger finger A state when finger flexion or extension is accomplished with a jerk due to tenosynovitis.

Trigger zone Any area of hyperexcitability in the body which when stimulated precipitates a specific response, e.g. epileptic fit or an attack of neuralgia.

Triglyceride Combination of glycerol with three different fatty acids.

Trigone A triangular area at the base of bladder, i.e. between the two openings of ureter and internal urinary meatus.

Trigonitis Inflammation of mucous membrane of the trigone of bladder.

Trihexyphenidyl hydrochloride An anticholinergic drug used in parkinsonism.

Tri-iodothyronine T_3, the active form of thyroid hormone.

Trikates A mixture of potassium acetate, potassium bicarbonate and potassium citrate.

Trilabe A three pronged forcep for removing foreign body from bladder.

Trilaminar Three layered.

Trilobate Having three lobes.

Trilocular Having three compartments.

Trilogy A series of three events.

Trimeprazine tartarate Antipyretic agent.

Trimester A block of 3 months.

Trimetazidine Antianginal coronary vasodilator.

Trimethadione An anticonvulsant.

Trimethaphan Ganglion blocking agent used for treatment of hypertension.

Trimethobenzamide An antiemetic drug.

Trimethoprim Antibacterial agent used for urinary tract infection; when combined with sulfamethoxazole causes sequential block in enzyme synthesis within a wide range of bacteria.

Trimethylene Cyclopropane, the general anesthetic agent.

Trimipramine Tricyclic antidepressant.

Trimmer Instrument used to cut and shape things like gingiva, dental plaster.

Trimorphous Having three different forms like larva, pupa and adults as in insects.

Trinitroglycerol Nitroglycerin, the vasodilator.

Trinitrophenol *SYN* − Picric acid, reagent.

Trinitrotoluene *SYN* – TNT, an explosive.

Triose A monosaccharide with 3 carbon atoms.

Trioxsalen Agent that induces repigmentation, hence used in vitiligo.

Trip Hallucinatory experience produced by various drugs.

Tripelenamine citrate An antihistaminic agent.

Tripier's amputation Amputation of foot with part of calcaneus.

Triple response The three basic response of skin to injury like redness, flare and wheal.

Triplet Three children in one pregnancy.

Triploidy Having three supports or legs.

Tripod Having three sets of chromosomes.

Tripolidine hydrochloride An antihistaminic drug.

Tripotassium dicitrato bismuthate Bismuth compound used in peptic ulcer.

Triptorelin GnRH analog.

Triquetrum Three cornered or triangular, e.g. cuneiform bone.

Triradiate Radiating in three directions.

Trismus Tonic spasm of jaw muscles as in tetanus.

Trisomy Having three homologous chromosomes instead of two.

T13 Trisomy of chromosome 13 manifest with hypertelorism, low set ears, mental retardation and death during infancy.

T21 Down's syndrome with simian crease, sloping forehead, epicanthic folds, Brush field's spots, flat nose and mental retardation.

Trisulfapyrimidines A combination of sulfamerazine, sulfamethazine and sulfadiazine.

Tritanopia Blue blindness.

Tritium Heavier form of hydrogen.

Trituration The act of making a substance into powdered form.

Trivalent Combining with or replacing three hydrogen atoms.

Trocar The instrument which is contained within the cannula for removal of fluid from body cavity.

Trochanter Bony processes. *t. greater* Outward projection at upper end of femur below its neck. *t. lesser* Conical tuberosity at the inner and posterior surface of upper end of femur at the junction of shaft and neck (*see* Figure on page 734).

Troche Solid cylindrical form containing medicine. *SYN* – Lozenge.

Trochlea 1. The smooth articular surface of bone upon

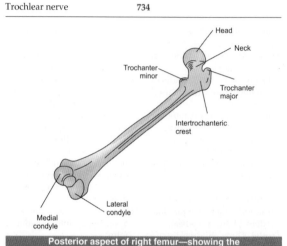

Posterior aspect of right femur—showing the greater and lesser trochanters

which glides another bone. 2. A structure having the function of pulley.

Trochlear nerve The fourth cranial nerve emerging from dorsal surface of midbrain and supplying superior oblique muscle.

Trombicula A genus of mite that may serve as vectors for various diseases.

Tromethamine *SYN*—THAM. A systemic alkalizer used in lactic acidosis.

Trophic Relating to nutrition of a part particularly when denervated.

Trophoblast The outermost layer of developing embryo consisting of inner cytotrophoblast and outer syntrophoblast that comes in contact with uterine endometrium.

Trophocyte The supporting cells of Sertoli which nourish the developing spermatozoa.

Trophology The science of nutrition.

Trophozoite The active mobile feeding state of protozoa.

Tropia Deviation of eyes away from visual axis: esotropia means inward; exotropia outward; hypertropia upward and hypotropia downward.

Tropicamide An anticholinergic drug used for producing mydriasis as 2% lotion.

Tropin When suffixed indicates stimulating effect especially of a hormone on target tissue.

Tropism Involuntary response of an organism like turning towards or away from a stimu-lus.

Tropomyosin A muscle protein involved in the formation of cross bridges during muscle contraction.

Troponin A muscle protein that attaches to actin and myosin. It binds to calcium and inhibits actin-myosin cross bridge formation. Elevated troponin T/I occurs in myocardial infarction.

Trousseau's sign Muscle spasm or tetany induced by pressure on the nerve, indicative of latent tetany (*see* Figure).

True conjugate (diameter of pelvic inlet) The distance from posterior surface of symphysis pubis to sacral promontory (11 cm).

Truncus A general term in anatomical nomenclature for a major, undivided and usually short portion of nerve, blood vessel, lymphatic vessel

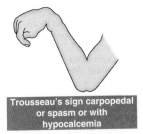

Trousseau's sign carpopedal or spasm or with hypocalcemia

or duct. *t. arteriosus* the embryonic vessel that forms aorta and pulmonary arteries. *t. bronchomediastinalis* right and left lymphatic vessels in chest draining lungs and parasternal lymph nodes, the left ending in thoracic duct and right into right lymphatic duct. *t. costocervicalis* an artery arising from subclavian dividing into deep cervical and intercostal arteries. *t. coeliac* arises from aorta and divides into left gastric, common hepatic and splenic arteries. *t. jugular* right and left draining deep cervical lymph nodes, ending on right side into right lymphatic duct and on left side into thoracic duct. *t. sympathetic* two nerve trunks on either side of vertebral column extending from base of skull to coccyx.

Trunk The main stem of lymphatic, nerve or blood vessel.

The middle portion of body without head and limbs.

Truss Device to occlude hernial orifica.

Trypanosoma A genus of flagellate protozoa found in blood, e.g. *T cruzi* causing Chaga's disease and *T. rodesiense* causing African sleeping sickness.

Tryparsamide An arsenic compound used in sleeping sickness.

Trypsin Proteolytic enzyme formed by action of enterokinase on pancreatic trypsinogen.

Trypsinogen Inactive form of trypsin found in pancreatic juice.

Tryptophan An essential amino acid, the precursor of serotonin.

Tsetse fly Blood sucking fly of genus glossina, transmitter of trypanosomiasis.

Tsutsugamushi fever Scrub typhus. *t. tube* A tube placed in common bile duct after cholecystectomy for bile drainage and cholangiography.

Tube A long hollow cylindrical structure. *t. endotracheal* A tube usually with an inflatable cuff put into trachea for airway during anesthesia. *t. nasogastric* Rubber tube passed into stomach for aspiration/ decompression of stomach. *t. stomach* A wide bore tube for stomach wash in poisoning.

Tubectomy Surgical removal of a part or whole of fallopian tube.

Tuber A swelling or enlargement.

Tuber cinereum A part of base of hypothalamus connected to posterior lobe of pituitary by an infundibulum.

Tubercle 1. A small rounded elevation on bone or skin. 2. Tubercular granuloma.

Tuberculin A preparation from human tubercle bacilli, used for diagnostic test of previous exposure to tubercular infection.

Tuberculin test A test to know if a patient has been exposed to tubercle bacilli in the past. 5 or 10 TU is injected intradermally and induration is measured after 72 hours. When induration exceeds 10×10 mm the test is termed positive.

Tuberculoma A tuberculous abscess.

Tuberculum A small emience. *t. adductor* A projection from medial condyle of femur to which adductor magnus is attached. *t. dental* Elevation on crown of a tooth due to excess enamel formation. *t. epiglottis* Posterior projection of epiglottic cartilage. *t. gracile* An enlargement of nucleus gracilis in the medulla oblongata on lateral border of fourth ventricle. *t. iliac* A prominence on iliac crest 2" behind anterior superior iliac spine. *t. labriaus superioris* Tubercle of upper lip, the central prominent. *t. major humerus*. Greater tubercle of humerus giving attachment to supra and infraspinatus. *t. mental* Prominence on either side of mental protruberance of mandible. *t. scaphoid* Scaphoid tubercle giving attachment to transverse carpal ligament. *t. quadrate* Quadrate tubercle of femur giving attachment to quadratus femoris. *t. trigeminal* An elevation on caudal posterior medulla oblongata due to descending spinal tract of trigeminal nerve.

Tuberculosis An infectious disease caused by *Mycobacterium tuberculosis* having propensity to infect lungs, bone, GU tract, meninges and the GI tract.

Tuberosity An elevated bony process, e.g. ischial tuberosity.

Tuberous sclerosis A neurocutaneous disorder with adenoma sebaceum, seizure, mental retardation, periventricular nodules.

Tubocurarine A skeletal muscle relaxant used during anesthesia and in convulsive states and to treat black-widow spider bite.

Tubo-ovarian Relates to fallopian tube and the ovary.

Tuboplasty Plastic surgery or repair of fallopian tubes inorder to restore fertility.

Tubule A small tube. *t. collecting* Tubules having transport function in renal medulla. *t. convoluted* The constituent parts of a nephron of kidney. *t. seminiferous* Very small tubules in testis in which the spermatozoa develop and leave the testis to enter the epididymis.

Tubulin A protein present in the microtubules of cell.

Tubulodermoid A dermoid tumor in the persistent remnant tubular structure.

Tuft A small coiled mass or cluster.

Tugging Drag or pull e.g., tracheal tug, the sign of aortic aneurysm.

Tularemia A plague like illness caused by *Francisella tularensis*, transmitted to man by bite of infected tick or direct contact with infected animal (Tulare: a place in California).

Tumescence Swelling.

Tumor A swelling or enlargement. *t. benign* That lacks properties of invasion and metastasis, is encapsulated with less anaplasia. *t. Brenner* Solid benign tumor of ovary resembling fibroma. *t. brocon* Giant cell granuloma of bone occurring in osteitis fibrosa cystica of hyperparathyroidism. *t. carcinoid* Vascular tumor of bronchus or GI tract, often invasive and malignant. *t. carotid body* Chemodectoma of carotid body, a benign tumor often causing dizziness. *t. germ cell* Group of tumors arising from primitive germ cell of testis or ovary. *t. glomus* Benign painful tumor of glomus body, usually at nail bed. *t. Grawitz* Renal cell carcinoma; gland containing large cells, usually benign. *t. Hurthle cell* Tumor of thyroid. *t. Klatskin's* Hilar cholangiocarcinoma. *t. Krukenberg* A form of carcinoma of ovary metastatic from stomach. *t. Leydig cell* Most common nongerminal tumor of testes. *t. phylloides* Large fibroadenoma of breast with sarcoma like stroma. *t. Pott's puffy* Edema surrounding osteomyelitis of skull. *t. Wilms'* Malignant mixed tumor of kidney occurring in children.

Tumor angiogenesis factor A protein factor present in all cancerous tissue which stimulates capillary growth.

Tumoricidal Having killing effect on tumor cells.

Tumor markers Certain substances present in blood that indicate possible presence of malignancy, e.g. carcinoembryonic antigen in tumors of colon, lungs and breast; alfa-fetoprotein in hepatoma, acid phosphatase in prostatic malignancy.

Tumor necrosis factor A lymphokine produced by macrophages.

Tumor viruses Viruses causing malignant neoplasms, e.g. EB virus linked to Burkitt's lymphoma; HSV_2 in cancer cervix, AIDS virus in Kaposi sarcoma.

Tunga A genus of fleas.

Tungsten A metallic element used in X-ray tube.

Tunica A covering. *t. adventia* The outer fibrous coat of blood vessels. *t. intima* The innermost layer of endothelial cells and the basement membrane including the internal elastic lamina of blood vessels. *t. media* The middle layer in the wall of a blood vessel containing circular smooth muscle and elastic fibers. *t. serosa* The mesothelial lining of the pleura, peritoneum and pericardium. *t. vaginalis* The serous membrane surrounding the testes.

Tuning fork A vibrating metallic instrument for testing hearing and sensation of vibration.

Tunnel A narrow channel. *t. carpal* The fibro osseous canal in the wrist through which pass the flexor tendons and the median nerve. *t. tarsal* The osteofibrous canal bounded by flexor retinaculum and tarsal bones giving way to posterior tibial vessels, tibial nerve and flexor tendons.

Tunnel vision 1. Severe constriction of visual field as in chronic glaucoma 2. A condition in hysterics where the field of vision remains the same irrespective of the distance from the visual screen.

Tuohy needle A needle used for inserting epidural catheters. It is slightly curved at the end.

Turbid Cloudy.

Turbidity The quality of not having transparency of liquid

due to contamination or suspended particles.

Turbinate Shaped like inverted cone.

Turgor Normal tension in a tissue, swelling.

Turner's syndrome 45 (XO) chromosomal pattern in girls manifested with amenorrhea, infertility, short stature and poor sexual maturation (*see* Figure).

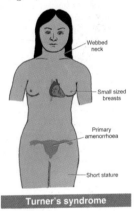

Webbed neck

Small sized breasts

Primary amenorrhoea

Short stature

Turner's syndrome

Turpentine A pine plant derivative containing mixture of terpenes and other hydrocarbon used in liniments and counter irritants.

Tutamen Tissue with protective action, e.g. tutamen oculi, i.e. eyebrows, eyelashes, etc. *t wave* The positive or negative wave representing repolarisation of heart muscle in electrocardiogram.

Twig A final branch of a nerve or vessel.

Twilight sleep A state of partial anesthesia where perception of pain is greatly reduced.

Twin Two fetuses developing within uterus in one pregnancy. *t. dizygotic* Twins developed from two separate ova. *t. monozygotic* Twins developing from a single fertilized ovum; hence have identical genetic makeup, are of same sex, have common placenta and one chorion sac. *t. siamese* Symmetrically united twins.

Twitch Sudden spasmodic muscle contraction.

Tyloxapol A detergent used to reduce viscosity of bronchopulmonary secretions.

Tympanic membrane Membrane at the junction middle ear and external ear.

Tympanitis Inflammation of middle ear.

Tympanography Radiographic examination of eustachian tubes and middle ear after introducing contrast material.

Tympanometry Procedure for objective evaluation of mobility of tympanic membrane

and diagnosis of middle ear diseases.

Tympanoplasty Surgical procedure for middle ear disease or reconstruction.

Tympanum The middle ear or tympanic cavity.

Tympany 1. Abdominal distension with gas. 2. Tympanic resonance on percussion.

Typhlectomy Excision of cecum.

Typhlitis Inflammation of cecum.

Typhlology Study of blindness and its causes.

Typhlopexy Suturing of movable cecum to anterior abdominal wall.

Typhloureterostomy Implantation of ureters into cecum.

Typhoid Resembling typhus.

Typhoid fever Acute infectious fever with inflamed Peyer's patches and mesenteric glands, enlarged spleen and continuous fever; caused by *Salmonella typhi*.

Typhoid vaccine Vaccine containing killed *Salmonella typhi*.

Typhus A group of acute infectious fevers with severe headache, prostration, maculopapular rash, and some neurologic involvement caused by Rickettsia organisms. *t. epidemic* Caused by *R. prowazekii*, transmitted by body louse. *t. endemic* Caused by *R. mooseri,* transmitted by rat flea. *t. scrub* Caused by *R. tsutsugamushi,* transmitted by mites.

Typing Identification of types, e.g. 1. Bacteriophage typing, i.e. determination of bacterial species by bacteriophages. 2. Tissue typing, i.e. testing for histocompatibility of tissues to be used in transplant or graft.

Tyramine An intermediate product during conversion of tyrosine to epinephrine, found in cheese, beer, yeast, beans, wine and chicken liver.

Tyrosinage An enzyme that converts tyrosine into melanin.

Tyrosine An amino acid serving as precursor for epinephrine, thyroxine and melanin.

Tyrosinemia Increased tyrosine concentration in blood due to deficiency of enzyme tyrosine aminotransferase manifested with mental retardation, keratitis, dermatitis, etc.

Tyrothricin Antibacterial agent.

Tyson's glands Modified sebaceous glands in prepuce secreting smegma.

Tzanck test Examination of tissue from base of an intact bulla to demonstrate degenerative changes as in pemphigus.

U

Ubiquinone Coenzyme Q, important for intracellular respiration.

Ulcer Discontinuity in the skin or mucous membrane with sloughing. *u. Curling* Stress induced peptic ulcer as in post-burn or cerebrovascular accident patient. *u. decubitus* Ischemic necrosis and tissue ulceration over bony prominence in bedridden patients. *u. Hunner's* Painful slowly healing ulcer in urinary bladder. *u. rodent* Deeply infiltrating ulcer with undermined edges as in basal cell carcinoma.

Ulceration Formation of ulcer on surface such as skin, cornea or mucous membrane.

Ulna The inner and larger bone of forearm (see Figure).

Ultrafiltration A filtration process that separates colloidal particles from the suspending liquid.

Ultrasonic Sound frequency above 20,000 cycles per second, not audible to human ear.

Ultrasonography Use of ultrasound to image body organs.

Ultrasound Sound frequency in the range of 20,000 to 10^9 cycles per second, employed

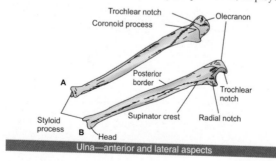

Ulna—anterior and lateral aspects

to image body organs and for therapeutic purposes (ultrasonic ablation/stone dissolution).

Ultrastructure Structure of tissue as visible only under electron microscope but not to normal eye.

Ultraviolet rays Light rays in the spectrum of 3900-1800 angstroms.

Ultraviolet therapy Treatment with ultraviolet radiation.

Umbilical cord The cord consisting two arteries and one vein embedded in Wharton's jelly attaching fetus to placenta.

Umbilication Formation at the apex of a vesicle or pustule a depression (e.g., in smallpox), any depression resembling the navel.

Umbilicus The navel or depression in the center of abdomen.

Umbo Projecting center of a round surface.

Umbrella filter A filter placed in a vein to prevent passage of emboli as in prevention of pulmonary infarction in deep vein thrombosis.

Uncal herniation Transtentorial herniation of uncus.

Unciform Shaped like a hook.

Unciform fasciculus The bundle of fibers connecting frontal lobes with temporal lobes (uncinate fasiculus).

Unciform process Anterior end of hippocampal gyrus.

Uncinate Hook shaped.

Uncinate bundle of Russel Fibers from cerebellum passing into vestibular nuclei via superior cerebellar peduncle.

Uncinate fits Periodic episodes of olfactory and gustatory hallucinations usually disagreeable or loss of taste and smell.

Uncinate gyrus Rostral portion of hippocampal gyrus.

Unconditioned reflex Natural reflex which is independent of previous experience or training.

Unconscious Lacking awareness of surrounding.

Uncus Hooked anterior end of hippocampal gyrus.

Undecylenic acid A fungistatic 11-carbon acid.

Undernutrition Malnutrition occurring either due to inadequate food intake or body's inability to utilize the nutrients.

Underweight Weight more than 10% less than the ideal weight for height and age.

Undine A small glass or metal flask for irrigation of eyes.

Undine curse Sleep apnea.

Undulant fever See brucellosis.

Undulation Continuous wave like motion or pulsation.

Ungual Resembling nails.

Unguentum Ointment.

Unicorn Having a single horn or cornu as in uterus.

Unicuspid Having a single cusp, e.g. tooth or valve.

Unilateral Affecting or occurring at one side.

Uninucleated Having a single nucleus.

Uniocular Pertains to one eye.

Union Meeting of two or more things at one point.

Uniparous Giving birth to one offspring at a time.

Unipolar Having a single process, e.g. unipolar neurone.

Unit A standard of measurement. *u. angstrom* Wave length of 1/10,000, 000 of a millimeter. *u. CH50* amount of complement that will lyse 50% of sheep RBCs coated with antibody. *u. Hounsfield* Unit of X-ray attenuation used for CT scan where air is-1000, water is 0 and compact bone is 1000. *u. motor* A neurone and the muscle cells innervated by it. *u. Todd* The reciprocal of the highest dilution that inhibits hemolysis as in measurement of antistreptolysin O titre in rheumatic fever.

Univalent Capable of combining with or replacing one atom of hydrogen.

Universal antidote Two parts of activated charcoal, one part magnesium oxide and one part tannic acid used in poisoning by unknown agents by oral route.

Universal cuff An adaptive device fitted on the palm to hold items such as utensils when normal grasp is not present.

Universal donor A person of blood group 'O' Rh-ve.

Universal recipient A person of blood group AB, Rh positive.

Unmedullated A nerve without myelin sheath. *SYN* – unmyelinated.

Unna's paste 15% Zinc oxide in glycogelatin base.

Unsaturated Not combined to the full extent or capable of dissolving or absorbing more.

Upper motor neuron lesion Damage to corticospinal or pyramidal tracts in the brain or spinal cord causing paraplegia, hemiplegia or quadriplegia upon location of lesion.

Upper respiratory infection Infection involving nasopharyngeal tissues and bronchi.

Uptake Absorption of nutrient or radioactive material.

Urachus A fibrous cord extending from apex of bladder to umbilicus. Often urachus remains patent resulting in an umbilical urinary fistula.

Uracil A pyrimidine base of ribonucleic acids.

Uranium A radioactive element.

Urate A salt of uric acid.

Urea The diamide of carbonic acid derived from ammonia by deamination representing 80-90% of total urinary nitrogen.

Urea cycle The metabolic process of urea formation from metabolism of nitrogen containing foods.

Urea frost Deposits of urea particle on skin in patients of advanced uremia.

Urea plasma A microorganism is sexually transmitted and causes urogenital infection in both partners.

Urease An enzyme that breaks down urea into ammonia and carbondioxide.

Uremia A complex biochemical abnormality in kidney failure, characterized by azotemia, acidosis, anemia and many systemic symptoms. *u. prerenal* Uremia occurring not primarily due to kidney disease but due to fluid loss.

Ureter 28-34 cm fibromuscular tubes conveying urine from kidney to urinary bladder (see Figure).

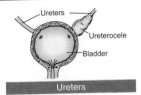

Ureters

Ureterocele Dilatation of ureter near its opening into bladder.

Ureteroileostomy Anastomosis of ureter into a segment of small intestine.

Ureterolithiasis Formation of stone in ureter.

Ureterovesicostomy Reimplantation of ureters into bladder.

Urethane Compound with diuretic, hypnotic and cytostatic properties, often used in leukemia.

Urethra The canal extending from bladder neck to exterior for discharge of urine.

Urethritis Inflammation of urethra. *u. anterior* Inflammation of anterior portion of urethra (portion anterior to triangular ligament).

Urethroplasty Repair of urethra as in stricture.

Urethroscope An instrument for visualization of interior of urethra.

Urgency A sudden, irresistible need to urinate.

Uric acid An end product of purine metabolism responsible for clinical manifestations of gout.

Uricase An enzyme present in most mammals excluding man that breaks uric acid into allantoin and carbon dioxide.

Uricemia Excess uric acid in blood.

Uricosuria Excessive excretion of uric acid in urine.

Uricosuric Agents that potentiate excretion of uric acid in urine.

Uridine A nucleoside of ribonucleic acids, consisting of uracil and D ribose.

Urinalysis Diagnostic analysis of urine sample.

Urinary calculus Concretions formed in urinary passage of calcium carbonate/phosphate/oxatate, uric acid and cystine.

Urinary incontinence Inability to control urination.

Urinary pigments Urochrome, urosilin, uroerythrin and hematoporphyrin.

Urinary retention Inability to empty the bladder of urine.

Urinary sediment Deposits in urine like bacteria, phosphates, uric acid, calcium oxalate/phosphate/carbonate, etc.

Urinary tract infection Infection involving urethra, bladder, ureter and renal pelvis.

Urination The act of voiding urine.

Urine The fluid excreted by kidneys with a specific gravity of 1005-1030, acidic in reaction and amber colored; 24 hour urine contains nearly 75 grams of solids, i.e., 25% as urea, 25% as chloride, 25% as sulfates.

Urinoma A cyst containing urine.

Urinometer Device for measuring specific gravity of urine.

Urobilin A brown pigment formed by oxidation of urobilinogen, a breakdown product of bilirubin.

Urobilinogen A colourless degradation product of bilirubin formed by action of intestinal bacteria.

Urobilinuria Excess of urobilin in the urine.

Urocele Swelling of scrotum with urine.

Urochesia Act of passing urine from the anus.

Urochrome A yellow pigment in urine derived from urobilin.

Urocyanin A blue pigment in urine in certain diseases like scarlet fever.

Urodynamics Study of bladder function both neural and muscular.

Urodynia Pain while passing urine.

Uroerythrin A red pigment found in urine.

Uroflavin A fluorescent compound present in persons taking riboflavin.

Urofuscin A red-brown pigment in urine of patients of porphyria.

Urogastrone A polypeptide present in urine that inhibits gastric acid secretion.

Urogenital diaphragm The sheet of tissue stretching across the pubic arch, formed by deep transverse perineal and sphincter urethrae muscles. *SYN* – triangular ligament.

Urography X-ray study of urinary tract after introduction of radiopaque dye. Can be ascending type: dye is injected into bladder or descending type: the dye is given IV and is excreted by the kidneys.

Urokinase An enzyme obtained from human urine used for coronary, pulmonary and peripheral thrombolysis.

Urolithiasis Formation of calculi in urinary tract and the associated symptoms thereof.

Urology The branch of medicine concerned with diseases of urinary tract.

Uroporphyrin A red pigment present in urine and feces in porphyria.

Urticaria Eruption of itchy wheals on skin. *u. pigmentosa* Brown itchy eruptions of mastocytosis. *u. solaris* Urticaria on exposure to sunlight.

Usher's syndrome Congenital deafness and retinitis pigmentosa progressing to complete blindness.

Uta Infection with *Leishmania braziliensis* causing nasopharyngeal and mucocutaneous lesions.

Uterine souffle The sound of blood flow in uterine vessels in gravid uterus.

Uterine subinvolution Failure of uterus to return to its normal size after childbirth.

Uterus The womb, the seat of embryo's imbedment and growth; a hollow muscular pelvic organ (*see* Figure on page 748).

Utricle 1. One of two sacs of the membranous labyrinth in the bony vestibule of inner ear, communicating with semicircular ducts, sacculus and endolymphatic duct. 2. Any small sac. *u. of prostate* A small blind pouch of urethra extending into substance of prostate, a remnant of embryonic mullerian duct.

Uvea The vascular pigmented coat of the eye lying beneath

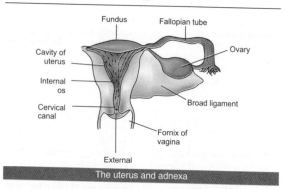

The uterus and adnexa

the sclera and consisting of iris, ciliary body, choroid.

Uveitis Inflammation of uvea or any part of it. *u. anterior* Inflammation of iris and ciliary body. *u. posterior* Choroiditis.

Uveoparotitis Inflammation of uvea and parotid glands as in sarcoidosis.

Uviometer An instrument for measuring the intensity of ultraviolet light.

Uvula A small fleshy structure hanging from soft palate (*see* Figure).

Uvulotome Instrument for performing uvulotomy.

U wave A low-amplitude positive wave that follows T-wave

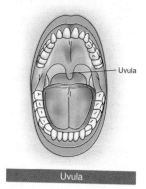

Uvula

in ECG. U-wave inversion indicates coronary artery disease.

V

Vaccination Inoculation with a vaccine to achieve resistance against an infectious disease.

Vaccine A suspension of live attenuated/killed infectious agent or its products/parts for achieving immunity against that infectious agent. *v. BCG Bacille Calmette-Guérin,* a preparation of dried live-culture of *Mycobacterium tuberculosis* whose virulence has been reduced by repeated cultures on glycerinated ox bile. *v. DPT* A preparation of diphtheria and tetanus toxoid and killed pertussis organisms given intramuscularly. *v. hepatitis B* Vaccine containing recombinant viral capsular antigen of hepatitis B virus. *v. human diploid cell* An inactivated rabies virus vaccine prepared in human diploid cell tissue culture. *v. influenza* A polyvalent vaccine containing inactivated antigenic variants of the virus for rendering immunity in chronically ill and aged. *v. measles* A live attenuated virus vaccine. *v. mumps* A live attenuated virus vaccine. *v. pneumococcal* A polyvalent vaccine effective against 23 strains of pneumococci, given to children under 2 years of age and to those who have undergone splenectomy. *v. polio* Oral poliovaccine containing 3 types of live attenuated (v. Sabin) or inactivated viruses (v. Salk).

Vaccine therapy A therapy in which infectious organisms, particles, or antigens are injected in body to develop immunity against a disease.

Vaccinia Cowpox, the vesicopustular disease of cattles.

Vacuole A clear space in the cell protoplasm.

Vacuum Empty space.

Vacuum extractor A device with a suction cup which is placed on fetal head for applying traction during delivery.

Vacuum aspiration A method of termination of pregnancy by applying suction to a catheter placed in uterine cavity.

Vagabond's disease Body louse infection causing itching and skin discoloration.

Vagal tone Cardiac inhibitory effect by vagus.

Vagina The musculomembranous passage between the cervix and vulva.

Vaginal bulb Small erectile tissue on each side of vestibule.

Vaginal hysterectomy Surgical removal of uterus through vagina.

Vaginal lubricant An ointment or cream which is used for reduction of dryness in vagina.

Vaginal vibrator A vibrator placed in vagina for erotic stimulation.

Vaginismus Painful spasm of vagina often preventing coitus; may be idiopathic, following trauma, vaginitis or psychological aversion to coitus.

Vaginitis Inflammation of vagina causing purulent malodorous discharge, itching, pain in perineum, and during coitus and painful micturition. *v. atrophic* Atrophy of vagina in post-menopausal women with reduced introitus and dryness. *v. Trichomonial* Vaginitis due to Trichomonas causing red frothy discharge with fishy odor.

Vaginodynia Pain in vagina.

Vaginoplasty Plastic surgery of the vagina.

Vagitus First cry of a newborn child.

Vagotomy Section of vagus nerve in treatment of peptic ulcer syndrome *V. super selective* section of vagal branches supplying gastric mucosa.

Vagus See tenth cranial nerve.

Valacyclovir L-valyl ester of acyclovir, antiviral for herpes.

Valdecoxib Anti-inflammatory, analgesic.

Valenthamate Uterine relaxant.

Valgus Outward bending; V-cubitus – the forearm in deviated outwards.

Valproic acid Anticonvulsant.

Valsalva maneuver Forcible expiration against closed glottis, nose, and mouth; used to increase pressure within middle ear to correct retracted ear drum.

Valsalva sinuses The dilatations in the root of aorta behind the semilunar cusps where the coronary arteries originate.

Valsartan ACE receptor inhibitor.

Valve Membranous structures that allow flow of fluid in one direction (see Figure on page 751).

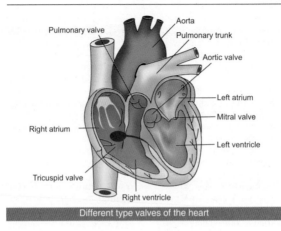

Different type valves of the heart

Valves of Houston Mucosal folds of rectum. *v. ileocecal* Valve between ileum and large intestine (cecum) composed of two membranous folds. *v. thebesian* Valves at the entrance of coronary sinus into right atrium.

Valvoplasty Dilatation of valve.

Valvotomy Incision into a valve to dilate it.

Valvulae conniventes Circular membranous folds in the lumen of small intestine that retard the passage of food thereby promoting absorption of nutrients. *SYN*—plica circularis.

Vancomycin hydrochloride Antibiotic given IV 1-2 gm daily, specific for resistant staphylococcal infection.

Van den Bergh's test Blood test for detection of bilirubin.

Vanilla Obtained from tropical orchid, an aromatic substance used for flavoring.

Vanilylmandelic acid (VMA) Metabolite of epinephrine and norepinephrine in urine, amount increased in pheochromocytoma.

Vapor Gaseous state of a substance.

Variance In statistics, the square of standard deviation.

Variant Having some different characteristic from the original.

Varicella Chickenpox, the viral disease with polymorphic maculo-vesico-pustular eruptions.

Varicella-zoster immune globulin An immunoglobulin isolated from human volunteers with high antibody titer against varicella-zoster virus.

Varicocele Dilated pampiniform plexus in the spermatic cord, commonly on left side, feeling like a bag of worms.

Varicose Means distended, tortuous and knotted.

Varicose veins Dilated tortuous veins as developing in legs due to venous incompetence or the development of esophageal varices in portal hypertension.

Varicosity The condition of varicose.

Varicotomy Excision of varicose vein.

Variola *SYN*—smallpox, the vesicopustular generalized eruptive viral disease that has disappeared from the globe for past two decades.

Varix Dilatation of a vein, artery or lymphatic channel.

Varus Turned inward.

Vas A duct. *v. deferens* The 18″ long excretory duct of testis transporting sperm to urethra.

Vasa Pleural of vas. *v. recta* 1. Straight collecting tubules of kidney. 2. Tubules that become straight prior to entering the mediastinum testis. *v. vasorum* The tiny blood vessels supplying the fibromuscular coats of arteries and larger veins.

Vascularity A condition of being vascular.

Vascularization Growth of new blood vessels in a structure.

Vascular ring A form of congenital anomaly where an arterial ring surrounds trachea and esophagus often causing compression.

Vasculature The arrangement and interrelationship of blood vessels.

Vasculitis Inflammation of blood or lymph vessels.

Vasculopathy Any disease of blood vessels.

Vasectomy Removal of a segment of vas deferens bilaterally to induce male sterility.

Vasoactive Causing either constriction or dilation of blood vessels.

Vasoactive intestinal polypeptide (VIP) A peptide of G.I. tract that inhibits gastric acid secretion but promotes intestinal secretion, excess secretion causing diarrhea.

Vasoconstriction Spasm or temporary narrowing of blood vessels.

Vasodepressor An agent that depresses circulation, i.e. lowers blood pressure by dilating blood vessels.

Vasodilator Agent causing relaxation of blood vessels.

Vasointestinal polypeptide A gut hormone increasing gut moility and secretion.

Vasomotor Pertains to or regulating the contraction and relaxation of blood vessels.

Vasomotor system Part of the nervous system which controls the constriction or dilation of blood vessels.

Vasopressin A posterior pituitary hormone having antidiuretic, and vasopressor effect (causes coronary spasm, hence not used to raise blood pressure).

Vasopressor Agent bringing about contraction of blood vessels.

Vasospasm Spasm of blood vessels.

Vasovagal syncope Sudden fainting due to hypotension caused by emotional stress, pain or trauma.

Vasovasostomy Rejoining of torn vas deferens of testis.

Vastus Large or great; one of the three muscles of thigh.

Vector 1. A carrier or disease transmitting living organism like arthropod or insect. 2. A force having a magnitude and direction.

Vectorcardiography Analysis of direction and magnitude of electrical forces of cardiac contraction by a continuous series of loops (Vectors), especially useful in diagnosing infarction in the presence of left bundle branch block.

Vecuronium Neuromuscular blocking agent.

Vegan A strict vegetarian who even abstains from milk and milk products.

Vegetate 1. To lead a passive existence either mentally or physically 2. Luxuriant growth.

Vegetation Wart like luxuriant growth from heart valves; consisting of fibrin mesh with enmeshed blood cells.

Vegetative Quiscent, passive.

Vehicle A therapeutically inactive substance that carries the active ingredient.

Vein Vessel carrying unsaturated blood towards the heart except for pulmonary veins that carry saturated oxygenated blood to left atrium.

Velamentous Expanding like a veil or sheet.

Velamentum Membranous covering.

Vellus The fine hair left on the body after the lanugo hairs disappear in the newborn.

Velpeau's bandage A special form of roller bandage incorporating shoulder, arm and forearm.

Veneer In dentistry, materials like acrylic resin which is bonded to surface of tooth.

Venereal Resulting from sexual intercourse.

Venereal disease Disease acquired by sexual intercourse. It includes gonorrhea, syphilis, AIDS, viral hepatitis B, trichomoniasis, chlamydia infection, granuloma inguinale and lymphogranuloma venereum (LGV).

Venereal wart Moist reddish elevations on genitals and anus.

Venereologist A specialist of study of the causes and treatments of sexually transmitted diseases.

Venereology The branch of medical science dealing with diagnosis and treatment of venereal disease.

Venesection Surgical incision into a vein for draining out blood or introducing blood/colloids.

Venipuncture Puncture of a vein for drawing out blood or introducing any substance.

Venlafaxine Antidepressant.

Venogram X-ray of the vein by introduction of contrast material.

Venom Poisonous secretion expelled by some animals, reptiles. *v. snake* The poisonous secretion of labial glands of snake containing neurocytolysins, hemolysins, hemocoagulants.

Venomous Poisonous.

Venoocclusive Pertains to obstruction of veins, e.g. venoocclusive disease of liver.

Venotomy Act of making incision in vein.

Venous hum A continuous murmur heard on veins of neck.

Vent An opening in any cavity.

Ventilation Circulation of fresh air in lung alveoli. *v. continuous positive pressure* Mechanical method of artificial ventilation where the respirator delivers air to the lungs under a continuous positive pressure. *v. intermittent positive pressure* The respirator delivers air under positive pressure to initiate inspiration but expiration is passive.

Ventilation coefficient The amount of air that must be respired for each liter of oxygen to be absorbed.

Ventilator A mechanical device to ventilate the lungs (*see* Figure).

Ventouse Cup shaped.

Ventral Anterior or front side or lower or underneath.

Ventral hernia Hernia through anterior abdominal wall.

Ventricle A small cavity or pouch, e.g. in the heart and in the brain. *v. third* The median cavity of brain bounded by thalamus and hypothalamus on either side, anteriorly by optic chiasm; communicating with lateral ventricles and fourth ventricle. *v. fourth* The CSF containing cavity at base of brain extending between upper end of spinal canal and cerebral aqueduct. Its roof is formed by cerebellum and floor by rhomboid fossa. *v. lateral* The ventricle in each cerebral hemisphere with triangular shaped body, inferior and posterior horns; communicating with third ventricle by interventricular foramen.

Ventricular escape Temporary assumption of pacemaker function by the ventricles either due to complete AV block or sinus standstill.

Ventricular folds The false vocal cords or folds of mucous

Endotracheal tube goes through patient's mouth and into the windpipe

Nasogastric tube goes through patient's nose and into the stomach

Mechanical ventilator blows air, with increased oxygen, through tubes into the patient's airways

Nurse periodically checks the patient

Air flowing to the patient passes through a humidifier, which warms and moistens the air

Exhaled air flowing away from the patient

Ventilator

membrane parallel or above true vocal cords.

Ventricular septal defect A congenital defect in the inter-ventricular septum of heart leading to passage of blood from left ventricle into right ventricle.

Ventriculitis Inflammation of ependymal lining of cerebral ventricles.

Ventriculoatriostomy Establishment of communication between cerebral ventricle and right atrium by placement of a shunt to treat hydrocephalus.

Ventriculocisternostomy Establishing communication between cerebral ventricle and cisterna magna.

Ventriculography Visualization of size and shape of cerebral ventricles by air injection or visualization of size, shape and contraction of ventricles of heart after contrast injection.

Ventriculostomy Establishing communication between third ventricle and cisterna interpeduncularis to treat hydrocephalus.

Ventrolateral Both ventral and lateral.

Ventromedial Both ventral and medial.

Ventrosuspension Fixation of displaced uterus to anterior abdominal wall.

Venturi mask A mask for controlled administration of O_2.

Venule A tiny vein continuous with capillary.

Verapamil Calcium channel blocker; antiarrhythmic agent.

Verbigeration Repetition of meaningless words.

Verge An edge or margin, e.g. anal verge, i.e. the transitional area between smooth perianal area and the hairy skin.

Vermicidal Capable of destroying intestinal worms or parasites.

Vermicular Resembling a worm, e.g. vermicular movement.

Vermiform Shaped like a worm.

Vermiform appendix The long narrow worm shaped tube arising from cecum closed at the distal end.

Vermifuge Agents that expel intestinal worms.

Vermilion border The junction between the skin and oral mucous membrane at the lips.

Vermin Small insects and animals.

Vermination Infestation with worms.

Vermis A worm, median lobe of cerebellum between the lateral lobes.

Vernet's syndrome Paralysis of 9th, 10th and 11th cranial nerves due to injury to jugular foramen.

Vernix caseosa A sebaceous deposit covering the fetus, abundant on creases and flexor surfaces, consisting of sebaceous secretion, lanugo and exfoliated skin.

Verruca *SYN* – wart.

Versicolor Having many colours or change in colors.

Version Change in position of fetus within uterus. *v. bipolar* A combination of both external and internal manipulation to bring a change in fetal position. *v. cephalic* Turning of the fetus so that head becomes the presenting part. *v. external* Version of fetus with both hands placed on abdomen. *v. internal* Version of fetus with one hand placed inside vagina. *v. podalic* Version by holding feet of the fetus to make the presenting part breech.

Vertebra One of the 33 bony segments making up the spinal column, consisting of 7 cervical, 12 thoracic (dorsal), 5 lumbar, 5 sacral and 4 coccygeal (see Figure).

Vertebral canal The cavity within spinal column containing the spinal cord.

Vertebral pedicle The portion of bone projecting backward from each side of body of vertebra and connecting the lamina with body.

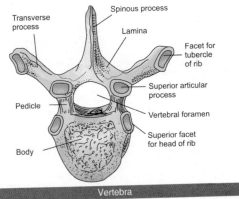

Vertebra

Vertebrate Those having a vertebral column.

Vertex The top portion of head.

Vertical Perpendicular to the horizontal plane, upright.

Vertiginous Afflicted with vertigo.

Vertigo The sensation of moving around in space (subjective vertigo) or experiencing the surrounding objects moving around oneself (objective vertigo).

Verumontanum An elevation on the floor or the prostatic urethra where seminal ducts open.

Very low-density lipoprotein (VLDL) The least dense plasma lipid.

Vesica A bladder.

Vesical Shaped like a bladder.

Vesical reflex Desire to urinate once bladder is distended.

Vesicant Agent that produces blisters.

Vesicle Elevated skin lesions containing serous fluid. *v. seminal* Membranous sacculated tubes at the base of bladder acting as reservoir of semen.

Vesicopustule A vesicle in which pus has formed.

Vesicostomy Surgical opening into bladder.

Vesicouterine pouch Extension of peritoneal cavity downwards between bladder and uterus.

Vesicovaginal Concerning urinary bladder and vagina.

Vesiculectomy Partial or complete excision of seminal vesicle.

Vesiculitis Inflammation of seminal vesicle.

Vesiculogram X-ray of seminal vesicles.

Vessel A duct or canal to carry fluids.

Vestibular apparatus The anatomical parts including saccule, utricle, semicircular canals, vestibular nerve and nuclei, concerned with body equilibrium.

Vestibular area A triangular area lateral to sulcus limitans, beneath which lie the terminal nuclei of vestibular nerve.

Vestibular bulbs Two sacculated collection of veins lying on either side of vagina homologous to male corpus spongiosum.

Vestibular nerve The main division of eighth cranial nerve, arising from vestibular ganglion and concerned with body equilibrium.

Vestibule Small cavity or space at the beginning of a canal.

Vestige A small incompletely developed structure.

Veterinary Pertains to animal diseases and their treatment.

Viability Ability to live or capable of living, e.g. a fetus reaching 24 weeks gestation or 500 gms of weight can live outside uterus.

Vial A small glass bottle for medicines and chemicals.

Vibrator Device that produces vibration or shaking.

Vibratory sense The ability to perceive vibrations or that transmitted through skin and bone from a vibrating tuning fork.

Vibrio A genus of comma shaped motile gram-negative bacilli, e.g. *V. cholerae,* the organism causing cholera.

Vibrometer 1. A device that produces rapid vibrations of tympanic membrane, a form of massage to treat deafness. 2. Device used to measure vibratory sensation threshold, useful in judging clinical status of peripheral neuropathy.

Vicarious Acting as alternative or substitute.

Vicarious menstruation Blood loss during menstruation at sites other than vagina like nose, breast.

Vidarabine Antiviral agent effective against herpes simplex and zoster.

Vidian artery Artery passing through pterygoid canal.

Vidian canal A canal in the medial pterygoid plate of sphenoid bone for passage of vidian vessels and nerve.

Vidian nerve A branch from sphenopalatine ganglion.

Vigil Wakefulness.

Vigilant Being attentive, watchful and alert.

Vigor Force or strength of body and mind.

Villiferous Having villi or tuft of hair.

Villus Short slender filamentous processes found on some membranous surfaces. *v. arachnoid* Protrusion of arachnoid into dural venous sinus. *v. chorionic* Tiny branching processes on surface of chorion that become vascular and form placenta. *v. intestinal* The projecting structures into lumen of small intestine that help to absorb fluid and nutrients (*see* Figure on page 760).

Vinblastine An extract from plant vinca rosea having cytotoxic properties.

Vincent's angina Acute necrotising gingivitis.

Vincristine sulfate A cytotoxic agent extracted from plant vinca rosea.

Vindesine Vinca alkaloid, antineoplastic agent.

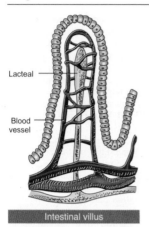

Intestinal villus

Vinegar A weak solution of acetic acid.

Vinorelbine Anticancer agent.

Vinyl chloride A chemical often causing lung malignancy.

Violaceous Violet, said of a discoloration of skin.

Violent Great force, fierceness.

Viomycin Antibiotic produced by *Streptomyces griseus*, used in tuberculosis.

Vipoma A rare tumor of pancreas secreting vasoactive polypeptide causing diarrhea, achlorhydria.

Virchow cell Lepra cell.

Virchow's node Supraclavicular lymphnode.

Virchow-Robin space Perivascular spaces.

Virchow's angle The angle formed by joining the naso-frontal suture and the most prominent point on superior alveolar process with the line joining the same point and superior border of external auditory meatus.

Viremia Presence of viruses in bloodstream.

Virgin Woman who has had no sexual intercourse; uncontaminated, fresh.

Virginity The state of being virgin.

Viricide Destructive to viruses.

Virile reflex Contraction of bulbocavernosus muscle on percussing dorsum of penis or compressing the glans penis.

Virilism Appearance of male secondary sexual characteristics in female.

Virility Sexual potency in male; state of possessing masculine qualities.

Virilization Masculine changes in female like appearance of moustache and beard, atrophy of breast, enlarged clitoris, male voice and male type baldness.

Virion A complete virus particle.

Viroids Small naked virus genome without a dormant phase.

Virology The study of viruses and viral diseases.

Virulence Degree of pathogenicity.

Virulent Highly infectious.

Virus Minute submicroscopic organisms with a central core of DNA or RNA and a capsid but no cell wall. They utilize the cell metabolic processes for their nutrition and replication. *v. cytomegalic (CMV)* A member of the herpes virus group transmitted transplacentally from mother to fetus with mental retardation and hepatosplenomegaly in the newborn. *v. enterocytopathogenic human orphan (ECHO)* Virus responsible for epidemic pleurodynia, meningoencephalitis, myocarditis, etc. *v. immunodeficiency* The RNA virus containing reverse trancryptase that confers its capacity to change the antigenicity indefinitely and hence the difficulty in producing a successful vaccine. It causes the dreaded disease AIDS for which there is no cure. *v. respiratory syncytial* The virus causing lower respiratory infection in infancy and childhood and that produces large syncytial masses in cell cultures.

Viscera Internal body organs.

Visceral Relating to viscera.

Visceroptosis Downward displacement of a viscus.

Viscid Sticky, adhering, gummy.

Viscosity 1. The state of being sticky or gummy. 2. Resistance of a fluid medium to changeability due to existing intermolecular force.

Vision Act of seeing external objects; sense by which light and color are perceived.

Visual acuity A measure of the resolving power of eye. A normal person is able to read letters at a distance of 20 feet that subtend angle of 5°.

Visual evoked response A test for entactness of visual pathway from retina to visual cortex through analysis of latency and amplitude of waves recorded in response to visual stimuli.

Vital capacity The quantity of air that can be expelled following deep inspiration.

Vitality The state of being alive, vigor.

Vital signs The traditional signs of life: like pulse, blood pressure, respiration, urination.

Vital statistics Statistics relating to birth, death, marriage, sickness, etc.

Vitamin Micronutrients essential for metabolism, growth and development.

Vitamin A Fat soluble vitamin derived from carotenes (alpha, beta and gamma) in food, responsible for growth, development and integrity of epithelial tissues, and functioning of Rhods, the visual sensory cells that contain visual purple for dim vision.

Vitamin B$_1$ Thiamine, an essential coenzyme for decarboxylation of pyruvate to acetyl coenzyme.

Vitamin B$_2$ Riboflavin; constituent of flavoproteins responsible for tissue oxidation.

Vitamin B$_6$ Pyridoxine, a coenzyme for over 60 different enzyme systems, required for heme synthesis and neuroexcitability.

Vitamin B$_{12}$ Cyanocobalamin, essential for cytoplasmic maturation of red cells and intactness of neurones.

Vitamin C Ascorbic acid, a factor essential for integrity of intercellular cement in many tissues, especially capillaries.

Vitamin D One of several vitamins (D$_2$, D$_3$, D$_4$, D$_5$) that have antirachitic property. Vitamin D$_2$ (calciferol) D$_3$ (irradiated 7 dihydrocholesterol), D$_4$ irradiated 22 dihydro ergosterol, D$_5$ (irradiated dehydrositosterol), all are essential for calcium and phosphorus metabolism.

Vitamin E Tachysterol (alpha tocopherol), which prevents oxidation of polyunsaturated fatty acids in cell membranes.

Vitamin K Naphthoquinone derivative that helps in synthesis of prothrombin in liver.

Vitamin supplement A tablet or capsule comprising of one or several vitamins.

Vitellin An egg yolk protein containing lecithin.

Vitelline duct The duct connecting yolk sac with the embryonic gut.

Vitelline veins Two veins carrying blood from yolk sac.

Vitellus The yolk of an ovum.

Vitiligo A skin depigmentary disorder of unknown etiology.

Vitrectomy Removal of vitreous.

Vitreous Transparent jelly like mass that fills the posterior chamber, enclosed by hyaloid membrane.

Viviparous Giving birth to young alive offspring rather than larvae or embryo.

Vocal apparatus Parts of human body that produce speech. These include the lips, tongue, teeth, hard and soft palates, uvula, larynx and pharynx.

Vocal cord Two thin mucous folds in larynx enclosing vocal ligaments responsible for production of sound.

Vocal fold The thin edges of vocal cords.

Vocal fremitus Palpable vibration on chest wall while patient speaks.

Vocal muscle The inner portion of thyroarytenoid muscle which lies in contact with vocal ligament.

Vocal process The part of arytenoid cartilage to which are attached the vocal cords.

Voice Sound produced in human beings by vibration of vocal cords.

Void To evacuate bladder and bowel.

Volar Relates to palm of hand and sole of foot.

Volatile Easily evaporable.

Volition The act or power of willing or choosing.

Volkmann's canals Vascular channels in compact bone, not surrounded by concentric lamellae as are haversian canals.

Volkmann's contracture Fibrosis, shortening and atrophy of muscles following ischemia.

Volley The discharge of a number of nerve stimuli in quick succession.

Volsella Forceps with one or more hooks at the end of each blade.

Volt The unit of electromotive force which when applied to a conductor with resistance of one ohm produces a current of one ampere.

Voltage Difference in potential expressed in volts.

Volume The space occupied by a substance. *v. expiratory reserve* The maximal amount of air that can be expelled after normal expiration. *v. inspiratory reserve* The maximal amount of air that can be inspired after end of normal inspiration. *v. mean corpuscular* The mean volume of an average erythrocyte, 80-90 fentoliter. *v. minute* Amount of air inspired in one minute. *v. packed cell* The volume of packed RBCs in a centrifuged sample of blood. *SYN*—hematocrit, normal range—42-47%. *v. residual* Volume of air remaining in the lungs after maximal expiration. *v. stroke* Amount of blood ejected from ventricle per one beat. *v. tidal* Volume of air inspired and expired in one normal respiratory cycle.

Voluntary muscle Any muscle whose contraction and relaxation is controlled by will.

SYN – Stripped, Skeletal muscles.

Voluptuous Pleasures of senses.

Volvulus Twisting of bowel upon itself causing obstruction to lumen and even blood supply of the segment leading to necrosis (*see* Figure).

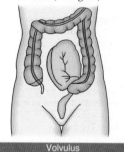

Volvulus

Vomer A thin plate of vertical bone forming posterior part of nasal septum, articulating with ethmoid and sphenoid bones.

Vomit Ejected material from stomach, the act of ejecting such material. *v. bilious* Bile ejected in vomits. *v. coffee ground* Blood mixed gastric content vomited as in bleeding peptic ulcer and erosive gastritis.

Vomiting The act of ejection of gastric contents through mouth.

Vomitus Material ejected by vomiting.

Von Gierke's disease Glycogen storage disease due to absence of glucose-6-phosphates resulting in hypoglycemia and acidosis.

Von Graefe's sign Failure of lid to roll downward on looking down as in thyrotoxicosis.

Von Recklinghausen's disease 1. Neurofibromatosis. 2. Hemochromatosis. 3. Generalized osteitis fibrosa cystica.

von-Willebrand's disease A congenital bleeding disorder due to factor VIII deficiency.

Voracious Having insatiable appetite.

Voriconazole Antifungal.

Vorinostat Antilymphoma drug.

Vortex A structure having whorled or spiral appearance.

Vorticose veins Four veins receiving all blood from choroid and emptying into posterior ciliary and superior ophthalmic veins.

Voyeurism Satisfaction obtained from observing nude persons or sexual activity of others.

Vuerometer Apparatus for measuring interpupillary distance.

Vulgaris Common or ordinary.

Vulnerable Susceptible to injury of any kind.

Vulnerate To wound.

Vulsellum A forcep with hook on each blade.

Vulva The external genital organ in female consisting of labia majora, labia minora, clitoris, vestibule and vaginal opening.

Vulvectomy Excision of vulva.

Vulvitis Inflammation of vulva.

Vulvodynia Nonspecific pain around vulva with itching and difficult intercourse.

Vulvovaginitis Inflammation of vulva and vagina; most commonly in diabetes.

W

Waardenburg syndrome A congenital pigmentary disorder with vitiligo, heterochromic irides, and often congenital deafness.

Wafer A flat vaginal pessary.

Waist The part of human body between trunk and hips.

Wakefulness Sleeplessness.

Wald cycle Metabolic cycle of breakdown and synthesis of rhodopsin.

Waldenstrom's disease Osteochondritis deformans juvenilis.

Waldeyer's ring The lymphatic tissue encircling nasopharynx and oropharynx, consisting of two palatine tonsils, lingual and pharyngeal tonsils.

Walk Locomotion in upright posture.

Wall The limiting material/substance of a cell, artery, vein, bladder.

Wallenberg's syndrome Occlusion of posterior inferior cerebellar artery syndrome manifest with dysphagia, cerebellar dysfunction, sensory-motor disturbances.

Wallerian degeneration Degeneration of nerve fiber along with myelin sheath. The neurillema does not degenerate but forms a tube to guide growth of severed axons.

Wandering Not fixed, moving about.

Warburg apparatus A capillary manometer employed for O_2 consumption and CO_2 production studies.

Ward A large hospital room accommodating more than 4 patients.

Warfarin Anticoagulant drug (Cumadin).

Wart Hypertrophied epidermis due to papilloma virus infection.

Wash The process of cleaning the body by using water or other liquid.

Wasp A form of insects.

Wasp sting Injection of wasp venom into skin.

Wasserman reaction A complement fixation test for diagnosis of syphilis.

Waste Loss of strength; refuse no longer useful to the body; waste product.

Wasting A process of loss of weight and decreased physical vigor, appetite and mental activity.

Water bed A rubber bed filled partially with water to prevent bedsore formation.

Waterborne disease A disease caused by consumption of contaminated water.

Water hammer pulse Pulse marked by a forceful beat but sudden collapse.

Waterhouse-Friderichsen syndrome Acute adrenal insufficiency due to hemorrhage into its substance occurring in meningococcal infection.

Watson-Schwartz test A test used in acute porphyria to differentiate porphobilinogen from urobilinogen.

Watt Unit of electrical power. i.e., power produced by one ampere of current flowing with electromotive force of one volt.

Wave An undulating or vibrating motion; an oscillation seen in ECG, EEG or other graphic recordings. *w. 'a'* A wave in jugular venous pulse produced by atrial contraction and absent in atrial fibrillation. *w. 'c'* A wave in jugular venous pulse that reflects closure of tricuspid valve. *w. excitation* The excitatory impulse originating from SA node of heart and spreading to ventricles via A-V node. *w. pulse* The ejection of blood into root of aorta that causes the impact to be transmitted along the arterial wall.

Wavelength The distance of a single wave cycle measured from top of one wave to top of next wave.

Wax Any substance of animal, plant or mineral origin consisting a mixture of high molecular weight fatty acids, high molecular weight monohydric alcohols, esters of fatty acids and alcohols and solid hydrocarbons. Waxes are usually hard, brittle solid that become pliable on warming and melt on further heating.

Waxy cast Dense highly refractile urinary cast composed of amyloid material as in chronic renal disease.

Waxy degeneration 1. Amyloid degeneration. 2. Zenker's degeneration.

Waxy flexibility In psychiatry, a form of stereotypy in which the patient maintains a posture in which he is placed with wax like rigidity for a much longer period than normally tolerable as in catatonic schizophrenia.

Wean To cease to suckle or breast milk substitution by other forms of nourishment.

Web A membrane extending across a space, e.g. esophageal web causing dysphagia.

Webbed Having a membrane or tissue connecting adjacent structures, e.g. toes of duck's feet.

Webbed neck A condition in which a thick triangular fold of loose skin extends from each lateral side of neck across the upper aspect of shoulder as in gonadal dysgenesis.

Weber's test A tuning fork test for unilateral deafness. A vibrating tuning fork is placed on middle of forehead. In conductive deafness the diseased ear perceives the vibrations better.

Wegener's syndrome Glomerulitis, vasculitis, granulomatous lesions of respiratory tract which respond to corticosteroids and cyclophosphamide.

Weil-Felix test Agglutination test for diagnosis of rickettsial diseases.

Weil's disease *Leptospira ictero hemorrhagica*.

Wenckebach's phenomenon A form of incomplete heart block where there is progressive lengthening of P-R interval ending in a dropped beat.

Werdnig-Hoffmann disease Hereditary progressive infantile muscular dystrophy resulting from degeneration of anterior horn cells.

Wermer's syndrome Multiple endocrine neoplasia.

Wernicke's encephalopathy Encephalopathy with memory deficit, ocular palsy, delirium associated with thiamine deficiency of chronic alcoholism.

Wernicke's syndrome Disorientation, memory loss and confabulation often due to old age.

Western blotting A technique for analyzing protein antigens and detecting small amount of antibodies as in test of AIDS.

Westphal-Edinger nucleus A parasympathetic nucleus rostral to motor nucleus of third nerve in midbrain whose efferent fibers innervate the ciliary muscles of eye.

Wet dream Nocturnal emission of semen.

Wharton's duct Duct of submandibular salivary gland opening by side of frenum linguae.

Wharton's jelly A gelatinous connective tissue constituent of umbilical cord.

Wheal An elevation of skin with white center and pale

red periphery accompanied by itching as seen in urticaria, anaphylaxis, insect bite.

Wheelchair A chair with four wheels—two small and two big for mobility of partially paralyzed patient or transporting sick.

Wheeze A whistling or sighing sound resulting from narrowing of airway.

Whiplash injury Injury to cervical vertebra and adjacent soft tissues due to sudden jerking.

Whipple's disease Intestinal lipodystrophy characterized by abnormal skin pigmentation, fatty stool, arthritis, etc.

Whipworm *Trichuris trichura.*

Whirl To feel giddy, to revolve rapidly.

Whisky An alcoholic drink with ethyl alcohol content of 45-50%.

Whisper To speak in a low, soft voice.

Whitfield ointment Benzoic acid + salicylic acid, keratolytic, antifungal.

White cell A white blood cell.

White line The midline (linea alba) of abdomen representing the white tendinous attachments of external oblique and transversus muscles.

White matter Part of central nervous system composed of myelinated nerve fibers.

White softening Softening of any tissue in which affected area becomes white and anemic.

Whitlow Suppurative inflammation involving pulp of finger or toe often extending to bone.

Whole bowel irrigation Flushing large volumes of fluid through the gastrointestinal tract; done for treatment of poisoning.

Whoop The inspiratory crowing sound following the cough paroxysm in whooping cough.

Whooping cough Acute infectious disease caused by *Bordetella pertussis.*

Whorl 1. A type of fingerprint. 2. Spiral arrangement.

Widal test Agglutination test for diagnosis of typhoid and paratyphoid.

Will The mental faculty for control of one's actions, emotions, thoughts and deciding the actions.

Willi's circle An arterial arrangement at base of brain encircling the optic chiasma and hypophysis formed by internal carotids, anterior cerebrals, posterior cerebrals and basilar arteries.

Wilm's tumor Embryonic tumor of kidney occurring in children.

Wilson's disease Autosomal recessive hereditary disease due to disorder of copper metabolism with accumulation of copper in liver, kidney, brain and cornea producing cirrhosis of liver, brain degeneration and Kayser-Fleischer ring in cornea.

Window An aperture for admission of light and air. *w. oval* The fenestra vestibuli. *w. round* The fenestra cochleae.

Wind pipe See trachea.

Wine Fermented juice of any fruit with alcohol content of 1-5%.

Wing Any structure resembling wings of bird, e.g. greater and lesser wings of sphenoid.

Winking jaw Involuntary simultaneous closure of the eyelids as the jaw is moved.

Wintergreen oil Methyl salicylate used as counter irritant.

Wire Kirschner Steel wire placed through long bone for traction.

Wisdom tooth Third molar.

Wiskott-Aldrich syndrome Sexlinked recessive disorder of immune function with impaired T and B-cell activity, thrombocytopenia, eczema and propensity to infection.

Witche's milk Milk secreted from breast of newborn infant from stimulation by maternal LH.

Withdrawal syndrome Tachycardia, insomnia, hypotension, etc. due to abrupt abstinence from alcohol and opiates in addicts.

Wolffian body An embryonic organ on each side of vertebral column, the mesonephros.

Wolffian cyst A cyst present in the broad ligament.

Wolffian duct Duct from mesonephros to cloaca in fetus.

Wolff-Parkinson-White syndrome A cardiac rhythm disorder with short P-R interval, delta wave and propensity to supraventricular tachycardia.

Wolman's disease An inherited metabolic disease in infants with hepatosplenomegaly, adrenal calcification and foam cells in bone marrow.

Womb Uterus, the female reproductive organ for nourishing the fetus.

Wood alcohol Methyl alcohol distilled from wood is highly poisonous causing blindness.

Wood's light Ultraviolet light.

Wool fat Anhydrous lanolin obtained from sheep wool, used as base for ointment.

Woolsorter's disease Pulmonary anthrax.

Word blindness A form of aphasia where patient is

unable to comprehend written words.

Word salad Use of words with no apparent meaning or relationship to each other as in schizophrenia.

Wormian bone Small irregular bones along cranial sutures.

Wound Break in continuity of skin or any tissue caused by trauma, infection. *w. incised* Any sharp clean cut wound. *w. lacerated* Wound with ragged unhealthy margins. *w. perforating* The object causing the wound penetrates the skin, subcutaneous tissue. *w. puncture* Wound made by sharp pointed instrument. *w. tunnel* Wound with equal size entrance and exit points.

Wright's stain Combination of eosin and methylene blue to stain blood slides.

Wright's syndrome A neuromuscular syndrome caused by prolonged hyperabduction of arm leading to occlusion of subclavian artery and stretching of trunks of brachial plexus.

Wrinkles A furrow or ridge on skin.

Wrist drop Inability to extend the wrist due to paralysis of radial nerve.

Writer's cramp Cramp affecting muscles of thumb and two adjacent fingers.

Wryneck *SYN* – Torticollis, due to spastic contraction of one or more neck muscles.

Wuchereria A genus of filarial worms. *w. bancrofti* The causative agent of elephantiasis, spread by bite of culex mosquito. *w. malayi* The causative agent of filariasis in south India.

Wylie's operation Shortening of round ligament of uterus for retroflexion in combating prolapse uterus.

X

Xanthelasma Yellowish raised plaques occurring around eye lids resulting from lipid filled cells in the dermis.

Xanthine An intermediary product in transformation of adenine and guanine into uric acid.

Xanthine calculi Brown to red, hard and laminated calculi in urinary tract.

Xanthine oxidase A flavo-protein enzyme catalyzing oxidation of certain purines.

Xanthochromia Yellow discoloration of CSF due to hemolysis of RBC within it.

Xanthoderma Yellow coloration of skin.

Xanthodont Yellowness of teeth.

Xanthogranuloma A tumor having characteristics of both xanthoma and granuloma.

Xanthoma Flat, slightly elevated rounded plaque or nodule on the eyelids due to cholesterol accumulation.

Xanthomatosis Appearance of multiple xanthomas in skin due to cholesterol deposit within histiocytes and reticuloendothelial cells.

Xanthophyll The yellow pigment of egg yolk.

Xanthosis Yellow discoloration of skin in hypercarotinemia.

Xanthuria Excretion of excess of xanthine in urine.

X-chromosome The chromosome responsible for female sexual characteristic.

X-disease Poisoning caused by ingestion of nuts contaminated with aspergillus aflatoxin.

Xenobiotic An antibiotic not produced by body, i.e. foreign antibiotic.

Xenograft Graft from one species to another *SYN*—heterograft.

Xenology Study of parasites, their relationship to each other.

Xenomenia Menstruation from a part other than vagina.

Xenon An inert gas whose radio-isotope (Xe^{133}) is used for photoscintiscanning of lungs.

Xenophobia Abnormal fear for strangers.

Xenophthalmia Inflammation of the eye due to presence of foreign body.

Xephoiditis Inflammation of the xiphoid process.

Xenopsylla A genus of fleas whose member X. cheopis is a vector for asylvatic plague, endemic typhus and *Hymenolepsis nana*.

Xerasia A condition of abnormal dryness and brittleness of hair resulting in hair loss.

Xerocheilia Dryness of lips.

Xeroderma Roughness and dryness of skin. *x. pigmentosum* Pigment discoloration, cutaneous atrophy and ulcers often causing death in infancy.

Xeromammography Xeroradiography of mammary glands.

Xerophthalmia Dry conjunctiva with keratinization as in vitamin A deficiency.

Xeroradiography A X-ray technique involving a dry process where selenium covered plates are altered by the X-ray producing the image.

Xerosis Abnormal dryness of skin and mucous membrane.

Xerostomia Dryness of mouth due to poor salivary secretion.

Xerotocia Dry labor caused due to diminished amount of amniotic fluid.

Xiphisternum The pointed lower end of sternum.

Xiphoid Sword shaped.

Xiphoid process The lowest portion of sternum with a sword shaped cartilaginous process supported by bone.

X-linked disorder A disease caused due to genes located on X chromosome.

X-ray An electromagnetic radiation in wavelength of 1-100 angstrom, produced by bombarding a tungsten target within vacuum tube by fast moving electrons.

Xylene Dimethyl benzene, used as a solvent and cleansing agent in microscopy.

Xylenol Dimethyl phenol, used in preparation of coaltar disinfectants.

Xylitol An alcohol with chemical properties similar to sucrose.

Xylocaine Lidocaine, a local anaesthetic.

Xylometazoline A vasoconstrictor used in nasal decongestant drops.

Xylose A pentose sugar, nonfermentable.

Xylulose A pentose sugar occurring in nature.

Xyrospasm Spasm of wrist and forearm muscles in professionals like barbers.

Xysma The flocculent pseudomembrane seen in diarrheal stool.

XYY male A super male with tall stature and tendency for criminal behavior.

Y

Yale brace An orthotic device used for stabilizing cervical spine.

Yawning Deep inspiration with widely opened mouth induced by drowsiness, boredom.

Yaws Nonvenereal spirochaetal disease caused by *Treponema pertenue.* *y. cartilage* The cartilage connecting pubis, ileum and ischium and extending into acetabulum. *y. chromosome* The sex chromosome responsible for male sex.

Yeast Unicellular fungi of genus Saccharomyces. *S. cerevisiae* is a source of proteins and vitamin B complex.

Yellow body Corpus luteum.

Yellow fever An acute mosquito borne viral disease with fever, jaundice and hemorrhagic tendency.

Yellow spot 1. anterior end of vocal cord. 2. central point of retina, the sight of clearest vision.

Yersinia A genus of gram-negative bacteria. *y. entero colitica* Producing mesenteric lymphadentis and dysentery. *y. pestis* Causative agent of plague. *y. pseudotuberculosis* Produces pseudotuberculosis. *y. ligament* The y-shaped ligament on anterior capsule of hip joint.

Yersiniosis Infection caused due to Yersinia organisms.

Yin-yang In Chinese philosophy, opposing but complementary forces sustaining life.

Yoga A system of beliefs and practices for union of self with supreme reality.

Yogurt A form of curdled milk by lactobacilli, useful in patients with lactase deficiency.

Yohimbine A poisonous alkaloid having alpha-adrenergic blocking properties, often used as aphrodisiac and antianginal agent.

Yolk The content of ovum. *y. sac* Membranous sac surrounding food yolk in the embryo.

Young Helmoholtz theory Theory stating that retinal

colour perception depends upon 3 different sets of fibers responsible for red, green and violet.

Young's rule The formula for calculating dose of a medicine for child from known adult dose, i.e. Age/Age + 12 × adult dose.

Z

Zaleplon Benzodiazepine anti-anxiety agent.

Z axis Anteroposterior axis.

Z disk In striated muscle the dark band that bisects I bands. Actin filament is attached to Z disk and area between two Z disks in the sarcomere.

Zein A maize protein deficient in tryptophan and lysine.

Zeis' gland Sebaceous glands on eyelid margin.

Z. line A thin dark line that transversely bisects the clear zone of a muscle fiber; the distance between two z lines constitutes a sarcomere.

Zafirlukast Leukotriene antagonst for asthma.

Zenker degeneration A waxy hyaline degeneration of skeletal muscles in acute infectious diseases like typhoid fever.

Zenker's diverticula Herniation of mucous membrane of esophagus through a defect in its wall often swelling with food to cause esophageal obstruction.

Ziehl-Neelsen method A method for staining acid-fast organisms like *Tubercle bacillus* with boiled carbol fuschin followed by rinsing with alcohol.

Zieve's syndrome Transient hyperlipidemia, hemolytic anemia and jaundice following consumption of large amounts of alcohol.

Zinc A bluish white metal found as carbonate and silicate, astringent and antiseptic used in eye drops and as mineral supplement. Deficiency causes delayed ulcer healing, impaired epithelial growth, diminished fertility and acrodermatitis enteropathica. Commonly used salts are carbonate, chloride, oxide, stearate, sulfate and undecylenate.

Zinc-eugenol cement Used in dentistry for impression material, cavity liner, temporary restoration.

Zinc ointment 20% zinc oxide ointment for external application.

Zinn's ligament Connective tissue in eye to which recti are attached.

Ziprosidone Anticonvulsant.

Zirconium A metallic element used as a white pigment in dental procelain.

Zollinger-Ellison syndrome Gastrin secreting tumors causing resistant peptic ulceration at unusual site; 60% of gastrinomas are malignant.

Zona 1. A bond or girdle. 2. *SYN* – herpes zoster. *z. fasciculata* The inner layer of adrenal cortex. *z. glomerulosa* The outer layer of adrenal cortex. *z.pellucida* Inner thick membranous covering of ovum. *z. reticularis* The innermost layer of adrenal cortex.

Zonary placenta Placenta arranged like a broad ring around the chorion.

Zone An area or belt. *z. ciliary* The peripheral part of the anterior surface of iris. *z. transitional* That area of lens where the capsular epithelium changes into lens fibers.

Zonesthesia Constricting cord like sensation.

Zonular cataract Cataract where opacity is limited to certain layers of lens.

Zonule A small zone.

Zonules of zin Suspensory ligament of the lens.

Zoogeny The development and evolution of animals.

Zoogony Animal breeding.

Zoology The science dealing with animal life.

Zoonoses Diseases communicable to man from animals.

Zoonotic Concerning zoonoses.

Zoophilia Sexual gratification by intercourse with animals.

Zoophilism Abnormal love for animals.

Zoophobia Abnormal fear for animals.

Zuclopenthixol Antipsychotic agent.

Zygoma 1. The malar bone. 2. The long arch joining zygomatic processes of temporal and malar bones.

Zygomaticoauricularis Muscle that draws pinna of ear forwards.

Zygomatic process 1. A thin projection from temporal bone at its squamous portion, articulating with zygomatic bone. 2. A strong prominent lateral projection from the supraorbital margin of the frontal bone articulating with maxillary process of zygomatic bone.

Zygomatic reflex When zygoma is percussed the lower jaw moves towards percussed side.

Zygomycosis A form of mycoses that predominantly affects the face, the lungs and paranasal sinuses with thrombosis of blood vessels and infarction, common to diabetics. *SYN*—mucormycosis.

Zygospore The spore resulting from union of two similar gametes, as in certain algae and fungi.

Zygote The fertilized ovum before cleavage.

Zymase An enzyme found in yeast, bacteria and plants that can convert carbohydrate into H_2O and CO_2 aerobically or ferment it to alcohol anaerobically.

Zyme An enzyme or ferment.

Zymogen The inactive precursor of an enzyme.

Zymologist The person who specializes in the study of enzymes.

Zymology The science of fermentation.

Zymosis 1. Fermentation 2. Process by which infectious disease is supposed to develop.

Zymosterol A sterol from yeast.

Appendices

Appendix 1

Abbreviations used in prescriptions

Abbreviation	Latin	English
a.c.	ante cibum	before food
ad lib.	ad libitum	to the desired amount
b.d. or b.i.d.	bis in die	twice a day
c.	cum	with
o.m.	omni mane	every morning
o.n.	omni nocte	every night
p.c.	post cibum	after food
p.r.n.	pro re nata	whenever necessary
q.d.	quaque die	everyday
q.d.s.	quaque die sumendum	four times daily
q.i.d.	quater in die	four times a day
q.q.h.	quater quaque hora	every four hours
R	recipe	take
s.o.s.	si opus sit	if necessary
stat.	statim	at once
t.d.s	ter die sumendum	three times a day
t.i.d.	ter in die	three times a day

Appendix 2

Abbreviations for diseases, investigations and procedures

AC	Air conduction
AFB	Acid-fast bacillus
ALT	Alanine aminotransferase
ANA	Antinuclear antibodies
ANF	Antinuclear factor
APB	Atrial premature beat
AR	Aortic regurgitation
ARF	Acute rheumatic fever
AS	Aortic stenosis
ASD	Atrial septal defect
ASO	Antistreptococcal `O' titer
AST	Antistreptozyme titer
	Aspartate transaminase
ATT	Antitubercular treatment
AVM	Arteriovenous malformation
BC	Bone conduction
BPH	Benign hypertrophy of prostate
CABG	Coronary artery bypass grafting
CAD	Coronary artery disease
CHF	Congestive heart failure
CMV	Closed mitral valvotomy, cytomegalovirus
CNS	Central nervous system
COPD	Chronic obstructive lung disease
CP	Creative protein
CPK	Creatine prosphokinase
CT	Computerised tomography
Cx	Circumflex
DAT	Differential agglutination test
DCM	Dilated cardiomyopathy
DIC	Disseminated intravascular coagulation
DLC	Differential leukocyte count
ECE	Extracapsular cataract extraction
ECT	Electroconvulsive therapy

EF	Ejection fraction
ELISA	Enzyme linked immunosorbent assay
ERCP	Endoscopic retrograde cholangiopancreatography
FEV	Forced expiratory volume
FVC	Forced vital capacity
G6PD	Glucose 6-phosphate dehydrogenase
HAV	Hepatitis A virus
HBcAg	Hepatitis B core antigen
HBsAg	Hepatitis B surface antigen
HBV	Hepatitis B virus
HIV	Human immunodeficiency virus
HOCM	Hypertrophic obstructive cardiomyopathy
HSV	Herpes simplex virus
ICCE	Intracapsular cataract extraction
ICCU	Intensive coronary care unit
ICT	Intracranial tension
ICU	Intensive care unit
IHD	Ischaemic heart disease
INO	Internuclear ophthalmoplegia
ITP	Idiopathic thrombocytopenic purpura
JVP	Jugular venous pressure
LA	Left atrium
LAD	Left anterior descending artery
LDH	Lactate dehydrogenase
LIMA	Left internal mamary artery
LMN	Lower motor neurone palsy
LP	Lumbar puncture
LV	Left ventricle
LVEDP	Left ventricular end-diastolic pressure
LVEDV	Left ventricular end-diastolic volume
LVH	Left ventricular hypertrophy
MCP	Metacarpophallangeal joint
MDM	Mid diastolic murmur
MND	Motor neurone disease
MR	Mitral regurgitation, mental retardation
MRCP	Magnetic resonance cholangiopancreatography

MS	Mitral stenosis
MTP	Metatarsophallangeal joint, medical termination of pregnancy
MVI	Multivitamin infusion
MVP	Mitral valvoplasty, mitral valve prolapse
NMR	Nuclear magnetic resonance
NSAID	Nonsteroidal anti-inflammatory drugs
OS	Opening snap
PaO_2	Partial pressure of oxygen
PCWP	Pulmonary capillary wedge pressure
PDA	Patent ductus arteriosus
PIP	Proximal interphallangeal joint
PKP	Penetrating keratoplasty
PNH	Paroxysmal nocturnal haemoglobinuria
PS	Pulmonary stenosis
RA	Right atrium
RIND	Reversible ischaemic neurologic deficit
RK	Radial keratotomy
RV	Right ventricle
SAH	Subarachnoid haemorrhage
SBE	Subacute bacterial endocarditis
SCAT	Sheep cell agglutination test
SGOT	Serum glutamic oxaloacetic transaminase
SGPT	Serum glutamic pyruvic transaminase
TB	Tuberculosis
TCA	Transient ischaemic attack
TGV	Transposition great vessels
TIPS	Transjugular intrahepatic portohepatic shunting
TLC	Total leukocyte count
TOF	Tetralogy of Fallot
TR	Tricuspid regurgitation
TS	Tricuspid stenosis
TTP	Thrombotic thrombocytopenic purpura
UMN	Upper motor neurone palsy
VPB	Ventricular premature beat
VSD	Ventricular septal defect

Appendix 3

Child and infant resuscitation

Infant younger than 1 year		Child older than 1 year
Shake, pinch gently. Shout for help	Check conscious level ↓	Shake, pinch gently. Shout for help.
Head tilt. Chin tilt (jaw thrust)	Open airway ↓	Head tilt. Chin tilt (jaw thrust)
Look, listen, feel.	Check breathing ↓	Look, listen, feel.
Five breaths (mouth to mouth and nose).	Breathe ↓	Five breaths (mouth to mouth).
Feel brachial pulse. Start compression if < 60/min.	Check pulse ↓	Feel carotid pulse. If no pulse start chest compressions.
Two fingers, over sternum Rate 100/min, depth 2 cm. Five compressions: one breath.	Chest compressions	Heel of one hand, over sternum. Rate 100/min, depth 3 cm. Five compressions: one breath

Appendix 4

Cardiopulmonary resuscitation

Every nursing staff is to be well-versed with cardiopulmonary resuscitation. Many precious lives can be saved if CPR is instituted at appropriate time. The sequence of CPR is

1. Recognition of cardiopulmonary arrest
2. Activation of emergency medical system
3. Basic CPR
4. Defibrillation
5. Intubation
6. IV medications.

The nursing staff is essentially involved in the first three steps of CPR. CPR can be divided to basic life support (BLS) and advanced cardiac life support (ACLS).

Basic Life Support

ABC of basic life support is airway, breathing and circulation. Its aim is to provide oxygen to brain and heart till ACLS is delivered.

- Put the patient on a firm flat surface.
- Remove dentures if any, and extend the patient's head and lift the chin that helps to open the airway.
- Suck out any secretion in mouth. Close patient's nose and give mouth to mouth respiration.
- Continue mouth to mouth breathing for 10-12 minutes and palpate carotid pulse.
- If carotid pulse is absent, continue mouth to mouth breathing and proceed for artificial external cardiac massage.
- Place heel of one hand on dorsum of another positioned 1" above xiphoid process and compress the sternum by 1-2" for 80-100 per minute.
- If only one trained hand is available 15 chest compressions should be performed followed by two ventilations.

Advanced Cardiac Life Support (ACLS)

- When breathing is present but pulse is not palpable give a precordial blow which may convert the verticular flutter or fibrillation to a more stable rhythm.
- When patient is unconscious and breathing and pulse are not recognizable—proceed for endotracheal intubation, oxygen therapy and defibrillation. Epinephrine is well-absorbed when given through endotracheal tube.
- Try for subclavian/internal jugular vein access and start IV fluids
- Take ECG and look for the arrhythmia.

Further management is by trained CPR team with IV drugs, pacing. The decision to discontinue CPR is with the doctor.

Appendix 5

A. Food sources of water-soluble vitamins

Vitamin	Food sources
C (ascorbic acid)	Fruit—especially citrus fruit, blackcurrants Green vegetabls—especially frozen peas, tomoatoes, capsicums New potatoes
B_1 (thiamin)	Meat—especially pork, duck Cereal products—especially brown and wholemeal bread, breakfast cereals, wheatgerm Yeast, yeast extract Pulses, nuts
B_2 (riboflavin)	Dairy products, eggs Bread, fortified breakfast cereals Wheatgerm, wheatbran Mushrooms, yeast extract Liver, kidney Pulses
B_6 (pyridoxine)	Meat, fish, milk, eggs, liver Wholegrain cereals Peanuts, walnuts Bananas, avocados
B_{12} (cobalamin)	Meat—especially liver, kidney, rabbit Sardines, oysters Dairy produce, eggs
Niacin (nicotinic acid)	Meat—especially offal Fish Brewer's yeast, yeast extract Wholemeal wheat, bran peanuts, pulses, coffee
Folate (folic acid)	Liver, kidney Dark green leafy vegetables (easily destroyed by cooking) Beetroot, bran, peanuts

Vitamin	Food sources
	Avocados, bananas, oranges
	Wholemeal bread
	Eggs, chocolate
	Some fish

B. Food sources of fat-soluble vitamins

Vitamin	Food sources
A	β-carotene—orange and green vegetables, apricots, melon, egg yolk
	Preformed vitamin A—offal, dairy produce, fortified margarine, oily fish, fish liver oils
D	Fish liver oils, oily fish
	Fortified margarine
	Liver, egg yolk
	Full cream milk, cheese, butter
E	Vegetable oils—especially wheatgerm oil
	Margarine
	Eggs, butter
	Wholemeal cereals
	Broccoli
K	Green vegetables
	Liver oils
	Potatoes

C. Food sources of minerals

Mineral	Food sources
Calcium	Dairy products
	Green leafy vegetables
	Cereal products, especially wheat flour products
	Pulses
Iron*	Red meat, egg yolk
	Green vegetables,
	Wholemeal, cereal products
	Pulses

Mineral	Food sources
Sodium	Milk, table salt and in all food products except oil and sugar. Tends to be high in readymade and tinned foods
Potassium	Oranges, bananas, dried fruit Vegetables and most other foods High in instant coffee, chocolate
Iodine	Drinking water, iodized salt Seafish and shellfish Bread, spinach
Fluoride	Tea, seafish, drinking water (depending on the area)

*Absorption enhanced in the presence of vitamin C.

Appendix 6

Duration of isolation in communicable diseases

Disease	Period of communicability
Cholera	7-14 days (till stool culture –ve)
Influenza	1 week from onset
Diphtheria	2-4 weeks after onset or 2 –ve consecutive throat cultures
Yellow fever	3-4 days during illness
Typhoid	Till stool culture –ve
Chickenpox	Up to 6 days after appearance of rash
Rubella	7 days from onset
Measles	4 days before and 5 days after appearance of rash
Hepatitis A	3 weeks
Polio	2 weeks adults, 6 weeks children
Mumps	uptill the swelling subsides
Whooping cough	uptill 3 weeks after whoop appears

Appendix 7

Centigrade and Fahrenheit scales

The Centigrade (Celsius) scale is preferred.

The following table shows the relationship of the Centigrade and Fahrenheit scales, as far as is likely to be required in clinical work.

Centigrade	Fahrenheit	Centigrade	Fahrenheit
110	230	36.5	97.7
100	212	36	96.8
95	203	35.5	95.9
90	194	35	95
85	185	34	93.2
80	176	33	91.4
75	167	32	89.6
70	158	31	87.8
65	149	30	86
60	140	25	77
55	131	20	68
50	122	15	59
45	113	10	50
44	111.2	5	41
43	109.4	0	32
42	107.6	−5	23
41	105.8	−10	14
40.5	104.9	−15	5
40	104	−20	− 4
39.5	103.1	−	−
39	102.2	0.54	1
38.5	101.3	1	1.8
38	100.4	2	3.6
37.5	99.5	2.5	4.5
37	98.6		

To convert Fahrenheit to Centigrade: $X°F - 32 \times 5/9 = Y°C$
To convert Centigrade to Fahrenheit: $X°C \times 9/5 + 32 = Y°F$

Appendix 8

Birth Through	Ability to suck, swallow, gag, cry, and maintain eye contact with a person.
1st Month	The head needs to be supported. Loud noises may cause a startle reflex.
2nd Month	May turn to either side when on their backs; will follow moving objects, able to lift head but not for a sustained period; begin to smile, frown, and turn away.
3rd Month	Greater movement and vocal response to stimuli; notice own hands and suck on them; head will be steady while in a supported position.
4th and 5th Months	Able to life head higher when lying on stomach; will reach for objects and may be able to encircle a bottle with both hands; may drool a lot; attempt to put all kinds of objects in mouth.
6th-9th Month	Develop ability to grasp and pick up food; are able to pull themselves up to a sitting position and eventually will crawl; they begin to make noises that sound like words and to recognize certain words; will play peek-a-boo.
9th-11th Month	Develop ability to handle food and to drink from a cup; may imitate sounds and say certain words; crawl by pulling body along with arms, and pull themselves to a standing position; they will point at objects and throw things; they want to feed themselves and to help with dressing and undressing; they will walk while holding a person's hand.
12th Month	Can eat food alone and drink from a cup with assistance; able to move around easily, and crawl up stairs, and out of crib.

Appendix 9

Items of mini-mental state examination

Maximum Score	
	Orientation
5	What is the (year) (season) (date) (day) (month)?
5	Where are we (state) (country) (city) (hospital) (floor)?
	Registration
3	Name three objects: One second to say each. Then ask the patient all three after you have said them. Give one point for each correct answer. Repeat them until he learns all three.
	Number of trials
	Attention and calculation
5	Begin with 100 and count backwards by 7 (stop after five answers). Alternatively, spell "world" backwards.
	Recall
3	Ask for three objects repeated above. Give one point for each correct answer.
	Language
2	Show a pencil and a watch and ask subject to name them.
1	Repeat the following: "No `if's,' `and's,' or `but's.'"
3	A three-stage command. "Take a paper in your right hand; fold it in half and put it on the floor."
1	Read the obey the following: (show subject the written item). CLOSE YOUR EYES
1	Write a sentence.
1	Copy a design (complex polygonas in Bender-Gestalt).
30	Total score possible

Reprinted from Folstein MF, Folstein S, and McHugh PR. Mini-mental state: A practical method for grading the cognitive state of patients for the clinician. Journal of Psychiatric Research 1975; 12: 189-198 with permission from Pergamon Press Ltd., Headington Hill Hall, Oxford OX3 OBW, UK.

Appendix 10

Geriatric depression scale (GDS)

Choose the best answer for how you felt this past week.

*1.	Are you basically satisfied with your life?	YES	NO
2.	Have you dropped many of your activities and interests?	YES	NO
3.	Do you feel that your life is empty?	YES	NO
4.	Do you often get bored?	YES	NO
*5.	Are you hopeful about the future?	YES	NO
6.	Are you bothered by thoughts you can't get out of your head?	YES	NO
*7.	Are you in good spirits most of the time?	YES	NO
8.	Are you afraid that something bad is going to happen to you?	YES	NO
*9.	Do you feel happy most of the time?	YES	NO
10.	Do you often feel helpless?	YES	NO
11.	Do you often get restless and fidgety?		
12.	Do you prefer to stay at home, rather than going out and doing new things?	YES	NO
13.	Do you frequently worry about the future?	YES	NO
14.	Do you feel you have more problems with memory than most?		
*15.	Do you think it is wonderful to be alive now?	YES	NO
16.	Do you often feel down hearted and blue?	YES	NO
17.	Do you feel pretty worthless the way you are now?	YES	NO
18.	Do you worry a lot about the past?	YES	NO
*19.	Do you find life very exciting?	YES	NO
20.	Is it hard for you to get started on new projects?	YES	NO
*21.	Do you feel full of energy?	YES	NO
22.	Do you feel that your situation is hopeless?	YES	NO
23.	Do you think that most people are better off then you are?	YES	NO
24.	Do you frequently get upset over little things?	YES	NO
25.	Do you frequently feel like crying?	YES	NO

26.	Do you have trouble concentrating?	YES	NO
*27.	Do you enjoy getting up in the morning?	YES	NO
28.	Do you prefer to avoid social gatherings?	YES	NO
*29.	Is it easy for you to make decisions?	YES	NO
*30.	Is your mind as clear as it used to be?	YES	NO

*Appropriate (nondepressed)   Score: (Number of "depressed"
answers = yes, all other = no   answers)

	Norms
Normal	5 ± 4
Mildly depressed	15 ± 6
Very depressed	23 ± 5

Yesavage J et al. Development and validation of a geriatric screening scale: A preliminary report. Journal of Psychiatric Research 1983; 17. (Reprinted with permission from Pergamon Press PLC, Headington Hill Hall, Oxford OX3 OBW, UK)

Appendix 11

Postanesthesia recovery room chart

Postanesthesia recovery room
scoring

Patient: Final Score:
Room: Surgeon:
Date: R.R. Nurse:

Area of assessment	Point score	Upon admission	After 1 hr	After 2 hr	After 3 hr
Respiration • Ability to breathe deeply and cough • Limited respiratory effort (dyspnea or splinting) • No spontaneous effort	2 1 0				
Circulation: Systolic arterial pressure • >80% of preanesthetic level • 50% to 80% of preanesthetic level • < 50% of preanesthetic level	2 1 0				
Consciousness Level • Verbally responds to questions/oriented to location • Aroused when called by name • Failure to respond to command	2 1 0				
Color • Normal skin color and appearance • Altered skin color: pale, dusky, blotchy, jaundiced • Frank cyanosis	2 1 0				

Muscle Activity	
Moves spontaneously or on command:	
• Ability to move all extremities	2
• Ability to move 2 extremities	1
• Unable to control any extremity.	0
Totals	

Required for Discharge from Recovery Room: 7-8 points

Time of Release   Signature of Nurse

Appendix 12

Characteristics of burns according to depth

Depth of burn and causes	Skin involvement	Symptoms	Wound appearance	Recuperative course
Superficial (First-Degree)				
Sunburn Low-intensity flash	Epidermis	Tingling Hyperesthesia (super sensitivity). Pain that is soothed by cooling.	Reddened; blanches with pressure Minimal or no edema	Complete recovery within a week Peeling
Partial-Thickness (Second-Degree)				
Scalds Flash flame	Epidermis and part of dermis	Pain Hyperesthesia Sensitive to cold air.	Blistered, mottled red base; broken epidermis; weeping surface Edema	Recovery in 2 to 3 weeks. Some scarring and depigmentation Infection may convert it to third-degree
Full-Thickness (Third-Degree)				
Flame Prolonged exposure to hot liquids Electric current	Epidermis, entire dermis, and sometimes subcutaneous tissue	Pain free Shock Hematuria (blood in the urine) and possibly, hemolysis (blood cell destruction). Possible entrance and exit wounds (electrical burn)	Dry, pale white leathery, or charred Broken skin with fat exposed Edema	Eschar sloughs Grafting necessary Scarring and loss of contour and function Loss of digits or extremity possible

Appendix 13

A. Nutrition ready reckoner for international foods

	Calories (Kcal)	Proteins (g)	Fats (g)	Carbo-hydrates (g)	Fibre (mg)	Calcium (g)	Iron (mg)	Caro-tene (mcg)	Retinol (mcg)	Vit B_1 (mg)	Vit B_2 (mg)	Niacin (mg)	Vit C (mg)	Serving Portion
BEVERAGES														
Hot tea	34	0.6	1.0	5.7	0.0	31.0	0.0	0.0	7.00	0.01	0.01	0.0	0	1 Tea cup
Instant coffee	149	1.0	13.3	6.3	0.0	31.0	0.0	0.0	7.00	0.01	0.01	0.0	0	1 Tea cup
Cold coffee (with cream)	279	3.9	17.0	27.7	0.0	144.0	0.3	487.0	183.00	0.06	0.23	0.1	2	1 Tall glass
Banana milk Shake	228	6.2	7.5	33.8	0.0	223.0	0.5	40.0	101.00	0.11	0.37	0.4	7	1 Tall glass
Mango milk Shake	237	6.2	7.7	35.6	0.8	227.0	1.3	2067.0	608.00	0.15	0.41	9.0	16	1 Tall glass
Lemonade	107	0.3	0.3	25.7	0.5	21.0	0.1	0.0	0.00	0.01	0.00	0.0	12	1 glass
BREAKFAST CEREALS														
Cracked wheat Porridge	292	10.0	10.4	39.7	2.5	296.0	1.5	152.0	39.00	1.29	0.49	1.3	5	1 bowl
Oat meal Porridge	217	6.6	6.6	32.8	2.0	154.0	1.0	70.0	18.00	0.80	0.26	0.3	2	1 bowl
Cornflakes with milk	291	9.8	10.8	38.7	1.2	290.0	0.9	157.0	41.00	1.28	0.48	0.6	5	1 bowl

Contd...

Contd...

Contd...

	Calories (Kcal)	Proteins (g)	Fats (g)	Carbo-hydrates (g)	Fibre (mg)	Calcium (g)	Iron (mg)	Caro-tene (mcg)	Retinol (mcg)	Vit B₁ (mg)	Vit B₂ (mg)	Niacin (mg)	Vit C (mg)	Serving Portion
EGGS														
Boiled egg	87	6.7	6.7	0.0	0.0	25.0	0.7	300.0	180.00	0.05	0.20	0.1	0	1 Egg
Poached egg	87	6.7	6.7	0.0	0.0	25.0	0.7	300.0	180.00	0.05	0.20	0.1	0	1 Egg
Fried egg	160	6.7	14.8	0.0	0.0	25.0	0.7	620.0	260.00	0.05	0.20	0.1	0	1 Egg
Scrambled egg	172	6.7	15.8	0.8	0.0	57.0	0.7	620.0	267.00	0.06	0.22	0.1	0	1 Egg
Baked egg	124	6.7	10.8	0.0	0.0	25.0	0.7	460.0	220.0	0.05	0.20	0.1	0	1 Egg
Fluffy omelette	160	6.7	14.8	0.0	0.0	25.0	0.7	620.0	260.00	0.05	0.20	0.1	0	1 Egg
Cheese and Mushroom omelette	308	12.9	27.1	3.0	0.0	182.0	1.3	780.0	373.00	0.09	0.42	1.5	1	1 Egg
SOUPS														
Minestrone soup	90	1.4	5.2	9.4	1.2	43.0	0.7	491.0	123.00	0.07	0.03	0.5	17	1 Bowl
Chicken sweet Corn soup	322	25.5	13.5	24.6	6.0	23.0	2.6	107.0	93.00	0.21	0.34	8.6	6	1 Bowl
French onion Soup	208	4.8	11.6	21.1	2.4	102.0	0.8	321.0	110.00	0.08	0.05	0.6	8	1 Bowl
Tomato soup	82	2.1	4.5	8.3	2.3	101.0	1.3	862.0	216.00	0.25	0.21	0.8	55	1 Bowl
Green pea soup	186	9.0	6.4	23.1	2.2	70.0	1.9	375.0	109.00	0.28	0.08	1.1	11	1 Bowl

Contd...

	Calories (Kcal)	Proteins (g)	Fats (g)	Carbohydrates (g)	Fibre (mg)	Calcium (g)	Iron (mg)	Carotene (mcg)	Retinol (mcg)	Vit B_1 (mg)	Vit B_2 (mg)	Niacin (mg)	Vit C (mg)	Serving Portion
Spinach soup	561	3.9	8.9	116.2	5.9	81.0	1.5	5902.0	1475.00	0.06	0.27	0.08	29	1 Bowl
Mixed vegetable soup	146	3.3	9.2	12.5	1.4	124.0	0.9	779.0	225.0	0.11	0.16	0.6	23	1 Bowl
Cream with tomato soup	245	5.4	16.6	18.5	2.3	180.0	1.5	984.0	287.00	0.32	0.25	1.0	45	1 Bowl
Cream with spinach soup	307	8.5	23.2	16.0	5.1	200.0	2.2	6214.0	1644.00	0.20	0.52	0.9	32	1 Bowl
Cream with carrot soup	250	4.6	16.2	21.5	2.0	172.0	1.4	1935.0	531.00	0.17	0.17	0.9	6	1 Bowl
Cream with mixed vegetable soup	263	7.5	13.4	28.0	3.2	179.0	2.0	1160.0	331.00	0.33	0.24	1.5	45	1 Bowl
Cream with mushroom soup	308	6.6	22.4	19.9	0.7	136.0	1.5	554.0	189.00	0.13	0.41	2.9	6	1 Bowl
Hot and sour Soup	181	11.2	9.3	13.2	1.6	65.0	2.8	86.0	22.00	0.22	0.25	23	6	1 Bowl
CEREALS														
Boiled rice	277	6.0	0.8	61.4	3.6	8.00	2.6	2.0	0.40	0.17	0.13	3.1	0	1
Beans and macaroni	352	12.1	16.8	38.0	3.7	243.0	2.2	673.0	242.00	0.20	0.20	1.5	40	1 Plate

Contd...

Contd...

	Calories (Kcal)	Proteins (g)	Fats (g)	Carbohydrates (g)	Fibre (mg)	Calcium (g)	Iron (mg)	Carotene (mcg)	Retinol (mcg)	Vit B$_1$ (mg)	Vit B$_2$ (mg)	Niacin (mg)	Vit C (mg)	Serving Portion
Spaghetti shallow dish bolognese	346	14.6	14.9	38.3	33.0	174.0	3.2	867.0	236.00	0.28	0.21	4.8	30	1
Chicken shallow dish chowmein	542	31.4	24.2	49.6	3.9	104.0	5.6	9.8	333.00	0.39	0.36	8.1	59	1
MEATS														
Shepherd's pie	486	23.8	34.5	20.0	2.2	206.0	3.5	339.0	98.00	0.31	0.18	9.2	15	1 Bowl
Roast chicken	297	25.3	21.8	0.0	0.0	18.0	2.0	334.0	166.00	0.13	0.20	10.0	0	1 Bowl
Chilli chicken	464	27.3	35.5	8.8	1.9	46.0	3.1	222.0	135.00	0.35	0.31	10.9	50	1 Bowl
Chicken sweet and sour	420	27.0	33.3	3.1	0.8	39.0	2.7	270.0	181.00	0.28	0.35	10.6	30	1 Bowl
Fried fish with chips	443	26.3	26.2	25.4	2.2	307.0	3.3	165.0	94.00	0.09	0.11	0.9	9	1 Bowl
Fish in coconut milk	371	27.0	17.1	27.2	3.2	150.0	3.2	4.0	1.00	0.06	0.03	0.5	7	1 Bowl
Prawn curry	342	30.1	19.9	10.5	2.7	509.0	9.3	3.0	0.80	0.05	0.18	7.5	4	1 Bowl
Crispy baked fish	390	32.3	15.1	31.2	4.1	461.0	4.1	496.0	153.00	0.13	0.13	1.3	16	1 Bowl
VEGETABLES														
Egg curry	314	15.5	17.6	23.3	2.8	85.0	2.8	483.0	237.00	0.38	0.25	1.2	21	1 Bowl
Stuffed tomatoes	233	6.0	15.6	17.1	2.8	138.0	1.5	829.0	228.00	0.27	0.08	1.1	41	2 Tomatoes

Contd...

Contd...

	Calories (Kcal)	Proteins (g)	Fats (g)	Carbohydrates (g)	Fibre (mg)	Calcium (g)	Iron (mg)	Carotene (mcg)	Retinol (mcg)	Vit B₁ (mg)	Vit B₂ (mg)	Niacin (mg)	Vit C (mg)	Serving Portion
Stuffed okra	132	2.3	10.2	7.7	5.9	79.0	0.5	62.0	16.00	0.08	0.12	0.7	16	1 Bowl
Roast potatoes	191	2.4	5.0	34.0	3.8	15.0	0.8	228.0	57.00	0.15	0.01	1.8	26	1-2 Potatoes
Stuffed baked	334	7.1	18.8	34.0	3.8	33.0	1.3	698.0	248.00	0.19	0.16	1.8	26	1-2 Potatoes
Creamed spinach	429	21.4	29.8	18.8	9.3	458.0	3.5	11812.0	3195.00	0.25	1.00	1.4	58	1 Small Bowl
Creamed spinach and mushrooms	363	13.4	25.8	19.2	7.1	366.0	2.9	8692.0	2284.00	0.23	0.90	3.5	45	1 Bowl
SALADS														
Russian salad	959	19.7	85.6	27.5	3.3	100.0	3.8	879.0	333.00	0.38	0.33	5.4	39	1 Small Bowl
Beetroot and egg salad	366	8.9	30.8	13.4	3.6	62.0	2.1	300.0	180.00	0.12	0.29	0.6	15	1 Small Bowl
Tossed creen salad	153	1.5	12.2	9.2	2.0	50.0	0.9	225.0	57.00	0.18	0.04	0.5	43	1 Small Bowl
Cucumber and yogurt salad	29	1.3	1.3	2.9	1.0	53.0	0.5	10.0	4.00	0.04	0.05	0.2	6	1 Small Bowl
French dressing	722	0.0	80.0	0.4	0.0	1.0	0.0	0.0	0.00	0.00	0.00	0.01	1	3/4 Cup
Mayonnaise	1220	7.1	131.8	1.3	0.0	56.0	1.4	380.0	229.00	0.08	0.26	0.0	4	1 Cup

Contd...

Contd...

	Calories (Kcal)	Proteins (g)	Fats (g)	Carbohydrates (g)	Fibre (mg)	Calcium (g)	Iron (mg)	Carotene (mcg)	Retinol (mcg)	Vit B$_1$ (mg)	Vit B$_2$ (mg)	Niacin (mg)	Vit C (mg)	Serving Portion
Mayonnaise without eggs	886	7.7	90.1	11.0	0.0	288.0	0.5	139.0	36.00	1.20	0.46	0.3	6	1 Cup
DESSERTS														
Vanilla ice cream	288	2.3	22.9	18.2	0.0	90.0	0.2	415.0	139.00	0.03	0.14	0.1	0	1 Ice Cup Cream
Strawberry ice cream	288	2.3	22.9	18.2	0.0	90.0	0.2	415.0	139.00	0.03	0.14	0.1	0	1 Ice Cup Cream
Chocolate ice cream	288	2.3	22.9	18.2	0.0	90.0	0.2	415.0	139.00	0.03	0.14	0.1	0	1 Ice Cup Cream
Fruit ice cream	323	2.6	23.0	26.5	0.3	95.0	0.4	832.0	246.00	0.05	0.16	0.3	5	1 Sundae Glass
Cold lemon Souffle	534	6.9	41.9	32.3	0.4	41.0	0.8	1000.0	355.00	0.05	0.20	0.1	8.8	1 Souffle Dish
cold orange Souffle	594	7.8	42.0	46.2	1.5	64.0	1.2	2656.0	769.00	0.05	0.20	0.1	45	1 Souffle Dish
cold pine-appple Souffle	525	6.7	42.0	30.00	0.0	25.0	0.7	1000.0	355.00	0.00	0.20	0.1	0	1 Souffle Dish
cold vanila Souffle	536	7.3	42.7	30.6	0.0	57.0	0.7	1000.0	362.00	0.06	0.20	0.1	0.2	1 Souffle Dish
cold chocolate Souffle	536	7.3	42.7	30.6	0.0	57.0	0.7	1000.0	362.00	0.06	0.20	0.1	0.2	1 Souffle Dish
bread and butter pudding	222	7.4	11.3	22.7	1.0	124.0	0.7	316.0	177.00	0.08	0.27	0.2	2	1 Small Plate

Contd...

Contd...

	Calories (Kcal)	Proteins (g)	Fats (g)	Carbohydrates (g)	Fibre (mg)	Calcium (g)	Iron (mg)	Carotene (mcg)	Retinol (mcg)	Vit B$_1$ (mg)	Vit B$_2$ (mg)	Niacin (mg)	Vit C (mg)	Serving Portion
SANDWICHES														
Tomato and cheese	268	7.2	11.8	33.3	4.6	88.0	0.9	460.0	145.00	0.09	0.06	0.6	11	2 Pcs
Tomato and cucumber	231	5.2	8.6	33.1	4.9	28.0	1.0	460.0	115.00	0.10	0.02	0.6	12	2 Pcs
Tomato grilled	313	9.6	15.0	34.8	5.0	160.0	1.2	530.0	192.00	0.12	0.12	0.6	16	4 Pcs
French toast	443	14.6	27.6	34.0	4.6	144.0	1.7	1088.0	407.00	0.15	0.20	0.6	11	2 Pcs
Cheese open	340	11.7	18.6	31.5	7.4	196.0	1.1	328.0	168.00	0.14	0.11	1.5	0	2 Pcs
Danish luncheon	350	16.2	17.5	31.9	4.6	42.0	2.1	620.0	260.00	0.24	0.22	1.2	3	2 Pcs
Chicken and corn open	340	15.6	15.0	35.6	5.5	18.0	1.8	362.0	124.0	0.12	0.11	4.6	3	2 Pcs
CAKES														
Sponge cake	177	6.2	4.6	27.8	0.5	20.2	0.9	202.0	120.00	0.05	0.14	0.4	0	1 Pc
Sponge chocolate cake	156	5.5	4.5	23.3	0.3	18.8	0.7	201.0	120.00	0.05	0.14	0.3	0	1 Pc
Pineapple pastry	279	7.1	13.2	32.9	0.6	23.1	1.0	390.0	176.00	0.06	0.16	0.5	0	1 Pastry
Chocolate pastry	228	5.5	12.5	23.3	0.3	19.0	0.7	361.0	160.00	0.05	0.14	0.3	0	1 Pastry
Chocolate cream cake	223	3.1	13.1	23.2	0.4	9.0	0.5	526.0	158.00	0.03	0.06	0.3	0	1 Pc

B. Fishes and sea food

Food	Protein (gm)	Fat (gm)	Carbohydrate	Calories	Calcium (mg)	Iron (mg)
Anchovy	19.4	9.5	0.2	165	142	1.5
Cat fish	21.2	—	—	88	550	0.4
Blue mussel	9.9	2.0	3.6	70	1130	8.0
Crab small	11.2	5.8	3.3	59	1370	20.4
Crab mussel	8.9	1.1	3.7	109	590	—
Lobster	20.5	0.9	—	90	16	—
Shrimp small dried	68.1	8.5	—	349	4380	—
Silver belly	19.2	1.6	—	91	715	2.2

C. Animal food

Food	Protein	Fat	Carbohydrate	Calories	Calcium (mg)	Iron (mg)
Beef meat	79.2	10.3	0.2	410	6	18.8
Beef mussel	22.8	2.5	—	114	10	0.8
Duck	21.6	4.8	0.1	130	4	—
Buffalo meat	19.4	0.9	—	86	3	—
Fowl	21.8	0.6	—	109	24	—
Goat meat	21.4	3.6	—	118	12	—
Liver goat	2.0	3.0	—	107	17	—
Liver sheep	19.5	7.5	1.3	150	10	6.3
Mutton	18.5	13.3	—	195	148	2.3
Pigeon	23.3	4.9	—	114	3	2.2
Snail small	12.6	1.0	3.7	75	1320	—
Snail big	10.5	0.5	12.4	98	870	—
Turtles meat	16.5	1.5	1.5	88	7	—
Finch	26.6	3.0	—	133	90	—

Appendix 14

Normal hematological values

Test	Normal Values
Total WBC Count (TLC)	0–1 year: 10,000–25,000/cmm 1–3 years: 6,000–18,000/cmm 4–7 years: 6,000–15,000/cmm 8–12 years: 4,500–13,500/cmm Adults: 4,000–11,000/cmm
Differential WBC Count (DLC)	Polymorphonuclear cells: 50–70% Lymphocytes: 20–40% Monocytes: 4–8% Eosinophils: 0–2% Basophils: 0–1%
RBC Count	4.5–5.5 million/cmm
Hemoglobin	At birth: 18 g% *Adults* Men: 13–16 g% Women: 12–15 g%
Erythrocyte Sedimentation Rate (ESR)	Men: 0–9 mm/hour Women: 0–20 mm/hour
Bleeding Time (BT)	1–6 minutes
Coagulation Time (CT)	5–18 minutes
Blood Urea	20–40 mg/dL
Blood Glucose	Fasting: < 110 mg/dL Post-prandial: < 140 mg/dL Random: 80–120 mg/dL (after waking up) 100–140 mg/dL (at bedtime)
Total Bilirubin	0.1–1.0 mg/dL
Thyroxine	4.5–11.5 µg/dL
Uric Acid	2.5–8 mg/dL
Aspartate Transaminase (AST) or Serum Glutamic Oxaloacetic Transaminase (SGOT)	5–40 IU/L

Test	Normal Values
Alanine Transaminase (ALT) or Serum Glutamic Pyruvic Transaminase (SGPT)	7–56 IU/L
Alkaline Phosphatase	25–100 IU/L
Total Cholesterol	< 200 mg/dL
Triglycerides	< 150 mg/dL
Serum Creatinine	1–2 mg/dL

Appendix 15

Normal values in urinalysis

Test	Normal Values
Color	Pale yellow to deep amber color
Specific Gravity	1.015–1.025
pH	4.5–8
Protein (albumin)	Negative
Sugar	Negative
Bilirubin	Negative
RBCs	Nil
WBCs	Nil
Creatinine	0.8–8 g/24 hours
Urobilinogen	Random: < 25 mg/dL
	24-hour urine: 4 mg/24 hours
Uric Acid	250–750 mg/24 hours

Appendix 16

Precautions against complications associated with immobility

1. Assessment of the initial signs of complications associated with prolonged immobility like pressure sore (redness on the areas under pressure), deep vein thrombosis (DVT; redness and swelling in lower extremities), pneumonia (tachypnea, fever, noisy breathing), contractures (stiffness in joints, muscles, and tendons), and constipation (distention in the abdomen, infrequent and hard stools) should be done primarily.
2. For preventing the pressure sores, use pressure-relieving accessories like air cushions, pillows, foam pads, etc. Changing of positions is highly recommended every 2 hours without dragging and pulling the patient, along with skin care to pressure-prone areas every 4 hours.
3. For DVT, monitoring for the presence of redness and swelling should be done at regular intervals. Elevation of lower extremities above the heart level intermittently for 20 minutes, performing passive range of motion exercises every 4 hours, and using elastic stockings can be done to avoid DVT.
4. For pneumonia (hypostatic or aspiration), suctioning of the airway at regular intervals and changing position every 2 hours should be done. Chest physiotherapy and postural drainage can be initiated, if not contraindicated. Patient must be monitored for regurgitation of food and vomiting.
5. For contractures and joint deformity, one must assist the patient in keeping his body in the anatomical position by using footrest, sand bags, etc. that helps in keeping it properly aligned and hence, prevents contractures. After removing the support devices, motion exercises must be performed every 4 hours.
6. For the prevention of constipation, adequate fluid intake, changing position every 2 hours, and administering stool softness and enema are highly indicated.
7. Along with all the specific measures, one must also pay attention towards maintain adequate nutrition and fluid intake of the patient.

Appendix 17

Glasgow's coma scale

S.No.	Test	Score
1.	Eye opening	
	Spontaneous	4
	To speech	3
	To pain	2
	No response	1
2.	Verbal Response	
	Oriented	5
	Confused	4
	Inappropriate words	3
	Incomprehensible sound	2
	No response	1
3.	Motor Response	
	Obeys commands	6
	Localizes	5
	Withdraws	4
	Flexes	3
	Extends	2
	No response	1

Appendix 18

APACHE II severity of disease classification

Physiologic Variable	High Abnormal Range			0	+1	+2	+3	Low Abnormal Range	
	+4	+3	+2	+1	0	+1	+2	+3	+4	Points

Physiologic Variable	+4	+3	+2	+1	0	+1	+2	+3	+4	Points
Temperature - rectal (°C)	≥ 41°	39 to 40.9°		38.5 to 38.9°	36 to 38.4°	34 to 35.9°	32 to 33.9°	30 to 31.9°	≤ 29.9°	
Mean Arterial Pressure - mm Hg	≥ 160	130 to 159	110 to 129		70 to 109		50 to 69		≤ 49	
Heart Rate (ventricular response)	≥ 180	140 to 179	110 to 139		70 to 109		55 to 69	40 to 54	≤ 39	
Respiratory Rate (non-ventilated or ventilated)	≥ 50	35 to 49		25 to 34	12 to 24	10 to 11	6 to 9		≤ 5	
Oxygenation: A-aDO₂ or PaO₂ (mm Hg) a. FIO₂ ≥ 0.5 record A-aDO₂ b. FIO₂ < 0.5 record PaO₂	≥ 500	350 to 499	200 to 349		< 200 PO2 > 70	PO2 61 to 70		PO2 55 to 60	PO2 < 55	
Arterial pH (preferred)	≥ 7.7	7.6 to 7.69		7.5 to 7.59	7.33 to 7.49		7.25 to 7.32	7.15 to 7.24	< 7.15	
Serum HCO3 (venous mEq/l) (not preferred, but may use if no ABGs)	≥ 52	41 to 51.9		32 to 40.9	22 to 31.9		18 to 21.9	15 to 17.9	< 15	

Contd...

Contd...

Physiologic Variable	High Abnormal Range				0	Low Abnormal Range				Points
	+4	+3	+2	+1		+1	+2	+3	+4	
Serum Sodium (mEq/l)	≥ 180	160 to 179	155 to 159	150 to 154	130 to 149		120 to 129	111 to 119	≤ 110	
Serum Potassium (mEq/l)	≥ 7	6 to 6.9		5.5 to 5.9	3.5 to 5.4	3 to 3.4	2.5 to 2.9		< 2.5	
Serum Creatinine (mg/dl)	≥ 3.5	2 to 3.4	1.5 to 1.9		0.6 to 1.4		< 0.6			
Double point score for acute renal failure										
Hematocrit (%)	≥ 60		50 to 59.9	46 to 49.9	30 to 45.9		20 to 29.9		< 20	
White Blood Count (total/mm3) (in 1000s)	≥ 40		20 to 39.9	15 to 19.9	3 to 14.9		1 to 2.9		< 1	
Glasgow Coma Score (GCS) Score = 15 minus actual GCS										

A. Total Acute Physiology Score (sum of 12 above points)

B. Age points (years) ≤ 44=0; 45 to 54=2; 55 to 64=3; 65 to 74=5; ≥ 75=6

C. Chronic Health Points (see below)

Total APACHE II Score (add together the points from A+B+C)

Chronic Health Points: If the patient has a history of severe organ system insufficiency or is immunocompromised as defined below, assign points as follows:

  5 points for nonoperative or emergency postoperative patients
  2 points for elective postoperative patients

Definitions: organ insufficiency or immunocompromised state must have been evident **prior** to this hospital admission and conform to the following criteria:

- **Liver** – biopsy proven cirrhosis and documented portal hypertension; episodes of past upper GI bleeding attributed to portal hypertension; or prior episodes of hepatic failure/encephalopathy/coma.
- **Cardiovascular** – New York Heart Association Class IV.
- **Respiratory** – Chronic restrictive, obstructive, or vascular disease resulting in severe exercise restriction (i.e., unable to climb stairs or perform household duties; or documented chronic hypoxia, hypercapnia, secondary polycythemia, severe pulmonary hypertension (> 40 mmHg), or respirator dependency.
- **Renal** – receiving chronic dialysis.
- **Immunocompromised** – the patient has received therapy that suppresses resistance to infection (e.g., immunosuppression, chemotherapy, radiation, long term or recent high dose steroids, or has a disease that is sufficiently advanced to suppress resistance to infection, e.g., leukemia, lymphoma, AIDS).

Interpretation of Score:

Score	Death Rate (%)
0–4	4
5–9	8
10–14	15
15–19	25
20–24	40
25–29	55
30–34	75
> 34	85

Appendix 19

Abbreviations used regarding the route of administration of medicine

Abbreviation	Meaning
AD	Right ear
AS	Left ear
AU	Each ear
H	Hypodermic
IM	Intramuscular
INJ	Injection
IV	Intravenous
IVP	Intravenous push
Rx	Take, prescription
OD	Right eye
Sc	Subcutaneously
SQ	Subcutaneous
OS	Left eye
OU	Both eyes
p or P	After, per
PO, per os	By mouth
EC	Enteric-coated
Elix	Elixir
Ext	External, extract
Os	Mouth

Appendix 20

Norton scale

Physical Condition		Mental State		Activity		Mobility		Incontinence		Total Score
Good	4	Alert	4	Ambulatory	4	Full	4	Not	4	
Fair	3	Apathetic	3	Walks with help	3	Slightly limited	3	Occasional	3	
Poor	2	Confused	2	Chairbound	2	Very limited	2	Usually urinary	2	
Very bad	1	Stuporous	1	Bed rest	1	Immobile	1	Double	1	

Appendix 21

Karnofsky's index

General Category	Percentage	Specific Criteria
Able to carry on normal activity and to work; no special care needed.	100	Normal no complaints; no evidence of disease.
	90	Able to carry on normal activity; minor signs or symptoms of disease.
	80	Normal activity with effort; some signs or symptoms of disease.
Unable to work; able to live at home and care for most personal needs; varying amount of assistance needed.	70	Cares for self; unable to carry on normal activity or to do active work.
	60	Requires occasional assistance, but is able to care for most of his personal needs.
	50	Requires considerable assistance and frequent medical care.
Unable to care for self; requires equivalent of institutional or hospital care; disease may be progressing rapidly.	40	Disabled; requires special care and assistance.
	30	Severely disabled; hospital admission is indicated although death not imminent.
	20	Very sick; hospital admission necessary; active supportive treatment necessary.
	10	Moribund; fatal processes progressing rapidly.
	0	Dead

Appendix 22

Differential diagnosis of abdominal pain

Region	Possible Causes
Generalized or diffuse abdominal pain	<ul><li>Perforation</li><li>Aortic aneurysm</li><li>Diabetic ketoacidosis</li><li>Bilateral pleurisy</li><li>Acute pancreatitis</li><li>Peritonitis</li><li>Severe pelvic inflammatory disease</li><li>Gastroenteritis</li></ul>
Central abdominal pain	<ul><li>Early appendicitis</li><li>Acute gastritis</li><li>Ruptured aortic aneurysm</li><li>Small bowel obstruction</li><li>Mesenteric thrombosis</li><li>Acute pancreatitis</li></ul>
Epigastric pain	<ul><li>Aortic aneurysm</li><li>Esophagitis</li><li>Acute pancreatitis</li><li>Gastric and duodenal ulcer</li></ul>
Right upper quadrant pain	<ul><li>Appendicitis</li><li>Hepatic and gall bladder diseases</li><li>Duodenal ulcers</li><li>Myocardial infarction</li><li>Acute pancreatitis</li><li>Duodenal ulcers</li><li>Acute pancreatitis</li><li>Basal pneumonia</li><li>Subphrenic abscess</li></ul>
Left upper quadrant pain	<ul><li>Gastric ulcer</li><li>Diaphragmatic pleurisy</li><li>Acute pancreatitis</li><li>Acute perinephritis</li></ul>

Appendix 23

Conditions leading to systemic or localized edema

Systemic Edema	• Congestive cardiac failure • Cirrhosis • Nephrotic syndrome or other conditions leading to hypoalbuminemia • Drug-induced • Idiopathic
Localized Edema	• Inflammation • Venous or lymphatic obstruction • Chronic lymphangitis • Resection of regional lymph nodes • Filariasis

Region	Possible Causes
	• Spontaneous splenic rupture • Aortic dissection • Ischemic colitis • Subphrenic abscess
Right lower quadrant pain	• Acute appendicitis • Mesenteric adenitis • Ruptured ectopic pregnancy • Perforated duodenal ulcer • Diverticulitis • Pelvic inflammatory disease • Salpingitis • Ureteric and biliary colic • Crohn's disease • Torsion of ovarian cyst or tumor
Left lower quadrant pain	• Diverticulitis • Constipation • Irritable bowel syndrome • Pelvic inflammatory disease • Rectal carcinoma • Ulcerative colitis • Ruptured ectopic pregnancy • Torsion of ovarian cyst or tumor • Salpingitis
Suprapubic pain	• Acute urinary retention • Urinary tract infection • Cystitis • Pelvic inflammatory disease • Ectopic pregnancy • Diverticulitis
Loin pain	• Muscle strain • Urinary tract infection • Renal stones • Pyelonephritis

Appendix 24

Common forms of drug preparation

Drug preparation	Description
Capsule	Powder or gel form of drug encased in a relatively stable and soluble shell, usually made of gelatin, to make it easily palatable
Elixir	A solution containing varying amounts of alcohol, a sweetening agent or flavor, and water and may or may not contain active medicine
Emulsion	Drug which is a mixture of 2 or more immiscible liquids
Enteric-coated tablet	Tablet coated with a substance that does not allow the absorption of drug anywhere in gastrointestinal tract, but small intestine
Lotion	A medicated liquid for external application on skin
Lozenge	Sweetened medicated candy that is intended to dissolve slowly in mouth to soothe the irritated tissues of throat
Ointment	Semisolid preparation of a drug that has a base of fatty or greasy material
Plaster	Medicated solid dressing used as an adhesive or a counterirritant
Poultice	Soft, moist mass often heated and medicated and used to treat painful and inflamed part of the body
Suppository	Solid base of drug (s) inserted into the body cavities, other than mouth like rectum and vagina, that melts slowly at body temperature to release the drug
Syrup	Drug dissolved in a thick, sweet, and sticky liquid intended to soothe the irritated membranes

Drug preparation	Description
Tablet	Small, flat pellet of drug to be taken orally
Transdermal patch	Medicated adhesive patch, placed on skin, to release a specific dose of medicine